Communications in Computer and Information Science 1400

More information about this series at http://www.springer.com/series/7899

Xuesong Ye · Filipe Soares ·
Elisabetta De Maria · Pedro Gómez Vilda ·
Federico Cabitza · Ana Fred ·
Hugo Gamboa (Eds.)

Biomedical Engineering Systems and Technologies

13th International Joint Conference, BIOSTEC 2020 Valletta, Malta, February 24–26, 2020 Revised Selected Papers

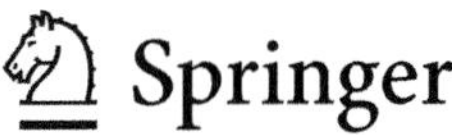
Springer

Editors
Xuesong Ye
Zhejiang University
Hangzhou, China

Elisabetta De Maria
Nice Sophia Antipolis University
Nice Cedex 2, France

Federico Cabitza
University of Milano-Bicocca
Milan, Italy

Hugo Gamboa
Universidade Nova de Lisboa
Caparica, Portugal

Filipe Soares
Fraunhofer Portugal Research Center for Assistive Information and Communication Solutions
Porto, Portugal

Pedro Gómez Vilda
Universidad Politécnica de Madrid
Madrid, Spain

Ana Fred
Instituto de Telecomunicações
University of Lisbon
Lisbon, Portugal

ISSN 1865-0929 ISSN 1865-0937 (electronic)
Communications in Computer and Information Science
ISBN 978-3-030-72378-1 ISBN 978-3-030-72379-8 (eBook)
https://doi.org/10.1007/978-3-030-72379-8

This Springer imprint is published by the registered company Springer Nature Switzerland AG
The registered company address is: Gewerbestrasse 11, 6330 Cham, Switzerland

Preface

The present book includes extended and revised versions of a set of selected papers from the 13th International Joint Conference on Biomedical Engineering Systems and Technologies (BIOSTEC 2020), held in Valetta, Malta, from the 24th to the 26th of February. BIOSTEC is composed of five co-located conferences, each specialized in a different knowledge area, namely BIODEVICES, BIOIMAGING, BIOINFORMATICS, BIOSIGNALS, and HEALTHINF.

BIOSTEC 2020 received 363 paper submissions from 56 countries, of which only 7% are included in this book. This reflects our care in selecting those contributions. These papers were selected by the chairs and their selection is based on a number of criteria that include the classifications and comments provided by the program committee members, the session chairs' assessment, and the program chairs' meta review of the papers that were included in the technical program. The authors of selected papers were invited to submit a revised, extended, and improved version of their conference paper, including at least 30% new material.

The purpose of the BIOSTEC joint conferences is to bring together researchers and practitioners, including engineers, biologists, health professionals, and informatics/computer scientists. Research presented at BIOSTEC includes both theoretical advances and applications of information systems, artificial intelligence, signal processing, electronics, and other engineering tools in areas related to advancing biomedical research and improving healthcare.

The papers selected to be included in this book contribute to the understanding of relevant trends of current research in the biomedical engineering field. This book contains chapters describing novel trends in biodevices and biosignals as well as a set of papers describing the current research on medical image analysis. Some book chapters devoted to bio-informatics focus on cutting-edge methods for predicting crucial dynamical properties of biochemical pathways and addressing the structure prediction problem for multiple RNAs. Finally, the health informatics contributions are the majority, accounting for almost half the chapters, and they express a high heterogeneity. The most frequent topics include eHealth applications, data mining, and predictive applications that embed some form of machine learning. However, also usability studies and certification issues are covered by some chapters: this can be taken as a sign of lively multidisciplinarity and of increasing attention to human-centered design and research.

We would like to thank all the authors for their contributions and also the reviewers, who have helped to ensure the quality of this publication.

February 2020

Xuesong Ye
Filipe Soares
Elisabetta De Maria
Pedro Gómez Vilda
Federico Cabitza
Ana Fred
Hugo Gamboa

Organization

Conference Co-chairs

Ana Fred	Instituto de Telecomunicações and University of Lisbon, Portugal
Hugo Gamboa	NOVA University Lisbon, Portugal

Program Co-chairs

BIODEVICES

Ye Xuesong	Zhejiang University, China

BIOIMAGING

Filipe Soares	Fraunhofer Portugal AICOS, Portugal

BIOINFORMATICS

Elisabetta De Maria	Université Côte d'Azur, CNRS, I3S, France

BIOSIGNALS

Pedro Gómez Vilda	Universidad Politécnica de Madrid, Spain

HEALTHINF

Federico Cabitza	Università degli Studi di Milano-Bicocca, Italy

BIODEVICES Program Committee

Carlos Abreu	Instituto Politécnico de Viana do Castelo, Portugal
Andreas Bahr	University of Kiel, Germany
Mohamed Bakr	CCIT-AASTMT, Egypt
W. Andrew Berger	University of Scranton, USA
Dinesh Bhatia	North-Eastern Hill University, India
Carlo Capelli	University of Verona, Italy
Wenxi Chen	The University of Aizu, Japan
JungHun Choi	Georgia Southern University, USA
Youngjae Chun	University of Pittsburgh, USA
Alberto Cliquet Jr.	University of São Paulo & University of Campinas, Brazil
Robert Day	Royal Perth Hospital, Australia
Heinz-Josef Eikerling	University of Applied Sciences Osnabrück, Germany
Pedro Estrela	University of Bath, UK

Maria Evelina Fantacci	University of Pisa and INFN, Italy
Mireya Fernández Chimeno	Universitat Politècnica de Catalunya, Spain
Bruno Gago	University of Aveiro, Portugal
Juan Carlos García	University of Alcalá, Spain
Miguel García González	Universitat Politècnica de Catalunya, Spain
Javier Garcia-Casado	Universitat Politècnica de València, Spain
Klas Hjort	Uppsala University, Sweden
Leonid Hrebien	Drexel University, USA
Emmanuelle Jacquet	Univ. Bourgogne Franche-Comté, FEMTO-ST Institute, France
Eyal Katz	Afeka Tel Aviv Academic College of Engineering, Israel
Ondrej Krejcar	University of Hradec Králové, Czech Republic
Dean Krusienski	Virginia Commonwealth University (VCU), USA
Vladimir Kublanov	Ural Federal University, Russian Federation
Hiroshi Kumagai	Kitasato University, Japan
Jung Lee	Seoul National University, Korea, Republic of
Rui Lima	Universidade do Minho, Portugal
Anita Lloyd Spetz	Linköpings Universitet, Sweden
Carlos Maciel	University of São Paulo, Brazil
Jordi Madrenas	Universitat Politècnica de Catalunya, Spain
Jarmo Malinen	Aalto University, Finland
Dan Mandru	Technical University of Cluj Napoca, Romania
Mohammad Mehrmohammadi	Wayne State University, USA
Joaquim Mendes	University of Porto, Portugal
Joseph Mizrahi	Technion, Israel Institute of Technology, Israel
Ana Moita	IN+ - Instituto Superior Técnico, Portugal
Raimes Moraes	Universidade Federal de Santa Catarina, Brazil
Umberto Morbiducci	Politecnico di Torino, Italy
Robert Newcomb	University of Maryland, USA
Mónica Oliveira	University of Strathclyde, UK
Abraham Otero	Universidad San Pablo CEU, Spain
Lionel Pazart	Tech4Health/ F-CRIN, Inserm, CHU Besançon, France
Nathalia Peixoto	George Mason University, USA
Marek Penhaker	VŠB - Technical University of Ostrava, Czech Republic
Saydulla Persheyev	University of St Andrews, UK
Wim Rutten	University of Twente, The Netherlands
Seonghan Ryu	Hannam University, Korea, Republic of
Michael Schöning	FH Aachen, Germany
Mauro Serpelloni	University of Brescia, Italy
Dong Ik Shin	Asan Medical Center, Korea, Republic of
Filomena Soares	Universidade do Minho, Portugal
John Tudor	University of Southampton, UK

Duarte Valério	Instituto Superior Técnico - Universidade de Lisboa, Portugal
Renato Varoto	University of Campinas, Brazil
Pedro Vieira	Universidade Nova de Lisboa, Portugal
Bruno Wacogne	FEMTO-ST, UMR CNRS 6174, France
Richard Willson	U of Houston, USA
Hakan Yavuz	Çukurova University, Turkey

BIOIMAGING Program Committee

Ahmet Ademoğlu	Boğaziçi University, Turkey
Péter Balázs	University of Szeged, Hungary
Virginia Ballarín	Universidad Nacional de Mar del Plata, Argentina
Richard Bayford	Middlesex University, UK
Alpan Bek	Middle East Technical University, Turkey
Obara Boguslaw	University of Durham, UK
Abdel-Ouahab Boudraa	Ecole Navale, France
Alberto Bravin	European Synchrotron Radiation Facility, France
Alexander Bykov	University of Oulu, Finland
Rita Casadio	University of Bologna, Italy
Julio César Ramírez San Juan	Instituto Nacional de Astrofisica, Optica y Electronica (INAOE), Mexico
Heang-Ping Chan	University of Michigan, USA
Mostafa Charmi	University of Zanjan, Iran, Islamic Republic of
Jyh-Cheng Chen	National Yang-Ming University, Taiwan, Republic of China
Giacomo Cuttone	INFN - Laboratori Nazionali del Sud Catania, Italy
Rachid Deriche	The French National Institute for Research in Computer Science and Control, France
Alexandre Douplik	Ryerson University, Canada
Edite Figueiras	Champalimaud Foundation, Portugal
Costel Flueraru	National Research Council of Canada, Canada
Carlos Geraldes	Universidade de Coimbra, Portugal
P. Gopinath	Indian Institute of Technology Roorkee, India
Dimitris Gorpas	Helmholtz Zentrum München, Germany
Mario Guarracino	National Research Council of Italy, Italy
Patricia Haro-González	Universidad Autònoma Madrid, Spain
Tzung-Pei Hong	National University of Kaohsiung, Taiwan, Republic of China
Ying Hu	Salk Institute, Nomis Center for Immunobiology and Microbial Pathogenesis, USA
Jae Youn Hwang	DGIST, Korea, Republic of
Xiaoyi Jiang	University of Münster, Germany
Jin Kang	Johns Hopkins University, USA
Eyal Katz	Afeka Tel Aviv Academic College of Engineering, Israel

Sinan Kockara	University of Central Arkansas, USA
Algimantas Krisciukaitis	Lithuanian University of Health Sciences, Lithuania
Pavel Kříž	University of Chemistry and Technology, Prague, Czech Republic
Roger Lecomte	Université de Sherbrooke, Canada
Hongen Liao	Tsinghua University, China
Ivan Lima Jr.	North Dakota State University, USA
Hua Lin	Shanghai Institute of Optics and Fine Mechanics, Chinese Academy of Sciences, China
Honghai Liu	Richard King Mellon Foundation Institute for Pediatric Research and Division of Cardiology, Children's Hospital of Pittsburgh of UPMC, USA
Lucia Maddalena	ICAR, National Research Council (CNR), Italy
Jan Mares	University of Chemistry and Technology, Prague, Czech Republic
Vaidotas Marozas	Kaunas University of Technology, Lithuania
Kunal Mitra	Florida Institute of Technology, USA
Konstantinos Moutzouris	University of West Attica, Greece
László Nyúl	University of Szeged, Hungary
Joanna Isabelle Olszewska	University of the West of Scotland, UK
Kálmán Palágyi	University of Szeged, Hungary
George Panoutsos	The University of Sheffield, UK
Tae Jung Park	Chung-Ang University, Korea, Republic of
Bahram Parvin	University of Nevada, Reno, USA
Gennaro Percannella	University of Salerno, Italy
Vadim Pérez	Instituto Mexicano del Seguro Social, Mexico
Jagath Rajapakse	Nanyang Technological University, Singapore
Alessandra Retico	Istituto Nazionale di Fisica Nucleare, Italy
Benjamin Risse	University of Münster, Germany
Sherif S. Sherif	University of Manitoba, Winnipeg, Canada
Olivier Salvado	CSIRO, Australia
Paula Sampaio	IBMC/i3S, Portugal
K. C. Santosh	The University of South Dakota, USA
Gregory Sharp	Massachusetts General Hospital, USA
Leonid Shvartsman	Hebrew University, Israel
Vijay Singh	Massachusetts Institute of Technology, USA
Magdalena Stoeva	Medical University of Plovdiv, Bulgaria
Chi-Kuang Sun	National Taiwan University, Taiwan, Republic of China
Piotr Szczepaniak	Institute of Information Technology, Lodz University of Technology, Poland
Pablo Taboada	University of Santiago de Compostela, Spain
Martin Tornai	Duke University, USA
Carlos Travieso-González	Universidad de Las Palmas de Gran Canaria, Spain
Benjamin Tsui	Johns Hopkins University, USA
Vladimír Ulman	Masaryk University, Czech Republic

Sandra Ventura	School of Health/ Escola Superior de Saúde do Politécnico do Porto, Portugal
Yuanyuan Wang	Fudan University, China
Wei Wei	LighTopTech Corp., USA
Quan Wen	University of Electronic Science and Technology of China, China
Xin Xie	Becton Dickinson and Company, USA
Hedi Yazid	LATIS, National School of Engineering of Sousse, Tunisia
Zeyun Yu	University of Wisconsin-Milwaukee, USA
Jun Zhao	Shanghai Jiao Tong University, China

BIOINFORMATICS Program Committee

Antonino Abbruzzo	Università degli Studi di Palermo, Italy
Mohamed Abouelhoda	Cairo University, Egypt
Carlos Abreu	Instituto Politécnico de Viana do Castelo, Portugal
Tatsuya Akutsu	Kyoto University, Japan
Jens Allmer	Hochschule Ruhr West, University of Applied Sciences, Germany
Emna Amdouni	University of Montpellier, France
António Anjos	Aberystwyth University, UK
Joel Arrais	Universidade de Coimbra, Portugal
Zafer Aydin	Abdullah Gül University, Turkey
Emiliano Barreto-Hernández	Universidad Nacional de Colombia, Colombia
Payam Behzadi	Shahr-e-Qods Branch, Islamic Azad University, Iran, Islamic Republic of
Shifra Ben-Dor	Weizmann Institute of Science, Israel
Gilles Bernot	Université Côte d'Azur, France
Paweł Błażej	University of Wrocław, Poland
Razvan Bocu	Transilvania University of Brasov, Romania
Rita Casadio	University of Bologna, Italy
Matthias Chung	Virginia Tech, USA
Amanda Clare	Aberystwyth University, UK
Jean-Paul Comet	Univesité Côte d'Azur, France
Federica Conte	National Research Council, Italy
Antoine Danchin	Institut Cochin INSERM U1016 - CNRS UMR8104 - Université de Paris, France
Thomas Dandekar	University of Würzburg, Germany
Sérgio Deusdado	Instituto Politécnico de Bragança, Portugal
Santa Di Cataldo	Politecnico di Torino, Italy
Richard Edwards	University of New South Wales, Australia
François Fages	Inria, France
Maria Evelina Fantacci	University of Pisa and INFN, Italy

António Ferreira	Faculdade de Ciências da Universidade de Lisboa, Portugal
João Ferreira	Faculdade de Ciências da Universidade de Lisboa, Portugal
Giulia Fiscon	National Research Council (CNR), Italy
Alexandru Floares	SAIA, Romania
Liliana Florea	Johns Hopkins University, USA
Dmitrij Frishman	Technical University of Munich, Germany
Max Garzon	The University of Memphis, USA
Christopher Hann	University of Canterbury, New Zealand
Ronaldo Hashimoto	University of São Paulo, Brazil
Steffen Heber	North Carolina State University, USA
Volkhard Helms	Universität des Saarlandes, Germany
Asier Ibeas	Universitat Autònoma de Barcelona, Spain
Sohei Ito	Nagasaki University, Japan
Bo Jin	MilliporeSigma, Merck KGaA, USA
Giuseppe Jurman	Fondazione Bruno Kessler, Italy
Natalia Khuri	Wake Forest University, USA
Jirí Kléma	Czech Technical University in Prague, Czech Republic
Ivan Kulakovskiy	EIMB RAS, Russian Federation
Man-Kee Lam	Universiti Teknologi PETRONAS, Malaysia
Carlile Lavor	University of Campinas, Brazil
Matej Lexa	Masaryk University, Czech Republic
Cédric Lhoussaine	lab CRIStAL | University Lille, France
Chen Li	Monash University, Australia
Yiheng Liang	Bridgewater State University, USA
Paweł Mackiewicz	Wrocław University, Poland
Morgan Magnin	École Centrale de Nantes, France
Elena Marchiori	Radboud University, Netherlands
Andrea Marin	University of Venice, Italy
Johnny Marques	Instituto Tecnológico de Aeronáutica, Brazil
Majid Masso	George Mason University, USA
Giancarlo Mauri	Università di Milano-Bicocca, Italy
Ivan Merelli	ITB CNR, Italy
Paolo Milazzo	Università di Pisa, Italy
Chilukuri Mohan	Syracuse University, USA
José Molina	Universidad Carlos III de Madrid, Spain
Vincent Moulton	University of East Anglia, UK
Jean-Christophe Nebel	Kingston University, UK
Binh Nguyen	Victoria University of Wellington, New Zealand
José Oliveira	University of Aveiro, DETI/IEETA, Portugal
Hakan Orer	Koç University School of Medicine, Turkey
Marco Pellegrini	Consiglio Nazionale delle Ricerche, Italy
Matteo Pellegrini	University of California, Los Angeles, USA
Carla Piazza	University of Udine, Italy
Nadia Pisanti	Università di Pisa, Italy

Alberto Policriti	Università degli Studi di Udine, Italy
Gianfranco Politano	Politecnico di Torino, Italy
Junfeng Qu	Clayton State University, USA
Jagath Rajapakse	Nanyang Technological University, Singapore
Javier Reina-Tosina	University of Seville, Spain
Laura Roa	University of Seville, Spain
David Rocke	University of California, Davis, USA
Vincent Rodin	UBO, LabSTICC/CNRS, France
Simona Rombo	Università degli Studi di Palermo, Italy
Claudia Rubiano Castellanos	Universidad Nacional de Colombia - Bogotá, Colombia
Ulrich Rückert	CITEC, Bielefeld University, Germany
Jakob Ruess	Inria Paris, France
Carolina Ruiz	WPI, USA
J. Cristian Salgado	University of Chile, Chile
Alessandro Savino	Politecnico di Torino, Italy
Thomas Schmid	Universität Leipzig, Germany
Andrew Schumann	University of Information Technology and Management in Rzeszow, Poland
Noor Akhmad Setiawan	Universitas Gadjah Mada, Indonesia
João Setubal	Universidade de São Paulo, Brazil
Anne Siegel	CNRS, France
Christine Sinoquet	University of Nantes, France
Gordon Smyth	Walter and Eliza Hall Institute of Medical Research, Australia
Sylvain Soliman	Inria Saclay, France
Yinglei Song	Jiansu University of Science and Technology, China
Sérgio Sousa	University of Porto, Portugal
David Svoboda	Masaryk University, Czech Republic
Peter Sykacek	University of Natural Resources and Life Sciences, Vienna, Austria
Piotr Szczepaniak	Institute of Information Technology, Lodz University of Technology, Poland
Y-h. Taguchi	Chuo University, Japan
Arkadiusz Tomczyk	Institute of Information Technology, Lodz University of Technology, Poland
Takashi Tomita	Japan Advanced Institute of Science and Technology, Japan
Aydin Tozeren	Drexel University, USA
Sophia Tsoka	King's College London, UK
Juris Viksna	Institute of Mathematics and Computer Science, University of Latvia, Latvia
Malik Yousef	Zefat Academic College, Israel
Wen Zhang	Icahn School of Medicine at Mount Sinai, USA
Qiang Zhu	University of Michigan-Dearborn, USA

BIOINFORMATICS Additional Reviewers

Eugene Baulin	Institute of Mathematical Problems of Biology, Russian Federation
Mariella Bonomo	University of Palermo, Italy
Dmitry Penzar	VIGG RAS, Russian Federation
Cristina Serrao	University of Calabria, Italy
Cristian Versari	Lille University, France

BIOSIGNALS Program Committee

Jean-Marie Aerts	M3-BIORES, Katholieke Universiteit Leuven, Belgium
Eda Akman Aydin	Gazi University, Turkey
Raúl Alcaraz	University of Castilla-La Mancha, Spain
Robert Allen	University of Southampton, UK
Hasan Al-Nashash	American University of Sharjah, UAE
Agustín Álvarez-Marquina	Universidad Politécnica de Madrid, Spain
Joonbum Bae	UNIST, Korea, Republic of
Vlasta Bari	IRCCS Policlinico San Donato, Italy
Richard Bayford	Middlesex University, UK
Eberhard Beck	Brandenburg University of Applied Sciences, Germany
Philipp Beckerle	TU Darmstadt, Germany
Bethany Bracken	Charles River Analytics Inc., USA
Maurizio Caon	University of Applied Sciences and Arts Western Switzerland, Switzerland
Guy Carrault	University of Rennes 1, France
Maria Claudia Castro	Centro Universitário FEI, Brazil
Jan Cornelis	VUB, Belgium
Bruce Denby	Sorbonne Université, France
Petr Doležel	University of Pardubice, Czech Republic
Pier Luigi Emiliani	Italian National Research Council (CNR), Italy
Pedro Encarnação	Universidade Católica Portuguesa, Portugal
Javier Garcia-Casado	Universitat Politècnica de València, Spain
Arfan Ghani	Coventry University, UK
James Gilbert	University of Hull, UK
Gilson Giraldi	National Laboratory for Scientific Computing, Brazil
Didem Gökçay	Middle East Technical University, Turkey
Pedro Gómez Vilda	Universidad Politécnica de Madrid, Spain
İnan Güler	Gazi University, Turkey
Thomas Hinze	Friedrich Schiller University Jena, Germany
Junichi Hori	Niigata University, Japan
Roberto Hornero	University of Valladolid, Spain
Jiří Jan	University of Technology Brno, Czech Republic
Aleksandar Jeremic	McMaster University, Canada
Ákos Jobbágy	Budapest Univ. of Tech. and Econ., Hungary
Gordana Jovanovic Dolecek	Institute INAOE, Mexico

Natalya Kizilova	Warsaw University of Technology, Poland
Dagmar Krefting	Hochschule für Technik und Wirtschaft Berlin - University of Applied Sciences, Germany
Pavel Kříž	University of Chemistry and Technology, Prague, Czech Republic
Lenka Lhotská	Czech Technical University in Prague, Czech Republic
Diego Liberati	Consiglio Nazionale della Ricerche @ Politecnico di Milano, Italy
Ana Rita Londral	Universidade NOVA de Lisboa, Portugal
Harald Loose	Brandenburg University of Applied Sciences, Germany
Carlos Maciel	University of São Paulo, Brazil
Maheswaran S.	Kongu Engineering College, India
Luca Mainardi	Politecnico di Milano, Italy
Jan Mares	University of Chemistry and Technology, Prague, Czech Republic
Catherine Marque	Univ. of Technology of Compiègne, France
Michela Masè	University of Trento, Italy
Jiří Mekyska	Brno University of Technology, Czech Republic
Luciano Menegaldo	Federal University of Rio de Janeiro, Brazil
Roberto Merletti	Politecnico di Torino, Italy
Fernando Monteiro	Polytechnic Institute of Bragança, Portugal
Mihaela Morega	University Politehnica of Bucharest, Romania
Minoru Nakayama	Tokyo Institute of Technology, Japan
Joanna Isabelle Olszewska	University of the West of Scotland, UK
Rui Pedro Paiva	University of Coimbra, Portugal
Palaniappan Ramaswamy	University of Kent, UK
George Panoutsos	The University of Sheffield, UK
Gennaro Percannella	University of Salerno, Italy
Paolo Perego	Politecnico di Milano, Italy
Riccardo Pernice	University of Palermo, Italy
Esteban Pino	Universidad de Concepción, Chile
Vitor Pires	Escola Superior de Tecnologia de Setúbal - Instituto Politécnico de Setúbal, Portugal
Fabienne Poree	Université de Rennes 1, France
Shitala Prasad	NTU Singapore, Singapore
José Joaquín Rieta	Universidad Politécnica de Valencia, Spain
Marcos Rodrigues	Sheffield Hallam University, UK
Pedro Rodrigues	Universidade Católica Portuguesa, Porto, Portugal
Heather Ruskin	Dublin City University, Ireland
Tomasz Rutkowski	RIKEN, Japan
Giovanni Saggio	University of Rome Tor Vergata, Italy
Andrews Samraj	Mahendra Engineering College, India
Md Shohel Sayeed	Multimedia University, Malaysia
Gerald Schaefer	Loughborough University, UK
Reinhard Schneider	Fachhochschule Vorarlberg, Austria
Lotfi Senhadji	University of Rennes 1, France

Samuel Silva	Universidade de Aveiro, Portugal
Zdeněk Smékal	Brno University of Technology, Czech Republic
Jana Šnupárková	University of Chemistry and Technology, Prague, Czech Republic
H. So	City University of Hong Kong, China
Jordi Solé-Casals	University of Vic - Central University of Catalonia, Spain
John Soraghan	University of Strathclyde, UK
Diogo Soriano	Federal University of ABC - UFABC, Brazil
Alan Stocker	University of Pennyslvania, USA
Asser Tantawi	IBM, USA
Wallapak Tavanapong	Iowa State University, USA
António Teixeira	University of Aveiro, Portugal
Carlos Thomaz	Centro Universitário FEI, Brazil
Hua-Nong Ting	University of Malaya, Malaysia
Carlos Travieso-González	Universidad de Las Palmas de Gran Canaria, Spain
Athanasios Tsanas	University of Edinburgh, UK
Ahsan Ursani	Mehran University of Engineering & Technology, Pakistan
Egon L. van den Broek	Utrecht University, The Netherlands
Pedro Vaz	University of Coimbra, Portugal
Chen Wang	Xinhua Net, China
Yuanyuan Wang	Fudan University, China
Quan Wen	University of Electronic Science and Technology of China, China
Didier Wolf	CRAN UMR CNRS 7039-Université de Lorraine, France
Rafał Zdunek	Politechnika Wrocławska, Poland
Huiru Zheng	University of Ulster, UK

BIOSIGNALS Additional Reviewers

Rafael Orsi	FEI, Brazil
Estela Ribeiro	FEI, Brazil
Simon Ruffieux	University of Applied Sciences and Arts Western Switzerland, Switzerland

HEALTHINF Program Committee

Carlos Abreu	Instituto Politécnico de Viana do Castelo, Portugal
Elske Ammenwerth	UMIT University for Health Sciences, Medical Informatics and Technology, Austria
Michela Assale	University of Milano-Bicocca, Italy
Payam Behzadi	Shahr-e-Qods Branch, Islamic Azad University, Iran, Islamic Republic of

José Alberto Benítez-Andrades	Universidad de León, Spain
Daniela Besozzi	University of Milano-Bicocca, Italy
Sorana Bolboaca	Iuliu Hatieganu University of Medicine and Pharmacy, Cluj-Napoca, Romania
Claus Bossen	Aarhus University, Denmark
Alessio Bottrighi	Università del Piemonte Orientale, Italy
Andrew Boyd	University of Illinois at Chicago, USA
Klaus Brinker	Hamm-Lippstadt University of Applied Sciences, Germany
Qasim Bukhari	Massachusetts Institute of Technology, USA
Ann Bygholm	Aalborg University, Denmark
Andrea Campagner	University of Milano-Bicocca, Italy
Eric Campo	LAAS CNRS, France
Guilherme Campos	University of Aveiro, Portugal
Manuel Campos-Martinez	University of Murcia, Spain
Marc Cavazza	University of Greenwich, UK
James Cimino	University of Alabama at Birmingham, USA
Davide Ciucci	Università degli Studi di Milano-Bicocca, Italy
Malcolm Clarke	Ondokuz Mayis University, UK
Mihail Cocosila	Athabasca University, Canada
Emmanuel Conchon	XLIM, France
Carlos Costa	Universidade de Aveiro, Portugal
Liliana Dobrica	University Politehnica of Bucharest, Romania
George Drosatos	Athena Research Center, Greece
Farshideh Einsele	Bern University of Applied Sciences, Switzerland
Christo El Morr	York University, Canada
Gunnar Ellingsen	UIT - The Arctic University of Norway, Norway
Daniela Fogli	Università degli Studi di Brescia, Italy
Christoph Friedrich	University of Applied Sciences and Arts Dortmund, Germany
Sebastian Fudickar	University of Oldenburg, Germany
Ioannis Fudos	University of Ioannina, Greece
Henry Gabb	Intel Corporation, USA
Angelo Gargantini	University of Bergamo, Italy
Jonathan Garibaldi	University of Nottingham, UK
James Geller	New Jersey Institute of Technology, USA
Mauro Giacomini	University of Genoa, Italy
Yves Gourinat	ISAE-SUPAERO, France
David Greenhalgh	University of Strathclyde, UK
Tahir Hameed	Merrimack College, USA
Andrew Hamilton-Wright	University of Guelph, Canada
Jui-Chien Hsieh	Yuan Ze University, Taiwan, Republic of China
Cristina Jácome	CINTESIS – Centro de Investigação em Tecnologias e Serviços de Saúde, Portugal
Dragan Jankovic	University of Niš, Serbia

Bridget Kane	Karlstad University Business School, Sweden
Tomasz Karpiński	Poznan University of Medical Sciences, Poland
Spyros Kitsiou	University of Illinois at Chicago, USA
Josef Kohout	University of West Bohemia, Czech Republic
ilker Köse	Istanbul Medipol University, Turkey
Frank Kramer	University of Augsburg, Germany
Tomohiro Kuroda	Kyoto University Hospital, Japan
Elyes Lamine	University of Toulouse, IMT Mines Albi, CGI, France
Nekane Larburu Rubio	Vicomtech, Spain
Erwin Lemche	King's College London, Institute of Psychiatry, Psychology & Neuroscience, UK
Lenka Lhotská	Czech Technical University in Prague, Czech Republic
Guillaume Lopez	Aoyama Gakuin University, Japan
Martín López Nores	University of Vigo, Spain
Chi-Jie Lu	Fu Jen Catholic University, Taiwan, Republic of China
Xudong Lu	Zhejiang University, China
Alda Marques	University of Aveiro, Portugal
Ken Masters	Sultan Qaboos University, Oman
James McGlothlin	Fusion Consulting Inc, USA
Vincenzo Della Mea	University of Udine, Italy
Rebecca Meehan	Kent State University, USA
Stefania Montani	Università del Piemonte Orientale, Italy
Hammadi Nait-Charif	Bournemouth University, UK
Norbert Noury	University of Lyon, France
José Oliveira	University of Aveiro, DETI/IEETA, Portugal
Agnieszka Onisko	Bialystok University of Technology, Poland
Thomas Ostermann	Witten/Herdecke University, Germany
Nelson Pacheco da Rocha	University of Aveiro, Portugal
Rui Pedro Paiva	University of Coimbra, Portugal
Fabrizio Pecoraro	National Research Council, Italy
Liam Peyton	University of Ottawa, Canada
Antonio Piccinno	University of Bari, Italy
Enrico Piras	Fondazione Bruno Kessler, Italy
Silvana Quaglini	University of Pavia, Italy
Arkalgud Ramaprasad	University of Illinois at Chicago, USA
Grzegorz Redlarski	Gdańsk University of Technology, Poland
David Riaño	Universitat Rovira i Virgili, Italy
Ita Richardson	Lero, Ireland
Marcos Rodrigues	Sheffield Hallam University, UK
Alejandro Rodríguez González	Centro de Tecnología Biomédica, Spain
Valter Roesler	Federal University of Rio Grande do Sul, Brazil
Carolina Ruiz	WPI, USA
George Sakellaropoulos	University of Patras, Greece
Ovidio Salvetti	National Research Council of Italy - CNR, Italy
Akio Sashima	AIST, Japan

Bettina Schnor	Potsdam University, Germany
Andrea Seveso	University of Milano-Bicocca, Italy
Carla Simone	University of Milano-Bicocca, Italy
Kulwinder Singh	University of South Florida, USA
Jan Sliwa	Bern University of Applied Sciences, Switzerland
Åsa Smedberg	Stockholm University, Sweden
Jiangwen Sun	Old Dominion University, USA
Francesco Tiezzi	University of Camerino, Italy
Yi-Ju Tseng	Chang Gung University, Taiwan, Republic of China
Lauri Tuovinen	University of Oulu, Finland
Carolyn Turvey	University of Iowa, USA
Mohy Uddin	King Abdullah International Medical Research Center (KAIMRC), Saudi Arabia
Gary Ushaw	Newcastle University, UK
Aristides Vagelatos	CTI, Greece
Bert-Jan van Beijnum	University of Twente, The Netherlands
Egon L. van den Broek	Utrecht University, The Netherlands
Francisco Veredas	Universidad de Málaga, Spain
Justin Wan	University of Waterloo, Canada
Chien-Chih Wang	Ming Chi University of Technology, Taiwan, Republic of China
Szymon Wilk	Poznań University of Technology, Poland
Dimitrios Zarakovitis	University of the Peloponnese, Greece
André Zúquete	IEETA, IT, Universidade de Aveiro, Portugal

HEALTHINF Additional Reviewers

Vita Santa Barletta	University of Bari, Italy
Silvia Bordogna	University of Milano-Bicocca, Italy
Francis Faux	Ecole d'ingénieurs ISIS, France
Alessandro Fumagalli	, Italy
Jon Kerexeta	Vicomtech Research Centre, Spain
Rafika Thabet	Ecole d'ingénieurs ISIS, France

Invited Speakers

Roy Ruddle	University of Leeds, UK
Helena Canhão	Universidade NOVA de Lisboa, Portugal
Petia Radeva	Universitat de Barcelona, Spain
Silvana Quaglini	University of Pavia, Italy

Contents

Health Informatics

Biomedical Electronics and Devices

Uncertainty Modeling and Deep Learning Applied to Food Image Analysis

Eduardo Aguilar[1,2(✉)], Bhalaji Nagarajan[2], Rupali Khatun[2], Marc Bolaños[2], and Petia Radeva[2,3]

[1] Departamento de Ingeniería de Sistemas y Computación, Universidad Católica del Norte, Avenida Angamos 0610, Antofagasta, Chile
eaguilar02@ucn.cl

[2] Departament de Matemàtiques i Informàtica, Universitat de Barcelona, Gran Via de les Corts Catalanes 585, 08007 Barcelona, Spain
{bhalaji.nagarajan,rupali.khatun,marc.bolanos,petia.ivanova}@ub.edu

[3] Computer Vision Center, Cerdanyola, Barcelona, Spain

Abstract. Recognizing food images arises as a difficult image recognition task due to the high intra-class variance and low inter-class variance of food categories. Deep learning has been shown as a promising methodology to address such difficult problems as food image recognition that can be considered as a fine-grained object recognition problem. We argue that, in order to continue improving performance in this task, it is necessary to better understand what the model learns instead of considering it as a black box. In this paper, we show how uncertainty analysis can help us gain a better understanding of the model in the context of the food recognition. Furthermore, we take decisions to improve its performance based on this analysis and propose a new data augmentation approach considering sample-level uncertainty. The results of our method considering the evaluation on a public food dataset are very encouraging.

Keywords: Uncertainty modeling · Food recognition · Deep learning

1 Introduction

In the present fast-paced world, unhealthy food habits are the basis of most chronic diseases (like obesity, diabetes, cardiovascular related diseases, thyroid, etc.). All over the world, problems regarding nutritional habits are related to the lack of knowledge about what people are eating on a daily basis. Unhealthy habits can more easily be prevented if they have the awareness about the nutritional value of the food they consume in their daily meals (Alliance 2019). The problem is that more than 80% of people is not completely aware of how much they eat, what percentage of proteins, carbohydrates, salt, etc. are consumed in every plate. Moreover, it is quite difficult for people to calculate the nutritional aspects for every meal they consume (Sahoo et al. 2019). Manual calculation of this information is quite time-consuming and more often results in imprecise methods. This creates the need for automatic systems that would be able

X. Ye et al. (Eds.): BIOSTEC 2020, CCIS 1400, pp. 3–16, 2021.
https://doi.org/10.1007/978-3-030-72379-8_1

to log the food a person consumes everyday (Bruno and Silva Resende 2017). This would enable both the patients and the health care professionals to better manage chronic conditions related to nutrition (El Khoury et al. 2019).

Automatic food recognition is not only performed in the dietary management of patients, but has a wide variety of applications in the food and restaurant chains. Food detection in smart restaurants is becoming a practical application rather than a research problem (Aguilar et al. 2018). Automatic food recognition faces challenging computer vision and machine learning problems due to the nature of images that are used in this task (see Fig. 1).

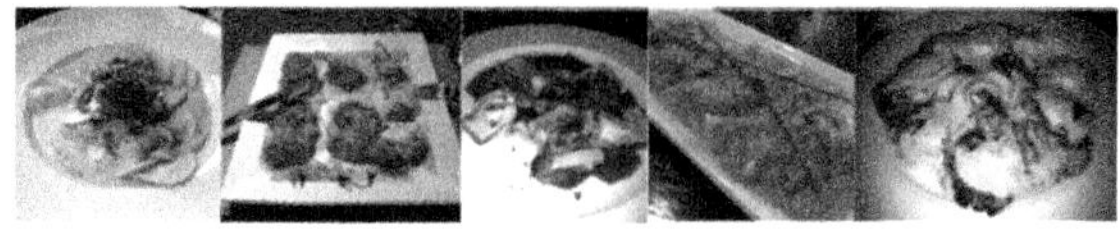

Fig. 1. Example of high within-class variability belong to the ravioli food class.

Deep learning algorithms have become very popular, and they own this popularity to their exceptional performance, enhanced processing abilities, large datasets, and outstanding classification abilities compared to the traditional machine learning methods (Subhi et al. 2019). However, despite the good performance shown, deep learning algorithms need huge amounts of data or they are prone to overfitting. To avoid it, one of the most difficult and general problems in this work is getting an adequate dataset, which not only means a large dataset, but also composed of very diverse and carefully curated samples.

Data augmentation is a popular strategy adopted to prevent deep learning methods from overfitting. It consists in applying transformations to the original data in order to increase the sample size and its variability. Examples of standard transformations in images are: random crops, image flips or reflections and color distortions. On the other hand, novel solutions have been provided by Generative Adversarial Network-based methods (GANs), which can generate synthetic, new and plausible images. However, the majority of data augmentation strategies have been applied indistinctly for all the images, without taking into account that in some cases, particular classes or images can be harder to classify and would require more particular data augmentation methods. On the other hand, uncertainty analysis can give us a good clue to understand what does the model learn and from this, we can expand the dataset to overcome the deficiencies we find. In this work, we propose to explore a combination of both fields: GANs and uncertainty modelling, with the aim of generating new data focusing on the samples that the model has not been able to learn well (with high uncertainty).

The major contributions of this work are as follows: a) to use Epistemic Uncertainty to find the samples that are the hardest for the model to learn; and b) to use Generative Adversarial Networks to perform data augmentation to create visually similar images to the hard samples in the dataset. The rest of the work is organized as follows. Next section details the recent relevant literature.

Section 3 explains the proposed methodology. Experimental details are provided in Sect. 4, followed by conclusions in the last Section.

2 Related Work

Food image analysis is an active area of research, which analyses food data from various sources and applies it to solve different food-related tasks. Here, the most relevant recent literature is discussed.

2.1 Food Recognition

Food recognition is a challenging computer vision task, due to the complex nature of food images. The images could contain dishes that are mixed or could contain many food items (Wang et al. 2019). The task is of a fine-grained nature, where the classes have high intra-class variability and high inter-class similarity.

The initial works related to the recognition task used different hand-crafted features such as color, texture and shape (Matsuda et al. 2012; Chen et al. 2009; Joutou and Yanai 2009; Bosch et al. 2011). These works were primarily concerned with tackling the problem in a constrained environment. The datasets during these studies had less number of images or classes and are restrictive in the conditions in which the images were taken (Ciocca et al. 2017a; Matsuda et al. 2012; Chen 2016).

With the advent of Convolutional Neural Networks (CNN), food recognition tasks of complex nature were also tackled. CNNs were able to massively outperform by far the traditional food recognition algorithms. The datasets started to have large numbers of images and a large number of dishes were being recognized (Bossard et al. 2014; Ciocca et al. 2017b; Donadello and Dragoni 2019; Kaur et al. 2019). Different CNNs have been successfully applied to food recognition task, as AlexNet (Yanai and Kawano 2015), GoogLeNet (Wu et al. 2016; Meyers et al. 2015; Liu et al. 2016a), Network-In-Networks (Tanno et al. 2016), Inception V3 (Hassannejad et al. 2016), ResNet-50 (Ming et al. 2018), Ensemble NN (Nag et al. 2017), Wide Residual Networks (Martinel et al. 2018), and CleanNet (Lee et al. 2018).

Food images in the wild often contain more than one food class. Therefore multi-label food recognition and detection have an increased complexity. Also, different food can be located very close to each other or even mixed. In this case, food recognition is usually preceded by food detection (Anzawa et al. 2019). Earlier works involved using colour and texture-based food segmentation (Anthimopoulos et al. 2014). (Aguilar et al. 2019) proposed a semantic food framework, covering food segmentation, detection and recognition. (Chen et al. 2017) focused on multi-label ingredient recognition, while a multi-task learning has been proposed in the works of (Aguilar et al. 2019; Zhou et al. 2016).

The high inter-class similarity of the food images makes it difficult to train models that could be used to recognize dishes in the wild. Although large datasets are created with more classes, the images do not represent the complex nature of the food. Therefore, generative models could be used to create new synthetic data that are similar to the real world data.

2.2 Generative Adversarial Network

A Generative Adversarial Network (Goodfellow et al. 2014) is a deep learning method that generates very realistic synthetic images in the domain of interest. In the GAN framework, two different networks compete with each other. And these two networks work as thief (generator) and police (discriminator). The Generator, as its name states, generates fake samples from random noise and tries to fool the Discriminator. On the other hand, the Discriminator has the role of distinguishing between real and fake samples.

They both compete with each other in the training phase. The steps are repeated several times in order for the Generator and Discriminator to get better in their respective jobs after each iteration.

One of the most popular extensions of Generative Adversarial Nets is the conditional model. Note that in an unconditioned generative model, there is no control over modes of the data being generated. However, in the Conditional GAN (CGAN) (Mirza and Osindero 2014), the generator learns to create new samples with a specific condition or set of characteristics. Such conditioning could be based on class labels, on some part of data for inpainting like (Goodfellow et al. 2013), or even on data from different modalities. Thus, in CGAN both the generator and the discriminator are conditioned on some extra information y, where y could be any kind of auxiliary information such as a label associated to an image or more detailed tag, rather than a generic sample from an unknown noisy distribution.

A further extension of the GAN architecture, which is built upon the CGAN extension, is the Auxiliary Classifier GANs (ACGAN) (Odena et al. 2017). In ACGAN, the input is the latent space along with a class label. Furthermore, every generated sample has a corresponding class label. The Generator model receives as input, a random point from the latent space and a class label, and gives as output the generated image. The Discriminator model receives as input an image and returns as output the probability that the provided image is real, or the probability of the image belonging to each known class. As well known, unbalanced data is a big problem for object recognition, where models tend to classify much better in the dominant classes. In the case of the GANs, this problem is also present producing low quality synthetic images in classes with few samples. Some proposals have addressed this problem (Mariani et al. 2018; Ali-Gombe and Elyan 2019), which are discussed in the following paragraphs.

In BAGAN (Mariani et al. 2018), an augmentation framework is proposed to restore balance in unbalanced datasets by creating new synthetic images for minority classes. The proposed approach requires two training steps: the first corresponds to initializing the GAN with the features learned by means of an autoencoder, and then the entire model is retrained. Another approach to restore balance is MFC-GAN (Ali-Gombe and Elyan 2019). Oppositely to BAGAN, MFC-GAN is simpler to train and just needs one training step. This model uses multiple fake classes to ensure a fine-grained generation and classification of the minority class instances.

A novel method titled SINGAN (Shaham et al. 2019) has been recently published. Differently to previous GANs, this model is an unconditional generative model that can be learned from a single natural image. SINGAN model is trained to capture the internal distribution of the image patches, then it generates high quality, diverse samples that contain the same visual content as the image. The pyramid structure of fully convolutional layers of SINGAN learns the patch distribution of the image at a different scale in each layer. This results in generating new samples of arbitrary size and aspect ratios that have significant variability, yet maintain both the global structure and the fine textures of the training image.

SINGAN requires to train a separate model for each new sample that one desires to generate from a particular image, thus, becoming a very expensive technique. However, this can be very useful if we only need to increase a small subset of the images. Uncertainty modeling can help us decide which subset is best suited to improve model performance.

2.3 Uncertainty Modeling

Uncertainty can be explained simply as a state of doubt about what the model has or has not learned from the input data. In Bayesian modeling, uncertainty mainly can be presented in two different ways (Kendall and Gal 2017): aleatory uncertainty, which captures noise inherent in the observations; and epistemic uncertainty, which can be explained away given enough data. The uncertainty can be captured from a Bayesian Neural Network (BNN). However, in a Deep Learning scheme it becomes intractable in this way (Blundell et al. 2015; Gal and Ghahramani 2016; Sensoy et al. 2018). Instead, variational Bayesian methods have been adopted in the literature (Blundell et al. 2015; Gal and Ghahramani 2016; Molchanov et al. 2017; Louizos and Welling 2017), where MC-dropout (Gal and Ghahramani 2016) is the most popular technique to estimate the uncertainty due to its simplicity regarding to the implementation.

Recent methods of image classification have adopted this technique to estimate the uncertainty in their scheme (Aguilar et al. 2019; Khan et al. 2019; Aguilar and Radeva 2019b; Aguilar and Radeva 2019a; Nielsen and Okoniewski 2019). In the case of (Aguilar et al. 2019), the aleatory uncertainty is used in order to weigh dynamically different kinds of losses for multi-label and single-label food-related tasks. On the other hand, in (Khan et al. 2019), the authors deal with the imbalanced object classification problem. They redefined the large-margin softmax loss (Liu et al. 2016b), incorporating uncertainty at the class-level and sample-level based on the Bayesian uncertainty measure to address the rarity of the classes and the difficulty level of the individual samples. Regarding (Aguilar and Radeva 2019b; Aguilar and Radeva 2019a), the analysis of the epistemic uncertainty has been applied for different purposes: to identify the best data augmentation that will be applied in a particular class (Aguilar and Radeva 2019a) and to judge when a flat or hierarchical classifier is used (Aguilar and

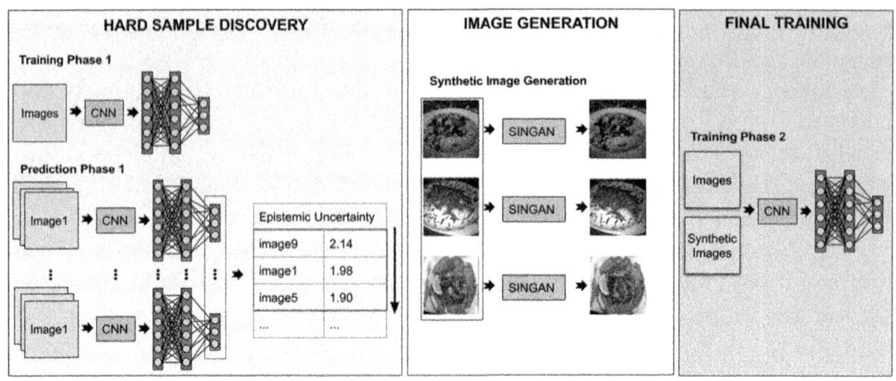

Fig. 2. Main scheme of the our UAGAN food recognition method.

Radeva 2019b). A work closer to our proposal, but not in the food recognition field, is that published by (Nielsen and Okoniewski 2019), that proposes an active learning scheme based on acquisition function sampling. This mechanism considers the prediction uncertainty of the classifier to determine the GAN samples to incorporate in the training set, which are labeled by an external oracle.

The main differences between our proposal and (Nielsen and Okoniewski 2019) are the following: a) our aim is completely different, we apply the uncertainty analysis to discover complex samples to perform data augmentation, and not to apply it after the data augmentation to select the sample that will be used during the training, b) our training scheme is done in two phases, and not several phases, which do not require an external oracle to do it, because the labels are automatically assigned, and c) we adopt a GAN that generates a new sample keeping a high quality content of the input image, instead of generating a sample by merging different input images that in some cases can be very noisy and insert a bias towards the most frequent content.

3 Uncertainty-Aware GAN-Augmented Food Recognition

In this section, we describe all phases involved in the Uncertainty-Aware GAN-Augmented (UAGAN) method to perform food recognition using uncertainty modeling and GANs. As you can see in Fig. 2, the method contemplates 3 main phases with the following purposes: a) hard samples discovery, b) synthetic image generation and c) final training.

3.1 Hard Sample Discovery

The first step of our proposed approach involves the analysis of the food images of the training set, with the aims of identifying those that are difficult to classify. To do this, our criterion is based on the analysis of Epistemic Uncertainty (EU) through the calculation of the entropy. The samples with high uncertainty are those in which the model has not been able to learn well their discriminant features and, therefore, are considered hard samples. On the other hand, we adopt the method called MC-dropout (Gal and Ghahramani 2016) for EU estimation, mainly due to its simple implementation. Basically, we need to add a dropout layer before each fully connected layer, and after the training, we perform K predictions with the dropout turned on. The K probabilities (softmax outputs) are averaged and then the entropy is calculated to reflect the EU. Finally, the images are ordered with respect to their EU, and we select the top n images with higher EU to perform the next step.

3.2 Image Generation

Once the images have been chosen, the next step corresponds to increasing the data with nearby images in terms of visual appearance. We believe that one of the determining factors that does not allow the model to learn the features of hard images corresponds to the fact that they differ from most images that represent a particular class. This hard images may be present in the training set due to the complexity of the acquisition and also after dividing the data for the training. The latter is due to the fact that during the generation of subsets only the sample size is considered and not the variability of the sample. Therefore, we propose to make new images by applying small changes to the original ones. The best method for this purpose is the recent GAN-based method called SINGAN (Shaham et al. 2019), which can learn from a single image and generate different samples carrying the same visual content of the input image. In this step, we adopt the SINGAN to generate one synthetic image for each chosen image according to the uncertainty criterion.

3.3 Final Training

Finally, in the last step, the whole CNN model is trained with both types of images: the synthetic images obtained with SINGAN and the original images.

4 Validation

In this section, we first describe the dataset used to evaluate the proposed approach, which is composed of public images of food belonging to Italian cuisine.

Next, we describe the evaluation metric and experimental setup. Finally, we present the results obtained with the baseline methods and our proposal.

4.1 Dataset

From the dataset MAFood-121 (Aguilar et al. 2019), we use all the images of the dishes that belong to the Italian cuisine. In total, 11 dishes were chosen, which are composed of 2468 images with a maximum, minimum and average of 250, 104 and 224 images, respectively. The data is distributed as 72% of the images for training, 11% for validation and 17% for test.

4.2 Metric

In order to evaluate our proposal, we use the standard metric used for object recognition named overall Accuracy (Acc). We evaluate our experiment 5 times and show the result in terms of average accuracy and the respective standard deviation.

4.3 Experimental Setup

For classification purposes, ResNet-50 (He et al. 2016) was adopted as the base CNN architecture. We adapted this model to be able to apply MC-dropout by removing the output layer, and instead, we added one fully connected layer of 2048 neurons, followed by a dropout layer with a probability of 0.5, and ended up with an output layer of 11 neurons with softmax activation. For simplicity, we call this architecture the same as the original (ResNet50). As for training, we use the categorical cross-entropy loss and the Adam optimizer to train all models during 40 epochs with a batch-size of 32, initial learning rate of 0.0002, decay of 0.2 every 8 epochs and patience of 10 epochs.

Three different training strategies of the same model are used for a benchmark purpose:

- ResNet50, baseline model training with the original images without data augmentation.
- ResNet50+SDA, baseline model with standard data augmentation applying during the training, like random crops and horizontal flips.
- UAGAN, ResNet50+SDA using the real and synthetic images.

With respect to the image generation, we use the default parameters proposed by the authors of SINGAN.

4.4 Results

In this section, we present the results obtained by the proposed method. The first step of our method corresponds to selecting those images difficult to classify (with high uncertainty). After training the model with the original images, we determine the EU and build a histogram for the training images (see Fig. 3). The right side of the histogram corresponds to all the images considered to generate the new ones. The criterion applied corresponds to selecting all images with EU equal to or greater than the uncertainty calculated by the average between the maximum and minimum uncertainty predicted for all images. A total of 120 images was selected.

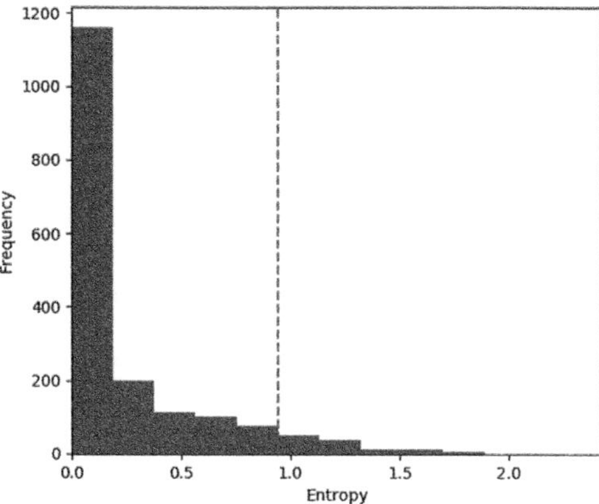

Fig. 3. Histogram for the entropy of the predicted images.

In Fig. 4, we can see the distribution of the training images along each dish, the average entropy in all the images, the proportion of the selected images and the average entropy for the selected images. Unlike the evidence shown in (Khan et al. 2019) for CIFAR-10, for this type of data, the frequency of the images is not a factor that determines a high or low uncertainty for a specific class. In our case, we believe that uncertainty occurs due to the great variability of visual appearance that may be present in the images belong to the same class of dish, where the factor to consider is the diversity of the collected sample and not only the size of the sample. To fill the gap of poorly represented sample for a class, we duplicate the presence of images with high uncertainty through a generation of synthetic images with the SINGAN method. In Fig. 5, some examples of the generated images are shown.

With a total of 1889 training images, 1679 originals and 120 synthetic ones, we train the final model. The results obtained by three different training strategies of the same model are shown in the Table 1. All models were fine-tuned from ImageNet (Krizhevsky et al. 2012) and retrained the whole network using the target training set. For each strategy, 5 models were trained with random initialization values and random order of images. Then, we calculated the average accuracy and the standard deviation achieved for the best model obtained on each iteration according to the performance on the validation set. For the results achieved, we can see that UAGAN improved the performance in terms of accuracy with respect to the rest of strategies. Specifically, the improvement is 3,17% on ResNet50 and 1,32% on ResNet50+SDA.

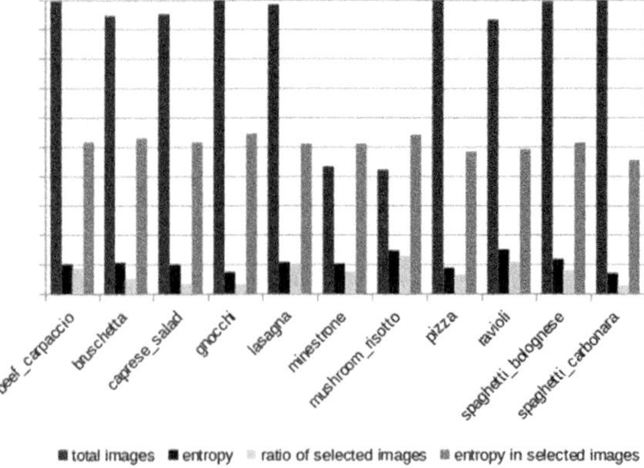

Fig. 4. Training images vs epistemic uncertainty.

Table 1. Results obtained on the test set in term of accuracy with the standard deviation.

Method	Acc	Std
ResNet50	79.15%	0,60%
ResNet50 + SDA	81.00%	0,78%
UAGAN (our proposal)	82.32%	0,96%

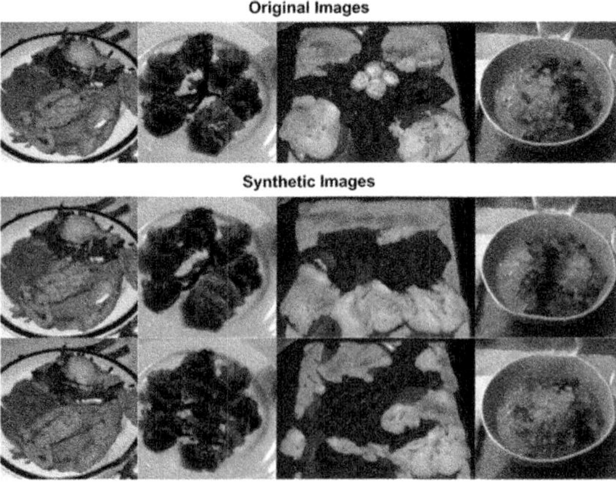

Fig. 5. Synthetic image generated on the selected images from the training set.

5 Conclusions

In this paper, we presented a novel method for sample-level uncertainty-aware data augmentation composed of three phases: 1) identification of hard samples, by means of analysis of the epistemic uncertainty; 2) generating new data from identified samples; and 3) performing the final training with the original and synthetic images. We demonstrated the effectiveness of the approach proposed on the Italian dishes from MAFood121 public dataset. The result obtained shows that our proposal outperforms the classification by incorporating only 120 synthetic images based on the uncertainty analysis (5% of the total). As future work, we will explore both sample-level and class-level uncertainty to increase deep learning datasets in an active learning framework.

Acknowledgements. This work was partially funded by TIN2018-095232-B-C21, SGR-2017 1742, Nestore ID: 769643, Validithi and CERCA Programme/Generalitat de Catalunya. E. Aguilar acknowledges the support of CONICYT Becas Chile. P. Radeva is partially supported by ICREA Academia 2014. We acknowledge the support of NVIDIA Corporation with the donation of Titan Xp GPUs.

References

Aguilar, E., Bolaños, M., Radeva, P.: Regularized uncertainty-based multi-task learning model for food analysis. J. Vis. Commun. Image Represent. **60**, 360–370 (2019)

Aguilar, E., Radeva, P.: Class-conditional data augmentation applied to image classification. In: Vento, M., Percannella, G. (eds.) CAIP 2019. LNCS, vol. 11679, pp. 182–192. Springer, Cham (2019a). https://doi.org/10.1007/978-3-030-29891-3_17

Aguilar, E., Radeva, P.: Food recognition by integrating local and flat classifiers. In: Morales, A., Fierrez, J., Sánchez, J.S., Ribeiro, B. (eds.) IbPRIA 2019. LNCS, vol. 11867, pp. 65–74. Springer, Cham (2019b). https://doi.org/10.1007/978-3-030-31332-6_6

Aguilar, E., Remeseiro, B., Bolaños, M., Radeva, P.: Grab, pay, and eat: semantic food detection for smart restaurants. IEEE Trans. Multimed. **20**(12), 3266–3275 (2018)

Ali-Gombe, A., Elyan, E.: MFC-GAN: class-imbalanced dataset classification using multiple fake class generative adversarial network. Neurocomputing **361**, 212–221 (2019)

Alliance, I.U.N.: National adult nutrition survey. Public Health (2019)

Anthimopoulos, M.M., Gianola, L., Scarnato, L., Diem, P., Mougiakakou, S.G.: A food recognition system for diabetic patients based on an optimized bag-of-features model. IEEE J. Biomed. Health Inform. **18**(4), 1261–1271 (2014)

Anzawa, M., Amano, S., Yamakata, Y., Motonaga, K., Kamei, A., Aizawa, K.: Recognition of multiple food items in a single photo for use in a buffet-style restaurant. IEICE Trans. Inf. Syst. **102**(2), 410–414 (2019)

Blundell, C., Cornebise, J., Kavukcuoglu, K., Wierstra, D.: Weight uncertainty in neural network. In: ICML, pp. 1613–1622 (2015)

Bosch, M., Zhu, F., Khanna, N., Boushey, C.J., Delp, E.J.: Combining global and local features for food identification in dietary assessment. In: 2011 18th IEEE International Conference on Image Processing, pp. 1789–1792. IEEE (2011)

Bossard, L., Guillaumin, M., Van Gool, L.: Food-101 – mining discriminative components with random forests. In: Fleet, D., Pajdla, T., Schiele, B., Tuytelaars, T. (eds.) ECCV 2014. LNCS, vol. 8694, pp. 446–461. Springer, Cham (2014). https://doi.org/10.1007/978-3-319-10599-4_29

Bruno, V., Silva Resende, C.J.: A survey on automated food monitoring and dietary management systems. J. Health Med. Inform. **8**(3) (2017)

Chen, L.-C., Papandreou, G., Kokkinos, I., Murphy, K., Yuille, A.L.: DeepLab: semantic image segmentation with deep convolutional nets, atrous convolution, and fully connected CRFs. IEEE Trans. Pattern Anal. Mach. Intell. **40**(4), 834–848 (2017)
Chen, M., Dhingra, K., Wu, W., Yang, L., Sukthankar, R., Yang, J.: PFID: Pittsburgh fast-food image dataset. In: 2009 16th IEEE International Conference on Image Processing (ICIP), pp. 289–292. IEEE (2009)
Ciocca, G., Napoletano, P., Schettini, R.: Food recognition: a new dataset, experiments and results. IEEE J. Biomed. Health Inform. **21**(3), 588–598 (2017a)
Ciocca, G., Napoletano, P., Schettini, R.: Learning CNN-based features for retrieval of food images. In: Battiato, S., Farinella, G.M., Leo, M., Gallo, G. (eds.) ICIAP 2017. LNCS, vol. 10590, pp. 426–434. Springer, Cham (2017b). https://doi.org/10.1007/978-3-319-70742-6_41
Donadello, I., Dragoni, M.: Ontology-driven food category classification in images. In: Ricci, E., Rota Bulò, S., Snoek, C., Lanz, O., Messelodi, S., Sebe, N. (eds.) ICIAP 2019. LNCS, vol. 11752, pp. 607–617. Springer, Cham (2019). https://doi.org/10.1007/978-3-030-30645-8_55
El Khoury, C.F., Karavetian, M., Halfens, R.J., Crutzen, R., Khoja, L., Schols, J.M.: The effects of dietary mobile apps on nutritional outcomes in adults with chronic diseases: a systematic review. J. Acad. Nutr. Diet. **119**, 626–651 (2019)
Gal, Y., Ghahramani, Z.: Dropout as a Bayesian approximation: representing model uncertainty in deep learning. In: ICML, pp. 1050–1059 (2016)
Goodfellow, I., Mirza, M., Courville, A., Bengio, Y.: Multi-prediction deep Boltzmann machines. In: Advances in Neural Information Processing Systems, pp. 548–556 (2013)
Goodfellow, I., et al.: Generative adversarial nets. In: Advances in Neural Information Processing Systems, pp. 2672–2680 (2014)
Hassannejad, H., Matrella, G., Ciampolini, P., De Munari, I., Mordonini, M., Cagnoni, S.: Food image recognition using very deep convolutional networks. In: Proceedings of the 2nd International Workshop on MADiMa, pp. 41–49. ACM (2016)
He, K., Zhang, X., Ren, S., Sun, J.: Deep residual learning for image recognition. In: Proceedings of the IEEE Conference on Computer Vision and Pattern Recognition, pp. 770–778 (2016)
Chen, J., Ngo, C.W.: Deep-based ingredient recognition for cooking recipe retrival. In: ACM Multimedia (2016)
Joutou, T., Yanai, K.: A food image recognition system with multiple kernel learning. In: 2009 16th IEEE International Conference on Image Processing (ICIP), pp. 285–288. IEEE (2009)
Kaur, P., Sikka, K., Wang, W., Belongie, S., Divakaran, A.: Foodx-251: a dataset for fine-grained food classification. arXiv preprint arXiv:1907.06167 (2019)
Kendall, A., Gal, Y.: What uncertainties do we need in Bayesian deep learning for computer vision? In: Advances in Neural Information Processing Systems, pp. 5574–5584 (2017)
Khan, S., Hayat, M., Zamir, S.W., Shen, J., Shao, L.: Striking the right balance with uncertainty. In: Proceedings of the IEEE Conference on Computer Vision and Pattern Recognition, pp. 103–112 (2019)
Krizhevsky, A., Sutskever, I., Hinton, G.E.: ImageNet classification with deep convolutional neural networks. In: Advances in Neural Information Processing Systems, pp. 1097–1105 (2012)
Lee, K.-H., He, X., Zhang, L., Yang, L.: CleanNet: transfer learning for scalable image classifier training with label noise. In: Proceedings of the IEEE Conference on Computer Vision and Pattern Recognition, pp. 5447–5456 (2018)

Liu, C., Cao, Yu., Luo, Y., Chen, G., Vokkarane, V., Ma, Y.: DeepFood: deep learning-based food image recognition for computer-aided dietary assessment. In: Chang, C.K., Chiari, L., Cao, Yu., Jin, H., Mokhtari, M., Aloulou, H. (eds.) ICOST 2016. LNCS, vol. 9677, pp. 37–48. Springer, Cham (2016a). https://doi.org/10.1007/978-3-319-39601-9_4

Liu, W., Wen, Y., Yu, Z., Yang, M.: Large-margin softmax loss for convolutional neural networks. In: ICML, vol. 2, p. 7 (2016b)

Louizos, C., Welling, M.: Multiplicative normalizing flows for variational Bayesian neural networks. In: ICML vol. 70, pp. 2218–2227. JMLR.org (2017)

Mariani, G., Scheidegger, F., Istrate, R., Bekas, C., Malossi, C.: Bagan: data augmentation with balancing GAN. arXiv preprint arXiv:1803.09655 (2018)

Martinel, N., Foresti, G.L., Micheloni, C.: Wide-slice residual networks for food recognition. In: 2018 IEEE Winter Conference on Applications of Computer Vision (WACV), pp. 567–576. IEEE (2018)

Matsuda, Y., Hoashi, H., Yanai, K.: Recognition of multiple-food images by detecting candidate regions. In: 2012 IEEE International Conference on Multimedia and Expo, pp. 25–30. IEEE (2012)

Meyers, A., et al.: Im2calories: towards an automated mobile vision food diary. In: Proceedings of the IEEE Conference on Computer Vision and Pattern Recognition, pp. 1233–1241 (2015)

Ming, Z.-Y., Chen, J., Cao, Yu., Forde, C., Ngo, C.-W., Chua, T.S.: Food photo recognition for dietary tracking: system and experiment. In: Schoeffmann, K., et al. (eds.) MMM 2018. LNCS, vol. 10705, pp. 129–141. Springer, Cham (2018). https://doi.org/10.1007/978-3-319-73600-6_12

Mirza, M., Osindero, S.: Conditional generative adversarial nets. arXiv preprint arXiv:1411.1784 (2014)

Molchanov, D., Ashukha, A., Vetrov, D.: Variational dropout sparsifies deep neural networks. In: ICML, vol. 70, pp. 2498–2507. JMLR.org (2017)

Nag, N., Pandey, V., Jain, R.: Health multimedia: lifestyle recommendations based on diverse observations. In: Proceedings of the 2017 ACM on International Conference on Multimedia Retrieval, pp. 99–106. ACM (2017)

Nielsen, C., Okoniewski, M.: GAN data augmentation through active learning inspired sample acquisition. In: Proceedings of the IEEE Conference on Computer Vision and Pattern Recognition Workshops, pp. 109–112 (2019)

Odena, A., Olah, C., Shlens, J.: Conditional image synthesis with auxiliary classifier GANs. In: ICML, vol. 70, pp. 2642–2651. JMLR.org (2017)

Sahoo, D., et al.: FoodAI: food image recognition via deep learning for smart food logging (2019)

Sensoy, M., Kaplan, L., Kandemir, M.: Evidential deep learning to quantify classification uncertainty. In: Advances in Neural Information Processing Systems, pp. 3179–3189 (2018)

Shaham, T.R., Dekel, T., Michaeli, T.: SinGAN: learning a generative model from a single natural image. In: Proceedings of the IEEE Conference on Computer Vision and Pattern Recognition, pp. 4570–4580 (2019)

Subhi, M.A., Ali, S.H., Mohammed, M.A.: Vision-based approaches for automatic food recognition and dietary assessment: a survey. IEEE Access **7**, 35370–35381 (2019)

Tanno, R., Okamoto, K., Yanai, K.: DeepFoodCam: a DCNN-based real-time mobile food recognition system. In: Proceedings of the 2nd International Workshop on MADiMa, p. 89. ACM (2016)

Wang, Y., Chen, J., Ngo, C.-W., Chua, T.-S., Zuo, W., Ming, Z.: Mixed dish recognition through multi-label learning. In: Proceedings of the 11th Workshop on Multimedia for Cooking and Eating Activities, CEA 2019, pp. 1–80. Association for Computing Machinery, New York (2019)

Wu, H., Merler, M., Uceda-Sosa, R., Smith, J.R.: Learning to make better mistakes: semantics-aware visual food recognition. In: Proceedings of the 24th ACM International Conference on Multimedia, pp. 172–176. ACM (2016)

Yanai, K., Kawano, Y.: Food image recognition using deep convolutional network with pre-training and fine-tuning. In: 2015 IEEE International Conference on Multimedia And Expo Workshops (ICMEW), pp. 1–6. IEEE (2015)

Zhou, B., Khosla, A., Lapedriza, A., Oliva, A., Torralba, A.: Learning deep features for discriminative localization. In: Proceedings of the IEEE Conference on Computer Vision and Pattern Recognition, pp. 2921–2929 (2016)

Novel Compact Robotic Flow Control Valve for Bioinspired Exosuit and Other Applications

Julia D'Agostino[1,2,3(✉)], Ellen Clarrissimeaux[2,3], Shannon Moffat[1,2,3], Juan D. Florez-Castillo[1,2], Felix Sanchez[1,2], Matthew Bowers[1,2], and Marko Popovic[1,2,4,5]

[1] Robotics Engineering Department, WPI, 100 Institute Road, Worcester, MA, USA
{jedagostino,smmoffat,jflorezcastillo,fasanchez, mpbowers,mpopovic}@wpi.edu

[2] Popovic Labs, WPI, 100 Institute Road, Worcester, MA, USA
eclarrissimeaux@wpi.edu

[3] Mechanical Engineering Department, WPI, 100 Institute Road, Worcester, MA, USA

[4] Physics Department, WPI, 100 Institute Road, Worcester, MA, USA

[5] Biomedical Engineering Department, WPI, 100 Institute Road, Worcester, MA, USA

Abstract. Currently, there are no low-cost commercially available fluid control valves that are suitable for a wide range of wearable robotics applications. To address this market shortcoming, the Compact Robotic Flow Control (CRFC) has been recently introduced. This 3-way 3-position proportional control valve utilizing a servo to implement a choking mechanism that proportionally lessens or widens the inlet opening takes up only 1/7th of the volume and 1/10th of the weight of the best on-off commercially available valve unit in the same "cost" range. It also exhibits relatively fast response times comparable to the response time of on-off valves priced roughly 10 times more than the CRFC valve manufacturing cost. The CRFC valve is reviewed in detail and ongoing work on several advanced applications including wearable exosuit is discussed.

Keywords: Exosuit · Wearable robotics · Valve · Hydro muscle · Fluid actuator

1 Introduction

Valves are necessary to operate pneumatic and hydraulic systems. The global industrial valves market size was valued at USD 48.1 billion in 2020 and is projected to reach USD 85.7 billion by 2025 [1].

Unfortunately, a gap exists in the current advanced valve market for valves that are suitable for wearable robotics systems [2]. Specifically, there are no electronically-controlled proportional flow control valves that are: small (<35 cm^3), compact,

---

J. D'Agostino, E. Clarrissimeaux, and S. Moffat—Contributed Equally.

X. Ye et al. (Eds.): BIOSTEC 2020, CCIS 1400, pp. 17–38, 2021.
https://doi.org/10.1007/978-3-030-72379-8_2

lightweight (<30 g), cost-effective ($\sim$\$10 USD), robust, easily-customizable, fast (<70ms to fully close or open), that can support flows ($\sim$2.5 l/min and $\sim$0.2 Ml/min for water and air respectively) and pressures ($\sim$100 PSI or 0.7 MPa).

The active exo-musculature or exosuit is a wearable soft robot actuated by a network of artificial muscles [3, 4]. Different types of muscles have been used in this milieu.

For example, Series Elastic Actuator (SEA) [5] represented by conventional linear or rotary motorized unit in series with an elastic element has been used to achieve variable impedance control characteristic of biological muscle [6, 7]. SEA has been also utilized in the context of cable-driven orthotic and prosthetic devices [8–14].

Non-SEA based solutions typically utilize fluidly actuated, soft and compliant muscles, like McKibben Muscles [15–17] or Hydro Muscles [2, 18–20]. Hydro Muscles have excellent strain and energy efficiency properties [21] and can closely mimic biological muscle dynamics [4]. In contrast, popular McKibben muscles invented about sixty years prior to Hydro Muscle, are not very efficient and cannot support a biologically realistic muscle strain [4, 19, 20].

A fluidly actuated muscle network has certain advantages over SEA based solution in the case of a larger number of artificial muscles. Fluid systems require only one strong (and likely heavy) motor unit, namely a pump, to provide enough force and joint torque. In contrast, SEA based solutions require one strong motor per each "muscle". The mass and size requirements critically impact wearable robotic design and hence fluidly actuated systems appear as a more promising direction. However, the fluidly actuated devices also require appropriate valves that are cost-effective, lightweight, compact, electronically controllable, and able to support a reasonable range of pressures.

The Compact Robotic Flow Control (CRFC) valve [2] was created to resolve previously mentioned valve market shortcomings and to work in conjunction with the Hydro Muscle. When integrated with one another, Hydro Muscles and the CRFC valve have the potential for implementation in a rehabilitative robotic system or a wearable assistive exosuit that is lightweight, low-cost, and has capabilities for fine control and customization.

Chronologically the research on Humanoid Walking Robot (HWR) utilizing Hydro Muscles [22, 23] brought a full understanding of insufficiencies characterizing commercially available valves. The network of 12 leg muscle groups required 12 large and heavy on-off valves that could maintain fluid flow causing biologically realistic gait patterns. The standalone fluidic system had an umbilical connection to the actual robot as robot legs were not able to upkeep its heavy mass. The research on HWR, briefly reviewed in Sect. 2 was critical for the realization of desired specifications for the better, practical valve including specifications on its mass, size, flow, open/close response times, and control aspects.

The CRFC valve that attained all desired specifications is reviewed in detail in Sect. 3. In Sect. 4, novel applications of the CRFC valve that are currently in development are discussed.

2 Previous Research

The inspiration for the development of the CRFC valve stemmed from the Humanoid Walking Robot (HWR) – a biologically-inspired legged robot [22, 23]. Through fluid actuation, the HWR can move through the stages of the human gait.

2.1 Humanoid Walking Robot: Modelling and Mechanics

The HWR was modeled using a 3B Scientific Lower Limb Skeletal Structure [24]. Lifelike degrees of freedom were possible through bungee cord ligaments that connected the bones of the model [2, 22, 23].

As seen in Fig. 1, each leg of the HWR had six Hydro Muscles groups that corresponded to the most active biological muscles used in the gait cycle. The muscles included the gluteus maximus, iliopsoas, tensor fasciae latae, quadriceps femoris, hamstrings, and gastrocnemius. The ischiofemoral/iliofemoral ligament and extensor hallucis longus were also modeled using passive string structures [22, 23].

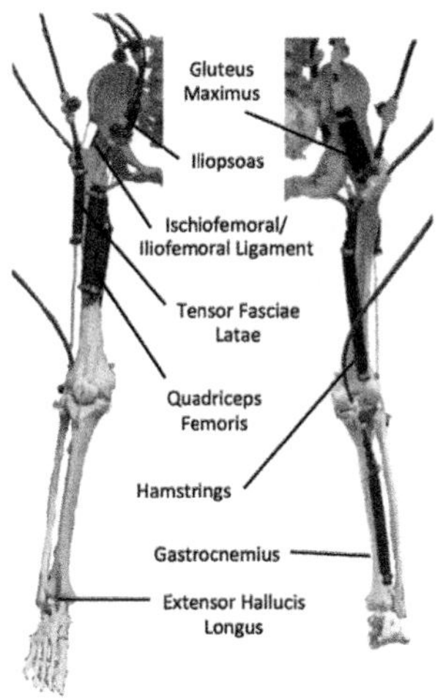

Fig. 1. HWR muscle model [22].

In order to direct flow in and out of the Hydro Muscles, Pneumatic Electric Solenoid Valves [25] were used in series with manual control Elbow Pneumatic Flow Control Valves [26]. PESVs are electronically controlled 5-way on-off pilot operated valves [22]. Pressurized air was supplied through an air tank that operated at 100 psi (0.69 MPa). After construction, the robot was suspended over a variable speed treadmill for testing [27].

2.2 HWR: Experiment

The Exacme 6400-0108BK Treadmill [27] was used to conduct testing. The HWR was powered through the stages of the gait cycle while the belt operated at a speed of 0.28 m/s. IMU sensors and a high-speed camera were used to record the movements of the HWR [22].

2.3 HWR: Results

In Fig. 2, the skeletal postures are compared to the biological postures of the gait [22]. The HWR displayed an average stride length of 0.78 m. The skeletal structure of the HWR was able to stand upright independently but required a tethering system for stability while walking. Based on inverted pendulum dynamics as well as the estimated center of pressure and center of mass locations, the tethering forces were calculated to be less than 20% of the weight of the skeletal system [22].

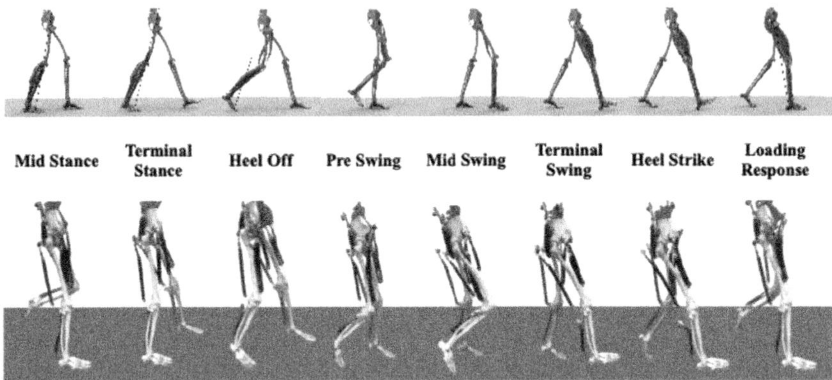

Fig. 2. The eight gait phases: top – numerical simulation and bottom – actual physical model in motion [22].

2.4 Previous Research: Discussion

The creation of the Humanoid Walking Robot showed that Hydro Muscles could be used to mimic the stages of the human gait cycle on a very detailed level. Due to the on-off nature of the digital solenoid valves used, the motions of the HWR were somewhat rigid [2]. Additionally, the valves used for the HWR were very heavy, which required the use of a suspension system.

The HWR showed that a biomimetic network of Hydro Muscles could be used to mimic the stages of the gait cycle, but that the size, weight, and controllability of the fluid control system would need to be improved for a wearable assistive device to be developed effectively. As a remedy to these requirements, a small, lightweight, fluid flow control valve was developed. The Compact Robotics Flow Control (CRFC) valve is a cost-effective solution to the shortcomings of valves currently on the market. The following section addresses the development, testing, and implications of the CRFC valve.

3 CRFC Valve

The Compact Robotic Flow Control (CRFC) valve [2] was designed, manufactured, and tested to fulfill the requirements of a wearable robotic system that utilizes fluid flow control.

3.1 CRFC Valve: Methods

The CRFC valve is a lightweight, small, and inexpensive method of utilizing pneumatics and hydraulics in robotic applications that allows for precise flow control. The CRFC valve is constructed using a servo motor that is positioned inside a 3D printed casing, with a 3D printed servo horn CAM mount attached. Two CAM-follower beads operate with the servo horn CAM mount (often referred to as the curved component) to choke two latex rubber tubes wrapped in fabric with string (Fig. 5 and 6) [28]. The two tubes act as bi-directional fluid flow channels, and at any given point in time either both are closed, or just one is closed. One tube acts as an input for fluid, while the other acts as an output (Fig. 3).

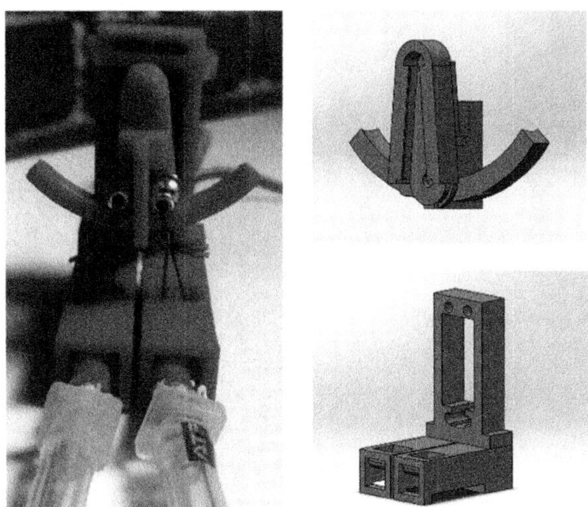

Fig. 3. CRFC valve: physical model (left) and CAD of motor casing (bottom right) and attachment (top right) [2, 23].

The valve alternates between three states (see Fig. 4, top). State 2 represents the resting state of the valve, where the servo motor has the curved component in the upright position. In this state, both Tube A and Tube B are constricted, and no flow can pass through. When the servo motor tilts the curved component counterclockwise, it switches to State 1. In this state, the string wrapped around Tube A will loosen, but the string around Tube B will continue to constrict it. Tube A will open, allowing fluid flow through Tube A, and Tube B will stay closed, and there will be no flow through Tube B. When the servo motor tilts the curved component clockwise, it switches to State 3. In this state, the string wrapped around Tube B will loosen, but the string around Tube A will continue to constrict it. Tube B will open, allowing fluid flow through Tube B, and Tube A will stay closed, and there will be no flow through Tube B.

The valve works by precisely controlling the opening and closing of the tubes. There are strings looped around each tube, which when tightened or untightened vertically, adjust the constriction of the flow. The strings are attached to a corresponding follower bead, which rolls along the smooth path of the curved component. When the curved component is rotated by the servo motor, the corresponding bead rolls, which shortens the distance from the bead and the tube. This gives the string some "slack" and allows the tube to expand due to the pressure inside the tube. This allows the valve to adjust the amount of flow through the servo motor angle. The string pulls the tubing upwards against the proximal portion of the casing, which is curved to provide a more gradual decline in the choking angle while preventing fluid flow [2].

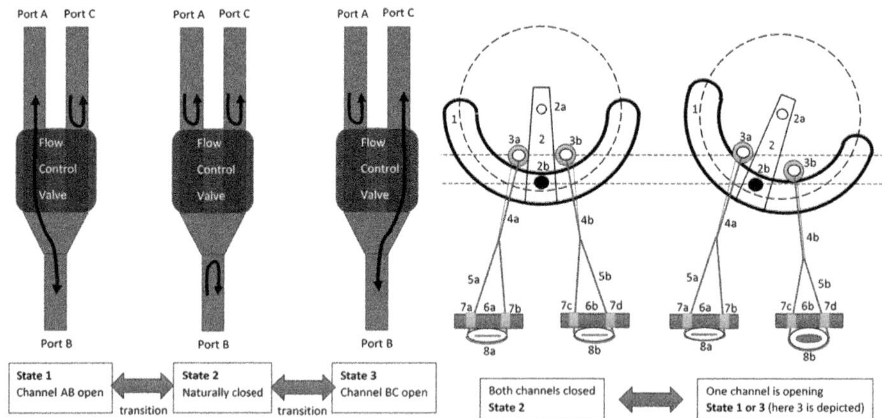

Fig. 4. CRFC valve: three states of the 3-port valve (top) and principle of operation, front view (bottom). Curved element (1, 2), CAM beads (3), Connecting strings (4, 5), Casing base with holes (6, 7), Tubes (8) [2, 23].

Optimized Geometric Model. The valve model is dependent on the necessary movement of the string to allow a tube to fully open, the strain on the string on a side that is already closed, and the desired dead-band angle for valve operation [2]. When the curved component is rotated, the tension of the string causes the bead to roll away from the center of rotation of the curved component, and this movement shortens the distance between the string's anchor position and the bead, which allows the tube to open [2].

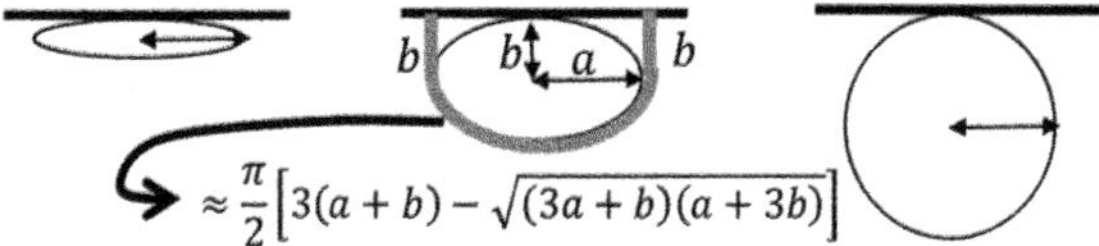

Fig. 5. Tube choking - simplified elliptical model [2, 23].

The equation from Fig. 5 to find the total change in length to allow the tube to fully open is demonstrated below:

$$\Delta l \approx \left\{2b + \frac{\pi}{2}\left[3(a+b) - \sqrt{(3a+b)(a+3b)}\right]\right\}_{b=0}^{b=a} \tag{1}$$

The general valve geometric model (Fig. 6, top) represents the valve in State 2, which is when the valve is in its resting state and the curved component is at a zero-degree angle. This model can be used to "relate string slackening, for the tube that is opening, and string strain, for the tube that is closed, to the servo angle for a set of specified valve parameters" [2]. In this current valve configuration, there are two separate, symmetric, curvature radii (of which only one R is shown in Fig. 6), and a dead band angle, which prevents the bead from rolling until points R, B, and A are collinear [2].

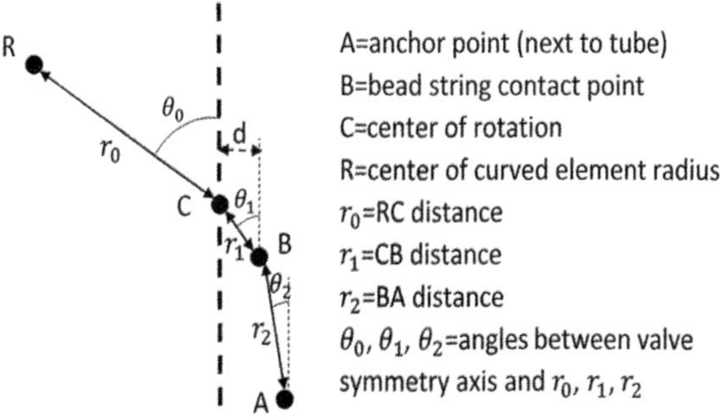

Fig. 6. The general valve geometric model [2, 23].

The optimized geometric configuration has coinciding R's (Fig. 6, top) positioned on the valve symmetry axis, i.e. $\theta_0 = 0°$, AB axis (r_2) parallel to the symmetry axis with $\theta_1 = 135°, \theta_2 = 0°$ θ. The values for r_0, r_1, r_2 are dependent on the dimension of the tube, overall valve, and moment that the servo motor can produce. As this model can be scaled, the optimization procedure can be easily reproduced with different tube diameters, fluid pressures, and desired valve dimensions for a given servo [2].

The geometric model was optimized to: (1) Minimize the volume of the valve, and allow that volume to be scalable, (2) the range of rotation of the servo motor can accomplish the slack needed for the string to allow the tube to fully open, (3) minimize the torque generated on the closed side, (4) account for servo motor error by including a dead band range in which there is no unwanted flow, but does not compromise the general control of the valve, (5) the torque needed to close the tube for whatever the desired pressure may be does not exceed the capabilities of the servo motor.

3.2 CRFC Valve: Experiments

For the following experiments, the specifications and components for the valve used were consistent, however, they are not the only configuration that could be used, and many aspects of the valve can be adjusted to accommodate a variety of devices and situations.

The servo motor used is rated at .08 s/60° at 6 V, .215 Nm, and is priced at around $10 USD [29]. Due to the specifications of the servo motor, the CRFC valve can process over 0.69 MPa (100 psi) of fluid pressure.

The latex tubing used is 5 mm in diameter, and 1 mm thick. Due to the soft and flexible nature of the tube, without any covering, the tube would be able to balloon outwards and burst when pressurized, and the friction of the string around the tube would be able to damage the tube. To prevent this, kite fabric was wrapped around the tube.

The dimensions of the CRFC valve used in these experiments are 6.00 cm × 5.00 cm × 1.75 cm, however, due to the L-shape of the valve it's volume only takes up 2/3 of that, measuring at a volume of only 35.00 cm^3 and a total mass, including the servo used, of only 28 g. The curvature radius of the curved component was 20 mm, and its total operational angle span to control the flow was 42° of rotation.

1) *Response Time*: To find the system response time for the CRFC valve, end-stops were used and positioned at the maximum of the CRFC valve's operational angle, 42°, and the neutral position of the valve. An internal timer was activated or stopped when the end-stops were triggered, which would time the movement of channel open and channel close rated at 100 psi of fluid pressure. This test was conducted ten times for both water and air.
2) *Flow Rate*: To test the relationship between the servo angle and the flow rate, steady-state flow rate readings were taken at 6-degree increments from the neutral position at 0°, where the tube being measured was fully closed, to the maximum operating angle of 42°, where the tube being measured was fully open. For the air tests, a compressed air reservoir at 100 psi was used and connected to the CRFC valve inlet, and then a digital anemometer was used at the outlet. For the water tests, a 12 V diaphragm pump connected to the CRFC valve inlet, and then a digital paddle-wheel flow meter was used at the outlet.
3) *Hydro Muscle Speed*: The CRFC valve angle's relationship with the elongation speed of a Hydro Muscle was determined by finding the rate of elongation at various rotation speeds and angles of the CRFC valve, and finding the time for a 10.4 cm Hydro Muscle to elongate fully from a contracted state.
4) *Controllability*: To test the controllability of the CRFC valve with water or air, the test setup (Fig. 7) can be seen below:

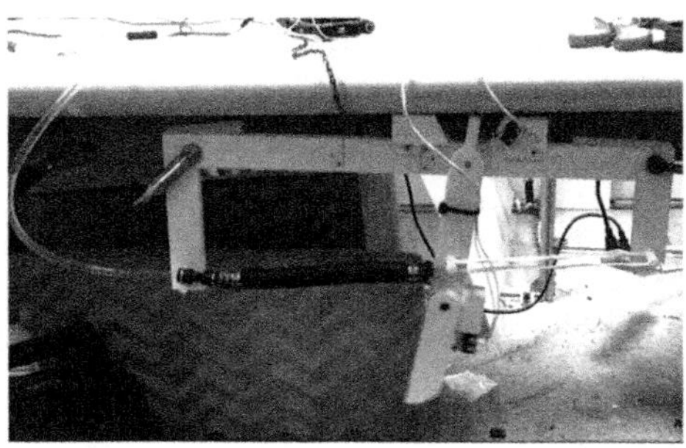

Fig. 7. Test setup for controllability of CRFC valve with 3D printed rigid element [2, 23].

The test setup involved a Hydro Muscle moving a simple 'leg' along with the desired sine wave angular trajectory over a period of time. The 'leg' angular displacement values were provided by a potentiometer. The same test was performed with a 5-way pneumatic solenoid valve, which utilized a custom, pseudo-analog, PWM loop with a cycle time of 5 ms and a tuned P-controller [2].

For the water test, a 12 V pump was used with an accumulator and was kept at steady fluid pressure in a closed-loop hydraulic system. For the air test, the air compressor used was kept at a constant pressure of 0.69 MPa (100 psi), and the exhaust was vented into the ambient space.

3.3 CRFC Valve: Results

1) *Response Time*: The average CRFC valve response times for water at 0.69 MPa (100 psi) were 75 ms and 70 ms for open to closed and then closed to open respectively. The average CRFC valve response times for air at the same pressure were 70 ms and 65 ms for open to closed and closed to open respectively. According to information obtained directly from the manufacturer, the specified solenoid valve has a response time between one and two seconds to fully shift between closed and open states [2] (Table 1).

Table 1. CRFC valve response time for full state transition [2, 23].

Response	Open to Closed	Closed to Open
Water	75 ms	70 ms
Air	70 ms	65 ms

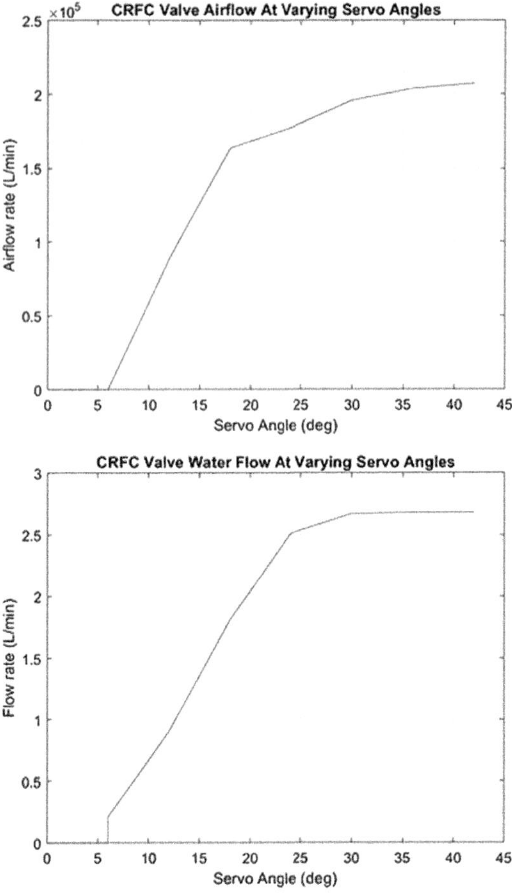

Fig. 8. Flow vs. angle; water (bottom) and air (top) [2, 23].

2) *Flow Rate*: The flow rate vs. Servo angle (Fig. 8).

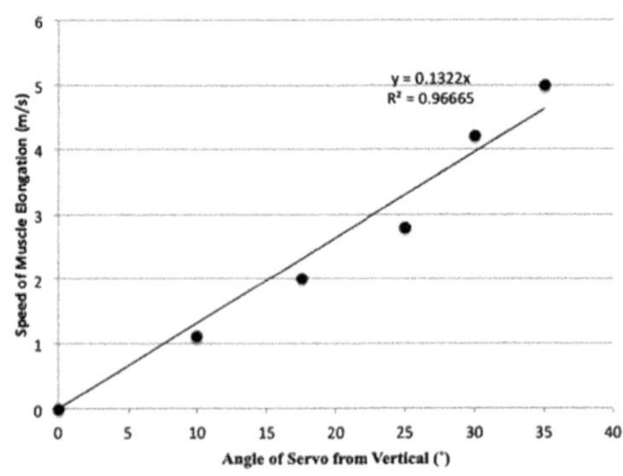

Fig. 9. Hydro Muscle speed vs. servo angle [2, 23].

3) *Hydro Muscle Speed*: The results of the test relating the CRFC valve angle to the speed of elongation of a Hydro Muscle had an R^2-value of 0.967 (Fig. 9).

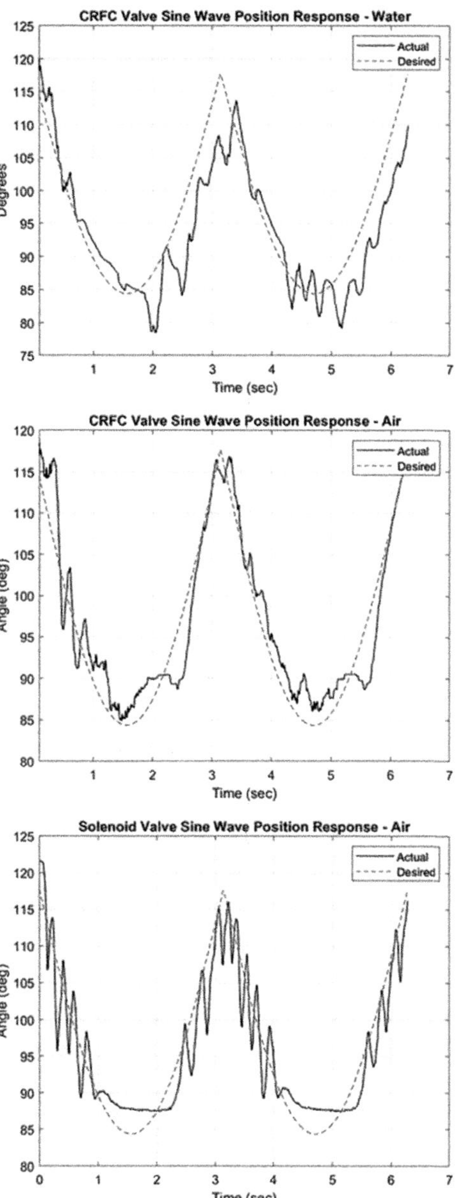

Fig. 10. Controllability tests: water CRFC valve (top), air CRFC valve (middle), air solenoid valve (bottom) [2, 23].

4) *Controllability*: The controllability test results (Fig. 10).

3.4 CRFC Valve: Similar Works

There are several ways of how flow control valves can be categorized. For example, valves can be classified as those with and those without an actuation mechanism, typically consisting of only mechanical elements, within the fluid conduit.

Ball valves and butterfly valves are standard examples of valves with the mechanical elements within the fluid conduit (submerged into fluid) [30]. For example, for ball valve, rotation of a ball with single or plurality of cylindrical holes within the ball allows for control of flow through single or plurality of possible fluid channels connecting various ports. The problem with this type of valve is that space between the ball and fluid conduit (e.g. pipe) needs to be tightly sealed as not to allow the passage of fluid outside of the ball. This is typically introduced with an elastic gasket which necessary introduces a large amount of friction such that a large portion of the energy used to turn the ball is lost on friction and it takes a large amount of torque to counteract friction and turn the ball. As a result, this class of flow control valves is not very energy efficient, it requires a strong motor to operate the valve, and therefore valves are typically very large and heavy. Heavy and non-compact valves are not suitable for many present-day robotics applications like wearable robotics.

The other class of fluid control valves has mechanical and/or pneumatic elements on the outside of the fluid conduit [30]. Here the fluid conduit is deformed in a controlled manner such to impede or allow flow. Diaphragm valve, pinch valve, and peristaltic (or roller) pump/valve are standard examples of this class of valves. Their mechanisms typically either detach mechanically/elastically sealed conduit to allow flow or vice versa press fluid conduit and create a seal to stop flow. In the former main resistive force is due to the fluid conduit that resists this deformation (this resistive force is by definition very large as it resists the fluid pressure even when no external actuation is present). In the latter, the main resistive force is directly due to fluid pressure. The actuator mechanism needs to perform work against this fluid pressure-induced force. Clearly, the smaller this force and displacement defining 0% to 100% flow range the smaller the work motor must perform and hence more energy efficient actuator. Moreover, large resistive force requires a large and heavy motor unit that is not suitable for many present-day robotics applications like wearable robotics.

The presented CRFC valve [2, 30] is best classified as the latter class of valves as the actuation mechanism is not submerged inside the fluid and the valve mechanism press and deform fluid conduit from the outside. The presented CRFC valve addresses challenges related to energy efficiency and the amount of force required for a complete seal and/or full opening by minimizing the fluid pressure-induced force. This is the result of the minimization of the fluid conduit wall area that is subject to an external force. Force is then equal to area multiplied with pressure. A very thin cord looped around a rubber (typically latex) tube is lengthwise actuated and this actuation cause squeezing of the tube. The rubber tube is covered with an inelastic element that prohibits ballooning of the rubber tube and provides a protective layer such that the thin cord does not cut through the rubber tube. The rubber tube is on one side also pressed against a slightly curved rigid wall on the outside of the rubber tube; as experimentally determined this curved extension stipulates the closing of the tube with less external cord tension force. Hence, the presented art is a very energy-efficient valve, requiring only a small amount of force to operate. Therefore, a small, lightweight, and cost-effective motor is only needed to provide fine fluid control. Similar as pinch valves, due to the high elasticity of the rubber that also helps to resist abrasion, this valve (although primarily designed for fluids, i.e. various gasses and liquids) can be also used on solids such as granules, powders, pellets, chippings, fibers, slivers, any kind of slurries and aggressive products.

3.5 CRFC Valve: Discussion

The commercially available valves used for the HWR discussed in Sect. 2 were heavy, large, and could only operate in on-off states. These aspects introduced major limiting factors for applications already discussed, and so the CRFC valve was made as a solution to the previous flow management system.

The CRFC valve used for the experiments was extremely small, lightweight, inexpensive, can be used in both pneumatic and hydraulic applications, and could utilize variable flow control.

In comparison to the original valve, the CRFC valve used was 1/7th the volume, 1/10th the weight, and costs only $10 USD to produce [30].

As seen by response times found in experiment 1, the CRFC can easily operate under both air and water conditions with minimal difference between the mediums with only 65 ms for air and 70 ms for water. This response time makes it optimal for robotics applications, specifically wearable robotic applications as a skeletal biological muscle takes about 250 ms to reach peak force.

As can be seen in experiment 2, the CRFC valve allows for roughly proportional continuous fine flow control before saturation and demonstrates a large flow of >2.5 L/min and >L/min for water and air respectively, for the specific tubing used in the tests. The flow can be easily adjusted by utilizing different sized tubing. The dead-band angle for the CRFC valve tested was 6°, which was found to be an optimal range for the specific servo motor inaccuracies.

The CRFC valve angle relationship with the speed of the elongation of the tested Hydro Muscle was largely linear, with an R^2-value of .967. This linear relationship can be attributed to the optimized geometric model and allows for much more biologically accurate movement potential than the original on-off solenoid valve.

Despite the type of fluid being used with the CRFC valve influencing the response time of the system, the valve still demonstrated controlled flow and achieve the trajectories set out by experiment 4. The test involving the water system could be improved with a higher quality diaphragm pump, as oscillatory behavior was observed from it and induced this behavior throughout the system. Because of this, it is likely that with improved components, the valve would demonstrate even more controllability than what was seen here.

Based on the fine flow control of fluids of the current CRFC valve, this design clearly has the potential to create robotic systems that are controllable and could demonstrate biologically accurate movement.

4 Current Development for CRFC Valve Applications

From here, further work was done to apply the design of the HWR and the CRFC valve to assist in our plans for a wearable exosuit as discussed in Sect. 4.1.

In addition, work has been done to apply the CRFC valve to relevant issues we face today, such as an inexpensive solution to oxygen concentrators and ventilators. With the emergence of Covid-19, oxygen concentrators are in high demand, but are expensive. According to the World Health Organization, a stationary oxygen concentrator can range from $1100 USD to $4000 USD, while a portable oxygen concentrator can range from $3,995 USD to $5,700 USD [31].

4.1 Wearable Exosuit: Objectives

As opposed to the HWR discussed in Sect. 2, this wearable exosuit would be used for a person instead of the lower legs of a skeleton model. Also, the wearable exosuit would utilize the CRFC valve as opposed to the Solenoid Valve discussed in Sect. 2.1 and 3.4.

The current goal for the exosuit is to create a portable system that would assist the user's legs to lower the metabolic cost for a walking gait cycle. The next step would be to adjust this system to lower the metabolic cost for a running gait cycle as well.

Wearable Exosuit: Key Similarities and Differences to Consider. The current development for the wearable exosuit has utilized the research done previously for the HWR discussed in Sect. 2.

Like the HWR, the wearable exosuit will use Hydro Muscles in place of the most active biological muscles during regular gait cycle: iliopsoas, tensor fasciae latae, quadriceps femoris, gluteus maximus, hamstrings (biceps femoris and semitendinosus), and gastrocnemius. The wearable exosuit will also follow the same actuation pattern and general placement of the Hydro Muscles as the HWR.

While we can draw a significant amount of insight from the research done for the HWR, the wearable exosuit has differences that need to be considered. The HWR was only actuating the lower limbs of a skeleton model, which greatly differs in weight than that of an actual person. The HWR could also screw in attachment points into the skeletal model for the Hydro Muscles, while the wearable exosuit will need to utilize different methods of attachment to the user as will be discussed in the next section. The wearable exosuit will be able to benefit from the user's own stability, while the HWR had to be tied to a wooden platform above it since it could not stand on its own. The wearable exosuit will be portable, as the user will be able to carry the power supply, valves, and potential other components discussed in Sect. 4.1.4. Another important consideration is the difference in the joint torques needed to actuate the joints in the skeleton model compared to a person. The peak joint torques for a walking gait cycle at 1.2 m/s in the hips, knees, and ankles, were 1.5 Nm/kg, .6 Nm/kg, and .9 Nm/kg respectively [3].

Wearable Exosuit: Securement. To help secure the wearable exosuit to the user, Velcro braces are being considered. There would be braces in four locations: an above the hip brace (AHB), a below the hip brace wrapped around the upper thighs (BHB), an above the knee brace (AKB) and a below the knee brace (BKB). These braces are indicated by the blue lines in Fig. 11.

These braces would be able to cover all the attachment points needed for the Hydro Muscles to pull against. There will be a strap above the ankle to allow the strings of the Hydro Muscle replacing the gastrocnemius a point to thread through.

However, due to the natural curvature of the legs, any force executed by the Hydro Muscles onto these braces will cause them to shift up and down the leg depending on the location. To prevent this, straps running along the sides of the legs, connecting to each of the braces are being considered. These straps would connect as follows: over the shoulders to the AHB, from the AHB to the BHB, from the BHB to the AKB, from the AKB to the BKB, and then finally from the BKB to wrap around underneath the heel of the user's foot. These straps are indicated by the black lines in Fig. 12.

This connection between the braces will prevent the movement of the braces along the user's legs, without needing to tighten the braces themselves.

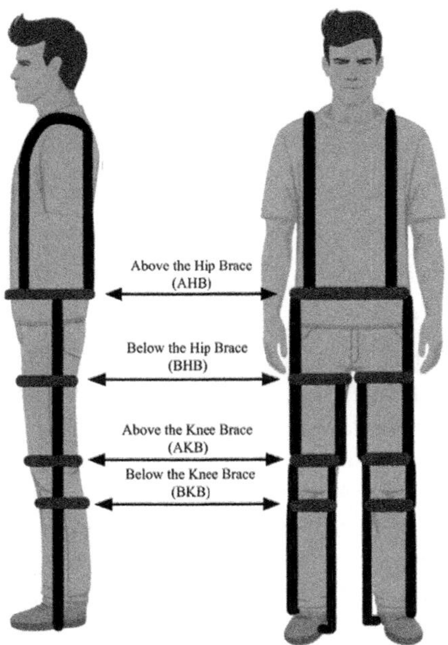

Fig. 11. Placement of Braces and Straps [32].

Wearable Exosuit: Component Carrying Methods. The extra weight of the exosuit system in addition to the user's own weight will also affect the required joint torques during the gait cycle.

The weight of all the components should be equally distributed across the front and the back of the user. To do this, a combination of a vest, a belt, and a backpack will allow the user to maintain balance in both directions.

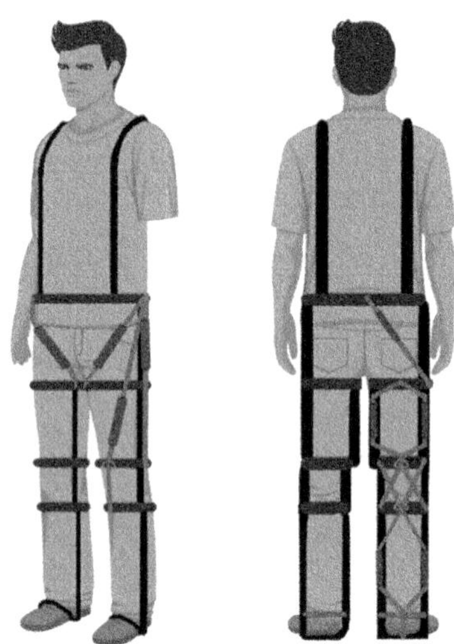

Fig. 12. Placement of Hydro Muscles [32].

4.2 Oxygen Concentrators and Ventilators: Demand Due to Recent Events

There exists number of other potential applications of the CRFC valve. For example, the recent COVID-19 pandemic caused an urgent need for large quantities of low-cost, medical grade oxygen concentrators and ventilators that are easy to manufacture. To address this global emergency several co-authors (M.P., E.C., and M.B.) employed the CRFC valve to design a new type of oxygen concentrator [33] that can be also used as an integral element of an automated ventilator. This design was included in the RepRap Ltd repository [34] containing useful links and notes on oxygen concentrators from all around the globe. Subsequently several companies contacted the co-authors with interest to use this design; most recently interest has been expressed by Sentient Bionics [35] based in Australia aiming to assist growing number of patients in Indonesia. Here we briefly overview the proposed oxygen concentrator design.

Oxygen Concentrators and Ventilators: Proposed Design. Oxygen concentration techniques can be based on air separation processes such as cryogenic techniques and membrane separation techniques that are typically preferred for larger scale industrial applications. For smaller scale applications other techniques are better suited [36] like pressure swing adsorption (PSA) method reviewed in [37] and pressure/vacuum swing adsorption (PVSA) method [38].

The proposed device, depicted in Fig. 13, inputs ambient air and outputs high-O2-concentrated air by utilizing pressure vacuum swing adsorption (PVSA) method. Nitrogen is first adsorbed by Zeolite at high pressure. The leftover high-O2-concentrated air is then passed to output. Nitrogen subsequently detaches from Zeolite by use of very low pressure (below atmospheric pressure) and high-nitrogen-concentrated air is vented out as exhaust.

Another approach popular for low scale portable devices is a pressure swing adsorption (PSA) method. The PSA method differs from the PVSA method as there is no application of very low pressure. Hence, PSA method requires more time for Zeolite to 'regenerate', that is for nitrogen to detach. Further still, the PSA method may leave more nitrogen trapped inside Zeolite micro-cracks after 'regeneration' is completed; this in turn affects the Zeolite's ability to capture more nitrogen during the next cycle. Hence, a device based on the PVSA method can have shorter cycle time and may provide better oxygen concentration.

The novelty of the proposed device is that it requires only one Zeolite molecular sieve instead of the commonly used pair. This is possible as very little time is required to complete an entire cycle for the PVSA method. This in turn allows for much simpler and more cost-effective device architecture requiring only 2 three-way valves instead of the typical 6 solenoid valves.

Another advantage of this device architecture is that it allows for quick real time control, that is stabilization of volume and/or pressure inside the variable volume and/or pressure oxygen storage, Fig. 13, anticipated to be an intermediary between oxygen concentrator and either (1) the patient breathing air directly or (2) the rest of the ventilator, for example, in the form of motorized Bag-Valve-Mask (BVM) type resuscitator. An additional pressure/volume sensor may be required to monitor the pressure/volume inside oxygen storage. For example, if there is accumulation/lack of oxygen the pressure may increase/decrease and the motorized low/high pressure pump will automatically slow down/speed up. The operation principle of the proposed device is as follows:

Step 1. Valve 1 BC open, valve 2 closed, pump closing, high pressure
Step 2. Valve 1 closed, valve 2 DF open, high-O2-concentration output
Step 3. Valve 1 BC open, valve 2 closed, pump opening, low pressure
Step 4. Valve 1 AB open, valve 2 closed, atmospheric pressure inside pump
Step 5. Valve 1 BC open, valve 2 DE open, pump closing, high-nitrogen-concentration output
Step 6. Valve 1 AB open, valve 2 closed, pump opening, atmospheric pressure inside pump

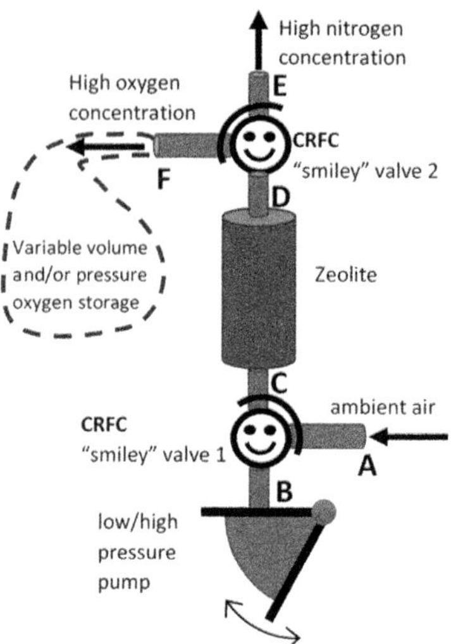

Fig. 13. Simple, easy-to-manufacture, low-cost Oxygen Concentrator anticipated to generate 90–95% medical-grade oxygen in a continuous fashion. The device can be employed as it is, or it may be part of a medical-grade ventilator. Its operation is based on a pressure vacuum swing adsorption (PVSA) method. Device consists of: 1 Zeolite molecular sieve, 1 low/high pressure pump, 2 CRFC "smiley" 3-way valves, (Arduino type) controller, tubing and tube connectors [39]. Manufacturing cost is estimated at not more than several hundred USD for system that could provide oxygen supply for in between 4 and 20 patients.

While there are several potentially good solutions for low/high pressure pumps, the simple motorized bellows pump is envisioned to be used here (Fig. 14). As discussed in more detail in "Low-cost Oxygen Concentrator, helping during the crisis," 2020, there is a $\sim$ \$100 motor solution that can be used to provide oxygen supplies to a number of patients (4 to 20) simultaneously and thus lower the overall manufacturing costs per patient. The pump speed can be finely tuned to provide optimal performance for the Oxygen Concentrator.

The device proposed here is anticipated to output high-O_2-concentrated air with a flow rate that should be at least in the regular range of 5 to 8 liters per minute per patient, that is 5.0 to 8.0 $\times 10^{-3}\mathrm{m}^3/\mathrm{min}$ or 0.8 to 1.3 $\times 10^{-4}\mathrm{m}^3/\mathrm{s}$. This flow rate should be sufficient for a patient inhaling high-O_2-concentrated air directly from the device (with intermediary variable volume and/or pressure oxygen storage). In the case of high-O_2-concentrated air even 4 liters per minute should be sufficient.

In the case of a motorized Bag-Valve-Mask (BVM) type resuscitator one may require factoring 2 or even 3 larger flows due to leaks and contamination with ambient air. Hence this universal device should preferably be capable of outputting up to 20 liters per minute, that is $3.2 \times 10^{-4} m^3/s$.

Based on calculations presented in "Low-cost Oxygen Concentrator, helping during the crisis," 2020 [33] a single low cost motor can produce up to 80 liters of high-O2-

low/high pressure pump
Option 1

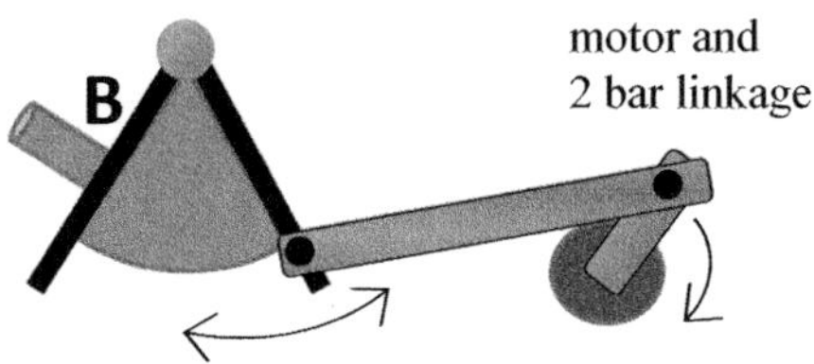

low/high pressure pump
Option 2

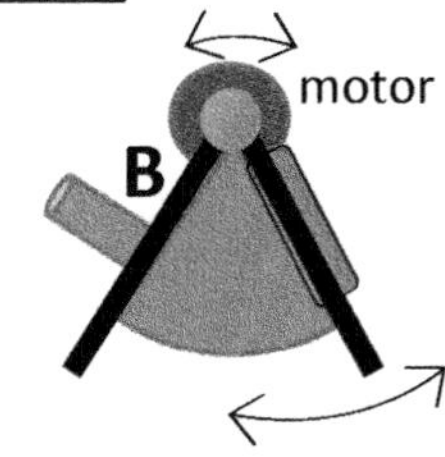

Fig. 14. Option 1: The pump motor may rotate in a single direction if added with a 2-bar linkage mechanism (similar to slider-crank) with one end attached to the main crankshaft bearing and the other end attached to one arm of the bellow pump. Option 2: the pump motor can be directly attached to one arm of the bellow pump requiring alternating direction of rotation; two switch sensors can be used to trigger change of direction and subsequent action of the 2 three-way valves.

concentrated air per minute which should be sufficient for 4 to 20 patients depending on how device is exactly used.

Furthermore, the Oxygen Concentrator may output high-O2-concentrated air after oxygen storage at desired pressure and in desired volume portions at desired time intervals if additional structure is added.

5 Conclusions

The Compact Robotic Flow Control (CRFC) valve, reviewed in detail here, was created to resolve market shortcomings in the context of valves suitable for the wearable and stand-alone robotics applications. Compared to other similar valves currently on the market, the CRFC valve allows for finer control and it is lighter, more compact, and less expensive. The CRFC valve also exhibits relatively fast response times with very little difference between water and air mediums.

The only commercially available, electronically controlled valves in the same "cost" range as the CRFC valve that can support similar flows ($\sim$2.5 l/min and $\sim$ 0.2 Ml/min for water and air respectively) and pressures ($\sim$100 PSI or 0.7 MPa) are simple on-off solenoid valves, for example, an electronically controlled, 5-way on-off solenoid, pilot operated valve [25] in series with a manual flow control valve [26]. In contrast, the CRFC valve's servo motor finely controls orifice size in a continuous fashion. Further, the CRFC valve occupies < 35 cubic centimeters (~ 2.1 cubic inches) volume and has a mass of only 28 g (~ 0.06lb); it takes up only 1/7th of the volume and 1/10th of the weight of the best on-off commercially available valve unit [3, 25, 26] in the same "cost" range. Finally, the CRFC valve exhibits relatively fast response times with very little difference between water and air mediums; the CRFC response time to fully close or to fully open is ~ 65 ms, which is comparable to the response time of on-off valves priced roughly 10 times more than the manufacturing cost of the CRFC valve.

The CRFC valve is a 3-way 3-position valve and utilizes a servo to implement a choking mechanism that proportionally lessens or widens the inlet opening of the latex tubing through which fluid flows.

The curved element attached to the servo is used similarly to a cam mechanism, with two spherical cam followers (beads). The two tubes serving as the flow channels, allow for bi-directional fluid flow. Of the two tubes, at least one or both are closed at any given point in time. One tube serves as a fluid input for an attached system, and the other tube is the release tube.

The CRFC valve can be configured to open or close the fluid tubes by any degree between fully closed and fully open. The degree of opening can be directly controlled by the rotation angle of the servo motor. The servo increases or decreases tension in the strings constricting flow through the fluid tubes. With an increase in tension, the opening size becomes smaller, and with a decrease in tension, the opening gets larger. The fluid flow is linearly related to the size of the opening and is, therefore, proportional to the angular rotation of the servo.

This highly efficient and affordable valve currently uses low-cost materials such as a 3D-printed casing, thin surgical latex tubing, canvas fabric, and a micro servo. It has a total mass of 28 g. The estimated average cost of the CRFC valve is around $10 USD [3, 28]. The CRFC valve can be also easily customized for a large range of various applications; it can be made of different materials, re-dimensioned, and utilize a variety of servo motor units.

Similar as pinch valves, due to the high elasticity of the rubber that also helps to resist abrasion, the CRFC valve (although primarily designed for fluids, i.e. various gasses and liquids) can be also used on solids such as granules, powders, pellets, chippings, fibers, slivers, any kind of slurries and aggressive products.

The CRFC valve can be used in fluid applications in wearable assistive, rehabilitation, and augmenting technologies, general robotics, aerospace and automotive industries, medical devices, pharmaceutical industry, pneumatic and hydraulic machines, agriculture, civil engineering, oil and gas, energy and power, water and wastewater treatment, etc. [3, 28].

The CRFC valve can work in junction with the Hydro Muscle. When integrated, Hydro Muscles and the CRFC valve may be utilized as modular building blocks for robots that can be rapidly assembled and utilized as either perform-alone or wearable robotic systems. The synergy of the CRFC valve with the cost-effectiveness, energy efficiency, and excellent strain properties of the Hydro Muscle opens a door into a new age of fascinating, useful, and accessible/affordable fluid-operated wearable robotic solutions.

Now that the CRFC valve has been developed, future work will be focused on constructing the proposed wearable exosuit with the CRFC valves as discussed in Sect. 4.1. Other applications for the CRFC valve will also be explored, as an example, the oxygen concentrator and ventilator discussed in Sect. 4.2.

References

1. MarketsandMarkets Research Private Ltd. https://www.marketsandmarkets.com/Market-Reports/industrial-valve-market-256097136.html. Accessed 26 Sept 2020
2. D'Agostino J., et al.: Development of bioinspired exosuit actuated with hydro muscles and novel compact robotic flow control valve. In: BIODEVICES 2020 - The 13th International Joint Conference on Biomedical Engineering Systems and Technologies, Valletta, Malta, 24–26 February 2020 (2020)
3. Popovic, M.B: Biomechanics and Robotics, 1st ed. Pan Stanford Publishing Pte. Ltd. (2013)
4. Popovic, M.B.: Biomechatronics, 1st ed. Academic Press/ Elsevier (2019)
5. Pratt, G.A., Williamson, M.M.: Series elastic actuators. In: 1995 IEEE/RSJ International Conference, no. 1, pp. 399–406 (1995)
6. Herr, H., Blaya, J.A., Pratt, G.A.: U.S. Patent No. 8,287,477. Massachusetts Institute of Technology (2012)
7. Blaya, J.A., Herr, H.: Adaptive control of a variable-impedance ankle-foot orthosis to assist drop-foot gait. IEEE Trans. Neural Syst. Rehabil. Eng. **12**(1), 24–31 (2004)
8. Asbeck, A.T., De Rossi, S.M., Galiana, I., Ding, Y., Walsh, C.J.: Stronger, smarter, softer: next-generation wearable robots. IEEE Robot. Autom. Mag. **21**(4), 22–33 (2014)
9. Asbeck, A.T., Dyer, R., Larusson, A., Walsh, C.J.: Biologically inspired soft exosuit. In: IEEE International Conference on Rehabilitation Robotics (ICORR), pp. 1–8 (2013)
10. Galiana, I., Hammond, F.L, Howe, R.D., Popovic, M.B.: Wearable soft robotic device for post-stroke shoulder rehabilitation: identifying misalignments. In: 2012 IEEE/RSJ International Conference on Intelligent Robots and Systems, Portugal, 7–12 October 2012 (2017)
11. Hunt, T., Berthelette, C., Iannacchione, G.S., Koehler, S., Popovic, M.B.: Soft robotics variable stiffness exo-musculature, one-to-many concept, and advanced clutches. In: IEEE ICRA 2012 WORKSHOP: Variable Stiffness Actuators Moving the Robots of Tomorrow, St. Paul, Minnesota, May, vol. 14. (2012)
12. Kesner, S.B., Jentoft, L., Hammond, F.L., Howe, R.D., Popovic, M.B.: Design considerations for an active soft orthotic system for shoulder rehabilitation. In: 33rd Annual International IEEE EMBS Conference, Boston, USA, 30 August–02 September 2011 (2011)
13. Mao, Y., Agrawal, S.K.: Design of a cable-driven arm exoskeleton (CAREX) for neural rehabilitation. IEEE Trans. Rob. **28**(4), 922–931 (2012)
14. Saint-Elme, E., Larrier, M.A., Kracinovich, C., Renshaw, D., Troy, K., Popovic, M.B.: Design of a biologically accurate prosthetic hand. In: IEEE RAS International Symposium on Wearable & Rehabilitation Robotics, Houston, TX, 5–8 November 2017 (2017)
15. Kurumaya, S., Suzumori, K., Nabae, H., Wakimoto, S.: Musculoskeletal lower-limb robot driven by multifilament muscles. ROBOMECH J. **3**(1), 1–15 (2016). https://doi.org/10.1186/s40648-016-0061-3
16. Park, Y.L., et al.: Design and control of a bio-inspired soft wearable robotic device for ankle–foot rehabilitation. Bioinspir. Biomim. **9**(1), 016007 (2014)

17. Ueda, J., Ming, D., Krishnamoorthy, V., Shinohara, M., Ogasawara, T.: Individual muscle control using an exoskeleton robot for muscle function testing. IEEE Trans. Neural Syst. Rehabil. Eng. **18**(4), 339–350 (2010)
18. McCarthy, G., Effraimidis, D., Jennings, B., Corso, N., Onal C., Popovic, M.B.: Hydraulically actuated muscle (HAM) exo-musculature. In: (RoMa) Workshop, the 2014 Robotics: Science and Systems Conference, Berkeley, CA, 12 July 2014 (2014)
19. Sridar, S., et al.: Hydro Muscle - a novel soft fluidic actuator. In: IEEE International Conference on Robotics and Automation (ICRA), pp. 4104–4021 (2016)
20. Bowers, M., Harmalkar, C., Agrawal, A., Kashyap, A., Tai, J., Popovic, M.B.: Design and test of biologically inspired multi-fiber Hydro Muscle actuated ankle. In: 2017 IEEE International Workshop on Advanced Robotics and its Social Impacts, 8–10, March 2017. University of Texas at Austin, Austin, TX, USA (2017)
21. Miriyev, A., Stack, K., Lipson, H.: Soft material for soft actuators. Nat. Commun. **8**(1), 596 (2017)
22. Curran, A., Colpritt, K., Moffat, S., Sullivan, M.: Humanoid walking robot. Major Qualifying Project, Worcester Polytechnic Institute (2018)
23. Moffat, S.: Biologically inspired legs and novel flow control valve toward a new approach for accessible wearable robotics. Master's thesis, Worcester Polytechnic Institute (2019)
24. Functional Physiological Skeleton Model - Frank. 3B Scientific. Human skeletal model
25. Pneumatic Electric Solenoid Valve. U.S. Solid. 1/4 5-way 2-position DC 24 V valve
26. Elbow Pneumatic Flow Control Valve. Utah Pneumatic. 1/4 OD 1/8 NPT Push-to-Connect Valve
27. Exacme 6400-0108BK Treadmill. Exacme. Combo 500W folding electric motorized treadmill
28. Spiderwire Stealth SCS50G-200. Spiderwire. 200yd, 50lb, braided fishing line
29. MG90D High Torque Metal Gear. Adafruit. Micro servo
30. Popovic, M., Moffat, S., D'Agostino, J., Clarrissimeaux, E.: Fluid flow control valve. PCT International Patent Application No. PCT/US2020/017302 filed February 7, 2020; U.S. Provisional Patent Application of Popovic, et al. Application No.: 62/802,933 Filed February 8, 2019, Title: WPI Ref. No.: W19-032 (2019)
31. World Health Organization, "Concentrator, Oxygen," UMDNS 12873 (2012)
32. Kowalska Art. iStock.com/kowalska-art. Accessed 16 June 2020
33. Low-cost Oxygen Concentrator > helping during the crisis, 01 April 2020. https://users.wpi.edu/~mpopovic/pages/OxygenConcentrator.html, Accessed 28 Sept 2020
34. RepRapLtd.: Oxygen-concentrator, v2.0 (2020). https://github.com/RepRapLtd/Oxygen-concentrator. Accessed 02 July 2020
35. BIONICS: Sentient Bionics. https://www.sentientbionics.com/bionics. Accessed 15 May 2020
36. Pan, M., Omar, H.M., Rohani, S.: Application of nanosize zeolite molecular sieves for medical oxygen concentration. Nanomat. (Basel, Switzerland) **7**(8), 195 (2019). https://doi.org/10.3390/nano7080195
37. Crittenden, B., Thomas, W.J.: Adsorption Technology and Design. Butterworth-Heinemann, Oxford (1998)
38. De, M.P.G., Daniel, D.: Process for separating a binary gaseous mixture by adsorption. 3,155,468. U.S. Patent. 1964 Nov 3
39. Arduino MEGA 2560. Arduino. Microcontroller

Towards the Development and Validation of a Smartphone-Based Pupillometer for Neuro-Ophthalmological Diseases Screening

Ana Isabel Sousa[1(✉)], Carlos Marques Neves[2], Luís Abegão Pinto[2], and Pedro Vieira[1]

[1] Department of Physics, Faculty of Science and Technology, NOVA University of Lisbon, Caparica Campus, 2829-516 Caparica, Portugal
ai.sousa@campus.fct.unl.pt

[2] Faculty of Medicine, University of Lisbon, 1649-028 Lisbon, Portugal

Abstract. Pupillometry allows a quantitative measurement of PLR and has been mainly used to assess patient's consciousness and vision function. The analysis of pupil light reflex (PLR) has been showing a renewed interest since the discovery of intrinsically photosensitive retinal ganglion cells (ipRGCs), that are sensitive to the blue light, as they have an important role in pupil response to a stimulus. Some researches have studied pupillometry, particularly chromatic pupillometry that uses blue and red stimuli, to be a screening tool for neuro-ophthalmological diseases. Automated pupillometers have been widely used, however they are either not portable or expensive, reason why this technique has been mainly used in academic research. A smartphone-based pupillometer could be a promising equipment to overcome these limitations and to be a widespread screening tool, due to its low price, portability and accessibility. This work shows our latest advances towards the development and validation of an Android system for pupillometry measurements. Pupillometric data was collected with the smartphone application in a group of five healthy individuals and used to test our proposed data processing algorithms. These tests showed that the data processing methods that we are proposing, although promising, did not behave as expected, indicating that new approaches, better validations and corrections should be made in the future to get a stable software for pupil detection. Nevertheless, preliminary pupillometric data indicate that this system has the potential to work as an inexpensive, easy-to-use and portable pupillometer.

Keywords: Pupil · Pupillometry · Smartphone · Neuro-ophthalmology · Neuro-ophthalmological diseases

1 Introduction

Pupil's main function is to control the quantity of light that enters the retina, by its constant size adjustments [16]. The way the pupil reacts to a certain stimulus

X. Ye et al. (Eds.): BIOSTEC 2020, CCIS 1400, pp. 39–52, 2021.
https://doi.org/10.1007/978-3-030-72379-8_3

is known as Pupil Light Reflex (PLR) which is regulated by the autonomic nervous system. PLR describes how the pupil rapidly constricts after a stimulus and sequentially dilates to its normal size. This response has been studied and used over the years to assess a subject's consciousness and visual system function.

Until recently, it was thought that PLR was primarily driven by rods and cones [1]. However, this perception changed with the discovery of intrinsically photosensitive retinal ganglion cells (ipRGCs) in the early 2000's [15,21]. These cells are a small percentage of the retinal ganglion cells (RGCs) (around 0.2% $\simeq$ 3000 cells) [5] and contain melanopsin photopigment that renders them photosensitive, particularly to the absorption of blue light [9]. Thereby, several studies [2,9,17,24,25] have shown that PLR consists in a combination of rod, cones and ipRGCs responses.

The discovery of ipRGCs in humans renewed the interest in PLR and pupillometry as it can be a non-invasive technique to assess the visual system function. With ipRGCs particularly sensitive to blue light [9] and considering that the exposure to different wavelengths stimulates differently each type of photoreceptor [3], colored stimuli started to gain interest in pupillometry. Referred as chromatic pupillometry, normally uses red or blue light stimuli, allowing the study of damages in rods, cones and ipRGCs [26]. Several studies have also shown pupillometry potential in relation to neuro-ophthalmological diseases, such as Parkinson [6,10,11,31], Alzheimer [6,13], Glaucoma [5,12,23,27] or Multiple Sclerosis [4], using both chromatic or white light stimuli. Thus, pupillometry has been showing potential to be used as a screening tool for this type of diseases.

The evaluation of a subject's PLR is usually referred as pupillometry, traditionally assessed by the clinicians with a penlight. Quantitative pupillometry, using a device normally referred as pupillometer, allows to objectively measure how pupil reacts to a certain stimulus. Since Lowenstein et al. [20] photoelectric pupillograph, several pupillometry equipments have been developed. This type of devices have evolved over the years allowing not only continuous video recording but also automatic data analysis. Pupillometers usually use infrared cameras, which give better image contrast and reduce the influence of external lights in pupil size. This characteristic is a main advantage of these pupillometers, as they allow more precise measurements of pupil size. However they are either expensive, not portable or both, which makes them hard to be widespread as a clinical tool for diseases screening and monitoring.

Smartphones interest for application in the medical field has been increasing over the years, as they have technological capabilities progressively similar to computers, are portable, accessible and have affordable prices. When compared to traditional pupillometry equipments, smartphones overcome their limitations, being a possible technology to develop a widespread tool for pupillometry.

Using a mobile phone for pupillometric measurements started in 2013 by Kim et al. [19], whose work used the smartphone camera for acquisition with an attached optical apparatus. This device had four infrared light emitting diodes (LEDs) three to improve the quality of the acquired images and a white one to work as stimulus. In this study, post processing and analysis of the acquired data was made in MATLAB® (Mathwords Inc., Natick, MA).

Shin et al. [28] also have used a smartphone to acquire pupillometric measurements, but instead of recording a video, this group acquired 5 steady pictures in different momentums of the experiment: before the flash, during the light stimulus and the last three after the stimulus. These images were not automatically post-processed and analyzed, instead a clinician evaluated them according to pupil size and compared the results with a penlight measurement in the same subjects and conditions. Although the smartphone usage in this case was only for the eye photographies, their results shown similar results for the smartphone application and the penlight experiment made by the clinician.

In 2018, an iPhone-based pupillometer was proposed by McAnany et al. [22], named Sensitometer, which uses the rear-facing camera and flash light to acquire a video of the pupil during constriction and redilation phases after the stimulus. This proposed system provides real time measurements of PLR, with all the acquisition and processing done in the iPhone. Results were compared with an infrared camera that was simultaneously recording pupil's response to the light stimulus and they were statistically correlated.

Recently, our team proposed an all-in-one smartphone-based pupillometer using a medium range Android device to acquire and process pupil response videos [29]. This proposed system uses the rear-facing camera and flash light of the smartphone to work as stimulus. Data processing is also performed in the smartphone, being all integrated in the same application. An algorithm for data processing was also proposed, based on Contrast Limited Adaptive Histogram Equalization (CLAHE) to increase image contrast and ElSe algorithm [7] for pupil detection. It is important to notice that the system was thought to allow chromatic pupillometry with a simple usage of a standard colored cellophane paper to work as filter to be applied in the flash light, which is relevant for neuro-ophthalmological diseases screening as previously referred.

This first proposal of the system [29] had only some preliminary results, with the application of the pupil detection algorithm to around 40 eye images, but no further testing and validation was performed. In the present work, data from 5 healthy individuals was acquired following a chromatic pupillometry protocol based in Park et al. [25] discoveries, to validate the acquisition part of the system. The data was then post-processed with the main goal to validate the algorithms proposed in [29] for pupil detection. This study also aims to understand the influence of CLAHE parameters in pupil detection by ElSe algorithm. Therefore, the data processing algorithms were applied to several frames from the videos acquired from the participant subjects. Basically, this work is a continuation of the work presented in [29] towards the validation of this smartphone-based pupillometer.

Thus, the main goal of the present work is to validate the proposed all-in-one smartphone-based pupillometer in healthy subjects. It is also intended to validate a medium range Android smartphone as a device for chromatic pupillometry allowing acquisition and running data processing algorithms.

2 Methods

This project intends to validate the low cost pupillometer system developed by our team as proposed in Sousa et al. [29]. The main goal is to use a medium range Android smartphone to acquire video of pupil response to a chromatic stimulus and post-process it to get the common parameters of PLR.

2.1 Study Participants

Five participants with no known visual abnormalities have been selected. All participants underwent a standard ophthalmic screening test to measure vision acuity, by autorefractor and Early Treatment Diabetic Retinopathy Study (ETDRS) 2 m exams, and intraocular pressure (IOP).

Pupillometry measurements were only made in the left eye in each subject, for the different conditions and types of experiments. All the recorded videos and participants data was anonymized and codified.

This study was approved by the Hospital Santa Maria ethics committee, and a written informed consent was obtained from all the individual participants.

2.2 Pupillometry System

The main goal of the proposed system is to use a medium range Android smartphone to allow acquisition and processing of pupillometric data, without the need of other equipments. For this purpose an Android application was developed that could support the desired functions. The device used in this study is a Nokia 7 Plus (Nokia Corporation, HMD Global, Finland), with Android operation system, version 9 Pie. This smartphone has front and two rear facing cameras but for this study only rear facing cameras were used, particularly due to the flash light that is linked to them, needed for light stimulus.

This system, summarized in Fig. 1, has two main sections: acquisition and data processing. As an all-in-one system, it contemplates different programming languages working together such as Java and C++, that communicate through Java Native Interface (JNI) framework which enables the integration of C or C++ code in Java Android application.

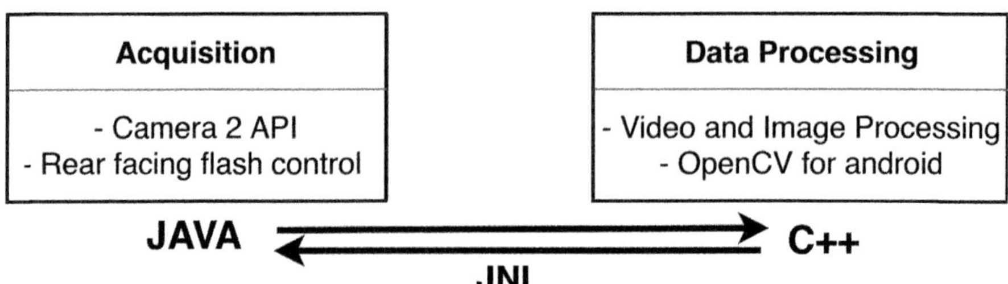

Fig. 1. Proposed system architecture, adapted from [29].

The acquisition part is mainly formed by the smartphone camera, the flash light and the application that controls their functioning. To do so, the Camera2 API is the Android interface used that allows proper control of smartphone cameras and flash and adjustment of the recording characteristics. The application that was developed for this system access the rear-facing cameras, starts recording, flashes a light stimuli automatically at a certain instant and stores the recorded video for post-processing. Recording duration and flash instant are parameters configurable in the application, allowing different experiments in terms of acquisition protocol.

The rear-facing flash allows a white light stimuli, however chromatic pupillometry is desired in this system to assess the influences of rods, cones and ipRGCs in pupil light reflex, as previously mentioned. To achieve this chromatic light stimuli, a standard grade cellophane paper is used as filter in front of the flash light, in both blue and red colors. Flash spectrum was acquired with a spectrometer in previous work, as referred in [29], indicating that these filters should be enough to get the desired light wavelengths in blue and red spectra.

2.3 Data Processing

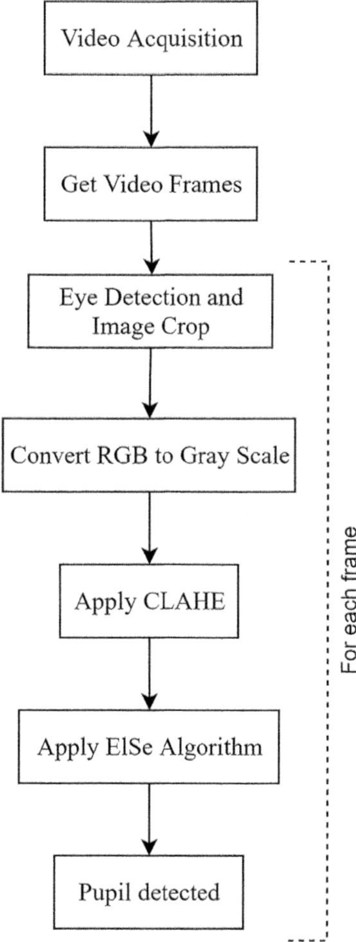

Fig. 2. Data processing algorithms flowchart, as referred in [29].

The second main section of this system is the data processing, that allows data extraction of the pupil videos. This process was developed using OpenCV for image processing, in both Java and C++, integrated in the Android application developed by the team. In this case, video processing is composed by getting all the frames, in each frame get the eye region and apply a pupil detection algorithm that will return its location and size. Having the pupil properly detected allows to build a graphic of the variation of the pupil size through time for a given experiment, which is used to understand PLR and compare between different experiments and protocols.

To detect the eye in each frame, OpenCV Haar-cascade eye detector, based in Viola and Jones Haar-cascade object detection algorithm [30], was used to reduce the area for pupil detection. The detected region area was verified and the regions with an area smaller area were automatically discarded, due to the cases where Haar-cascade algorithm fails to detect the eye.

Pupil detection in each eye frame is then the next data processing step. Each eye cropped image is converted to gray scale and image processing algorithms are applied to achieve the desired pupil detection. In [29] our team have proposed the application of Contrast Limited Adaptive Histogram Equalization (CLAHE) and then ElSe algorithm, developed by Fuhl et al. [7] for pupil detection is real world scenarios. A summary of this process is shown in Fig. 2.

Even though in our previous work [29] CLAHE didn't seem to make a difference in the pupil detection, as the results were similar to the images without any CLAHE application, the dataset used was small to take that conclusion. Therefore, we have tested again the influence of CLAHE in pupil detection in our system. With the goal to enhance image contrast, CLAHE is used as a way to overcome the low contrast between iris and pupil in images acquired by non-infrared cameras, such as the smartphone one. This method overcome simple histogram equalization or adaptive histogram equalization for iris recognition in Hassan et al. study [14]. OpenCV CLAHE function has two main parameters, the clipLimit, that represents the threshold from which the histogram is clipped and redistributed, and the tileGridSize, related to the tile size that the input will be sliced for the algorithm application. In the present work these two parameters of CLAHE were tested in order to better understand how this value influences the pupil detection in the videos acquired with our system. Tests were made with OpenCV CLAHE function default values, clipLimit = 4.0 and tileGridSize = (8,8), and clipLimit = 10.0 and tileGridSize = (10,10), that leads to a higher increase of the contrast in the images. This tests were made in 1071 eye frames acquired from different individuals.

After image enhancement, pupil detection is the main concern in this process. Although it is an apparently easy task, as the pupil is the black round area of the image, some difficulties need to be overcome such as low contrast between pupil and iris, blur, reflexes, illumination issues and other scenarios. Many algorithms have been developed over the years to achieve a proper pupil detection and ElSe algorithm, by Fuhl et al. [7], was considered the gold standard [8]. ElSe, that stands for Ellipse Selection, is an open source algorithm developed in C# that was targeted and tested in images acquired with infrared cameras in real world scenarios. As the name implies, this algorithm tries to find in a gray scale image the best suitable ellipse that could be the pupil. Very briefly, ElSe starts with the application of a Canny filter to get the image edges which are then filtered with straightening patterns. After this morphological operations, the straight lines are discarded and least square ellipse fitting is applied to get the best ellipse, after an ellipse evaluation to exclude unlikely pupils. If this process fails, a second approach is tried through a coarse positioning of the pupil. Image is downscaled and a convolution is applied with a surface and a mean filters. After multiplying the results of the convolutions, the resultant maximum value is defined as the starting point to be refined. This point surroundings are verified and the center of mass of the pixels under this threshold is the new pupil position. ElSe algorithm was tested in datasets acquired with infrared cameras, which is slightly different from the images acquired with a smartphone camera.

After pupil detection in each frame, pupil size variation through time should be normalized by the baseline, correspondent to the mean pupil size before the light stimulus. Pupil normalization was made based in the equation mentioned in [18], adapted for both pupil diameter or area variations, where 100% means pupil in its baseline size:

$$\text{pupil constriction} = 100 - \frac{\text{pupil baseline size} - \text{absolute pupil size}}{\text{pupil baseline size}} \times 100 \quad (1)$$

2.4 Chromatic Pupillometry Protocol and Preliminary Experiments

A pupillometry experiment needs to take into account a period for the pupil adaptation to the ambient light conditions, to get a proper measurement of PLR to the light stimulus, then recording should start for a short duration to get pupil size baseline, then a short colored light stimulus followed by a post-stimulus period after which the recording stops. In the present work a protocol for chromatic pupillometry is proposed, considering these intervals and based on the literature. Adapted from Park et al. [25] proposed pupillometry protocol, our protocol, showed in Figure 3, records the pupil for 5 s, then flashes the light stimulus, with 1 s duration, and continues recording for 30 s to get the pupil redilation phase. In the beginning of the experiment subjects were 7 min in the light ambient conditions, which in this case was a mesopic environment, to pupil adaptation. There was 5 min pause without recording, in the same light conditions, between experiments. This chromatic pupillometry protocol was applied in each participant, first for red light stimulus followed by the blue stimulus.

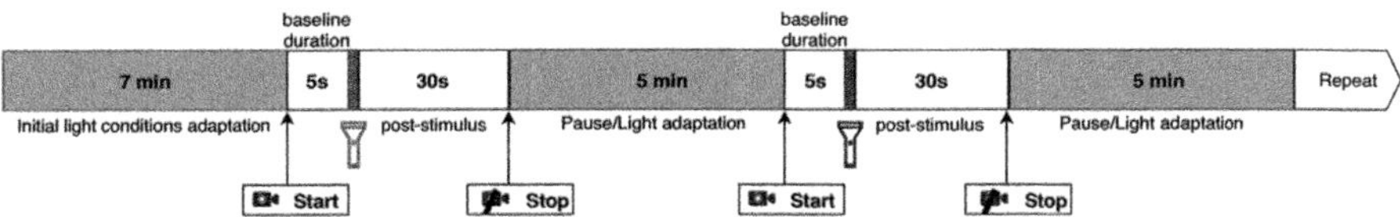

Fig. 3. Proposed protocol for chromatic pupillometry. Schema adapted from [29].

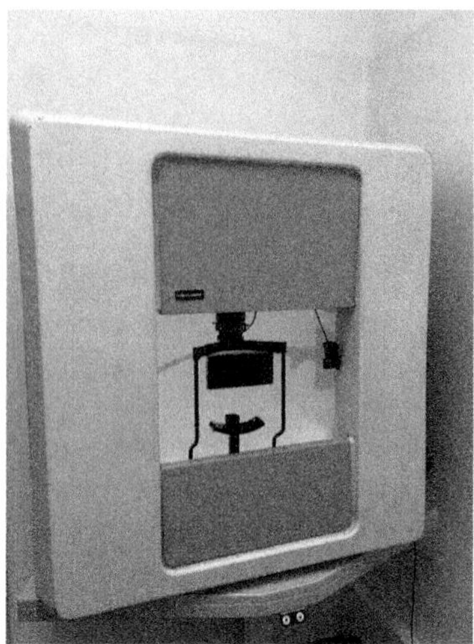

Fig. 4. Apparatus used to fix the smartphone in front of individual's face and to have a controlled ambient light.

The smartphone was fixed in a support in front of subject's face, which was resting in a face support common in ophthalmology equipments. The apparatus is shown in Fig. 4. During the acquisition time, subject's were focusing their vision in the center of an image usually used in autorefractors to avoid accommodation. In this way, the individuals eyes were focusing in that point, without moving all around, and the proximity of the smartphone to their face's and eye sight was overcome.

To each recorded video the data processing algorithm was applied in order to evaluate its efficiency in videos acquired with this proposed pupillometric system and in the light conditions they were acquired.

3 Results and Discussion

3.1 Study Participants

Five participants were included in this study, their demographic and ophthalmic characteristics are shown in Table 1. This group has an average age of 19.8, in a range of 18 to 23 years old. They present no known vision abnormalities or other kind of diseases, meaning it is considered a healthy group of participants. They were all cooperative and felt no discomfort during the experiments.

Table 1. Demographic characteristics of study participants.

Characteristics	Healthy participants data
Age	19.8 ± 2
Gender (F:M)	4:1
IOP (left eye)	13.9 ± 4.9

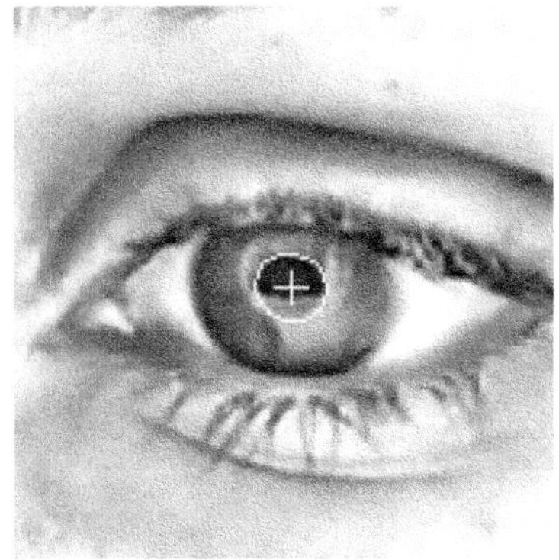

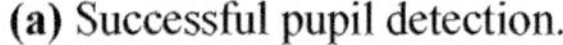
(a) Successful pupil detection.

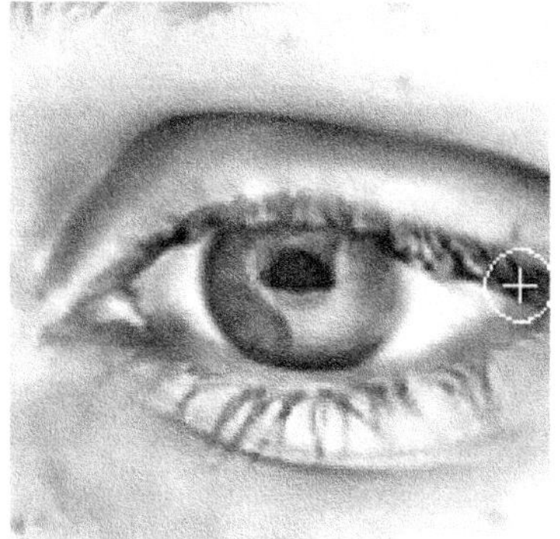
(b) Failed pupil detection.

Fig. 5. Examples of detection in images with default (clipLimit = 4.0 and tileGridSize = (8,8)) CLAHE parameters.

3.2 Data Processing Results and Discussion

The first validation of this system was in the acquisition part, with the proper working of the smartphone application during the recording period in the five participants. The application performed as expected, automatically applying the flash light at the desired instant and stopping the record 30 s after that. Each video was stored in the smartphone for post processing.

Video data processing was made as suggested in the flowchart presented in Fig. 2, testing different values of CLAHE, as referred in Sect. 2.3.

To test the detection algorithm and the influence of CLAHE parameters, 1071 frames from different subjects were analyzed with both default values (clipLimit = 4.0 and tileGridSize = (8,8)) and clipLimit = 10.0 and tileGridSize = (10,10). Some examples of images with successful and failed detection for both default values and 10.0 for CLAHE parameters are shown in Figs. 5 and 6, respectively. Pupil detection was manually verified. It is considered a success, cases in which the algorithm finds the center and the contours of the pupil correctly. A summary of number of successes and failures in the tested eye images is presented in Table 2.

In 1071 eye images tested, the algorithm had low success, being the error 88.4% for default CLAHE parameters and 93.6% for the others. This results were really low and not as expected. Although considering that ElSe algorithm [7] was tested in images acquired with infrared cameras, as the algorithm was developed for real world scenarios we were expecting better results, as the testing dataset of Fuhl et al. [7] had several images with poor quality, many reflexes and glares. However just applying CLAHE for image enhancement and then ElSe algorithm does not seem to be enough for our system.

Table 2. Results of variation in CLAHE parameters in pupil detection.

cutLimit	tileGridSize	Frames with success	Frames failed
4.0	(8,8)	124 = 11.6%	947 = 88.4%
10.0	(10,10)	69 = 6.4%	1002 = 93.6%
	Total frames	1071	1071

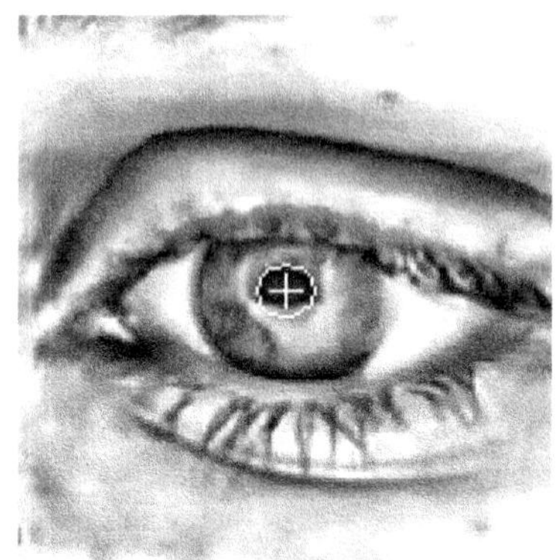

(a) Successful pupil detection.

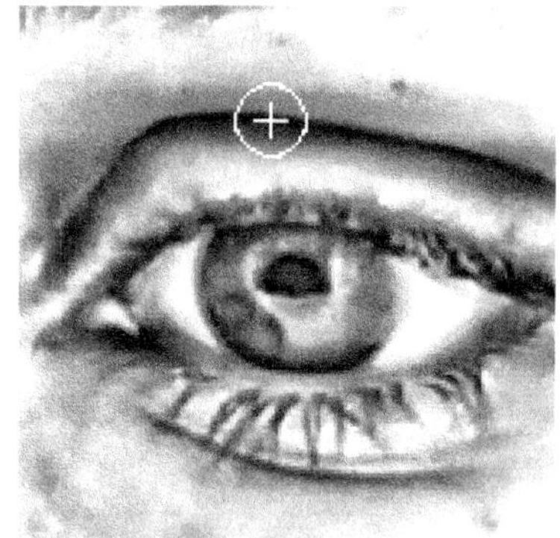

(b) Failed pupil detection.

Fig. 6. Examples of detection in images with clipLimit = 10.0 and tileGridSize = (10,10) CLAHE parameters.

3.3 Preliminary Pupillometry Results

As observed in last Sect. 3.2, the algorithm for pupil detection that our team proposed in [29] is not working in all frames and does not present enough stability for the acquisitions made with the participants. As the algorithms did not perform as expected, difficulties in constructing a PLR graphic, with pupil size variation in function of time, were suffered.

Nevertheless, with the goal and effort to see the typical pupillometry curve, the video of one of the participants in the case of a blue stimulus was used for some other try. After some enhancement of the results, we tried to filter some wrong measurements, for example, if the center of the pupil was much deviated from the previous one or the pupil didn't have a circular shape values were discarded. A median filter and a smoothing were applied. After doing this, the results were plotted in function of time and we obtained a graphic like the one shown in Fig. 7.

Even though the noticeable imperfections in the resultant graph and a decay in the pupil size between 15 and 25 s that is abnormal in a healthy patient and must be related to errors in pupil detection, one can see the expected PLR behavior: fast pupil constriction after the light stimulus until around half the size and a redilation after that. This constriction until around 50% of the baseline is concordant with what Park et al. [25] show in their study for 1 s flash stimulus for a healthy individual.

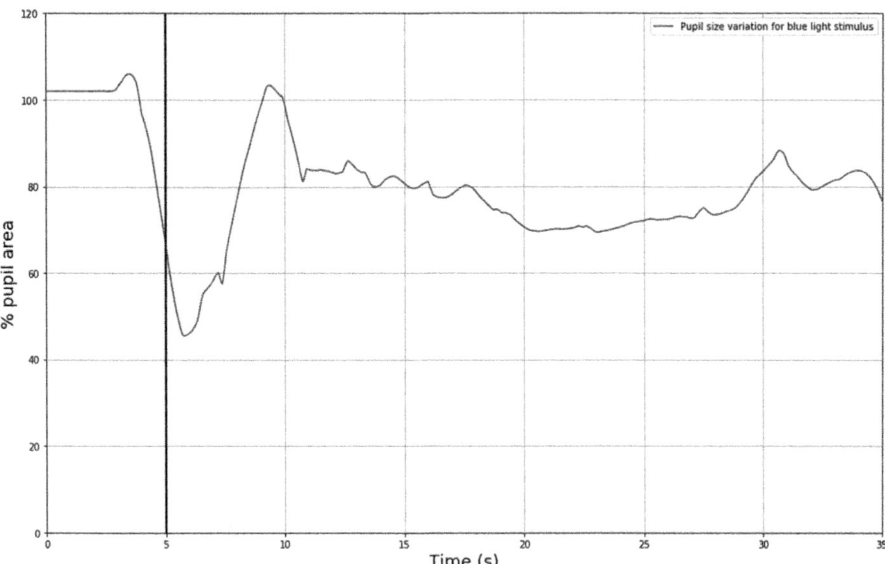

Fig. 7. Graphic showing some preliminary filtered results for one of the participants in the case of blue light stimulus. The vertical red line represents the flash instant. (Color figure online)

Despite the clear need for improvements in terms of data processing and pupil detection, it is visible that this system is in the right track to be a pupillometer tool. This preliminary pupillometric results showed that the rear-facing flash of the smartphone is capable enough of causing pupil reaction and the Nokia 7 Plus camera has enough quality for the acquisition process.

4 Conclusion

The possibilities of applications and usage for smartphones in the medical field are huge, due to their low price, easy access, portability and being used by everyone all over the world. This are great advantage in terms of pupillometry, that could allow to have a widespread screening and monitoring tool in diseases such as Parkinson's, Glaucoma or Alzheimer's, as previously mentioned.

Although there are some studies using a smartphone for pupillometry measurements, the system we proposed, first mentioned in [29] and the target of the present work, uses a medium range Android device and allows chromatic pupillometry which is necessary for diseases screening due to different color sensitivities of rods, cones and ipRGCs. We were able to prove functioning of the acquisition part of the system, showing that the Nokia 7 Plus flash light and camera are a sufficient equipment for pupillometric measurements. As for the data processing stage of the system, we are not yet with a stable and efficient method, particularly in the pupil detection part of the algorithm. There is a need to improve the algorithm that was proposed in [29] and further explored in this work, to define validations to automatically verify if the pupil was properly detected and possibly to develop alternative algorithms in case it fails.

The data acquired in this experiment allowed to have a proper knowledge of the acquired videos quality, the possible existant reflexes in each frame, as the smartphone is in front of subject's face and reflects in the eye, and other constraints. It also will allow the team to continue developing and improving the algorithms for pupil detection, clearly needed to properly validate the system as a whole.

Further work is then to improve the algorithms of pupil detection, so that this system can be prepared to severe illumination conditions and reflexes in the pupil. It is also important to make tests in different ambient light conditions to validate the algorithms and the system as a whole so that it can be used in different scenarios.

Finally, after the enhancement in data processing system and to proper validate the protocol in healthy individuals, the next steps include the validation of this smartphone-based pupillometer in patients with neuro-ophthalmological diseases. The main interest is to validate that this is an interesting and potential tool for early screening pathologies such as Parkinson's, Alzheimer's or Glaucoma.

Despite the need of improvements and more validation, the present work added some validation steps needed to show the potential of the proposed system. Smartphones seem to be promising devices for pupillometry, particularly to take this technique more close to clinical application, to be used as a screening tool for neuro-ophthalmological diseases.

Acknowledgments. This work is funded by National Funds through FCT - Portuguese Foundation for Science and Technology and Compta S.A. under the PhD grant with reference PD/BDE/135002/2017. A special acknowledgment to Compta S.A. team and to the Ophthalmology Department of Hospital Santa Maria for all the support given.

References

1. Alpern, M., Campbell, F.W.: The spectral sensitivity of the consensual light reflex. J. Physiol. **164**(3), 478–507 (1962). https://doi.org/10.1113/jphysiol.1962.sp007033
2. Barrionuevo, P.A., Nicandro, N., McAnany, J.J., Zele, A.J., Gamlin, P., Cao, D.: Assessing rod, cone, and melanopsin contributions to human pupil flicker responses. Invest. Ophthalmol. Vis. Sci. (2014). https://doi.org/10.1167/iovs.13-13252
3. Dacey, D.M., et al.: Melanopsin-expressing ganglion cells in primate retina signal colour and irradiance and project to the LGN. Nature (2005). https://doi.org/10.1038/nature03387
4. de Rodez Benavent, S.A., et al.: Fatigue and cognition: pupillary responses to problem-solving in early multiple sclerosis patients. Brain Behav. **7**(7), 1–12 (2017). https://doi.org/10.1002/brb3.717

5. Feigl, B., Mattes, D., Thomas, R., Zele, A.J.: Intrinsically photosensitive (melanopsin) retinal ganglion cell function in glaucoma, pp. 4362–4367 (2011). https://doi.org/10.1167/iovs.10-7069
6. Fotiou, D.F., Stergiou, V., Tsiptsios, D., Lithari, C., Nakou, M., Karlovasitou, A.: Cholinergic deficiency in Alzheimer's and Parkinson's disease: evaluation with pupillometry. Int. J. Psychophysiol. **73**(2), 143–149 (2009). https://doi.org/10.1016/j.ijpsycho.2009.01.011
7. Fuhl, W., Santini, T.C., Kuebler, T., Kasneci, E.: ElSe: ellipse selection for robust pupil detection in real-world environments (2015). https://doi.org/10.1145/2857491.2857505, http://arxiv.org/abs/1511.06575
8. Fuhl, W., Tonsen, M., Bulling, A., Kasneci, E.: Pupil detection for head-mounted eye tracking in the wild: an evaluation of the state of the art. Mach. Vis. Appl. **27**(8), 1275–1288 (2016). https://doi.org/10.1007/s00138-016-0776-4, http://arxiv.org/abs/1405.0006, http://link.springer.com/10.1007/s00138-016-0776-4
9. Gamlin, P.D., McDougal, D.H., Pokorny, J., Smith, V.C., Yau, K.W., Dacey, D.M.: Human and macaque pupil responses driven by melanopsin-containing retinal ganglion cells. Vis. Res. **47**(7), 946–954 (2007). https://doi.org/10.1016/j.visres.2006.12.015
10. Giza, E., et al.: Pupillometry and 123I-DaTSCAN imaging in Parkinson's disease: a comparison study. Int. J. Neurosci. **122**(1), 26–34 (2012). https://doi.org/10.3109/00207454.2011.619285
11. Giza, E., Fotiou, D., Bostantjopoulou, S., Katsarou, Z., Karlovasitou, A.: Pupil light reflex in Parkinson's disease: evaluation with pupillometry. Int. J. Neurosci. **121**(1), 37–43 (2011). https://doi.org/10.3109/00207454.2010.526730, http://www.tandfonline.com/doi/full/10.3109/00207454.2010.526730
12. Gracitelli, C.P.B., et al.: A positive association between intrinsically photosensitive retinal ganglion cells and retinal nerve fiber layer thinning in glaucoma. Invest. Ophthalmol. Vis. Sci. **55**(12), 7997–8005 (2014). https://doi.org/10.1167/iovs.14-15146
13. Granholm, E.L., et al.: Pupillary responses as a biomarker of early risk for Alzheimer's disease. J. Alzheimer's Dis. **56**(4), 1419–1428 (2017). https://doi.org/10.3233/JAD-161078, https://www.ncbi.nlm.nih.gov/pmc/articles/PMC5808562/
14. Hassan, R., Kasim, S., Jafery, W.A.Z.W.C., Shah, Z.A.: Image enhancement technique at different distance for Iris recognition. Int. J. Adv. Sci. Eng. Inf. Technol. **7**(4–2 Special Issue), 1510–1515 (2017)
15. Hattar, S., Liao, H.W., Takao, M., Berson, D.M., Yau, K.W.: Melanopsin-containing retinal ganglion cells: architecture, projections, and intrinsic photosensitivity. Science **295**(5557), 1065–1070 (2002). https://doi.org/10.1126/science.1069609
16. Kardon, R.: Regulation of light through the pupil (Chap. 26). In: Kaufman, P.L., Alm, A. (eds.) Adler's Physiology of the Eye, 11th edn. pp. 502–525. Elsevier, Mosby, St Louis (2011)
17. Kardon, R., Anderson, S.C., Damarjian, T.G., Grace, E.M., Stone, E., Kawasaki, A.: Chromatic pupil responses. Preferential activation of the melanopsin-mediated versus outer photoreceptor-mediated pupil light reflex. Ophthalmology **116**(8), 1564–1573 (2009). https://doi.org/10.1016/j.ophtha.2009.02.007
18. Kelbsch, C., et al.: Standards in pupillography. Front. Neurol. **10** (2019). https://doi.org/10.3389/fneur.2019.00129, https://www.frontiersin.org/article/10.3389/fneur.2019.00129/full

19. Kim, T.H., Youn, J.I.: Development of a smartphone-based pupillometer. J. Opt. Soc. Korea **17**(3), 249–254 (2013). https://doi.org/10.3807/JOSK.2013.17.3.249
20. Lowenstein, O., Loewenfel, I.E.: Electronic pupillography; a new instrument and some clinical applications. A.M.A. Arch. Ophthalmol. **59**(3), 352 (1958). https://doi.org/10.1001/archopht.1958.00940040058007
21. Lucas, R.J., Douglas, R.H., Foster, R.G.: Characterization of an ocular photopigment capable of driving pupillary constriction in mice. Nat. Neurosci. **4**(6), 621–626 (2001)
22. McAnany, J.J., Smith, B.M., Garland, A., Kagen, S.L.: IPhone-based pupillometry: a novel approach for assessing the pupillary light reflex. Optom. Vis. Sci. **95**(10), 953–958 (2018). https://doi.org/10.1097/OPX.0000000000001289, http://insights.ovid.com/crossref?an=00006324-201810000-00007
23. Najjar, R.P., et al.: Pupillary responses to full-field chromatic stimuli are reduced in patients with early-stage primary open-angle glaucoma. Ophthalmology **125**(9), 1362–1371 (2018). https://doi.org/10.1016/j.ophtha.2018.02.024
24. Park, J.C., McAnany, J.J.: Effect of stimulus size and luminance on the rod-, cone-, and melanopsin-mediated pupillary light reflex. J. Vis. **15**(3), 1–13 (2015). https://doi.org/10.1167/15.3.13
25. Park, J.C., Moura, A.L., Raza, A.S., Rhee, D.W., Kardon, R.H., Hood, D.C.: Toward a clinical protocol for assessing rod, cone, and melanopsin contributions to the human pupil response. Invest. Ophthalmol. Vis. Sci. **52**(9), 6624 (2011). https://doi.org/10.1167/iovs.11-7586
26. Rukmini, A.V., Milea, D., Gooley, J.J.: Chromatic pupillometry methods for assessing photoreceptor health in retinal and optic nerve diseases. Front. Neurol. **10**(FEB), 1–20 (2019). https://doi.org/10.3389/fneur.2019.00076
27. Rukmini, A.V., et al.: Pupillary responses to high-irradiance blue light correlate with glaucoma severity. Ophthalmology **122**(9), 1777–1785 (2015). https://doi.org/10.1016/j.ophtha.2015.06.002
28. Shin, Y.D., Bae, J.H., Kwon, E.J., Kim, H.T., Lee, T.S., Choi, Y.J.: Assessment of pupillary light reflex using a smartphone application. Exp. Ther. Med. **12**(2), 720–724 (2016). https://doi.org/10.3892/etm.2016.3379, https://www.spandidos-publications.com/10.3892/etm.2016.3379
29. Sousa, A.I., et al.: Development of a smartphone-based pupillometer for neuro-ophthalmological diseases screening. In: BIODEVICES 2020–13th International Conference on Biomedical Electronics and Devices, Proceedings; Part of 13th International Joint Conference on Biomedical Engineering Systems and Technologies, BIOSTEC 2020 (Biostec), pp. 50–56 (2020). https://doi.org/10.5220/0008962600500056
30. Viola, P., Jones, M.: Rapid object detection using a boosted cascade of simple features. In: Proceedings of the 2001 IEEE Computer Society Conference on Computer Vision and Pattern Recognition. CVPR 2001, vol. 1, pp. I-511–I-518. IEEE Computer Society (2001). https://doi.org/10.1109/CVPR.2001.990517, http://ieeexplore.ieee.org/document/990517/
31. Wang, C.A., McInnis, H., Brien, D.C., Pari, G., Munoz, D.P.: Disruption of pupil size modulation correlates with voluntary motor preparation deficits in Parkinson's disease. Neuropsychologia **80**, 176–184 (2016). https://doi.org/10.1016/j.neuropsychologia.2015.11.019, https://linkinghub.elsevier.com/retrieve/pii/S0028393215302347

Optical Spectroscopy Methods to Monitor Cells and Bacteria Concentrations and to Detect Contamination During Cell Culture: Application to the Fabrication of ATMPs

Bruno Wacogne[1,2(✉)], Déborah Legrand[1], Charles-Louis Azzopardi[1], Christian Pieralli[1], and Annie Frelet-Barrand[1]

[1] FEMTO-ST Institute, Univ. Bourgogne Franche-Comte, CNRS, 15B Avenue des Montboucons, 25030 Besançon, Cedex, France
bruno.wacogne@univ-fcomte.fr

[2] Centre Hospitalier Universitaire de Besançon, Centre d'Investigation Clinique, INSERM CIC 1431, 25000 Besançon, France

Abstract. Currently, the production of Advanced Therapy Medicinal Products is highly sensitive to any contamination sources and therefore takes place in clean and sterile environments. Several days are required for each production, making these products extremely expensive. Throughout the process, numerous quality controls must be performed. This is especially true during the expansion phase in order to monitor cell growth and to detect any contamination. Bioreactor's content must periodically be sampled to perform these controls. Two major drawbacks can be identified: a delayed knowledge of the quality control result and an additional risk of new contaminations due to sampling. In this work, we present optical spectroscopy methods which can be used to drastically reduce the risk of contamination. They provide a real time control of what happens in the bioreactor in a closed system manner. Cell concentrations are measured with an accuracy below 5% and contamination can be detected about 3 h after it occurred. The real time operation leads to several tens of thousand dollars' savings because it allows stopping the production as soon as a problem arises. Consequently, the price of these products should be greatly reduced and they may be proposed to more patients.

Keywords: Optical spectroscopy · Advanced therapy medicinal product · Cell growth monitoring · Contamination detection

1 Introduction

New treatment solutions for patients with no further therapeutic options have recently emerged. They are called ATMPs (Advanced Therapy Medicinal Products). Some of them are based on the use of "drug" cells derived from genetic modification or tissue and cell engineering. Cells acquire new physiological functions, biological characteristics or reconstruction properties to the expense of substantial manipulations. Indeed,

X. Ye et al. (Eds.): BIOSTEC 2020, CCIS 1400, pp. 53–75, 2021.
https://doi.org/10.1007/978-3-030-72379-8_4

natural processes of the body such as the use of stem cells for tissue regeneration, lymphocytes for cancer immunotherapy or apoptotic cells for anti-inflammatory purposes have inspired studies concerning these new biological drugs.

However, the production of these drugs requires the implementation of complex technologies of cell sorting, amplification, genetic transduction, amplification-division, activation, and this at several stages of production in sterile clean room type environment and in complex facilities. Also, the time needed to complete the production and the complex quality control processes further increase the fabrication costs. A schematic description of the fabrication process of CAR-T cells is given in Fig. 1 (adapted from [18]). It also applies to other ATMP productions.

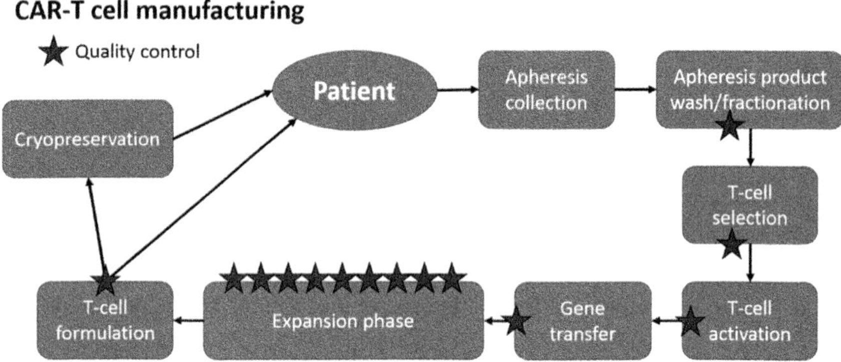

Fig. 1. Fabrication process of CAR-T cells. Adapted from [18].

Basically, the patient's blood is sampled and cells of interest (T cells for Fig. 1) are extracted/isolated and transduced to acquire the desired therapeutic properties. At this step, only well-transduced T cells are conserved. Now, these genetically modified cells are amplified/expanded in a bioreactor for a period that can extend up to 1 week. Eventually, the ATMP can be either injected to the patient or cryo-preserved before injection. Among others, one of the main constraints that must be addressed is the following.

Working in a controlled environment and preserving the closed system as necessary is crucial to meet the requirement of no contamination of the products. Frequently, the absence of containers, reagents or materials adapted to the protocol makes it difficult. Quality controls (red stars in Fig. 1) imply repeated samplings during the production, especially to control cell multiplication (expansion phase) and to detect any possible bacterial contamination (throughout the process). This increases the risk of contamination, the time of completion and requires increased traceability. Because these evaluations are time consuming, the production process still continues in parallel. In some cases, the production is stopped after several days when a contamination is detected. Obviously, this actually increases the cost and delay or even stop the delivery of the drug to the patient.

The work presented in this paper addresses the constraint of closed system and real time control of what happens in the bioreactor during the expansion phase. The goal is to provide an easygoing/soft/simple method to monitor the cell growth and to detect contaminations as early as possible. In-line or real time measurement techniques have been widely studied either for cell culture or contaminant development monitoring, very rarely for both.

Various spectroscopic coupled to chemometric techniques were presented in Teixeria review [14] concerning cell culture. In addition, other methods based on ultrasonic measurements [12] or capacitive techniques [7] have been proposed. Impedance monitoring, either in a bulk system [1] or in a microfluidic chip [8] has also been presented. But, in these references, indications whether or not the proposed method can be adapted in a closed system configuration were not discussed.

Concerning bacteria detection or monitoring, different sensors have been proposed to detect *Escherichia coli* (hereafter *E. coli*) by Ikonen [5]. Modified Field Effect Transistors have been experimented to detect the same bacteria [15]. Detecting several contaminants with a single device is challenging. However, it has been demonstrated by using optical absorption spectroscopy [16], fiber optic Fourier Transform Infra-Red spectroscopy [4], quartz crystal sensors [3] and electrochemistry [13]. More generally, recent reviews concerning electrochemical biosensors [2] and impedimetric immunosensors [9] for pathogen detection have been published.

Simultaneous cell monitoring and contaminant detection has only been the subject of very few papers. For example, Liu proposed advanced signal processing applied to Raman spectroscopy [10]. Together with normal condition monitoring, authors demonstrated the detection of growth problems 5 h after they stopped feeding the cells. They also detected effects of contamination with their monitoring algorithm. However, the nature of the contamination and the time required to detect it was not specified.

In this paper, we propose a proof of concept based on different optical spectroscopy methods to continuously monitor the evolution of cell concentration in a bioreactor and to issue an alarm signal shortly after a contamination occurred. The next section describes the experimental set-up, biological samples used in this study and spectroscopy methods employed. Section 3 presents the results obtained using several ways of exploiting information contained in transmission or absorption spectra of solution containing cells or bacteria (lymphocyte B cell and *E. coli*). Optical characterizations of the concentrations are based on colorimetric estimations of lymphocyte and *E. coli* solutions. These methods, together with the measurement of the maximum of the absorption spectra, can be used to monitor cell growth in real time. Other methods can be used for early detection of contamination. They are based on spectra shape analysis and Principal Component Analysis (PCA) respectively. Short discussions of these early results and aspects concerning socio-economic impacts will be given in Sect. 4.

2 Materials and Methods

For this proof of concept, measurements are not performed in a closed system configuration. Adaptation of the method in this particular environment is shortly discussed in Sect. 4.

2.1 Lymphocytes and *E. Coli* Preparation

Lymphocyte cell lines (Ramos, ATCC, USA) were cultured in X-Vivo (Lonza, Switzerland) with 5% FBS (Gibco™ 10270106) and 10% streptomycine/penicillin (100 µg/mL + 100 UI/mL, CABPES01-0U, Eurobio) in a humidified 37 °C, 5% CO_2 incubator. Cells were recovered after 2–3 days culture by centrifugation at 700 g, 10 min, 25 °C. Different cell concentrations ($10^4 \times$ [1, 2, 4, 6, 8, 10, 20, 30, 40, 50, 60, 70, 80, 90, 100] cells/mL) were prepared after dilution in autoclaved PBS 1x pH7.4 (Sigma, USA).

Escherichia coli DH5α (NEB, USA) were cultured in Luria Bertani overnight at 37 °C, 180 rpm in a MaxQ incubator. They were recovered by centrifugation at 5000 g, 15 min, 20 °C and re-suspended in autoclaved PBS 1x pH7.4 (Sigma, USA). Optical density of the re-suspension was measured in a spectrophotometer Shimadzu at 595 nm. Afterwards, different bacteria concentrations ($10^6 \times$ [1, 2, 4, 6, 8, 10, 20, 30, 40, 50, 60, 70, 80, 90, 100] bacteria/mL) were prepared for experiments.

2.2 Experimental Set-Up

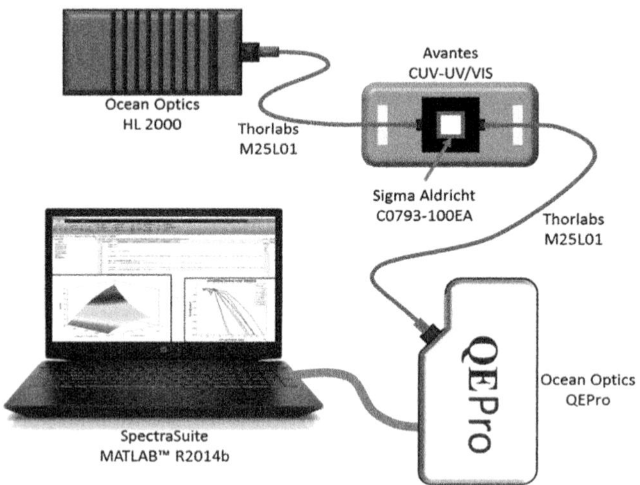

Fig. 2. Description of the experimental set-up.

The extremely simple experimental set-up is schematically presented in Fig. 2. The set-up was composed of a white light source (Ocean Optics HL 2000) connected to a cuvette holder (Avantes CUV-UV/VIS) via conventional step index optical fibers (Thorlabs M25L01). After propagation through the cuvette, light was launched into a spectrometer for transmission/absorption spectra acquisition (Ocean Optics QE-Pro). Fluorimeter polymethacrylate cuvettes were filled up to 3 mL with solutions of cells or bacteria (Sigma-Aldricht C0793-100EA). Spectra were measured using the specific feature available in the SpectraSuite software from Ocean Optics. Reference was obtained with a cuvette filled with PBS only. After transfer to PC, data processing was performed using MATLAB™ R2014b version. Spectra were truncated between 450 nm and 1120 nm in order to remove noisy data due to the transmission calculation in the SpectraSuite software.

2.3 Color Based Analysis of Transmission Spectra

The associated colors of the solutions were computed from transmission measurements. They do not actually correspond to the true colors of the solutions as discussed in Sect. 4. However, they are expressed in different color spaces in order to study the evolution of colorimetric parameters with species concentrations.

Tristimulus values (CIE XYZ) were calculated from spectral distribution with a CIE 1931 standard colorimetric standard observer 2° and a CIE standard illuminant D65. Color of the sample expressed in tristimulus color space was then converted in other color spaces: CIELAB (CIE Lab 1976), sRGB (standard RGB) and HSV. HSV coordinates were determined from sRGB. Color space conversion were performed using the open source Python package "Colour" dedicated to color science [11].

2.4 Analysis of Absorption Spectra

Absorption spectra used in Sect. 3.3 were slightly smoothed using a cubic spline algorithm in order to maximize the R^2 of the spectra fittings. Principal Component Analysis was performed with smoothed and normalized spectra.

In this work, so-called "contaminated spectra" presented below are artificial and made by adding spectra of lymphocytes and *E. coli*. This aspect will be discussed in Sect. 4.

3 Experimental Results

3.1 Measuring Concentrations of Both Species with Colorimetric Description of Transmission Spectra

Examples of transmission spectra recorded with lymphocytes and *E. coli* for different concentrations are given in Fig. 3. Transmission data are used because they are more consistent with a colorimetric description of the spectra than absorption data.

As previously mentioned, colors of the solution are described in several color spaces. Among them, we arbitrarily chose the following color spaces: XYZ, Lab, sRGB and HSV. The goal is to describe each parameter of these color spaces as a function of species concentration. Figure 4 shows the evolution of these colorimetric components as a function of the lymphocyte concentrations. In this figure, "star markers" correspond to experimental values. When the experimental data can be used to determine species concentrations, mathematical fitting of the experimental data is performed and displayed as continuous lines in the figure. In other cases, fitting is not performed.

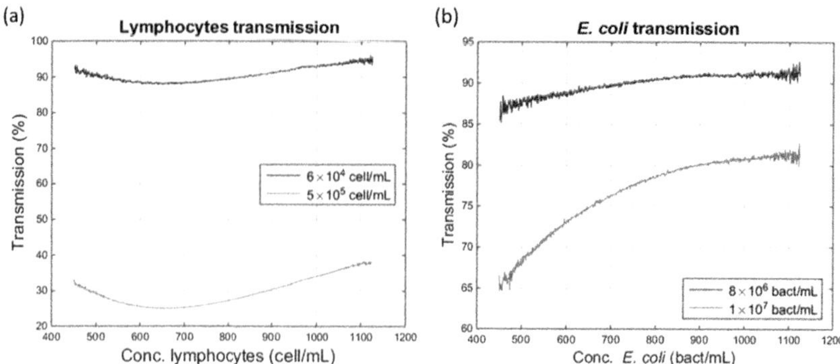

Fig. 3. Examples of transmission spectra of lymphocytes and *E. coli.* (a) Lymphocytes at 6×10^4 and 5×10^5 cell/mL, (b) *E. coli* at 8×10^6 and 1×10^7 bact/mL.

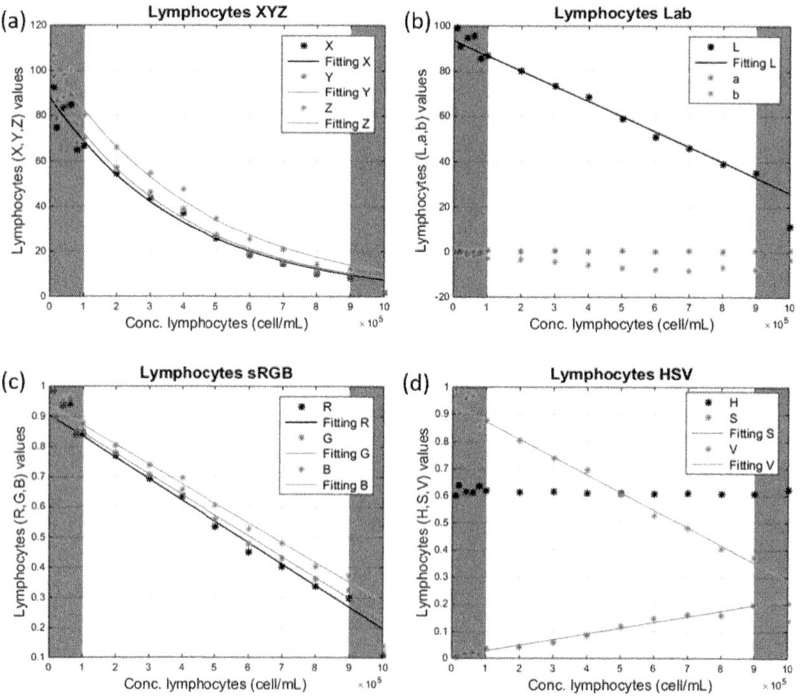

Fig. 4. Evolution of the colorimetric components with lymphocyte concentrations. (a) XYZ space, (b) Lab space, (c) sRGB space and (d) HSV space. (Color figure online)

XYZ components of the transmission spectra can easily be described by an exponential function. However, and as it is depicted on the Fig. 4 with the light red areas, fitting XYZ only works in a reduced range: [1×10^5–9×10^5] cell/mL. For low concentrations, transmission is of the order of 100% and no real difference can be observed in the transmissions spectra corresponding to these concentrations.

Conversely, for high concentrations, the transmission approaches 0% and no coherent information can be extracted from the spectra.

The situation is slightly different for the Lab components. Here, only the "L" component is useful. It can be described with a linear regression. The "a" component is almost zero for any lymphocyte concentration and contains no exploitable information. The "b" component shows a non bijective evolution with the concentration. Therefore, it cannot be used to compute lymphocyte concentrations. For these two components, no attempts were made to describe their behavior. For the Lab space again, the useful measurement range is [1×10^5–9×10^5] cell/mL.

The 3 components of the sRGB space can be used to compute the concentration using linear regressions in the above mentioned useful range. The HSV space only shows 2 exploitable components: "S" and "V". They are described with linear regression in the same useful range.

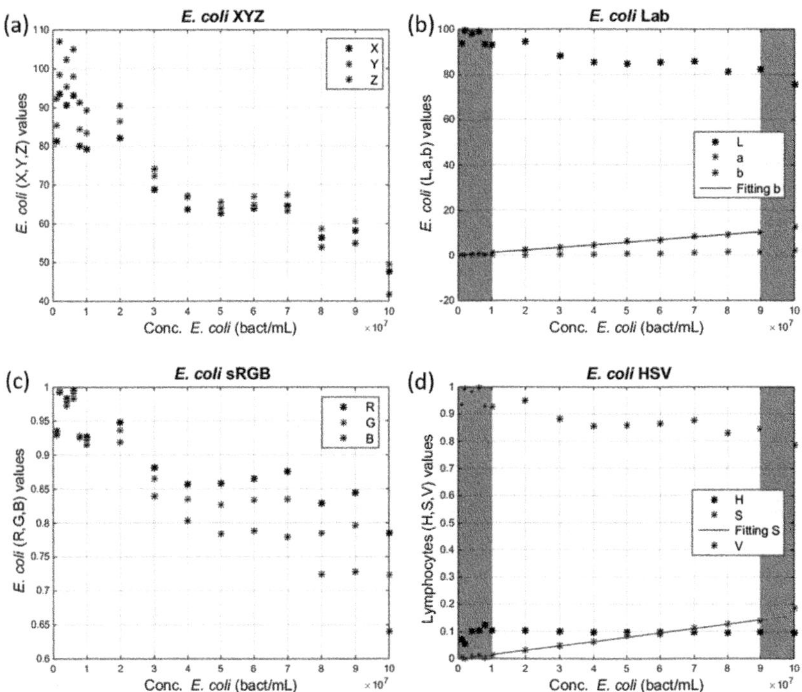

Fig. 5. Evolution of the colorimetric components with *E.* coli concentrations. (a) XYZ space, (b) Lab space, (c) sRGB space and (d) HSV space. (Color figure online)

The same analysis can be conducted with transmission spectra of *E. coli*. The result is given in Fig. 5. In this case, much less components can be used to compute bacteria concentrations. Indeed, for the XYZ and sRGB spaces, the evolutions of the components with the concentrations are non-bijective. This is also the case for the "L" and "V" components in corresponding color spaces. Concentrations can only be computed from the behavior of "b" and "S". Evolutions of the components with the concentration are linear. Again, the useful range of the usable colorimetric components is [1 × 10^5–9 × 10^5] bact/mL.

In order to define components offering the best accuracy when computing the concentration, we calculated the R^2 of each possible fitting. This is summarized in Table 1.

Table 1. Summary of the methods used to describe the evolution of the lymphocyte and *E. coli* concentrations, type of function used to fit the experimental data, values of the fitting R^2 and useful ranges. "pol deg 2": second order polynomial function, "exp": exponential function, "linear": linear regression. NA: not applicable. Light red highlighted rows correspond to non-exploitable components.

Lymphocytes				*E. coli*			
Method	**Fit type**	**R^2**	**Range (cell/mL)**	**Method**	**Fit type**	**R^2**	**Range (bact/mL)**
X	exp	0,9881	1×10⁵ - 9×10⁵	**X**	NA	NA	NA
Y	exp	0,988	1×10⁵ - 9×10⁵	**Y**	NA	NA	NA
Z	exp	0,9873	1×10⁵ - 9×10⁵	**Z**	NA	NA	NA
L	linear	0,9939	1×10⁵ - 9×10⁵	**L**	NA	NA	NA
a	NA	NA	NA	**a**	NA	NA	NA
b	NA	NA	NA	**b**	linear	0,9904	1x10⁷ - 9×10⁷
R	linear	0,9903	1×10⁵ - 9×10⁵	**R**	NA	NA	NA
G	linear	0,992	1×10⁵ - 9×10⁵	**G**	NA	NA	NA
B	linear	0,9936	1×10⁵ - 9×10⁵	**B**	NA	NA	NA
H	NA	NA	NA	**H**	NA	NA	NA
S	linear	0,9662	1×10⁵ - 9×10⁵	**S**	linear	0,9901	1x10⁷ - 9×10⁷
V	linear	0,9936	1×10⁵ - 9×10⁵	**V**	NA	NA	NA

R^2 values are all relatively high. The highest values are obtained with the "L" component of the lymphocyte transmission spectra (R^2 = 0.9939) and with the "b" component of the *E. coli* transmission spectra (R^2 = 0.9904). For these two examples, fitting functions $L_{lym}(\boldsymbol{C})$ for the lymphocyte L component and $b_{E.coli}(\boldsymbol{C})$ for the *E. coli* "b" components are given by:

$$L_{lym}(\boldsymbol{C}) = m1.\boldsymbol{C} + m2 \quad (1)$$

$$b_{E.coli}(\boldsymbol{C}) = n1.\boldsymbol{C} + n2 \quad (2)$$

Where $m1 = -6.735 \times 10^{-5}$, $m2 = 93.56$, $n1 = 1.147 \times 10^{-7}$ and $n2 = 0.1295$.

Using Eqs. (1) and (2) allows estimating the species concentrations as presented in Fig. 6. Blue diamonds correspond to the real concentrations and red crosses correspond to the concentrations calculated using Eqs. (1) and (2). Standard deviations reported in the figure correspond to 1.89×10^4 cell/mL for the lymphocytes (3.8% at the center of the concentration range) and 2.37×10^6 bact/mL for *E. coli* (4.7% at the center of the concentration range).

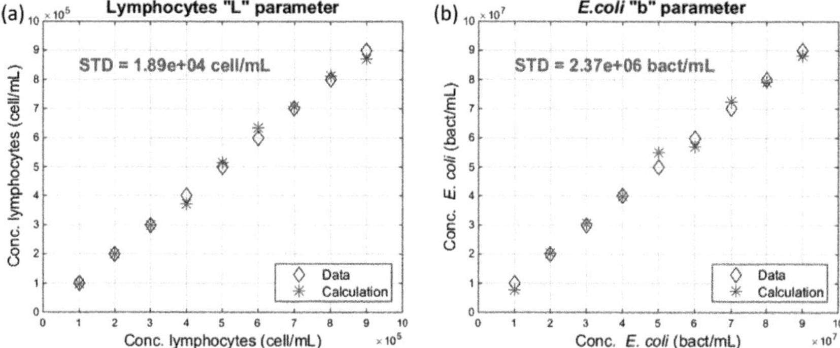

Fig. 6. Calculating the species concentrations from colorimetric parameters. (a) Lymphocytes concentrations using the "L" component in the Lab color space. (b) *E. coli* concentrations using the "b" component in the same color space. (Color figure online)

STDs obtained using fitting equations corresponding to exploitable color spaces shown in Table 1 are reported in Table 2.

Table 2. Values of the Standard Deviation for the different fitting possibilities.

Lymphocytes			*E. coli*		
Method	**Fit type**	**STD (cell/mL)**	**Method**	**Fit type**	**STD (bact/mL)**
X	exp	$4{,}19\times10^4$	X	NA	NA
Y	exp	$3{,}84\times10^4$	Y	NA	NA
Z	exp	$4{,}27\times10^4$	Z	NA	NA
L	linear	$1{,}89\times10^4$	L	NA	NA
a	NA	NA	a	NA	NA
b	NA	NA	b	linear	$2{,}37\times10^6$
R	linear	$2{,}39\times10^4$	R	NA	NA
G	linear	$2{,}17\times10^4$	G	NA	NA
B	linear	$1{,}94\times10^4$	B	NA	NA
H	NA	NA	H	NA	NA
S	linear	$4{,}51\times10^4$	S	linear	$2{,}41\times10^6$
V	linear	$1{,}94\times10^4$	V	NA	NA

To summarize this section, concentrations of lymphocytes and *E. coli* can be measured over a large concentration range using the color associated to transmission spectra ([1×10^5–9×10^5] cell/mL). Table 2 shows that the “L” component of the Lab color space leads to the lowest STD for cell concentration measurements (1.89×10^4 cell/mL, i.e. 3.78% at the center of measurement range). For *E. coli* the lowest STD is obtained with the “b” component of the same Lab color space (2.37×10^6 bact/mL, i.e. 4.74% at the center of measurement range). Aspects concerning the use of colorimetric analysis of transmission spectra will be shortly discussed in Sect. 4.

Often in biology laboratories, concentration is measured using the absorption of a solution at a fixed wavelength. Measured solutions are diluted in order to obtain optical densities in a range which ensures a reliable measurement. In the next section, we show how the information contained in the whole absorption spectrum can be used to measure concentrations. This will also introduce Sect. 3.3 where the possibility to exploit the shapes of absorption spectra can be used to detect culture contaminations.

3.2 Measuring Concentrations with the Shapes of the Absorption Spectra

Examples of absorption spectra recorded with lymphocytes and *E. coli* for different concentrations are given in Fig. 7.

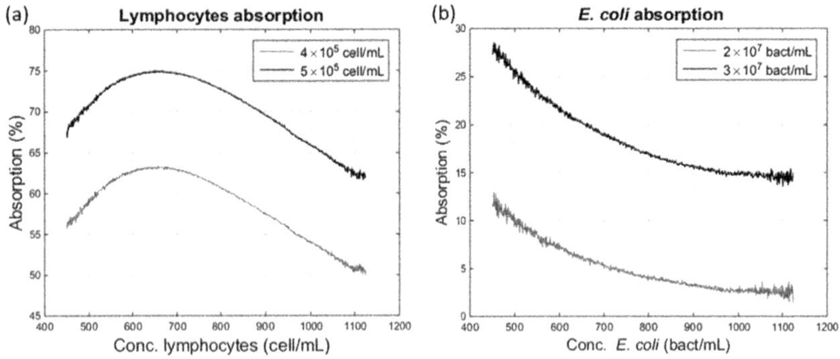

Fig. 7. Examples of absorption spectra of lymphocytes and *E. coli*. (a) Lymphocytes at 4×10^5 and 5×10^5 cell/mL, (b) *E. coli* at 2×10^7 and 3×10^7 bact/mL.

The shapes of spectral absorptions of the two species are completely different. The idea is, for each species, to model the evolution of the shapes of absorption spectra as a function of concentration and to use this mathematical description to calculate the concentration in species from any measured spectrum.

Indeed, the ulterior motive is to measure the absorption spectrum of the contents of the bioreactor continuously. For each recorded spectrum, the idea is to analyze the shape, to separate the part due to the contribution of lymphocytes from that due to *E. coli* and to calculate their respective concentrations. This would allow detecting a possible contamination in real time and stopping the fabrication of the ATMPs extremely early, i.e. before a large amount of money is lost and possibly reducing the final cost of the drug.

First, it is necessary to determine the evolution of the spectra of the two species as a function of the concentration. This is achieved using spectra mathematical fitting. We found a general equations which can be used for each of the species. We found that an exponential based function can be used to fit absorption spectra of lymphocytes while those of *E. coli* can be fitted with a 3rd order polynomial function. We then have:

$$Spec_{lym}(\lambda, \boldsymbol{C}) = p1.exp\left(-\left(\frac{\lambda - p2}{p3}\right)^2\right) + p4 \quad (3)$$

$$Spec_{E.Coli}(\lambda, \boldsymbol{C}) = q1\lambda^3 + q2\lambda^2 + q3\lambda + q4 \quad (4)$$

Here, λ is the wavelength, C is the concentration. The concentration dependence exists through the "pi" and "qi" parameters which can be expressed as follows.

$$p1(\boldsymbol{C}) = a1.exp\left(-\left(\frac{\boldsymbol{C} - a2}{a3}\right)^2\right) \quad (5)$$

$$p2(\boldsymbol{C}) = b1.\boldsymbol{C} + b2 \quad (6)$$

$$p3(\boldsymbol{C}) = c1.\boldsymbol{C}^2 + c2.\boldsymbol{C} + c3 \quad (7)$$

$$p4(\boldsymbol{C}) = d1.\boldsymbol{C}^2 + d2.\boldsymbol{C} + d3 \quad (8)$$

$$q1(\boldsymbol{C}) = e1.\boldsymbol{C}^2 + e2.\boldsymbol{C} + e3 \quad (9)$$

$$q2(\boldsymbol{C}) = f1.\boldsymbol{C}^2 + f2.\boldsymbol{C} + f3 \quad (10)$$

$$q3(\boldsymbol{C}) = g1.\boldsymbol{C}^2 + g2.\boldsymbol{C} + g3 \quad (11)$$

$$q4(\boldsymbol{C}) = h1.\boldsymbol{C}^2 + h2.\boldsymbol{C} + h3 \quad (12)$$

Coefficients used in Eqs. (5) to (12) are given in Table 3.

Table 3. Coefficients used in Eqs. (5) to (12).

$p1(\mathbf{C})$	a1 = 14.32	a2 = 4.1×10^5	a3 = 6.145×10^5
$p2(\mathbf{C})$	b1 = 7.21×10^{-5}	b2 = 647	
$p3(\mathbf{C})$	c1 = 1×10^{-10}	c2 = -1.9×10^{-5}	c3 = 325.7
$p4(\mathbf{C})$	d1 = -5×10^{-11}	d2 = 1.3×10^{-3}	d3 = 6.791
$q1(\mathbf{C})$	e1 = 1.2×10^{-23}	e2 = -1.6×10^{-15}	e3 = 1.2×10^{-9}
$q2(\mathbf{C})$	f1 = -3.3×10^{-20}	f2 = 5.1×10^{-12}	f3 = -1.7×10^{-6}
$q3(\mathbf{C})$	g1 = 2.8×10^{-17}	g2 = -5.5×10^{-09}	g3 = -8.3×10^{-4}
$q4(\mathbf{C})$	h1 = -1×10^{-14}	h2 = 2.4×10^{-6}	h3 = 1.234

Figures 8 and 9 show the evolutions of the pi and qi functions and Eqs. (5) to (12) are recalled in the figures.

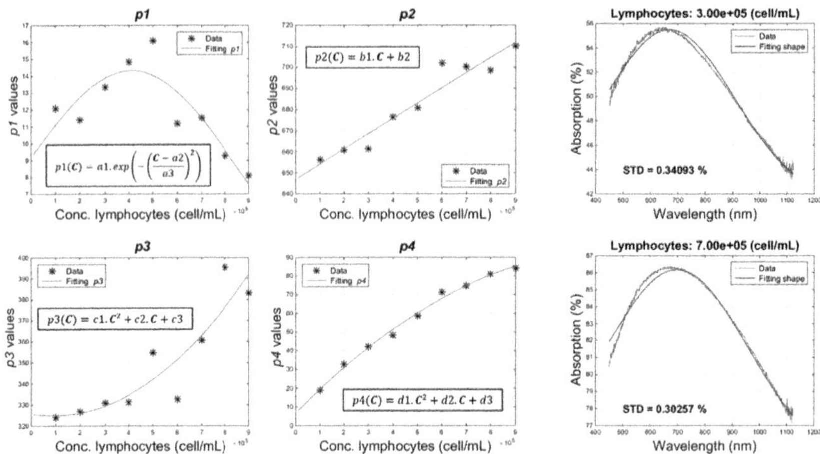

Fig. 8. Evolution of the *pi* functions with the lymphocyte concentration (left hand side). Examples of experimental absorption spectra fitted with the $\mathrm{Spec}_{\mathrm{lym}}(\lambda, \mathbf{C})$ function (right hand side).

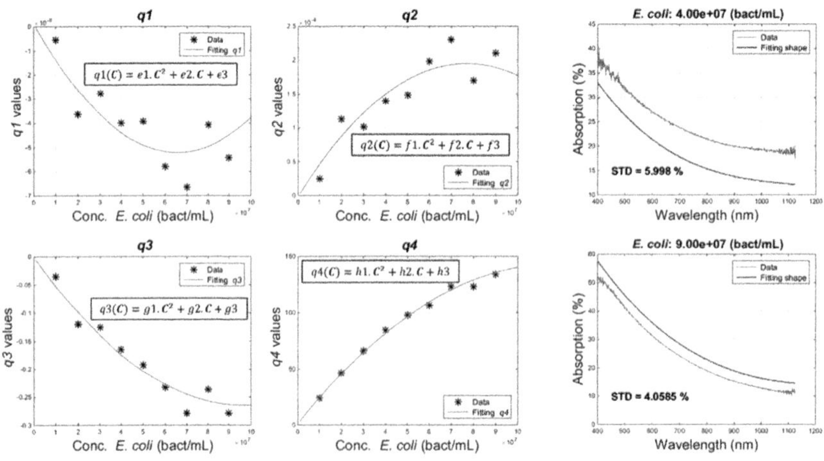

Fig. 9. Evolution of the *qi* functions with the *E. coli* concentration (left hand side). Examples of experimental absorption spectra fitted with the $\mathrm{Spec}_{E.Coli}(\lambda, \mathbf{C})$ function (right hand side).

Obviously, pi and qi data can hardly be fitted with mathematical function. Only p4 and q4 data can efficiently be modelled (this aspect will be discussed in Sect. 4). Despite this, shapes of the absorption spectra can be modelled with a relatively good accuracy. For the lymphocytes, the STD is of the order of 0.3%. For the *E. coli* however, the STD is larger: between 4% to 6%.

Functions $\text{Spec}_{\text{lym}}(\lambda, \mathbf{C})$ and $\text{Spec}_{E.Coli}(\lambda, \mathbf{C})$ are represented in Fig. 10.

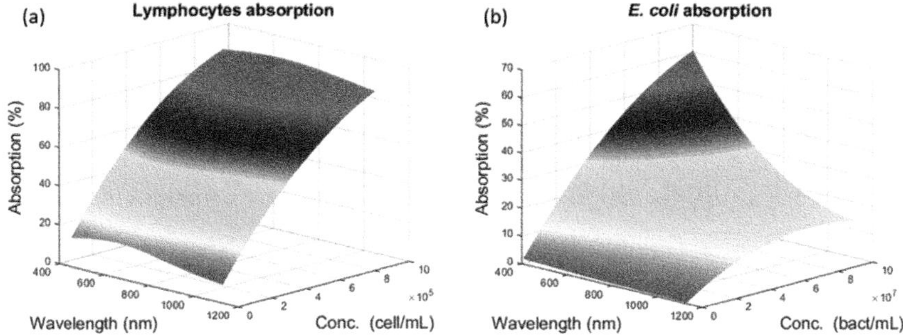

Fig. 10. Theoretical evolutions of the absorption spectra with species concentrations. (a) Lymphocytes, (b) *E. coli*. Adapted from [17].

These functions are used to calculate species concentrations from the shapes of the experimental absorption spectra. The result is shown in Fig. 11.

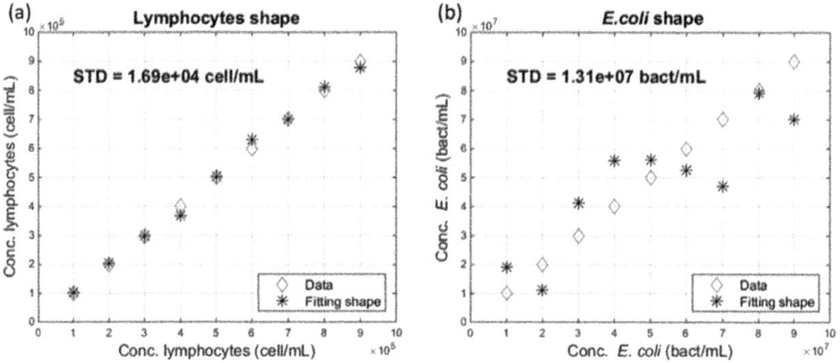

Fig. 11. Calculating the species concentrations from the shapes of the absorption spectra. (a) Lymphocytes concentrations. (b) *E. coli* concentrations. Adapted from [17].

The standard deviation for the lymphocytes is 1.69×10^4 cell/mL. This is lower than what was obtained using the "L" components in the Lab color space (1.89×10^4 cell/mL). For *E. coli* obviously, we failed measuring concentrations from the shape of the absorption spectra. Indeed, the standard deviation (1.31×10^7 bact/mL) is more than 5 times larger than what was obtained using the "b" component in the Lab color space (2.37×10^6 bact/mL). Therefore, the initial idea consisting in studying the shape of an absorption spectrum in real time in order to early detect any contamination seems impossible when trying to compute the actual concentrations values.

We now consider the evolution of the maxima of the lymphocyte absorption spectra with concentration. This evolution can be modelled with a second order polynomial function as depicted in Fig. 12(a). Here again, the useful range is [1×10^5–9×10^5] cell/mL. Maxima of the absorption spectra can be modelled as follows.

$$Max_{lym}(\boldsymbol{C}) = s1.\boldsymbol{C}^2 + s2.\boldsymbol{C} + s3 \quad (13)$$

Where: $s1 = -7.557 \times 10^{-11}$, $s2 = 1.527 \times 10^{-4}$ and $s3 = 16.74$.

Calculation of lymphocyte concentrations from the evolution of the spectra maxima is shown in Fig. 12(b). Here, a standard deviation as low as 1.39×10^4 cell/mL (2.78% at the center of the range) is obtained. This is the lowest values obtained so far in this study.

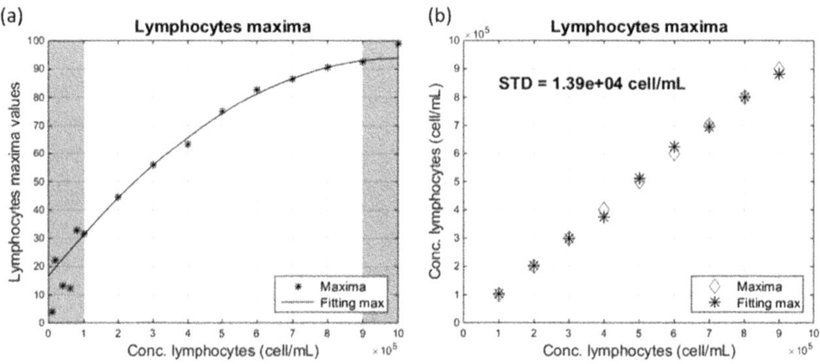

Fig. 12. Calculating the lymphocyte concentrations from the absorption maxima. (a) Evolution of the maxima with the lymphocyte concentrations. (b) Fitting concentrations using a second order polynomial function.

To summarize Sects. 3.1 and 3.2, concentrations of either lymphocyte or *E. coli* can be measured using white light spectroscopy. The best way to monitor lymphocyte concentration is to consider the evolution of the maxima of the absorption spectra. Concerning *E. coli*, the best method consists in measuring the "b" component in the Lab color space from the transmission spectra. Surprisingly, the evolution of the shape of the lymphocyte absorption spectra does not lead to a better accuracy than the simple measure of the absorption maximum.

However, estimating the shape of the absorption spectra can be used for another purpose. Indeed, the above described methods can be used to monitor the evolution of the concentrations of both species when only one species is present. When considering spectra of lymphocyte and *E. coli* mixtures, it is extremely difficult to separate their respective contributions. The problem becomes insoluble when several types of pathogens are considered.

We recall that the main goal is to measure the lymphocytes concentrations in a close–system environment and in real time. The goal is also to be able to detect any possible contamination in the same experimental environment. This can be achieved by considering things differently. This is the subject of the next section.

3.3 Monitoring Cell Concentrations and Detecting Contaminations: A New Approach

Fitting the Shape of the Absorption Spectra. As long as everything is normal (no contamination) during the expansion phase, cell concentration can be monitored using methods described above. Also, we know the equation which describes the shape of the absorption spectra (Eq. (5)). In case of contamination, the shape of the spectrum resulting from the contribution of the lymphocytes and the contaminant differs from the ones corresponding to lymphocyte alone. In this situation, Eq. (5) should no longer be usable to fit the shape of absorption spectrum.
Practically, during the expansion phase, absorption spectra are recorded and fitted with a function representing the shapes of the lymphocyte spectra when they are alone. At this stage, only the shape of the spectra is analyzed. Therefore, Eq. (5) can be used in a simpler way than what is presented in Sect. 3.2 where coefficients are expressed as a function of the concentration. This function is called $Abs_{lym}(\lambda)$. Here, the function only depends on the wavelength and coefficients are adjusted only to obtain the highest R^2. Therefore, an accurate fitting (high R^2) using $Abs_{lym}(\lambda)$ means no contamination, lymphocyte concentration is calculated using Eq. (13), content of the bioreactor is adjusted according to this concentration and fabrication continues. Conversely, an R^2 value less than a threshold to be determined is the sign of a contaminated culture. Fabrication must then be stopped. Figure 13 explain this process.

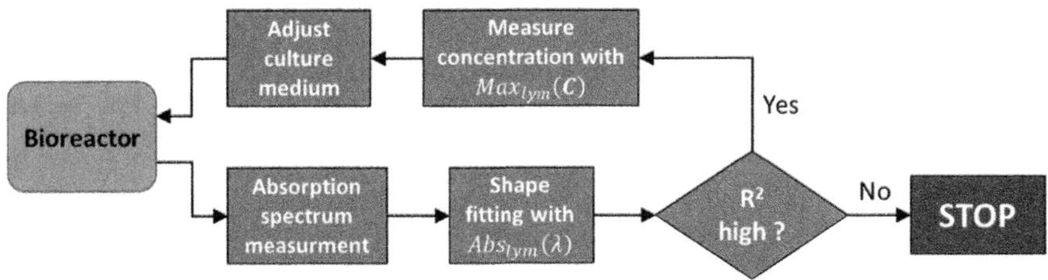

Fig. 13. In-line process to detect contaminations and to adjust the bioreactor composition as a function of the lymphocyte concentration.

As concentrations are not calculated, only the shape of the recorded spectrum is fitted. The following equation can efficiently be used.

$$Abs_{lym}(\lambda) = a.exp\left\{-\left(\frac{\lambda - b}{c}\right)^2\right\} + d \tag{14}$$

Here, constraints were put to coefficients a, b, c and d. Otherwise, the fitting algorithm ("trust region" in Matlab™ Curfitting toolbox) always finds a set of parameters to describe even contaminated spectra. The fitting bounds and starting points are summarized in Table 4.

Table 4. Lower bounds, upper bounds and starting points used to fit absorption spectra with Eq. (14).

Coefficient	Lower bound	Upper bound	Starting point
a (%)	0	200	100
b (nm)	600	750	675
c (nm)	0	500	250
d (%)	0	200	100

Figure 14 shows examples of absorption spectra fittings using Eq. (14). Spectra were slightly smoothed as mentioned above.

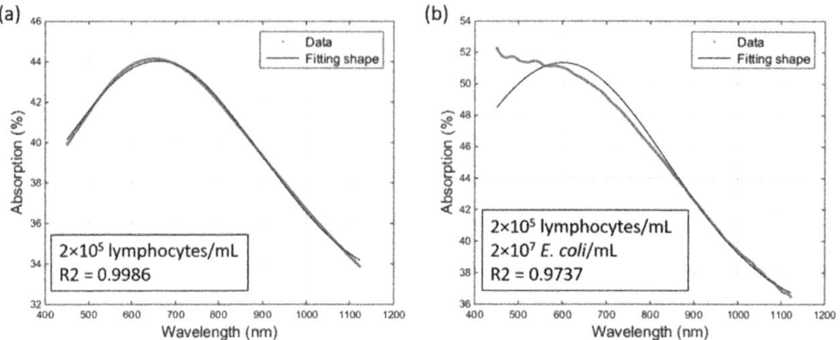

Fig. 14. Examples of spectra fitting using Eq. (14). (a) Lymphocyte concentration = 2×10^5 cell/mL, $R^2 = 0.9986$. (b) Lymphocyte concentration = 2×10^5 cell/mL, *E. coli* concentration = 2×10^7 bact/mL, $R^2 = 0.9737$.

In Fig. 14(a) fitting is performed with pure lymphocytes at 2×10^5 cell/mL. The R^2 value is quite high: $R^2 = 0.9986$. Indeed, with pure lymphocyte spectra, R^2 coefficients are always greater than 0.99 in the above mentioned useful range [1×10^5–9×10^5].

In Fig. 14(b) fitting is performed with the same lymphocyte concentration contaminated with 2×10^7 *E. coli*/mL. In this case and because the contamination modifies the shape of the recorded spectrum, R^2 decreases to 0.9737. Note that the so-called "contaminated spectra" are artificial and obtained by adding absorption spectra of both species as described in Sect. 2.4.

For different lymphocyte concentrations in the useful range, Fig. 15 shows the evolution of R^2 with increasing concentrations of *E. coli*. Each curve corresponds to one lymphocyte concentration. It is observed that, for any lymphocyte concentrations, the contamination detection limit is of the order of $2.5.10^7$ bact/mL. For this, we set a positivity threshold $R^2 = 0.988$ (arrows in the figure). Knowing that *E. coli* divides every 20 min and considering that the contamination is due to 1000 bact/mL, the warning signal can be issued 4 h 52 min post contamination.

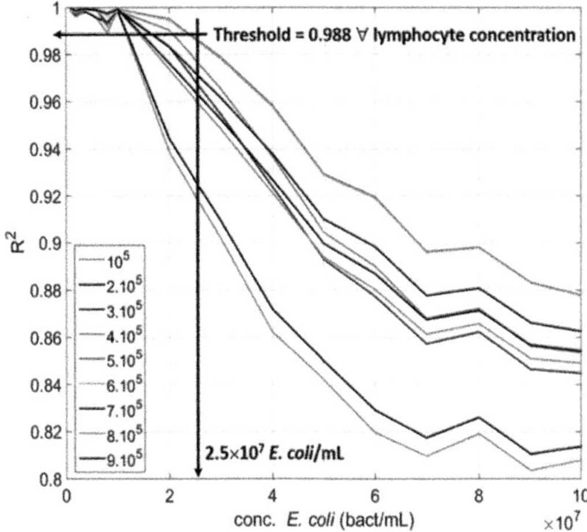

Fig. 15. Evolution of the R^2 coefficient with the concentration in *E. coli* for different lymphocyte concentrations. The legend corresponds to lymphocyte concentrations in cell/mL [17].

Using Principal Component Analysis. Analyzing the shape of the absorption spectra allows detecting a contamination when $2.5.10^7$ bact/mL are present in the bioreactor. But it is possible to further reduce the time required to issue the alert signal using Principle Component Analysis (PCA). In what follows, spectra are smoothed and normalized as mentioned above. PCA is conducted in two steps.

The first step consists in verifying that populations of both lymphocytes and *E. coli* can be distinguished. Figure 16(a) shows that plotting PC2 vs. PC1 allows separating biological populations. The black line represents the frontier between these populations. It is defined by either the analysis of the mean and variance of the two distributions or the minima of the coordinates of lymphocytes (circles) and maxima of *E. coli* (crosses). Taking into account these data, a straight line which separates the PC1-PC2 domain in two zones is defined [6].

The second step consists in checking where a so-called "contaminated spectrum" is located in the PC1-PC2 space. Indeed, the 30 data used to generate Fig. 16(a) form a base for the pure lymphocyte and pure *E. coli* populations. Contaminated spectra correspond to all possible combinations of lymphocyte spectra added to *E. coli* spectra. They are processed one by one. Each contaminated spectrum is considered as a 31rst data in the above mentioned base before a new PCA is performed. This is iterated for the 225 possible combinations. Indeed, in this PCA study, all *E. coli* spectra are considered and not only those corresponding to concentrations above 1×10^7 bact/mL as it was the case up to now. The result is shown in Fig. 16(b) with the contaminated spectra marked with red squares.

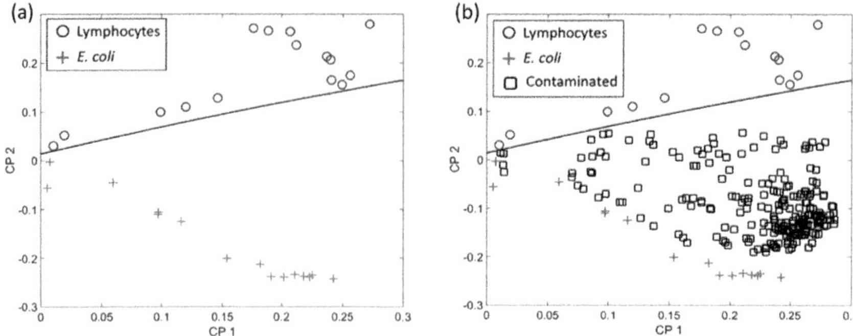

Fig. 16. Principal Component Analysis. Blue circles: lymphocytes, green crosses: *E. coli*, red squares: contaminated cultures and black line: separation between lymphocytes and *E. coli*. (a) ACP for pure lymphocyte and *E. coli*. (b) The same as (a) with contaminated cultures. (Color figure online) Adapted from [17].

Contaminated spectra of contaminated culture are all situated in the *E. coli* region. This means that the bacteria detection limit is at least 1×10^6 bact/mL (the minimum *E. coli* concentration considered in this study). The warning signal can now be issued only 3 h 19 min after a contamination with 1000 bact/mL occurred. Therefore, the in-line process proposed in Fig. 13 can now be modified as presented in Fig. 17.

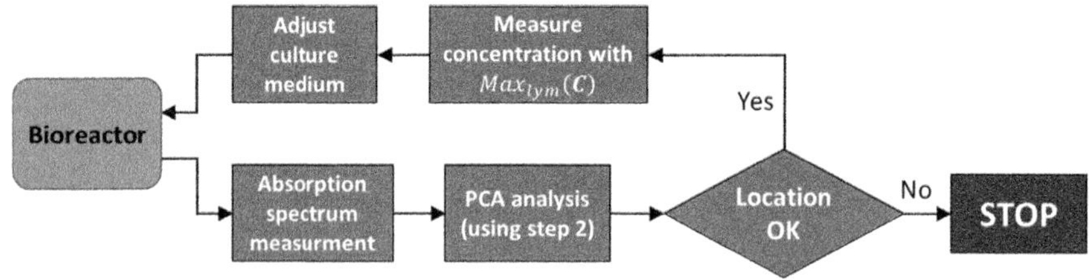

Fig. 17. In-line process to detect contaminations and to adjust the bioreactor composition based on Principal Component Analysis.

4 Discussion

4.1 Technical Aspects

Figures 4, 5, and 6 show that analyzing transmission spectra using the associated color proves to be efficient to measure both species concentrations. Indeed, according the results obtained in this study, this is the best way to measure *E. coli* concentration in real time and possibly in a closed system environment. In a general manner (for both lymphocyte and *E. coli*), we note that the "H" (Hue) and "a" (scale between green and red) parameters remain constant while the "b" (from blue to yellow) evolves very little. This means that the color of the solutions is not changing (or very little) with the concentration. The "L" (Luminance) and "V" (Value) parameters decrease with the concentration. This indicates that the intensity of the transmitted light decreases with the concentration. Although the color is not changing the associated color is reinforced with the concentration. This is observed with the increase of the "S" (Saturation parameter. "L" decreases but the color remains almost constant: this is confirmed by the fact that the "RGB" parameters decrease almost the same way with the concentration. Also, the relative values of the "RGB" parameters are constant which is consistent with a constant "H" parameter.

However, it is somehow inappropriate to talk of color when working with transmission spectra of biological solutions. Indeed, measuring the true color of the solutions would imply using a calibrated light source and studying the spectrum of the light reflected by the sample solution. Determining the true color of the solutions is not our purpose. Decomposition of the measured spectra in different color spaces is only a mathematical means of determining concentrations. For example, we also studied the entropy of the spectra. Estimating the quantity of information contained in the spectra using their entropy makes possible to measure concentration but in a reduced useful range which will not be presented in this paper.

Figures 8, 9, 10, 11 and 12 show that, during ATMPs production, analyzing the shape absorption spectra of lymphocytes allows monitoring the expansion phase. However, looking closer at Figs. 8 and 9 shows that most of the coefficients used to describe the shape of the absorption spectra cannot be efficiently fitted with mathematical functions. Indeed, for lymphocytes, only the p4 function can be efficiently described (this is the same for *E. coli* considering q4). This means that a better concentration determination could be obtained using p4 only instead of the whole spectrum shape. This was not investigated in this study but looking at Eq. (4), we understand that this p4 function somehow represents the baseline of the recorded spectra. Functions p2 and p3 describe the shape of the spectra while p1, together with p4 contribute to the amplitude of the spectra. This is why indeed, measuring the concentration using the maxima of the absorption spectra (Eq. (13)) is particularly accurate (Fig. (12)).

This does not mean that the shape itself contains no useful information. It also provides powerful a tool to issue an alert signal less than 5 h after a contamination with 1000 bact/mL occurred as it is shown in Fig. (15). Principal Component Analysis can be used to reduce the time required to issue a warning signal (Figs. (16)) the drawback being that it cannot be used to measure lymphocyte concentrations.

So-called "contaminated spectra" are artificial. They do not correspond to real lymphocyte and *E. coli* mixtures. These spectra consist of the addition of lymphocytes and *E. coli* spectra. Therefore, a bias could be introduced in the results presented here because adding absorption spectra may lead to artificial absorptions greater than 100%. The method described in Sect. 3.3 is still valid because only the shape is considered and not the actual value of the maximum absorptions. We recall that the R^2 coefficient is only used to issue an alert signal. Equation depicted in Fig. 10(a) remains valid to monitor the expansion phase as long as no contamination occurs. Because it is performed using normalized spectra, results obtained using Principal Component Analysis are not affected. However, an ongoing and more realistic study involves real spectra recorded with real mixture of lymphocytes and *E. coli*.

Although they are not the only ones, we mentioned methods based on spectro(photo) metry in the introduction. One, based on Fourier Transform Infrared Spectroscopy

(FTIR), was used to identify four types of bacteria [4]. This was not performed in solution but onto a sensor's surface. Also, Principal Component Analysis was used by the authors to successfully separate types of bacteria, to discriminate between Gram$^+$ and Gram$^-$ bacteria and to analyze mixtures. Another cited work presents the use of several sensors (Turbidity, particle counting, temperature, pH and spectrophotometry) to detect contaminants in drinking water [5]. However, methods described in this paper seem to be extremely difficult to automate. Also in this paper, analysis was performed using only 2 wavelengths which drastically reduces the amount of available information. Note that 2 reduced wavelength ranges were used by Hassan [4].

It should be noted that in our work, we exploit the total amount of information contained in the whole 450 nm to 1120 nm wavelength range (except for associated-color investigations) which represents over 900 data per spectrum with the spectrometer we used. Also, because measurements are performed in a cuvette and not on a biosensor's surface, the method can easily be used to provide a real time analysis of what happens in the bioreactor, in a closed-loop environment and without the need for any biosensor cleaning and/or regeneration.

From a practical point of view indeed, white light spectroscopy and conventional cuvettes makes possible an easy adaptation in a closed system configuration as illustrated in Fig. 18.

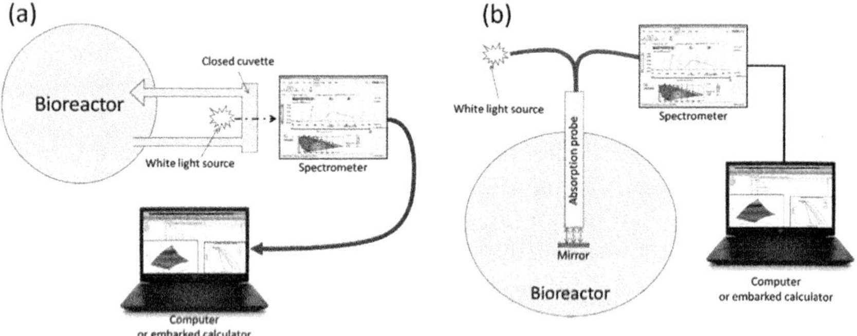

Fig. 18. Possible integrations of the method in a closed system environment. (a) Using a derivation. (b) Using a sterilized reflection probe coupled to a mirror. Adapted from [17].

In this work, only a contamination due to *E. coli* is considered. Cases of other bacteria or other types of containments like yeasts and fungi are currently being investigated. But as long as the shapes of the absorption spectra of contaminants are different enough from the ones of lymphocytes, the methods presented here should still be valid.

4.2 Socio-Economic Impacts

The expansion phase lasts several days and each day increases the price of ATMPs. The quality control imposes regular samplings, themselves risk of contamination.

Being able to monitor cell expansion and to perform quality controls without sampling is particularly interesting. In this way, expansion phase can be stopped rapidly which reduces the global cost of ATMPs. In this work, methods able to issue a warning signal about 3 h after a contamination with 1000 *E. coli*/mL are described.

ATMPs are likely to create a real therapeutic revolution in the coming years because they are designed to treat patients with pathologies that are currently incurable. It is right now difficult to estimate the number of pathologies that these medicines from the living can address and the number of patients likely to benefit.

Only a few ATMPs are available on the market. The enormous production cost also led to marketing authorization cancellation of some of them (Glybera, Sipuleucel-T, ChondoCelect). At the date of manuscript writing, only the following treatments are available (note the price for a single treatment):

- KYMRIAH ($ 475,000)
- YESCARTA ($ 373,000)
- Strimvelis ($ 594,000)

Included in these costs are losses due to fabrications, which are found to be contaminated during the final conformity test and those due to late-stage fabrication stops due to the scheduling of controls at precise times. Having a real-time and closed system monitoring and quality control method is of great interest in terms of research, industrial manufacturing and more importantly in terms of benefit to the patients.

5 Conclusion

In this paper, we have presented spectroscopic methods to continuously perform a quality control during the expansion phase of ATMP production. These methods are based on analyzing the transmission or absorption optical spectra of the content of a bioreactor. Colorimetric based techniques can be used to monitor lymphocyte multiplication during the expansion phase of ATMP production. They can also be used to monitor *E. coli* proliferation in other applications. However, the colorimetric method cannot be used to simultaneously monitor the concentration of lymphocytes and bacteria when a contamination occurs.

The originality of this work is that we do not need to measure the contaminant concentration but only to detect its presence. Consequently, spectral shape analysis can be used not only to monitor the lymphocytes multiplication but also to issue an alert signal about 4 h 52 min post contamination. Warning can even be issued earlier by using Principal Component Analysis. The warning signal can then be issued 3h19min post contamination. However, Principal Component Analysis cannot be used alone as it fails to measure lymphocyte concentrations when no contamination is detected. Note that the warning delays are calculated for a contamination due to 1000 *E. coli*/mL. Advantages of such methods can be summarized as follows.

- Regular sampling of the content of the bioreactor is no longer required. This further reduces the risk of sampling related contaminations.

- The use of planned sampling at a fixed date and time without even knowing whether contamination is avoided.
- The goal being to stop the production as soon as a contamination is detected and not to identify the pathogen responsible for it, this identification can be performed later.

As long as the culture is normal, the lymphocyte expansion is monitored in real time. Because contamination is detected extremely early the production can be stopped instantly which greatly contribute to reduce the production cost.

Indeed, in order to guarantee access of ATMPs to the largest number of patients, a new conception of the current mode of production and qualification of these living drugs is necessary. Currently, our studies are focused on the validation of these above described methods considering other types of pathogens.

Acknowledgements. This work was supported by the MiMedi project funded by BPI France (grant No. DOS0060162/00) and the European Union through the European Regional Development Fund of the Region Bourgogne-Franche-Comte (grant No. FC0013440).

References

1. Cacopardo, L., et al.: Real-time cellular impedance monitoring and imaging of biological barriers in a dual-flow membrane bioreactor. Biosens. Bioelectron. **140**, 111340 (2019). https://doi.org/10.1016/j.bios.2019.111340
2. Cesewski, E., Johnson, B.N.: Electrochemical biosensors for pathogen detection. Biosens. Bioelectron. **159**, 112214 (2020). https://doi.org/10.1016/j.bios.2020.112214
3. Chang, K.-S., Jang, H.-D., Lee, C.-F., Lee, Y.-G., Yuan, C.-J., Lee, S.-H.: Series quartz crystal sensor for remote bacteria population monitoring in raw milk via the Internet. Biosens. Bioelectron. **21**, 1581–1590 (2006). https://doi.org/10.1016/j.bios.2005.07.015
4. Hassan, M., Gonzalez, E., Hitchins, V., Ilev, I.: Detecting bacteria contamination on medical device surfaces using an integrated fiber-optic mid-infrared spectroscopy sensing method. Sensors Actuators B: Chem. **231**, 646–654 (2016). https://doi.org/10.1016/j.snb.2016.03.044
5. Ikonen, J., Pitkänen, T., Kosse, P., Ciszek, R., Kolehmainen, M., Miettinen, I.T.: On-line detection of Escherichia coli intrusion in a pilot-scale drinking water distribution system. J. Environ. Manage. **198**, 384–392 (2017). https://doi.org/10.1016/j.jenvman.2017.04.090
6. Janné, K., Pettersen, J., Lindberg, N.-O., Lundstedt, T.: Hierarchical principal component analysis (PCA) and projection to latent structure (PLS) technique on spectroscopic data as a data pretreatment for calibration. J. Chemom. **15**, 203–213 (2001). https://doi.org/10.1002/cem.677
7. Lee, S.-M., et al.: Real-time monitoring of 3D cell culture using a 3D capacitance biosensor. Biosens. Bioelectron. **77**, 56–61 (2016). https://doi.org/10.1016/j.bios.2015.09.005
8. Lei, K.F., Wu, M.-H., Hsu, C.-W., Chen, Y.-D.: Real-time and non-invasive impedimetric monitoring of cell proliferation and chemosensitivity in a perfusion 3D cell culture microfluidic chip. Biosens. Bioelectron. **51**, 16–21 (2014). https://doi.org/10.1016/j.bios.2013.07.031
9. Leva-Bueno, J., Peyman, S.A., Millner, P.A.: A review on impedimetric immunosensors for pathogen and biomarker detection. Med. Microbiol. Immunol. **209**(3), 343–362 (2020). https://doi.org/10.1007/s00430-020-00668-0

10. Liu, Y.-J., et al.: Multivariate statistical process control (MSPC) using Raman spectroscopy for in-line culture cell monitoring considering time-varying batches synchronized with correlation optimized warping (COW). Anal. Chim. Acta **952**, 9–17 (2017). https://doi.org/10.1016/j.aca.2016.11.064
11. Mansencal, T., et al.: Colour 0.3.15. Zenodo (2020)
12. Melchor, J., et al.: In-bioreactor ultrasonic monitoring of 3D culture human engineered cartilage. Sensors Actuators B: Chem. **266**, 841–852 (2018). https://doi.org/10.1016/j.snb.2018.03.152
13. Safavieh, M., Ahmed, M.U., Ng, A., Zourob, M.: High-throughput real-time electrochemical monitoring of LAMP for pathogenic bacteria detection. Biosens. Bioelectron. **58**, 101–106 (2014). https://doi.org/10.1016/j.bios.2014.02.002
14. Teixeira, A.P., Oliveira, R., Alves, P.M., Carrondo, M.J.T.: Advances in on-line monitoring and control of mammalian cell cultures: Supporting the PAT initiative. Biotechnol. Adv. **27**, 726–732 (2009). https://doi.org/10.1016/j.biotechadv.2009.05.003
15. Thakur, B., et al.: Rapid detection of single E coli bacteria using a graphene-based field-effect transistor device. Biosens. Bioelectron. **110**, 16–22 (2018). https://doi.org/10.1016/j.bios.2018.03.014
16. Theint, H.T., Walsh, J.E., Wong, S.T., Voon, K., Shitan, M.: Development of an optical biosensor for the detection of Trypanosoma evansi and Plasmodium berghei. Spectrochim. Acta Part A Mol. Biomol. Spectrosc. **218**, 348–358 (2019). https://doi.org/10.1016/j.saa.2019.04.008
17. Wacogne, B., Legrand, D., Pieralli, C., Frelet-Barrand, A.: Optical spectroscopy for the quality control of ATMP fabrication: a new method to monitor cell expansion and to detect contaminations. In: Proceedings of the 13th International Joint Conference on Biomedical Engineering Systems and Technologies - Volume 1: BIODEVICES. pp. 64–72. SciTePress (2020)
18. Wang, X., Rivière, I.: Clinical manufacturing of CAR T cells: foundation of a promising therapy. Mol. Ther. Oncolytics **3**, 16015 (2016). https://doi.org/10.1038/mto.2016.15

Non-invasive Optical Methods in Quantitative Minimal Erythema Dose Assessment in Vivo: Comparison of Preclinical and Clinical Data

Mikhail Makmatov-Rys[1(✉)], Irina Raznitsyna[1], Dmitriy Kulikov[1], Alexey Glazkov[1], Anton Molochkov[1,2], Marina Gureeva[2], Daria Mosalskaya[1], Maksim Bobrov[1], Ekaterina Kaznacheeva[3], Alexey Sekirin[1], and Dmitry Rogatkin[1]

[1] Moscow Regional Research and Clinical Institute "MONIKI", 61/2, Shchepkina Street, 129110 Moscow, RF, Russia

[2] Peoples' Friendship University of Russia, 6 Miklukho-Maklaya Street, 117198 Moscow, RF, Russia

[3] Cosmetological Clinic «Lemark», 32 Vladimir Nevsky Street, 394088 Voronezh, RF, Russia

Abstract. Even in modern dermatology clinics, the determination of the severity of ultraviolet (UV)-induced erythema and assessment of individual photosensitivity based on the calculation of minimal erythema dose (MED) is still performed visually, which is subjective, and associated with high variability of the results and frequent errors when it done be untrained personnel. The application of non-invasive quantitaitve methods such as laser fluorescence spectroscopy (LFS) and optical tissue oximetry (OTO) could be a solution of these problems. In is well known that acute UV skin damage is associated with structural alterations, vasodilatation and inflammatory response. Moreover, porphyrins which have well-known autofluorescent properties play a role in the chemoattraction of immune cells to the area of local inflammation caused by UV. Using LFS in the preclinical part of the study on ICR mice (N = 25) time-dependent dynamic changes in the fluorescence parameters of porphyrins were found. Optical parameters were in a good agreement with histological findings. Statistically significant correlation was found between the severity of inflammatory infiltrate and the tissue content index (η) of porphyrins. During the clinical part of the study on healthy volunteers (n = 14) the analysis of endogenous fluorescence and microcirculation characteristics by LFS and OTO revealed the correlation relationship between the intensity of endogenous fluorescence of porphyrins and oxygen consumption with a dose of UV radiation. The correlation of the porphyrins fluorescence with a dose of UV was also demonstrated. Overall results have fundamental value and should be investigated and applied in clinical practice to objectively assess and predict MED.

Keywords: Ultraviolet erythema · Minimal erythema dose · Inflammation · Fluorescence · Porphyrins · Immune infiltration · Saturation · Non-invasive · Diagnostics

X. Ye et al. (Eds.): BIOSTEC 2020, CCIS 1400, pp. 76–89, 2021.
https://doi.org/10.1007/978-3-030-72379-8_5

1 Introduction

Nowadays, the problem of precise assessment of the effects of ultraviolet radiation (UVR) on human skin is being actively discussed in photobiological studies. Traditionally, the extent of UV exposure applied to a biological organism in vivo is determined based on minimal erythema dose (MED) - amount of UV radiation required to cause a faint skin redness (erythema) with diffuse borders on untanned skin several hours (traditionally, 24 h) after exposure [2]. MED is usually measured in mJ/cm^2. The determination of photosensitivity using MED to date is widely implemented in scientific and clinical practice. For instance, when starting a course of phototherapy (in order to treat dermatoses such as psoriasis, morphea or atopic dermatitis) initial doses of UVA and UVB are determined based on the patient's MED [1]. Moreover, MED assessment is used in cosmetic industry to calculate sun protecting factor (SPF) and applied as essential diagnostic method in follow-up of patients with photodermatoses [3].

It is important to point that MED represents the degree of individual's acute response to the UVR which is described as nonspecific skin damage, associated with structural, vascular and immunological changes in the epidermis and dermis, and is clinically manifested as UV-erythema [4]. The cascade of immune reactions, molecules-mediators involved in the damage to the epidermis and vasodilatation, as well as the course of structural changes in the skin induced by acute UV exposure, are being actively investigated but yet no fully understood [5].

Even today MED is routinely determined visually, which is a is subjective and connected with errors due to high intrarater and interrater variability. Some authors point that MED reading is a serious challenge because traditional visual method lacks accuracy, quantification, reproducibility and [6]. Falk M. and Ilias M. showed that the agreement between observers was excellent for skin UV-erythema with a sharp border, but a significant inter-observer variability was detected for zones of skin hyperemia with diffuse and indistinct borders. Moreover, mistakes can occur during the visual assessment of the Fitzpatrick skin phototype especially in tanned patients or in individuals with dark skin when the evaluation is made by untrained observer [7].

Unfortunately, there are some adverse effects connected with incorrect estimation of MED: for instance, it could cause the overvaluation of the starting dose of UV in the phototherapy course and consequently lead to such complications as dry skin, erythema and burn, hyperpigmentation, herpes simplex reactivation and to worsening of the underlying dermatosis. On the other hand, described adverse reactions lead to a delay in the UV-treatment course, extra clinic appointments and additional economic losses. There is a further problem with the increasing risk of malignant cutaneous tumors and premature photoaging. The existing association between UV-erythema and molecular changes in the deoxyribonucleic acid (DNA) was described in literature, highlighting oncogenic risks [8].

The majority of available techniques aimed at detecting UV-induced erythema and MED (biochemical, molecular, pathomorphological) are invasive, time-consuming and not sensitive enough to early alterations [9]. A possible solution to these problems could be found in non-invasive optical methods. According to the literature such approaches as colorimetry [10], diffuse reflectance spectroscopy [11], laser doppler flowmetry [7], laser doppler visualization [12], optical coherent tomography [13] and confocal microscopy [14].

However, described methods also have serious limitations: some of them are difficult to master and operate, it is hard to achieve quantitative data, they mostly were used solely but not in combination with each other and the majority of them are not implemented in clinical particle and were used only for scientific purposes. In the abovementioned studies optical measurements were performed on fully developed UV erythema 24 h after the irradiation not allowing to predict erythema formation and MED. Moreover, existing methods don't reflect all dynamic skin changes involved in UV-induced skin damage pathogenesis. Some pathophysiologic markers of UV-induced skin damage were out of the scope of previous works.

One approach to solve these problems involves the use of laser fluorescence spectroscopy (LFS) and optical tissue oximetry (OTO) in MED assessment. Molecular markers which are accountable for oxidative stress, proteolysis, inflammation and hypoxia – processes, involved in the pathogenesis of UV-induced skin damage, - could be assessed by OTO and LFS in red and green spectrum range [15]. Several studies report the application of LPF and OTO in investigation of local inflammation [16], radiation skin damage [17] and skin fibrosis [18] in vivo. Additionally, some authors used LFS to skin alternations in course of chronic UV damage and photoaging [9, 19]. In one study it was found that fluorescence parameters correlated with tryptophan expression and cell proliferation and may indicate the presence of "sunburn cells" in the epidermis [9].

In our previous research we tried to assess the applicability and prospects of LFS and OTO in the assessment MED in healthy volunteers at different time periods after UV irradiation [20]. For this study, it was of interest to investigate changes in inflammatory and immune response in experimental model of acute UV-skin damage in mice using LFS and OTO and found the link between fluorescence characteristics and histology. The overall goal of this work was to analyze and compare preclinical and clinical data connected with quantitative assessment of UV-erythema and MED.

2 Materials and Methods

2.1 Animals and Ultraviolet Irradiation

The preclinical part of the research was carried out on male ICR mice aged 6–8 weeks (N = 25) weighing 28–35 g. The animals were kept under standard vivarium conditions at a temperature of 21–23 °C, humidity 50–65%, 14-h daylight. They received balanced granular food that did not contain fluorophores and had free access to drinking water. The animal quarantine period was 10 days. The experiment was conducted in compliance with the welfare of animals used in experiment (Declaration of Helsinki), EU Directive 86/609/EEC on the protection of animals used in experiments, and European Convention for the Protection of Vertebrate Animals Used for Experimental and other Scientific Purposes (ETS 123) Strasbourg, 1986).

In all experimental animals acute UVB-induced erythema was initiated using «Dr. Honle Dermalight» 500-1 series (manufactured by Dr. Honle Medical Technology GmbH, Germany), equipped with Phillips UV-B Narrowband PL lamps with a wavelength of 311 nm. The intensity of the UV lamps was measured at each stage of the experiment using a Waldmann Variocontrol spectroradiometer (UV-meter). Preliminary, 48 h before the irradiation, mice were denuded in the dorsal area (using veet depilatory cream). During the UV exposure, all animals were anesthetized to avoid unnecessary stress and movements.

In the course of the study mice were divided into 5 subgroups of 5 animals each. The intact subgroup (control, N = 5) was not irradiated. Other subgroups were exposed to an UVB irradiation in dose of 2 MED (1392 mJ/cm2) in the dorsal area. The distance between the surface of the skin and light source was 10 cm, the exposure period was 16 min Previously, in pilot experiments we've determined the MED for ICR mice using the method described by Gyöngyösi [21]. Finally, 24 h after irradiation, mice were visually examined in the back region and photographed.

2.2 Volunteers and Ultraviolet Irradiation

The clinical part of the study was conducted on a group of healthy volunteers (n = 14, 8 male and 6 female) aged 26 ± 3 years with Fitzpatrick skin phototypes II and III. Using traditional method (described by [2]. MED was estimated in all participants. Measurements were conducted on the skin of the upper back region or on abdominal skin. UVB irradiation was performed using light source «Dr. Honle Dermalight]2 500-1 series (manufactured by Dr. Honle Medical Technology GmbH, Germany), equipped with Phillips UV-B Narrowband PL lamps with a wavelength of 311 nm. During MED assessment hypoallergenic test patch (Daavlin DosePatch) with six square windows (a square size of 1 cm^2) was applied to the skin of the back or abdomen; the distance between UV source and surface of the skin was 30 cm. Before each session of irradiation UV intensity of lamps was measured using a Waldmann Variocontrol spectroradiometer (UV-meter). The dose of UV radiation was increased stepwise from window to window depending on the individual's phototype according to reference tables [22]. Thus, skin regions in the square cells were cumulatively exposed to UV radiation doses in range from 100 to 770 mJ/cm^2. Then, 24 h after UV-B exposure, the participants went through the visual assessment of MED performed by 2 observers. The erythema reaction was graded using a visual rating scale [23]. Based on the results of the visual examination, the square zone of skin with redness corresponding to the MED (barely noticeable erythema) was determined and the dose of UVB was calculated. Detailed characteristics of MED and phototype of the participants are presented in our previous study [20].

2.3 Optical Measurements and Data Processing

Optical diagnostics was conducted before UVB irradiation (intact skin) and 0.5, 3, 6, 24 h after it, on the dorsal denuded skin of experimental animals (preclinical part) and on the skin in each of 6 square windows and on the contralateral area in healthy volunteers (clinical part). The parameters of endogenous porphyrins fluorescence was evaluated by LFS and local blood flow characteristics was measured by OTO. Both methods are implemented in the LAKK-M system (SPE 'LAZMA' Ltd, Russia). The principal scheme of the device was described in our previous paper [20]. The process of registering optical parameters is presented in Fig. 1.

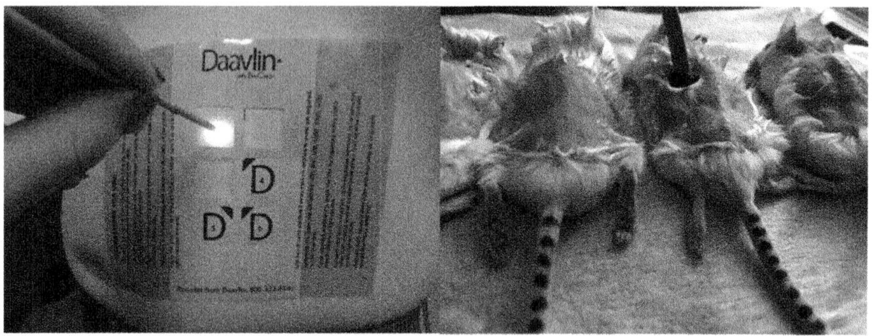

Fig. 1. The process of optical measurements on the abdomen skin in healthy volunteers (left) and on the dorsal skin in ICR mice (right) after the UVB-irradiation.

The choice of the above mentioned time points was based on an analysis of the literature on the pathogenesis of the of acute UV damage [8, 24].

The spectra of secondary radiation (backscattered and fluorescence) were recorded from each region of interest after selected (at wavelength of $\lambda_e = 635$ nm or $\lambda_e =$ 535 nm) low-power laser source irradiates the tissue.

Porphyrin has a two-hump fluorescence spectrum with maxima at wavelengths of 625–630 and 700–710 nm [25]. In the waveband of 650 - 750 nm, porphyrins are the major contributor to the endogenous fluorescence spectrum of biological tissue, but at λ = 625–630 nm porphyn fluorescence is most expressed.

The porphirin fluorescence intensities I_f were estimated at $\lambda_f = 710$ to verify theirs presence and at $\lambda_f = 630$ nm to quantitative assessment, respectively. Despite the fact that other fluorophores (for example, lipofuscin) can also fluoresce in the range of 625–630 nm, we believe that their contribution to the total intensity is minor.

To estimate the fluorescence quantitatively in mice skin, the tissue content index of fluorophore ηf was used, which is calculated by the formula:

$$\eta_f = \frac{I_f \cdot \beta}{I_f \cdot \beta + I_{bs}} \tag{1}$$

where If is the intensity at λ_f of a particular fluorophore, Ibs is the intensity at λ_e used to excite fluorescence, β is the attenuation coefficient of the used optical filter, $\beta \approx 1000$.

In the case of studies involving volunteers, the individual variability of the content of fluorophores in intact tissue plays a significant role. To minimize its influence we normalized the fluorescence to the intact region:

$$\mu(\lambda_f) = I(\lambda_f)/\, I_0(\lambda_f) \tag{2}$$

where $I(\lambda_f)$ is the fluorescence intensity from the iradiated area, $I_0(\lambda_f)$ is the fluorescence intensity from the intact area.

To evaluate the local blood flow, blood filling volume (V_b) and tissue oxyhemoglobin saturation (S_tO_2) were recorded for each region of interest for 20 s. Then, according to the time-averaged data the specific oxygen consumption of the tissues U characterized by the oxygen intake per tissue blood flow volume unit was calculated by the following formula [27]:

$$U = \left(S_pO_2 - S_tO_2\right)/V_b \tag{3}$$

where S_pO_2 is the functional pulse saturation of the oxyhaemoglobin fraction in the arterial peripheral blood. It was assumed equal to 98%.

2.4 Morphology and Staining

In order to investigate structural alteration in epidermis ad dermis caused by acute UV exposure all experimental animals were sacrificed before, 0.5, 3, 6, and 24 h after irradiation with subsequent biopsy of the dorsal skin (skin flap 1.0 cm2), material sampling and pathomorphogy (hematoxylin and eosin (H&E) strain). For each histological sample, the number of inflammatory cells (polymorphonucleocytes) was counted in 10 high-power fields (hpf). Further, the immune infiltrate was graded as - pronounced (400–600 cells), moderate (200–400 cells), weak – (less than 200 cells).

2.5 Statistical Analysis

Statistical analysis was performed in Microsoft Excel 2016 and Statistica 12 (Statsoft inc., USA). The analysis of dynamic changes in the optical parameters described above was carried out using the Wilcoxon test. The relationship between the obtained optical data and the dose of UV radiation was evaluated using the Spearman rank correlation coefficient. The probability of an error of the first kind was considered statistically significant to be less than 5% ($p < 0.05$).

3 Results and Discussion

3.1 Preclinical Study

Grouped-averaged fluorescence spectra assessed from on the dorsal skin of ICR mice before and in various time points after UV-irradiation are depictured in Fig. 2.

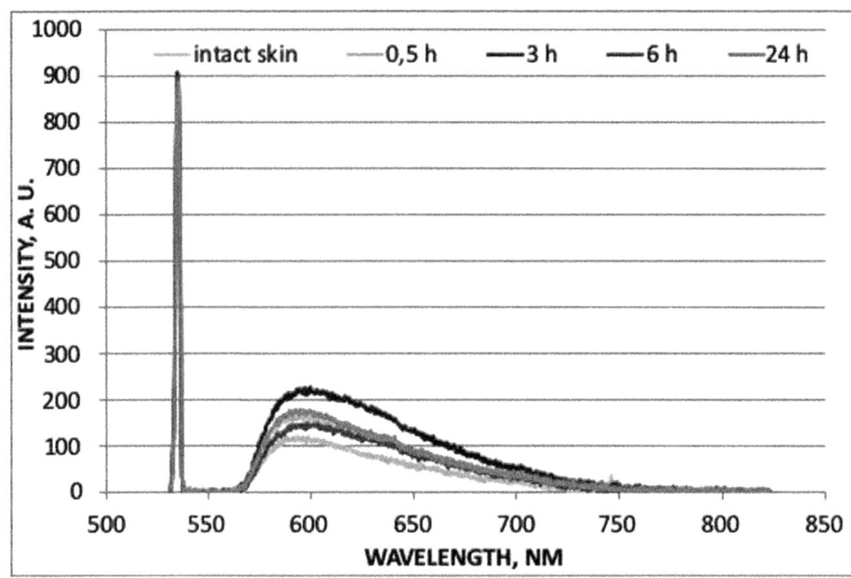

Fig. 2. Group-averaged fluorescence spectra for intact (without UV-exposure, 0 h) and irradiated skin 0,5, 3, 6, 24 h after UV-exposure. Excitation wavelength $\lambda_e = 535$ nm.

According to the results of LFS, dynamic changes in the fluorescence parameters of porphyrins over time were noted. The results of optical measurements are presented in the Fig. 3. Peak values of the tissue content index (η) of porphyrins were found after 3 h after UV exposure. Then a gradual decrease in η of porphyrins was observed - after 24 h its values closely approached normal levels (as in unirradiated skin).

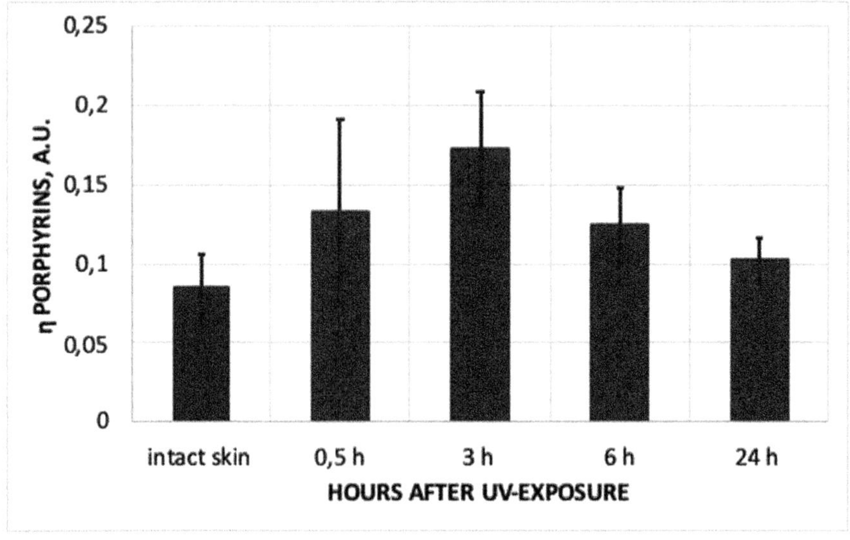

Fig. 3. Dynamic changes in the tissue content index of porphyrins, $\lambda_e = 535$ nm.

During the analysis of pathomorphological samples, dynamic structural, vascular and inflammatory changes at the different time points after UV exposure we detected. It was evident that 30 min after irradiation, the first signs of an acute inflammatory response were noted: vasodilation, an influx of neutrophilic leucocytes. At the point of 3 h, the inflammatory response reached its peak: abundant neutrophilic infiltration developed, and after 6 h the immune infiltrate became less pronounced and had mixed structure (neutrophils and histiocytes) and single «sunburn cells» were noted. After 24 h, the stabilization of the inflammatory reaction was observed: lymphocytic-histiocytic infiltrate was widely distributed in the skin, specific signs of UV damage appeared («sunburn cells», vacuolization of the basal cell layer) and were also uniformly distributed in the thickness of the epidermis. Figure 4 show the histological changes that occurred 3 h after UV exposure compared with unirradiated skin (hematoxylin and eosin staining).

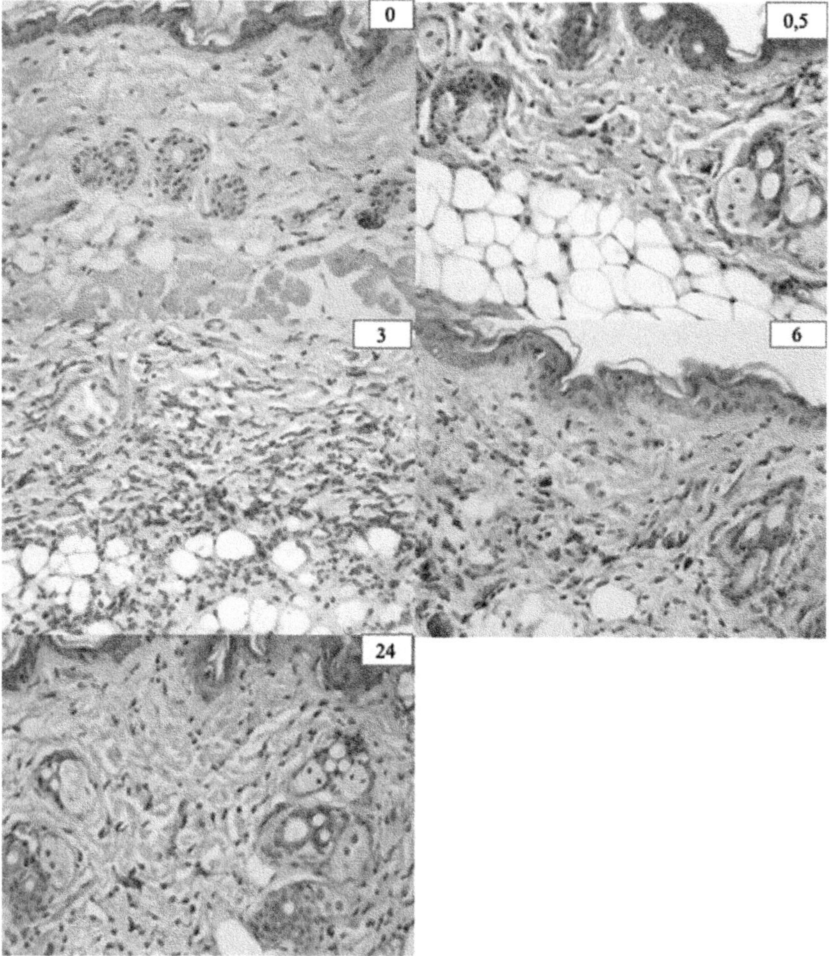

Fig. 4. Morphology of unirradiated dorsal skin of ICR mice (0), and animal skin 0,5, 3, 6, 24 h after UV-exposure (H&E stain, magnification of x 400).

Using Pearson correlation coefficient, we found a statistically significant relationship between the severity of inflammatory immune infiltrate and the tissue content index (η) of porphyrins ($r = 0.912$, $p = 0.031$).

The obtained preclinical data have certain fundamental value and could have potential clinical implementation. A number of studies have shown that porphyrins, nitrogen-containing orange-red fluorescent pigments, accumulate in inflamed tissues after mechanical, chemical, and radiation damage [16, 17]. In experiments conducted by Schneckenburger and colleagues using the LFS method, the accumulation of porphyrins in the area of artificially-induced skin inflammation in Wistar rats was shown [26]. It is believed that the source of porphyrins in tissues can be free heme, the concentration of which increases sharply in tissues due to hemolysis or excessive damage to cells induced by internal or external (e.g. high dose UV- exposure) stimuli. Hypotheses are put forward that porphyrin molecules play a role of chemoattractants and engage immune cells to come the site of inflammation and contribute to the formation of infiltrate [28].

Described association between fluorescence parameters of porphyrins and immune infiltrate can be explained from pathogenetic point of view: porphyrins, that are released from damaged and destructed skin cells and accumulated in area of UV-irradiated skin, play a role pf chemoattractants for neutrophilic granulocytes. It was found that the peak of neutrophilic infiltration 3 h after UV exposure coincided with the peak porphyrins fluorescence. In addition, a marked increase in porphyrins fluorescence may be associated with the pronounced vasodilation observed in the UV-injured skin.

3.2 Clinical Study

Examples of measured fluorescence spectra from the intact (non-irradiated) and irradiated skin sites at $\lambda_e = 535$ nm after 24 h after the UV-irradiation is shown in the Fig. 5.

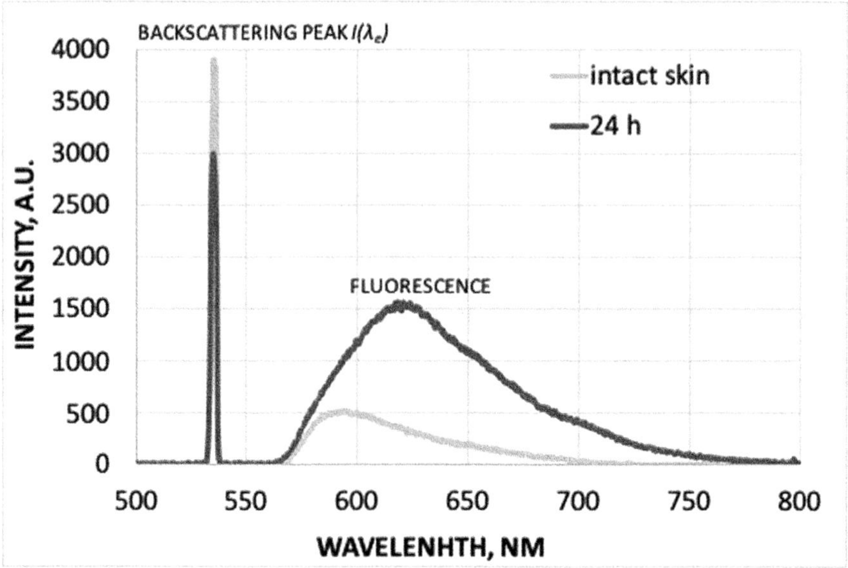

Fig. 5. The example of the fluorescence spectra in intact and irradiated skin after 24 h after UVB exposure; $\lambda_e = 535$ nm.

Correlation analysis was performed and associations were revealed between the dose of UV applied to square windows and the specific oxygen consumption of the tissues (U) normalized to intact skin 3 h (Spearman correlation coefficient [r] = −0.297; p = 0.01) and 24 h (r = −0.307; p = 0.0004) after the irradiation (Fig. 6). Moreover, a correlation was reveled between the degree of UV dose and the fluorescence intensity of porphyrins λ_e = 535 nm 6 h after UV irradiation normalized to intact skin (r = −0.249, p = 0.01).

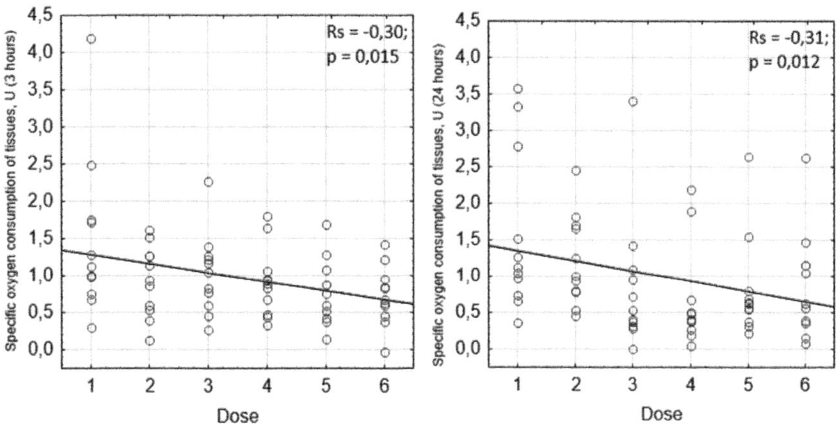

Fig. 6. Correlation relationships between U and UV dose 3 (left) and 24 h (right) after irradiation (1 - lowest dose, 6 - highest dose).

Abovementioned clinical results show the fluctuations in optical markers in the course of acute UV-induced skin damage and are consistent with preclinical data. Thus, the changes in U index reflects an alterations in the metabolic state epidermal and dermal cells altered by acute UV exposure. Moreover, high-dose UV radiation cause vascular endothelial damage, vasodilatation and mast cell degranulation and the release of vasoactive substances - nitric oxide, histamine, arachidonic acid derivatives, which also contribute to the formation of infiltrate from immune cells in the affected area [8]. One study showed that peak infiltration of leucocytes after UVB irradiation occurs at 4–6 h and the response concludes after 48 h [29]. It has also been shown that with increasing intensity and dose of UV radiation, skin damage becomes more pronounced [24].

In addition, according to the results of the study, it was found that normalized fluorescence intensity and tissue content index in all irradiated skin sites regularly changed stepwise over time. The most significant increase in the intensity of fluorescence of porphyrins in green light (λ_e = 535 nm), normalized to intact skin in all 6 cells was observed 24 h compared with 0,5 h after UV exposure (Fig. 7).

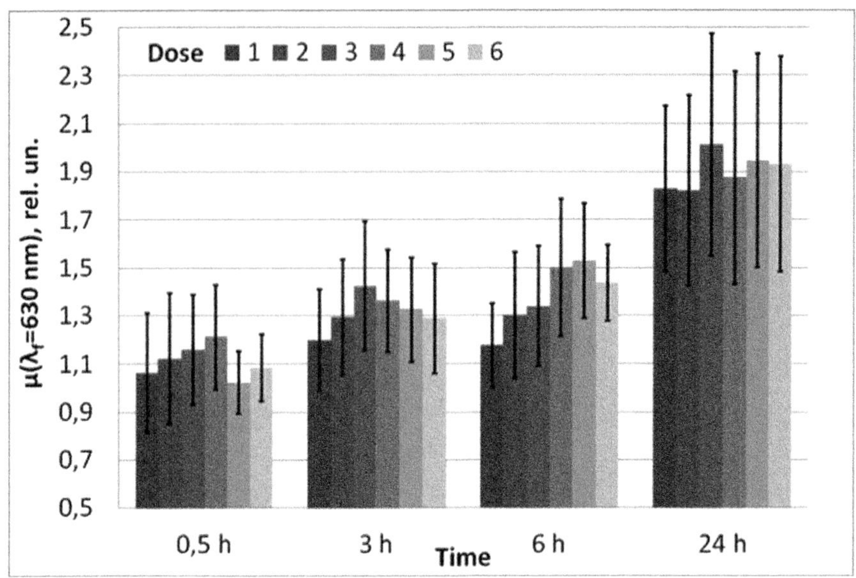

Fig. 7. The dynamics of the porphyrin's intensity normalized to intact tissue in skin sites irradiated with stepwise increasing doses of UVB (6 – lowest dose, 1 – highest dose) in 4 time points after UV-exposure; λ_e = 535 nm *(cited from* [20]*)*.

These results allow us to hypothesize that UV exposure affects the metabolism and accumulation of porphyrins in the skin and these patterns could be used in the future studies aimed to create new method of non-invasive quantitative method of MED assessment.

It is necessary to discuss major limitation of our research. In current study volunteers were not divided by the anatomical zone where the phototest was carried out and their diet and constitution of were not considered. We didn't divide participants according to the special skin characteristics (oily, seborrheic. Acne-prone skin). For instance, the number of studies showed that the presence of enlarged pores and comedones is associated with increased synthesis of porphyrins by Cutibacterium acnes and increased fluorescence intensity of porphyrins [30].

Also, since this study involved young patients of approximately the same age, it is also necessary to conduct the similar studies with subjects of different age groups. Lipofuscin age pigments accumulate in cells with age, also has fluorescent properties [31]. Therefore, it is necessary to evaluate its contribution to the total skin spectrum and the possibility of reliable identification of porphyrins in older people.

Subjects with darker skin phototypes (IV-VI) were not included in study population. It is known that melanin content is significantly higher in the skin of subjects with darker skin type [32]. Melanin is known to absorb the radiation of the visible spectrum, which reduces the registered signal significantly. In these cases, increasing the power of the laser radiation may increase the signal-to-noise ratio and solve the problem. But in further studies it is important to estimate the minimum laser power for skin phototypes IV-VI at which peaks of endogenous fluorophores can be distinguished.

4 Conclusions

To summarize, current study achieved several valuable results. First of all, in preclinical experiment it was shown that LFS and OTO can be applied for non-invasive quantification of UV-induced inflammatory response in the skin. Moreover, prospective markers of UV-damage (such as porphyrins, local blood flow characteristics) were described. During clinical part of the study interrelations were found between the dose of UV radiation, specific oxygen consumption of the tissues and porphyrins fluorescence parameters. These results demonstrate that the integrated application of the LFS and OTO methods for objective non-invasive assessment of erythema is pathophysiologically relevant and has prospects for further investigation in larger clinical studies. To gain more precise data, it is important to analyze optical parameters of the skin of different anatomical zones irradiated with UV (for example, back and abdomen) in a larger group of volunteers of different age groups including individuals with darker skin phototypes. It is interesting to additionally consider factors reflecting tissues biological age, local/systemic conditions and their influence on MED. Further, these developments may become the basis for the development of diagnostic systems for assessment of MED. Future device for this purpose should include a bunch of non-invasive methods and allow to gain quantitative data about the individual's skin characteristics and implement predictive algorithms.

References

1. Krutmann, J., Hönigsmann, H., Elmets, C.A., Bergstresser, P.R. (eds.): Dermatological phototherapy and photodiagnostic methods. Springer, Berlin (2009). https://doi.org/10.1007/978-3-540-36693-5
2. Heckman, C.J., et al.: Minimal erythema dose (MED) testing. JoVE (J. Visual. Exp.), (75), e50175 (2013)
3. Hönigsmann, H.: Polymorphous light eruption. Photodermatol. Photoimmunol. Photomed. **24**(3), 155–161 (2008)
4. Makmatov-Rys, M.B., Kulikov, D.A., Kaznacheeva, E.V., Khlebnikova, A.N.: Pathogenic features of acute ultraviolet-induced skin damage. Klinicheskaya dermatologiya i venerologiya **18**(4), 412 (2019). https://doi.org/10.17116/klinderma201918041412
5. Sklar, L.R., Almutawa, F., Lim, H.W., Hamzavi, I.: Effects of ultraviolet radiation, visible light, and infrared radiation on erythema and pigmentation: a review. Photochem Photobiol. Sci. **12**, 54–64 (2013)
6. Lock-Andersen, J., Wulf, H.C.: Threshold level for measurement of UV sensitivity: reproducibility of phototest. Photodermatol. Photoimmunol. Photomed. **12**(4), 154–161 (1996)
7. Falk, M., Ilias, M., Anderson, C.: Inter-observer variability in reading of phototest reactions with sharply or diffusely delineated borders. Skin Res. Technol. **14**(4), 397–402 (2008)

8. Clydesdale, G.J., Dandie, G.W., Muller, H.K.: Ultraviolet light induced injury: immunological and inflammatory effects. Immunol. Cell Biol. **79**(6), 547–568 (2001)
9. Papazoglou, E., Sunkari, C., Neidrauer, M., Klement, J.F., Uitto, J.: Noninvasive assessment of UV-induced skin damage: comparison of optical measurements to histology and MMP expression. Photochem. Photobiol. **86**(1), 138–145 (2010)
10. Jeon, S.Y., Lee, C.Y., Song, K.H., Kim, K.H.: Spectrophotometric measurement of minimal erythema dose sites after narrowband ultraviolet B phototesting: clinical implication of spetrophotometric values in phototherapy. Ann. Dermatol. **26**(1), 17–25 (2014)
11. Bodekær, M., Philipsen, P.A., Karlsmark, T., Wulf, H.C.: Good agreement between minimal erythema dose test reactions and objective measurements: an in vivo study of human skin. Photodermatol. Photoimmunol. Photomed. **29**(4), 190–195 (2013)
12. Wilhelm, K.P., Kaspar, K., Funkel, O.: Comparison of three techniques for evaluating skin erythemal response for determination of sun protection factors of sunscreens: high resolution laser Doppler imaging, colorimetry and visual scoring. Photodermatol. Photoimmunol. Photomed. **17**(2), 60–65 (2001)
13. Gambichler, T., et al.: Acute skin alterations following ultraviolet radiation investigated by optical coherence tomography and histology. Arch. Dermatol. Res. **297**(5), 218–225 (2005). https://doi.org/10.1007/s00403-005-0604-6
14. Yamashita, T., Akita, H., Astner, S., Miyakawa, M., Lerner, E.A., González, S.: In vivo assessment of pigmentary and vascular compartments changes in UVA exposed skin by reflectance-mode confocal microscopy. Exp. Dermatol. **16**(11), 905–911 (2007)
15. Franco, W., Gutierrez-Herrera, E., Kollias, N., Doukas, A.: Review of applications of fluorescence excitation to spectroscopy dermatology. Br. J. Dermatol. **174**(3), 499–504 (2016)
16. Petritskaya, E.N., Kulikov, D.A., Rogatkin, D.A., Guseva, I.A., Kulikova, P.A.: Use of fluorescence spectroscopy for diagnosis of hypoxia and inflammatory processes in tissue. J. Opt. Technol. **82**(12), 810–814 (2015)
17. Raznitsyna, I., et al.: Fluorescence of radiation-induced tissue damage. Int. J. Radiat. Biol. **94**(2), 166–173 (2018)
18. Chursinova, Y.V., et al.: Laser fluorescence spectroscopy and optical tissue oximetry in the diagnosis of skin fibrosis. Biomed. Photonics **8**(1), 38–45 (2019)
19. Tian, W.D., Gillies, R., Brancaleon, L., Kollias, N.: Aging and effects of ultraviolet a exposure may be quantified by fluorescence excitation spectroscopy in vivo. J. Invest. Dermatol. **116**(6), 840–845 (2001)
20. Makmatov-Rys, M., et al.: Optical technology for ultraviolet erythema assessment and minimal erythema dose determination in healthy volunteers. In: Proceedings of the 13th International Joint Conference on Biomedical Engineering Systems and Technologies, vol. 1 Biodevices: Biodevices, pp. 73–78 (2020)
21. Gyöngyösi, N., et al.: Photosensitivity of murine skin greatly depends on the genetic background: clinically relevant dose as a new measure to replace minimal erythema dose in mouse studies. Exp. Dermatol. **25**(7), 519–525 (2016)
22. Palmer, R., Garibaldinos, T., Hawk, J.: Phototherapy guidelines. St John's Institute of Dermatology/St Thomas' Hospital, London (2005)
23. Faurschou, A., Wulf, H.C.: European dermatology guideline for the photodermatoses. 2. Phototesting. EDF guidelines for dermatology in Europe. ABW Wissenschaftsverlag, Berlin (2009)
24. Hruza, L.L., Pentland, A.P.: Mechanisms of UV-induced inflammation. J. Invest. Dermatol. **100**(1), 35–41 (1993)
25. Croce, A.C., Bottiroli, G.: Autofluorescence spectroscopy and imaging: a tool for biomedical research and diagnosis. Eur. J. Histochem. **58**(4), 2461, 320–337 (2014)

26. Schneckenburger, H., Lang, M., Köllner, T., Rück, A., Herzog, M., Hörauf, H.: Fluorescence spectra and microscopic imaging of porphyrins in single cells and tissues. Lasers Med. Sci. **4**, 159–166 (1989). https://doi.org/10.1007/BF02032430
27. Rogatkin, D., Shumskiy, V., Tereshenko, S., Polyakov, P.: Laser-based non-invasive spectrophotometry–An overview of possible medical applications. Photonics Lasers Med. **2** (3), 225–240 (2013)
28. Porto, B.N., et al.: Heme induces neutrophil migration and reactive oxygen species generation through signaling pathways characteristic of chemotactic receptors. J. Biol. Chem. **282**, 24430–24436 (2007)
29. Logan, G., Wilhelm, D.L.: Vascular permeability changes in inflammation. I. The role of endogenous permeability factors in ultraviolet injury. British journal of experimental pathology, 47(3), 300 (1966).
30. Borelli, C., et al.: In vivo porphyrin production by P. acnes in untreated acne patients and its modulation by acnetreatment. Acta Derm. Venereol. **86**(4), 316–319 (2006)
31. Brunk, U.T., Terman, A.: Lipofuscin: mechanisms of age-related accumulation and influence on cell function. Free Radical Biol. Med. **33**(5), 611–619 (2002)
32. Lu, H., Edwards, C., Gaskell, S., Pearse, A., Marks, R.: Melanin content and distribution in the surface corneocyte with skin phototypes. Br. J. Dermatol. **135**(2), 263–267 (1996)

Bioimaging

Deep Learning for the Automated Feature Labelling of 3-Dimensional Imaged Placenta

Benita S. Mackay[1(✉)], James A. Grant-Jacob[1], Robert W. Eason[1], Rohan Lewis[2], and Ben Mills[1]

[1] Optoelectronics Research Centre, Faculty of Engineering and Physical Sciences, University of Southampton, Southampton SO17 1BJ, UK
b.mackay@soton.ac.uk

[2] Institute of Developmental Sciences, Faculty of Medicine, University of Southampton, Southampton SO16 6HW, UK

Abstract. 3-D visualisation of cellular structures within the placenta is important for advancing research into the factors determining fetal growth, which are linked to chronic disease risk and quality of lifelong health. 2-D analysis can be challenging, and spatial interaction between structures can be easily missed, but obtaining 3-D structural images is extremely labour-intensive due to the high level of rigorous manual processing required. Deep neural networks are used to automate this previously manual process to construct fast and accurate 3-D structural images, which can be used for 3-D image analysis. The deep networks described in this chapter are trained to label both single cell, a fibroblast and a pericyte, and multicellular, endothelial, structures from within serial block-face scanning electron microscopy placental imaging. Automated labels are equivalent, pixel-to-pixel, to manual labels by over 98% on average over all cell structures and network architectures, and are able to successfully label unseen regions and stacks.

Keywords: 3-D image processing · Deep learning · Placenta

1 Introduction

Previous work has been done on the automated 3-D labelling of fibroblasts and endothelial cells in scanning electron microscopy (SEM) imaged placentae via deep learning, specifically a U-Net architecture and trained on unlabelled-labelled pairs of 2-D image sections [1]. This chapter enhances this work with additional analysis of these techniques, a wider range of uses and comparing the performance of networks trained on 50%, 20% and 10% of images within a 3-D serial block-face scanning electron microscopy (SBFSEM) stack.

The placenta is the barrier interface between a mother and the fetus, mediating the transfer of nutrients and simultaneously performing as a barrier for the transfer of molecules that are toxic to the fetus. Poor placental function can impair fetal growth and development, affecting an individual's health over their whole life [2]. 3-D imaging approaches allow a much more effective characterisation of spatial heterogeneity of structures or proteins than 2-D techniques can provide [3]. Serial block-face scanning

X. Ye et al. (Eds.): BIOSTEC 2020, CCIS 1400, pp. 93–115, 2021.
https://doi.org/10.1007/978-3-030-72379-8_6

electron microscopy (SBFSEM) has emerged as an important tool revealing the nanoscale cellular and a cellular structures of the placenta in 3-D. While this technique is able to reveal novel structures and the spatial relationships between cells, it is limited by the time it takes to manually label the features of interest, which necessitates the labelling of hundreds of serial sections. This can take weeks if not months of dedicated time to label a single SBFSEM stack. Developing a deep learning-based approach dramatically speeds up this labelling process and enables more quantitative analytical approaches.

A deep neural network is trained on stacks of unlabelled and their associated labelled image pairs of a fibroblast, pericyte or endothelial cells within SBFSEM-imaged placental tissue. The network is subsequently used to generate automated labels on unlabelled images that were not used during training and therefore unseen by the network. Visual comparison between the automated labelling, achieved via the neural network, and manual labelling of the fibroblast shows excellent agreement, with quantitative analysis showing high pixel-to-pixel comparison accuracy. This deep learning approach enables the labelling of a variety of features, in this case, both single and multicellular, within the SBFSEM stacks, with the future possibility of other cell and tissue types, such as osteoblasts within bone, and different 3-D imaging techniques.

2 3-D Imaging of Placentae

2.1 Placenta

The placenta is a fetal organ which forms the interface with the mother. The placenta feeds the fetus, cleans its blood and secretes hormones which adapt the mother's physiology to support the pregnancy [3]. Placental function determines fetal growth, with poor placental function compromising development of the fetus predisposing it to perinatal and postnatal diseases [4]. It can therefore be considered a cornerstone of the reproductive success, especially as it is important for health in later life, as poor fetal growth is associated with higher chromic disease rates throughout life [5].

To fully investigate placental function, an understanding of its structure, physiology and biochemistry is required. The placentas of growth restricted fetus show alterations in structure and reduced transport capacity and these changes are thought to underlie the poor fetal growth. However the relationship between structure and transport is poorly understood. While changes in structure have been observed progress understanding how structure determines function has been limited by lack of good tools to study structure in 3-D [6].

While the overall structure of the placenta is well understood, this is not true of cellular anatomy is poorly understood especially at the ultrastructural level. Furthermore, while there has been much research into trophoblast, other cell types like fibroblasts, pericytes and endothelial cells have received less attention. In order to understand the function of the placenta it is necessary to understand the anatomy and spatial relationships of all placental cell types [7].

2.2 3-D Imaging

Studying the anatomy of the placenta has previously relied on 2-D images, which can be supported by SEM and vascular casting data for 3-D interpretation [5, 8]. The underlying 3-D structures within the placenta have also been developed from 2-D images using stereology [6]. However, these approaches are limited in the information they provide about placental structure, such as visual data illustrating the spatial relationship between cells, and whether there is regional heterogeneity in structure or even protein localisation [4].

3-D imaging has the potential to make more complex spatial information about the placental structures obtainable, including factors like villous and vascular branching. The associations between structures can be more clearly identified and it is possible to determine structures that are not readily visualised from 2-D imaging techniques, such as thin stellate processes of stromal fibroblasts embedded within surrounding features [2].

There are multiple techniques available for imaging biological tissue in 3-D, such as micro-computed tomography (micro-CT), where X-rays at multiple angles are used to construct a microscale resolution 3-D image, and SBFSEM, which is capable of producing nanoscale resolution 3-D images [9]. The latter is possible by taking a standard 2-D SEM image of a plastic-embedded contrast-enhanced tissue and then removing a thin slice of tissue from the top of the block using an ultramicrotome slicing. This creates a new surface typically 50 nm below the previous surface, although slices as thin as 10 nm are possible. Another 2-D SEM image is then taken of the new surface and these steps repeated until a large stack of 2-D images is obtained and then computationally joined into a 3-D image stack, with the z-resolution limited by the depth of the ultrathin slices removed at each step [10].

SBFSEM imaging has been used to identify novel structures in the human placenta, displaying the 3-D structures of different cell types, and the interaction between cell structures and their surrounding environment, including the positional interplay between cells [2, 11, 12]. However, while some cell types and structures can be relatively easily computationally rendered into 3-D through optimised heavy metal staining techniques [13], for many tissue samples, 3-D visualisation from a SBFSEM image stack is a time-consuming and hence expensive task. While application of conventional image segmentation for 3-D medical image data can be combined to more quickly extract important feature information, these approaches require intensive data processing or a distinctive contrast in features within the tissue sample, which can be difficult and sometimes impossible to obtain in SBFSEM images of tissue [14, 15].

For data and resolution to be maintained, each 2-D SEM image within the 3-D SBFSEM stack needs to be manually labelled to extract the desired feature(s). As it takes several minutes to an hour for an expert to accurately label each slice, due to the complexity of the images, and each stack can contain several thousand slices, this labelling can take a month, if not more, of dedicated work to complete. The complexity of the SBFSEM stacks means that standard programmatical rules cannot achieve computer automation of labelling. However, recent advances in the field of deep learning can provide a way to optimise the labelling process and dramatically reduce the time taken from several months to only hours to extract a labelled 3-D feature.

3 Deep Learning

3.1 ConvNets

Deep learning is a subsection of artificial neural networks, a common machine learning architecture, which have long been used for both medical tasks, such as optimal matching of patients and donors of kidney transplants for improvement of long-term survival [16]. In addition such networks have been used for the creation of patient-specific predictions for osteoarthritis [17], and for imaging tasks, such as those by Google for assigning keywords to an image for automatic image tagging [18] or detection of pollution particles in real-time through variations in light [19].

While a neural network must have an input layer and an output layer, the number of layers in-between is highly adjustable. These middle layers, generally known as hidden layers, are where most of the data transformations happen. The first hidden layer will process information directly from the input layer. However, the second hidden layer will process information only from the first hidden layer, which means the second can operate at a comparatively more abstract level. A third hidden layer may be more abstract still. Deep learning allows a machine to be supplied with unprocessed input data and uncover the representation needed for solutions at every layer, without representation design or interference from human engineers: the machine learns what features of the input data are relevant for itself at each layer.

As a result, deep learning is highly proficient with image-based problems [20]. While it can be susceptible to misclassification of images with relatively small perturbations of the input data [21], it is beating records in image recognition [20, 22, 23] and is highly adaptable to a range of applications, from general medical diagnostics [24–26] to identifying cancer [27, 28].

One type of deep network frequently utilised for a range of imaging tasks are Convolutional networks (ConvNets) [29–37]. From original models in 1990 for handwritten number recognition [38] to newer developments capable of ImageNet classification (15 million images with over 22000 categories) [20], this architecture dominates the imaging field [23]. An intrinsic part to ConvNets are the convolutional and pooling layers. These layers are partially inspired from archetypal concepts of simple and complex cells in visual neuroscience [39, 40]. The general architecture is similar to the hierarchy in the visual cortex ventral pathway, necessary for visual perception [41, 42].

To process an image, it is important to extract features only visible through the positional arrangement of the pixels. This is done by the convolution layer. A weight matrix, an array of numbers, convolves the image to extract specific features without losing important spatial data. A pooling matrix reduces the size of the image – the number of parameters. Consequently, this results in fewer parameters for the network to consider. A weight combination may extract a variety of features, with one focused on colour, another on edges and another blurring unimportant noise from the image, for example. As ConvNets are a type of deep learning, the weights are learned by the ConvNet and altered by the ConvNet to minimise loss. This means that it discovers what should be considered features and which features to focus on without human intervention. The deeper the network, the more complex the features extracted, therefore the more suited the ConvNet can be to a given problem. The role of the pooling layer is to merge semantically similar features and create invariance to small shifts and distortions, as well as reducing the size of the data. There are several variations on pooling but all variants will reduce the number of trainable parameters for the ConvNet.

3.2 U-Nets

ConvNets are not an all-purpose solution to image problems. Image-to-image translation requires a more advanced architecture – conditional generative adversarial networks (GANs) [43]. When a ConvNet is designed to minimise the difference between expected and generated pixels, blurry images will likely be produced due to the averaging of all statistically likely outputs [44]. To prevent this outcome, competition is added to the AI architecture in the form of a discriminator, trained solely on whether the generated output is thought to be real or fake: blurry images are swiftly eliminated as a viable output as they are evidently fake. A widely used architecture is the U-Net, where a generator works in parallel to a discriminator, which only focuses on small sections of the image, to produce a highly effective image-to-image network with multiple applications [45, 46].

U-Net architecture is an adaption of ConvNets first used for Biomedical Image Segmentation [47], and an improvement on the current Fully Convolutional Networks [48]. Capable of producing accurate predictions with relatively fewer training images, the large number of feature channels make it ideal for complex and high resolution situations, as the network only uses the valid part of each convolution without any fully connected layers. The name comes from the architectural design. Consisting of two paths, a contracting path of convolutions and max pooling, where the spatial information is reduced as feature information is increased, and an expanding path of up-convolutions and concatenations, joining sections together, combining spatial information with high-resolution features from the contracting path. While uses in GAN architecture broaden the uses of U-Nets, they remain prevalent in the biomedical field, with uses in cell counting, detection, and morphometry [49]. These new U-Net models utilise a cloud-based setup, completely eliminating the need for researchers to acquire potentially expensive graphics-processing units (GPUs) and allow for constant additions to the training data, adapting the U-Net and giving continual improvements.

Deep learning has already been applied in image processing and image labelling processes for enhancing microscopy resolution [19] and here this approach is developed for the automated feature labelling of cells, including fibroblasts and endothelial cells, in SBFSEM images of placentas. The purpose of this work is to fully automate the labelling of fibroblasts across all 2-D SEM images in a 3-D stack (roughly one thousand in total) so that data visualisation in 3-D can be more easily accomplished and utilised. Automation requires training a neural network to label the z-stack images without human involvement, such that the labels can then be isolated and converted using standard imaging software into 3-D projections, without requiring months of image processing.

4 Method

Labelling a desired feature from within a 3-D SBFSEM image was split into multiple steps, as seen in Fig. 1. The first step (1) was to isolate a 2-D section of the larger 3-D image for inputting into a deep network. The network was then trained to generate the same 2-D section containing an automated label of the desired feature (2). The third step (3) was to isolate the automated label from the 2-D section so that it could be collected with all other sections. The final step (4) was to project the collection of extracted labels into 3-D, resulting in a completely labelled feature (a 3-D projection), which can then be easily manipulated in standard imaging software (built-in functions in ImageJ were used) for simpler visual analysis of the feature.

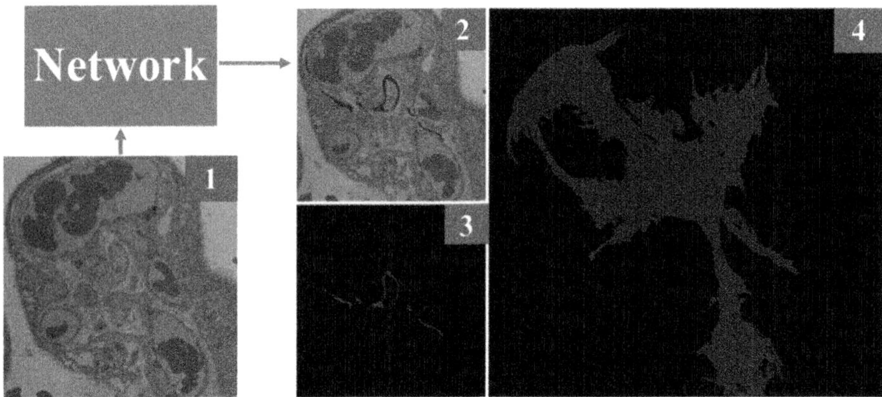

Fig. 1. Automation process for extracting desired 3-D features from a 3-D image dataset. Step 1 was isolation of a single unlabelled SEM image from a larger 3-D SBFSEM stack. Step 2 was inputting that image into a trained network to generate an automated labelled image. Step 3 was the extraction of the automated label from the SEM image, which was collected with all other automated labels. Step 4 was the 3-D projection, using the built-in functions in ImageJ, of the collection of automated labels.

A 3-D stack of SBFSEM-imaged placental tissue resulted in a sequence of high-resolution 2-D images of a placenta, and each z-stack position referenced a different depth within the 3-D stack. Three stacks were used in this chapter, with the first used for labelling fibroblasts and pericytes and consisted of over 1000 z-positions, of which 943 were used, and the second and third were used for the labelling of endothelial cells and consisted of 370 and 140 z-positions respectively. For labelling fibroblasts, the network was trained on 50% of the stack and then tested on the remaining 50%. To increase the amount of training data available to the network, image augmentation was utilised. This involved resizing the 2-D images into 2000 by 2000, cropping the resized images into a minimum of eight 512 by 512 images and then resizing again into 256 by 256. The reduction in resolution resulted in the network taking only six hours on an NVIDIA TITAN Xp GPU to perform 100 epochs (the network had every training image input 100 times).

The network consisted of a U-Net architecture, shown in Fig. 2. The encoder-decoder structure utilised standard backpropagation, but was also paired with a discriminator, which would have a random input of either an automated or manually labelled image. The discriminator would then determine whether it had been shown an automated image or manually labelled image. Both discriminator error, whether it could distinguish between automated or manual images, and generator error, comparing the automated and manually labelled image, were used to improve the network output after every training image (batch size was one image).

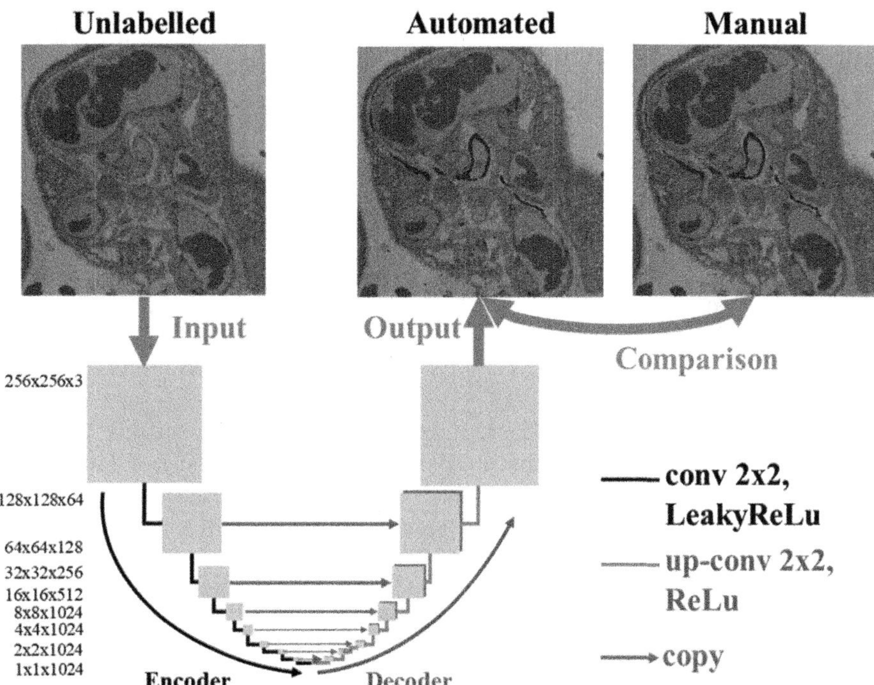

Fig. 2. Diagram of the network architecture used for automated labelling. It was based on a U-Net framework consisting of an encoder-decoder pair, which **resized** the image through multiple convolutional and deconvolutional/up-convolutional layers and utilised skip connections between mirror layers.

The U-Net contained 17 layers and each layer contained a convolution/deconvolution with a stride of 2, a 4 by 4 kernel size and used rectified linear unit activation functions. The effective size of the image was therefore resized from 256 by 256 to 1 by 1 before being resized back up to 256 by 256. The skip connections between the encoder and decoder allowed for spatially relevant information to pass across the architecture and resulted in more realistic output images. The discriminator was formed of a 4 layer convolutional network, which led to a single output, via a sigmoid activation function that labelled an image either automated or manually generated. Pixel-to-pixel comparison error (also known as the L1 loss) was given a weighting of 100 times the discriminator error, and this weighted error function was then used via standard backpropagation for the network to "learn" (the weights in the network altered to produce an output resulting in less error from this function).

Testing the network was similar in process to training the network shown in Fig. 1. However, the images input to the network were unseen and not part of the training dataset. Unlike in step 4 in Fig. 1, where the labels were 3-D projected, the automated labels were extracted and then compared to the corresponding manual labels so the difference could be analysed for each z-stack position (each 2-D SEM image within the 3-D SBFSEM stack). Post individual analysis, the automated labels were then projected in 3-D for a final visual comparison between automated and manual labelling. While this last step provided less quantitative analysis, deciding whether the network generated a realistic looking 3-D structure was an important final test for determining whether the network provides an automation method capable of being safely utilised in real-world situations.

The networks were given no background information of SBFSEM techniques or additional data beyond the unlabelled-labelled pairs, therefore the technique would not be limited to SBFSEM and could be applied to other 3-D imaging techniques.

5 Single Cell Labelling

5.1 Fibroblast

Fibroblast labelling was previously successfully automated [1], but this work was analysed in more detail for technique transfer and automated labelling of different 3-D single cell structures. The same error method was applied, where each individual pixel within a generated image was considered correct if it matched the same corresponding pixel value in the corresponding manually labelled image. A labelled pixel had the (RGB) value [0,0,255], visualised as blue on a standard three channel image, and any deviation from this value was not considered to be a labelled pixel. Therefore, a network-generated output that differed value by a single pixel value, for example [0,0,254], was an unlabelled pixel or incorrectly labelled. In other words, a pixel difference of ± 1 or greater in any of the three colour channels was considered incorrect when comparing automated and manual labels.

The total correlating pixels, the pixels that matched values for the same pixel position, as a percentage of total pixels in the extracted label was graphically depicted, shown in Fig. 3, by dark blue markers. One marker corresponded to one label comparison at each z-stack position which was unused in the training data, and therefore unseen by the network. The purple line that intersected the blue markers was the mean average pixel correlation over ten images, and the larger purple region showed the standard deviation, also across ten images, throughout the stack. The red markers showed the precision of each z-stack position (the ratio of correctly automated labelled pixels to the total labelled pixels); the orange markers showed the recall, also known as sensitivity, for each position (the ratio of correctly automated labelled pixels to the manually labelled pixels); the yellow markers showed the specificity (correct automated unlabelled pixels as a ratio to manually unlabelled pixels) and the light green markers showed the accuracy (the ratio of correctly automated labelled and unlabelled pixels to every pixel within the image). The F1 value, the harmonic mean average of precision and recall, was shown in dark green.

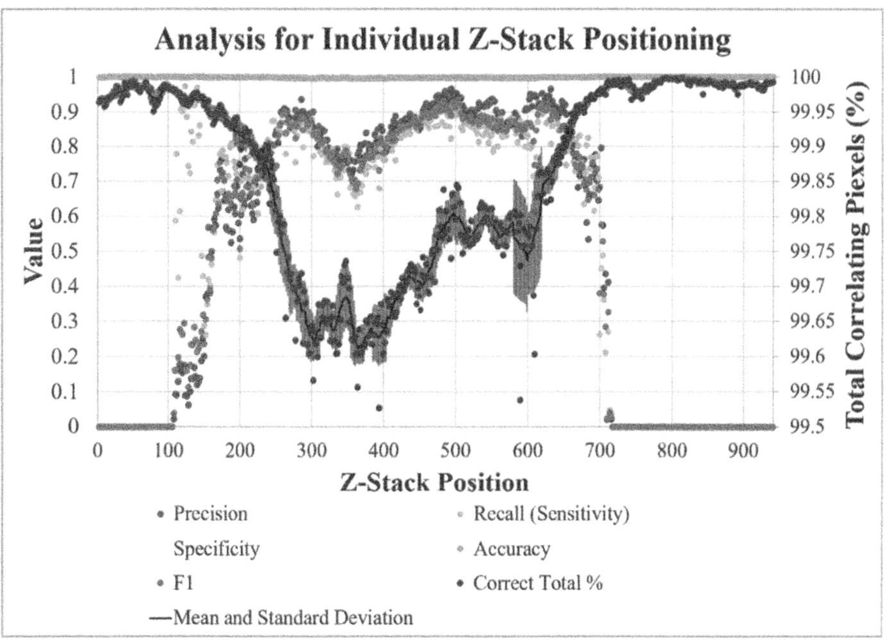

Fig. 3. Graph comparing automated and manual fibroblast labelling for individual z-stack positions. Precision (red), recall (orange), specificity (yellow), accuracy (light green) and F1 (dark green) are all measured using the standard 0–1 value of the primary axis on the left-hand side. The correct total as a percentage (blue), or the total correlating pixels, and the rolling mean and standard deviation over ten positions (purple) are plotted against the secondary axis on the right-hand side. (Color figure online)

The areas where the total number of corresponding pixels was highest, roughly the first 100 positions and the last 200 positions, had corresponding pixels of over 99.95%. This was also the region where the F1 value is lowest. This was because there were no manually labelled fibroblast pixels in these regions. However, the network still generated a few areas of labelled pixels because there were other fibroblasts besides the manually labelled feature-fibroblast in these regions. While the network was only trained to label the manually labelled fibroblast, some confusion over the partially labelled training data lead to an automation method unable to generate 100% accuracy in these regions. This 0.05% uncertainty was eliminated with a fully labelled dataset, shown in Sect. 5.2. The incompletely labelled dataset was the reason why there was such a large difference between specificity and recall. The accuracy and specificity were close to 1 (perfect value) across the entire dataset and false positives occurred in less than 0.2% of all unlabelled pixels. Specificity and recall were closer in value towards the centre of the z-stack because the singularly labelled fibroblast dominated the SBFSEM stack and the likelihood of other unlabelled fibroblasts being present was reduced.

The recall (the measure of how well the network has automatically labelled the pixels that were labelled manually) had two regions of large variation. The first region was where the fibroblast started to appear within the stack and there were very few pixels to label, and the second was where the fibroblast stopped appearing and, once again, the labelled pixel regions were a lot smaller. The precision also deviated around these areas for the same reason. Some variation in automated and manually labelled regions was due to subjective boundaries in which areas of the SEM images can be defined as fibroblast or not. These boundary regions were up to roughly ten pixels in size so, in areas of low quantity of labelled pixel, the percentage of corresponding pixels fluctuates and precision lowers. The smaller areas of variation, the dip between positions 300 and 400, are areas where the fibroblast labelling took up the highest proportion of image space compared to other regions in the SBFSEM stack. Therefore, there was a higher number of boundary regions and greater variability in the results. The standard deviation was only higher for the area around position 600. When inspected, this was due to two specific positions, 590 and 610, having much fewer correlating pixels. The position with the lowest correlating pixel percentage in this region, 590, was extracted for further visual comparison, as shown in Fig. 4.

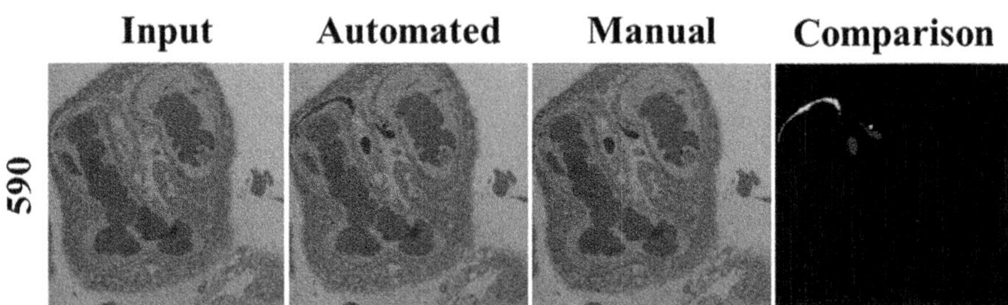

Fig. 4. A visual analysis of z-position 590. The input is the 2-D image extracted from the larger 3-D SBFSEM **stack**. The automated image is the network generated image with automated labelling. The manual image is the manually labelled image for the same position, which was used to test the network. The comparison image shows a visualisation of correlating pixels between the automated and manual labels. Blue indicates labelled pixels in both images and black are unlabelled pixels in both images, while red indicates pixels only labelled in the manual image and green indicates pixels only labelled in the automated image. (Color figure online)

The large green areas in the comparison image highlighted the difference between the automated and manually labelled image. These green pixels were where the automated image had labelled the fibroblast correctly, but the manual label was only outlined in this region and the filling of this labelled section had been missed. This showed that this automation method can not only be used to label 3-D stacks much faster than possible manually but can also be used as a method for checking manually labelled 3-D images for unfinished labels, which could have been missed by standard manual quality checks due to the high number of 2-D images within the larger 3-D stack.

Other visual analysis was completed for additional positions. Positions 278 and 398 were chosen for being areas of relatively lower correlating pixel percentage, both below 99.65%, while 498 was additionally chosen for being a position of relatively higher correlating pixel percentage, above 99.8%, (shown in Fig. 5). As with Fig. 4, Fig. 5 consisted of the 2-D unlabelled image input to the network, the automated labelled output image, the manually labelled image, and a comparison between the extracted labels of the automated and manually labelled images.

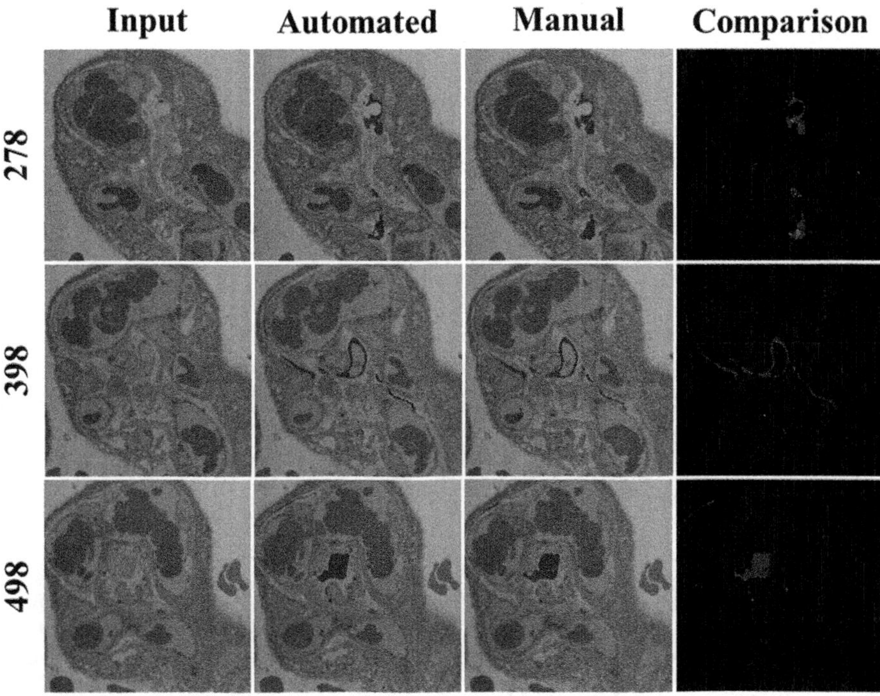

Fig. 5. A visual analysis of three z-positions throughout the stack, 278, 398, and 498. The input are the 2-D images extracted from the larger 3-D SBFSEM stack. The automated image are the network generated images with automated labelling. The manual images are the manually labelled images for the same position. The comparison image shows a visualisation of correlating pixels between the automated and manual labels. Blue indicates labelled pixels in both images and black are unlabelled pixels in both images, while red indicates pixels only labelled in the manual image and green indicates pixels only labelled in the automated image. (Color figure online)

Comparison images were used because differences between the automated and manually labelled images were difficult to see clearly. The vast majority of pixels, over 99.5%, were black (correct negative) or blue (correct positive), which were the colours for no difference between the automated and manual images. Black pixels outnumbered other colours and were the reason why overall error was low, less than 0.05%, across the stack, as the network correctly did not label areas which did not contain the desired feature – the labelled fibroblast. The green pixels (false positives), areas with automated labelling but without manual labelling, and the red pixels (false negative), the opposite, were in regions next to the labelled fibroblast, which could have been a result of uncertainty in the network and inaccuracies in human labelling. This showed that the network was capable of labelling the correct general shape of the fibroblast and provide the vital information required for a 3-D model. Figure 6 confirmed this, as it compared the 3-D projected automated and manually labelled fibroblast without any computational clean-up or post-network-generated output alterations. Computational alterations would include ignoring labelled pixels outside regions of interest and clumps of labelled pixels below a certain size threshold. There were small areas of false positives, shown by the regions of blue at various sporadic positions but mostly on the bottom right of the automated projection. The inclusion of fibroblasts in the stack that were not manually labelled was the likely cause of this comparative over-labelling. There were also small areas of false negatives, where detail on the edge of the fibroblast was lost. This boundary region was subject to the most variability and a wider range of training data would likely overcome this source of error.

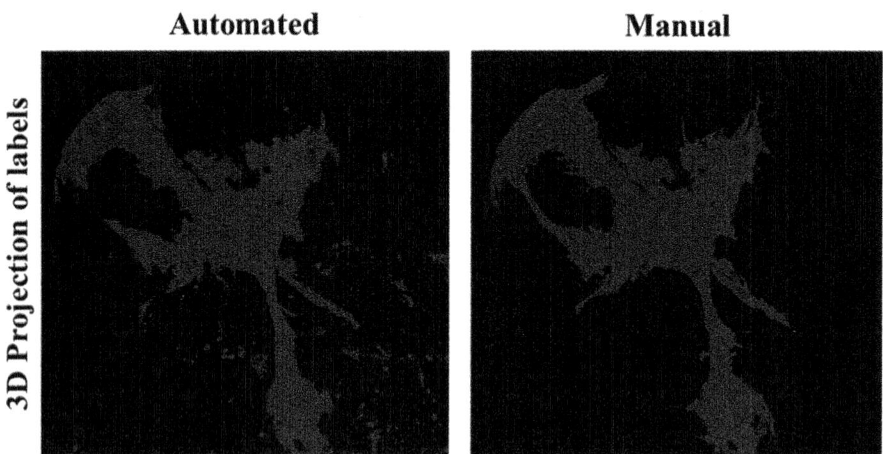

Fig. 6. Comparison of 3-D projections of automated and manually labelled fibroblast. Both were formed through projecting a **collection** of extracted 3-D labels via built-in ImageJ software. No computational or manual clean-up was done to alter the network generated labelling.

5.2 Pericyte

Pericytes are found wrapped around the endothelial cells which form the walls of blood vessels. Pericytes are believed to control vasculature stability and permeability. Pericytes communicate with endothelial cells through both direct physical contact and paracrine signalling (cell-to-neighbouring cell communication) [50, 51].

The method for labelling pericytes were identical to the method used for labelling fibroblasts, with a U-Net structure trained on manually labelled images within the same SBFSEM stack. However, the method was advanced in this section to determine if fewer images can be used to train a network without compromising accuracy. Therefore, the network was trained on only odd images (1 in 2), as with the fibroblast. Then the network was trained on 1 in 5 images, followed by 1 in 10. The remaining images were used for testing in each of the three networks to determine an optimal labelling amount for a single stack on an untrained network, where lowering manual labelling time was balanced against a reliable network output.

The total corresponding pixels, the percentage of pixels which were equal in value for both the extracted automated and manually labelled image, were plotted for each of the three networks, shown in Fig. 7. The blue pixels showed the testing of the network trained on 1 in 2 images of the 3-D SBFSEM stack and tested on the remaining images. The red and green pixels showed the testing of the networks trained on 1 in 5 and 1 in 10 images respectively. There was very little difference between the red and blue markers, with on average total correlating pixels for all tested positions differing by only 0.01%. The difference between the blue and green markers was on average six times greater than between blue and red.

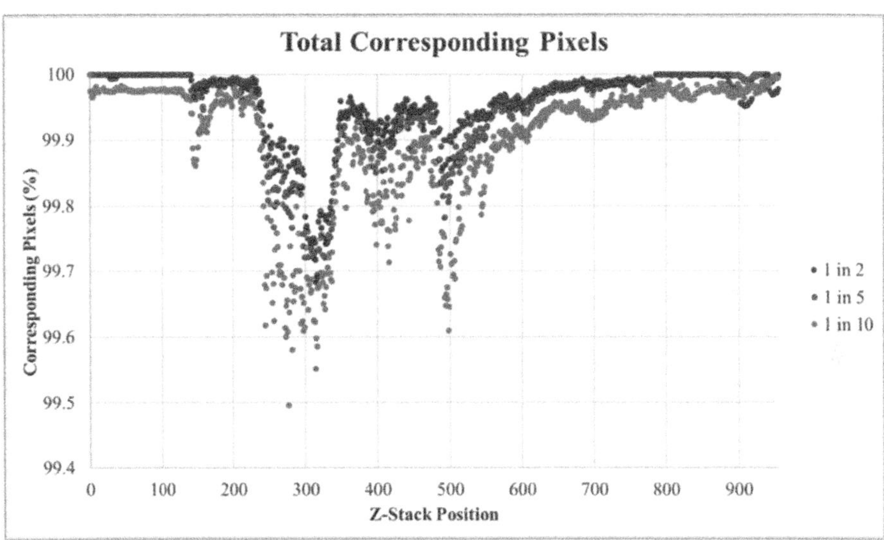

Fig. 7. Comparison graph for the testing of three networks trained to label pericytes. One is trained on 1 in 2 (blue), another trained on 1 in 5 (red) and the final on 1 in 10 images throughout the z-stack (green). (Color figure online)

In contrast to the partially labelled fibroblast dataset, where only one fibroblast was labelled in the stack containing multiple fibroblasts, there was only a single dominant pericyte labelled in the stack. This resulted in areas where the network was confident, when trained on 1 in 5 or more images throughout the stack, that there was no pericyte, and there are 100% corresponding pixels. This confirmed that there would be improvement in automated labelling of fibroblasts with a fully labelled training dataset. However, the network trained on 1 in 10 images throughout the stack was not capable of producing a labelled image that matched the manual label image at the level of 100%, and was considered a cut-off to training further networks on fewer images. To analyse the increase in pixel difference further, a visual comparison was conducted, shown in Fig. 8.

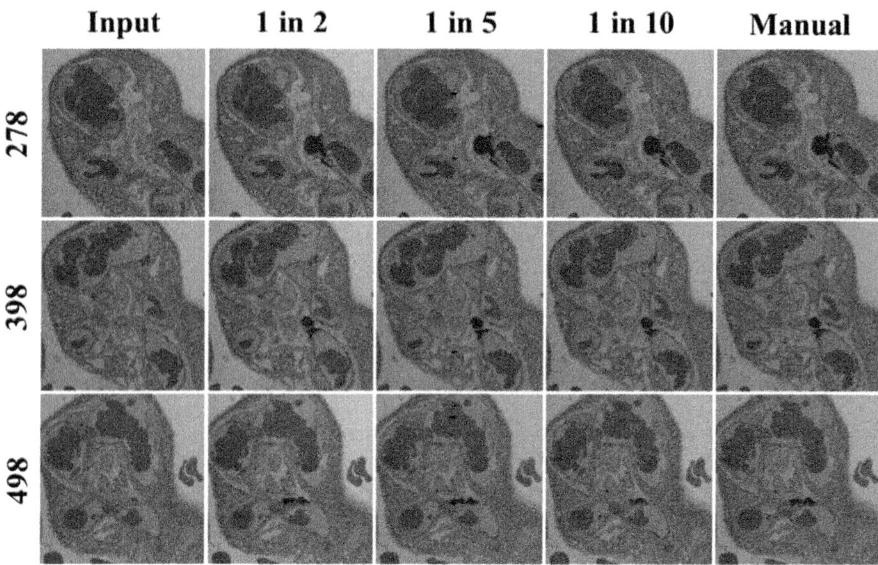

Fig. 8. A visual analysis of three z-positions throughout the stack, 278, 398, and 498 for labelling pericytes. The inputs are the 2-D **images** extracted from the larger 3-D SBFSEM stack. The automated images are the network-generated images with automated labelling for networks trained in 1 in 2, 1 in 5 and 1 in 10 images. The manual images are the manually labelled images for the same position.

Three positions were chosen, the z-positions 278, 398 and 498, which were areas of lower pixel correlation and the same positions as analysed for previous fibroblast feature extraction. Each network has small areas of difference when compared to manual labelling. The 1 in 2 network produced images which most closely matched the manual images, with some detail lost in boundary regions. This could be improved with a wider range of training data than a single stack, or more fine-tuning of the error function which altered the backpropagation and training of the network. The 1 in 5 network produced small black regions for all images, which did not contain red pixels and so would not have been classed as a labelled region, and the 1 in 10 image produced small blocks of randomised red, cyan and grey pixels, typically 10 to 20 pixels across, on apparently random areas of the image, which did contain red pixels and so would be classed as a labelled region. Both were likely due to overfitting, where the networks were less confident on the greater variation between testing and training data, and the lower amount of training data available to the networks hindered more adequate training. Training data comprising multiple labelled stacks would likely improve this overfitting in the 1 in 5 and 1 in 10 networks.

Not all additional pixel difference seen between 1 in 10 and 1 in 2 was due to overfitting-symptomatic pixel generation on small sections of the image. Most clearly seen for position 278 and 498, there were fewer labelled pixels as the networks decreased in training images available to them. Concentrating on 278, 1 in 2 contained almost all the labelled pixels as in the manual image. However, 1 in 5 lost some of the finer labelling, where the cell structure was thinnest, and 1 in 10 lost the entire upper labelled area. While Fig. 3 and Fig. 7 showed a network could be used to successfully automate the labelling process for feature extraction of a variety of single cell structures, with a pixel correlation between manual and automated labelling of over 99.5%, Fig. 8 arguably showed training on one stack required over 1 in 10 images to be manually labelled to maintain confidence in the resulting automated 3-D projection. Yet a variety of data, or more accurate human labelling would likely result in a more successful result for a scenario of 1 in 10 or fewer images used for network training, which was determined to be true in the next section.

6 Multi-cellular Structures

6.1 Endothelial Cells

The automation method of using a deep neural network to label a single cell, a fibroblast and pericyte, required a U-Net architecture. However, labelling larger structures, such as a multi-cellular ring of endothelial cells, required use of a W-Net [1], an architecture of serial U-Nets. Unlike the U-Net, which had 17 layers, the W-Net had 33 layers and contained two encoder-decoder pairs. The image was effectively resized down to 1 by 1 and upsized to 256 by 256 twice as data was processed through the network. The discriminator remained unchanged. Increasing the number of layers within the network increased the complexity of the network and therefore the amount of time in which the network needed to train. Approximately 24 h were required to train the W-Net, 50 epochs, compared to only ~6 h for the U-Net, even while all other parameters remained unchanged. Increases to number of layers, as opposed to increases in filter number, did not require an increase in the necessary GPU size requirements for the network to train and run.

The labelling of endothelial cells was conducted on a different set of SBFSEM stacks to the labelling of single cellular structures. This was to determine the adaptability of the network and therefore general usability. 50% of the images were extracted for testing, as was an additional 10% block in the centre of the stack. There was also a block of images that were not manually labelled at the end of the stack, beyond what the network would have seen in training. This was to determine how well the network could adapt to more varied input data without causing overfitting due to a lack of adequate training data, shown in Fig. 8.

A visual analysis of the automated endothelial labelling in comparison to manually labelled images showed promising results, shown in Fig. 9. The comparison showed that (as was the case for a single cell structure) the network was capable of matching the over 98% of pixels to the manually labelled image, shown by the blue and black pixels. Compared to the single cell structures, less detail in the boundary region appeared lost in the automation process. This was likely due to both the increase in layers allowing for greater complexity in network-generated output and the clear boundary of a blood vessel compared to the more complex regions of placental tissue. However, the boundary region was still not without subjective manual labelling, and close examination of the comparison images showed the location of the red and green pixels, where the automated and manual labelling differed, were virtually all around endothelial sections.

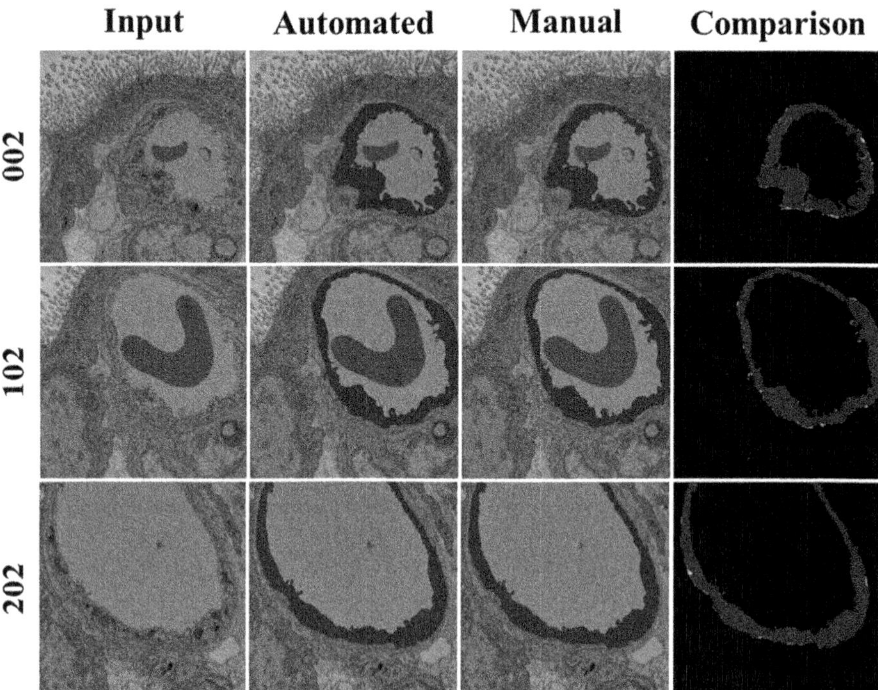

Fig. 9. A visual analysis of three z-positions throughout the stack, 002, 102, and 202. The inputs are the 2-D images extracted from the larger 3-D SBFSEM stack. The automated images are the network-generated images with automated labelling. The manual images are the images labelled by human experts for the same position. The comparison image shows a visualisation of correlating pixels between the automated and manual labels. Blue indicates labelled pixels in both images and black are unlabelled pixels in both images, while red indicates pixels only labelled in the manual image and green indicates pixels only labelled in the automated image. (Color figure online)

When the corresponding pixel percentage for every position in the stack was plotted (shown in Fig. 10) the rolling mean (the mean over ten positions centred at the plotted position) was almost 2% lower for the endothelial cells than for fibroblast and pericyte labelling. This was a direct result of the large boundary regions, especially large due to the increased labelling per image from the larger structure and also from the higher magnification on this stack. However, the precision (red markers) and recall (orange markers) were all much higher in value and more stable than for the single cell analysis in Fig. 3, never dropping below 0.75. This is a consequence of labelled regions being present in every portion of the stack, and the labelled regions were much larger than for the single cells. However, these relatively high and stable values also showed how successful the network was at automated endothelial labelling. The high specificity (yellow markers) showed the network was correctly ignoring undesired features and the accuracy (light green markers) remained above 0.96 for all regions of the stack throughout testing, even for the central extracted region.

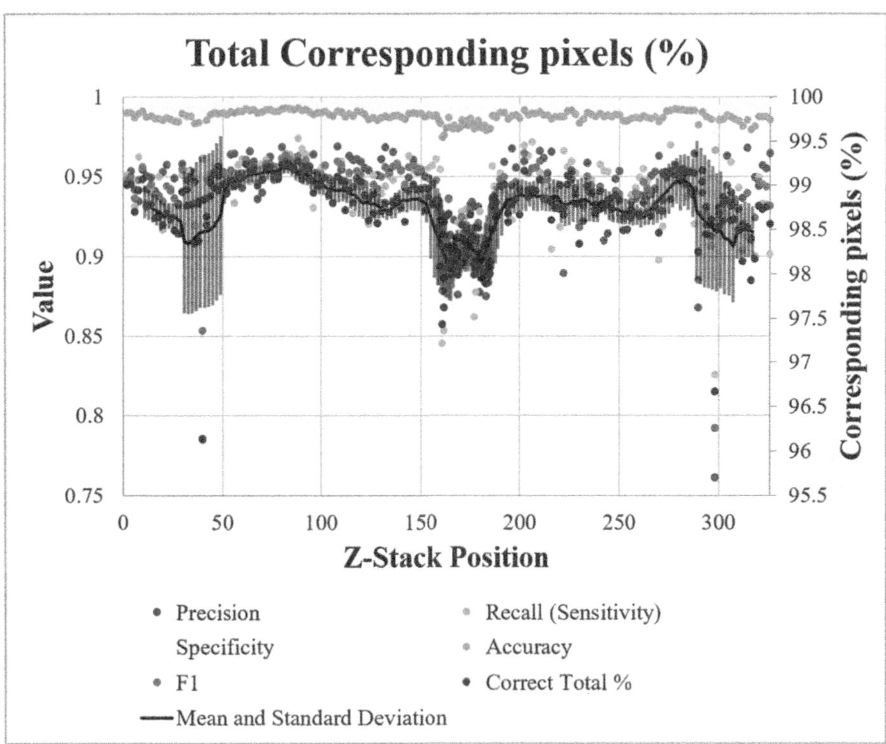

Fig. 10. Graph comparing automated and manual endothelial labelling for individual z-stack positions. Precision (red), recall (orange), specificity (yellow), accuracy (light green) and F1 (dark green) are all measured using the standard 0–1 value of the primary axis on the left-hand side. The correct total as a percentage (blue), or the total **correlating** pixels, and the rolling mean and standard deviation over ten positions (purple) are plotted against the secondary axis on the right-hand side. (Color figure online)

The centrally extracted region, positions 158–187, was the cause of the dip in both precision and recall, and therefore F1, but also in the total correlating pixels (dark blue markers), which was plotted against the secondary axis on the right-hand side. The mean over ten images (the purple line) and the standard deviation (the surrounding purple region) showed that, even though the percentage of corresponding pixels dropped by roughly 0.5%, the deviation between results was stable, without becoming larger towards the centre of the extracted region. This showed that the network was equally as capable of labelling images 15 positions away as 5 positions away. It can then be hypothesised that the network would be capable of successfully labelling stacks with fewer than 1 in 15 images manually labelled, as long as there were enough total images in the training set to avoid overfitting.

There are two positions on the graph that clearly showed increased deviation and reduced the mean for the surrounding regions. The first was position 040 and the second was position 298. These images were extracted for further analysis, shown in Fig. 11. The latter, 298, was the result of a similar manual labelling fault as in Fig. 4, where the manual labelling for that image was incomplete and it had been missed in standard human quality checking mechanisms, shown by the large green region in the comparison image. The endothelial cell was correctly labelled by the network but not manually, which made a sizable difference in the number of pixels that did not correspond and gave an (incorrectly) high false positive reading for position 298.

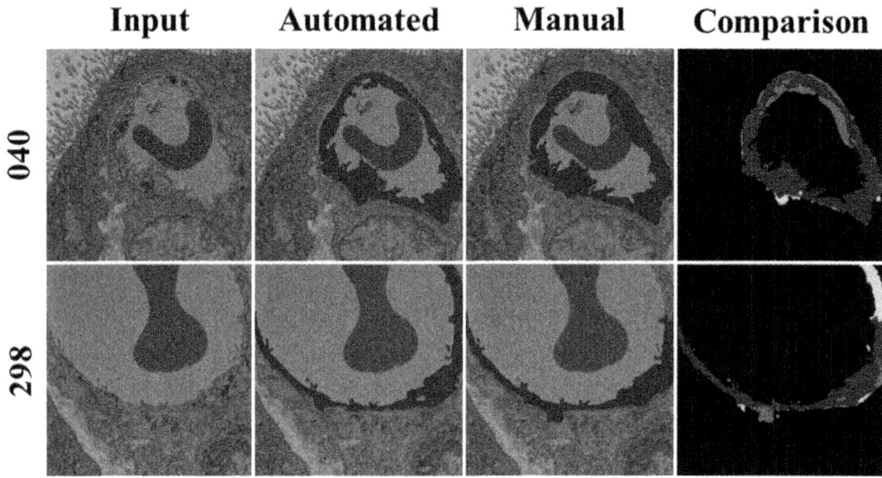

Fig. 11. A visual analysis of z-positions 040 and 298 showing automation outperforming manual labelling. The input is the 2-D image extracted from the larger 3-D SBFSEM stack. The automated image is the network-generated image with automated labelling. The manual image is the manually **labelled** image for the same position, which was used to test the network. The comparison image shows a visualisation of correlating pixels between the automated and manual labels. Blue indicates labelled pixels in both images and black indicates unlabelled pixels in both images, while red indicates pixels only labelled in the manual image and green indicates pixels only labelled in the automated image. (Color figure online)

The low percentage in corresponding pixels for position 040 was also due to a mistake in manual labelling but in a way more difficult to spot when quality checking manual labelling. The bottom half of the manual label was done relatively well, and the automated labelling matched this, shown by the large number of blue pixels in the comparison image. The large number of red pixels, an (incorrect) false negative, was the result of an inaccurate manual labelling which over-labelled the endothelial cells and led to an incorrect increase of labelling into the surrounding regions. The automated labelling was not similarly incorrect. Deep neural networks therefore have the ability to outperform manual labelling, even when trained on imperfect manually labelled data.

6.2 Labelling the Unseen

For automation to be easily used in a wider setting, the network must be able to label stacks, which it had not been trained on. Testing this was done in two stages. First, the network was input an image roughly 40 positions away from the training data, from the same stack which it had been trained on. Second, the network had an input of a completely unseen stack, in which it would also output labelled endothelial cells. For this to be achievable, the stack used for training data was augmented to contain a variety of contrast and brightness combinations to match the different variables at which an SBFSEM stack could be subjected when being produced. The result of these tests is shown in Fig. 12.

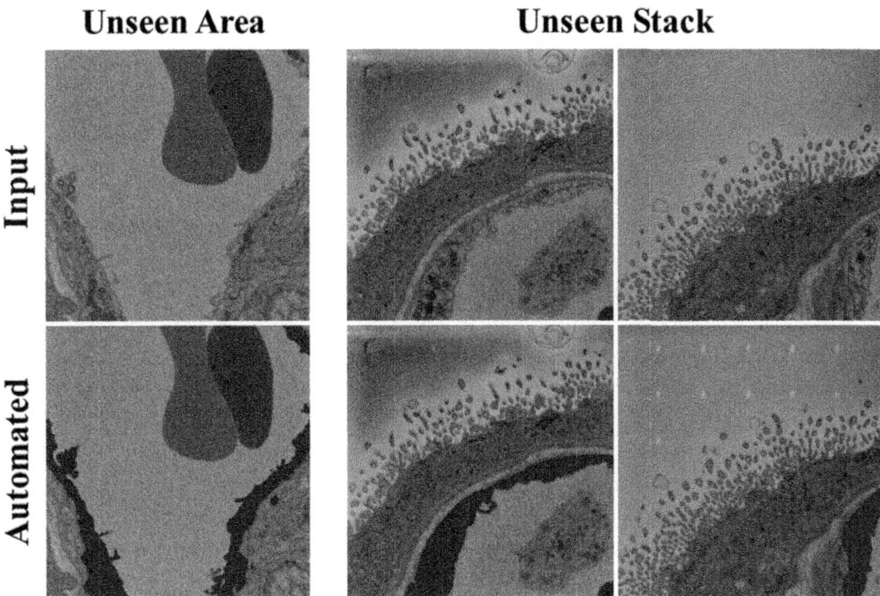

Fig. 12. Automated labelling outputs from the network for different input images. The first column shows the input and corresponding automated labelling for an unseen area of the stack used to train the network, 40 images away from the last "seen" **image**. The second and third column show the inputs and corresponding automated labelling for different positions in a completely unseen stack.

The first test, labelling an image from an unseen area of the stack 40 images away from the training data and therefore from the last "seen" image, produced a realistic appearing image with the endothelial cells fully labelled and minimal false positives. The second test produced a more interesting result, with the endothelial correctly labelled even with the stack and magnification being completely unseen by the network. This automated labelling of an unseen region and unseen stack shows that the network can be trained on previously labelled data to accurately automate the labelling of new and unseen 3-D stacks, potentially without any manual labelling being required. The inclusion of additional techniques, such as super-resolution techniques [52] or arrow detection [53], or other recent advances in region-of-interest labelling or upscaling in medical images, could be combined with this neural network labelling approach to both improve the mean accuracy of automated labelling but also to increase the range of features which could be extracted, with the aim of a single manual arrow on a feature of interest leading to an accurate and complete labelled stack.

7 Conclusion

The placenta is the interface between the mother and the fetus, mediating the transfer of nutrients, while acting as a barrier to the transfer of toxic molecules. Poor placental function can impair fetal growth and development, and affect its health across the lifecourse. SBFSEM has emerged as an important tool revealing the nanoscale structure of cellular placental structures in 3-D, and how the structures interact. While this technique is revealing novel structures, as well as the spatial relationships between cells, it is limited by the time it takes to manually label the structures of interest in hundreds of serial sections. This is restricting the ability to model the placenta computationally. Developing a machine learning-based approach dramatically speeds up this process, from several weeks to a few minutes to label an entire stack, and enables more quantitative analytical approaches.

The correlating pixels across all features and all network architectures averaged greater than 98%. This gave an effective error of less than 2%, with the ability to be lower with perfected training data across a wider range of SBFSEM stacks, with as few as 1 in 15 labelled manually. Training a network took 6–24 h, and testing a single image took less than a second, which was much faster than the month of dedicated time it took to manually label the individual stacks used in this chapter. This method did not sacrifice data and resolution for an increase in processing time, as the only data loss (resizing of the image) was due to restrictions of the GPU size available. GPU dependent, there is no need to limit the input resolution of standard SBFSEM generated images for this labelling technique. Inclusion of medical-imaging region-of-interest labelling in future work could provide consistent maximum accuracy with even fewer manual data processing steps.

Deep neural networks can be trained on stacks of unlabelled and their associated labelled images of a single desired cell type within placental tissue. This machine learning approach enabled can label different structures, with not only fibroblasts, pericytes and endothelial cells within the placenta a possibility, but also other cell and tissue types, such as osteoblasts within bone. There is potential therefore for automation of any labelled feature. The networks were given no information of SBFSEM besides the unlabelled-labelled pairs, therefore the technique is not limited to SBFSEM and could be applied to other 3-D imaging techniques.

References

1. Mackay, B., et al.: Automated 3-D labelling of fibroblasts and endothelial cells in SEM-imaged placenta using deep learning. In: Proceedings of the 13th International Joint Conference on Biomedical Engineering Systems and Technologies, BIOIMAGING 2020, INSTICC, vol. 2, pp. 46–53. SciTePress, Malta (2020)
2. Palaiologou, E., et al.: Human placental villi contain stromal macrovesicles associated with networks of stellate cells. J Anat. **236**(1), 132–141 (2019)
3. Lewis, R.M., Cleal, J.K., Hanson, M.A.: Review: placenta, evolution and lifelong health. Placenta **33**, S28–S32 (2012)
4. Lewis, R.M., Pearson-Farr, J.E.: Multiscale three-dimensional imaging of the placenta. Placenta. https://doi.org/10.1016/j.placenta.2020.01.016. (Article in press)
5. Burton, G.J.: Scanning electron microscopy of intervillous connections in the mature human placenta. J. Anat. **147**, 245–254 (1986)
6. Mayhew, T.M.: Morphomics: an integral part of systems biology of the human placenta. Placenta **36**(4), 329–340 (2015)
7. Wang, Y., Zhao, S.: Vascular Biology of the Placenta. Morgan & Claypool, San Rafael (2010)
8. Cahill, L.S., et al.: Feto- and utero-placental vascular adaptions to chronic maternal hypoxia in the mouse. J. Physiol **596**(15), 3285–3297 (2018)
9. Kherlopian, A.R., et al.: A review of imaging techniques for systems biology. BMC Syst Biol. **2**, 74 (2008)
10. Denk, W., Horstmann, H.: Serial block-face scanning electron microscopy to reconstruct three-dimensional tissue nanostructure. PLoS Biol. **2**(100), e329 (2004)
11. Kazemian, A., Hooshmandabbasi, R., Schraner, E.M., Boos, A., Klisch, K.: Evolutionary implications of fetal and maternal microvillous surfaces in epitheliochorial placentae. J. Morphol. **280**(4), 615–622 (2019)
12. Palaiologou, E., et al.: Serial block-face scanning electron microscopy reveals novel intercellular connections in human term placental microvasculature. J. Anat. **237**, 1–9 (2020)
13. Deerinck, T.J., Bushong, E.A., Lev-Ram, V., Shu, X., Tsien, R.Y., Ellisman, M.H.: Enhancing serial block-face scanning electron microscopy to enable high resolution 3-D nanohistology of cells and tissues. Microsc. Microanal. **16**(2), 1138–1139 (2010)
14. Zachow, S., Zilske, M., Hege, H.: 3-D reconstruction of individual anatomy from medical image data: segmentation and geometry processing. Konrad-Zuse-Zentrum für Informationstechnik Berlin, Berlin (2007)
15. Pugin, E., Zhiznyakov, A.: Histogram method of image binarization based on fuzzy pixel representation. In: Dynamics of Systems, Mechanisms and Machines 2017 (Dynamics), p. 17467698. IEEE, Omsk (2017)
16. Yoo, K.D., et al.: A machine learning approach using survival statistics to predict graft survival in kidney transplant recipients: a multicenter cohort study. Sci. Rep. **7**, 8904 (2017)
17. Jamshidi, A., Pelletier, J., Martel-Pelletier, J.: Machine-learning-based patient-specific prediction models for knee osteoarthritis. Nat. Rev. Rheumatol. **15**, 49–60 (2019)
18. Google Cloud: Vision AI| Derive Image Insights via ML. Google. https://cloud.google.com/vision/. Accessed 14 Nov 2019

19. Grant-Jacob, J.A., et al.: Real-time particle pollution sensing using machine learning. Opt. Express **26**(21), 27237–27246 (2018)
20. Krizhevsky, A., Sutskever, L., Hinton, G.: ImageNet classification with deep convolutional neural networks. In: Proceedings of the Advances in Neural Information Processing Systems 25, pp. 1090–1098 (2012)
21. Szegedy, C., et al.: Intriguing properties of neural networks. arXiv:1312.6199v4 (2014)
22. Schmidhuber, J.: Deep learning in neural networks: an overview. Neural Netw. **61**, 85–117 (2015)
23. Simonyan, K., Zisserman, A.: Very Deep Convolutional Networks for Large-Scale Image Recognition. arXiv:1409.1556v6 (2015)
24. Kermany, D.S., Goldbaum, M., Cai, W., Lewis, M.A., Xia, H., Zhang, K.: Identifying medical diagnoses and treatable diseases by image-based deep learning. Cell **172**(5), 1122–1131 (2018)
25. Litjens, G., et al.: A survey on deep learning in medical image analysis. Med. Image Anal. **42**, 60–88 (2017)
26. Esteva, A., et al.: Dermatologist-level classification of skin cancer with deep neural networks. Nature **542**, 115–118 (2017)
27. Haenssle, H.A., et al.: Man against machine: diagnostic performance of a deep learning convolutional neural network for dermoscopic melanoma recognition in comparison to 58 dermatologists. Ann. Oncol. **29**, 1836–1842 (2018)
28. Le Cun, Y., Huang, F. J., Bottou, L.: Learning methods for generic object recognition with invariance to pose and lighting. In: Proceedings of the 2004 IEEE Computer Society Conference on Computer Vision and Pattern Recognition, vol. 2, p. II-97 (2004)
29. Lo, S.B., Chan, H., Freedman, M.T., Min, S.K.: Artificial convolution neural network for medical image pattern recognition. Neural Netw. **8**(7–8), 1201–1214 (1995)
30. Le Cun, Y., Bengio, Y.: Convolutional Networks for Images Speech and Time-Series. The Handbook of Brain Theory and Neural Networks. MIT Press, Cambridge (1995)
31. Sermanet, P., Eigen, D., Zhang, X., Mathieu, M., Fergus, R., Le Cun, Y.: OverFeat: Integrated Recognition, Localization and Detection using Convolutional Networks. arXiv: 1312.6229v4 (2013)
32. Donahue, J., et al.: 2015 IEEE Conference on Computer Vision and Pattern Recognition (CVPR), pp. 2625–2634 (2015)
33. Zhang, X., Le Cun, Y.: Text Understanding from Scratch. arXiv:1502.01710v5 (2015)
34. Dong, A., He, K., Tang, X.: Image super-resolution using deep convolutional networks. IEEE Trans. Pattern Anal. Mach. Intell. **38**(2), 295–307 (2016)
35. Simard, D., Steinkraus, P.Y., Platt, J.C.: Best practices for convolutional neural networks. In: Proceedings of the Document Analysis and Recognition, pp. 958–963 (2003)
36. Vaillant, R., Monrocq, C., Le Cun, Y.: Original approach for the localisation of objects in images. Proc. Vis. Image Sig. Process. **141**, 245–250 (1994)
37. Nowlan, S., Platt, J.: A convolutional neural network hand tracker. In: Advances in Neural Information Processing Systems, pp. 901–908 (1995)
38. Le Cun, Y., et al.: Handwritten digit recognition with a back-propagation network. In: Advances in Neural Information Processing Systems (1990)23
39. Hubel, D.H., Wiesel, T.N.: Receptive fields, binocular interaction, and functional architecture in the cat's visual cortex. J. Physiol. **106**, 160 (1962)
40. LeCun, Y., Bengio, Y., Hinton, G.: Deep learning. Nature **521**, 436–444 (2015)
41. Fukushima, K., Miyake, S., Ito, T.: Neocognitron: a neural network model for a mechanism of visual pattern recognition. IEEE Trans. Syst. Man Cybern. **13**(5), 826–834 (1983)
42. Felleman, D.J., Essen, D.C.V.: Distributed hierarchical processing in the primate cerebral cortex. Cereb. Cortex **1**, 1–47 (1991)

43. Mirza, M., Osindero, S.: Conditional Generative Adversarial Nets. arXiv:1411.1784v1 (2014)
44. Pathak, D., Krahenbuhl, P., Donahue, J., Darrell, T., Efros, A. A.: Context Encoders: Feature Learning by Inpainting. arXiv:1604.07379v2 (2016)
45. Isola, P., Zhue, J., Zhou T., Efros, A.A.: Image-to-Image Translation with Conditional Adversarial Networks. arXiv:1611.07004v3 (2018)
46. Esteva, A., et al.: A guide to deep learning in healthcare. Nat. Med. **25**, 24–29 (2019)
47. Ronneberger, O., Fischer, P., Brox, T.: U-Net: convolutional networks for biomedical image segmentation. In: Navab, N., Hornegger, J., Wells, W.M., Frangi, A.F. (eds.) MICCAI 2015. LNCS, vol. 9351, pp. 234–241. Springer, Cham (2015). https://doi.org/10.1007/978-3-319-24574-4_28
48. Long, J., Shelhamer, E., Darrell, T.: Fully Convolutional Networks for Semantic Segmentation. arXiv:1411.4038 (2014)
49. Falk, T., et al.: U-Net: deep learning for cell counting, detection, and morphometry. Nat. Methods **16**, 67–70 (2019)
50. Barreto, R.S.N., Romagnolli, P., Cereta, A.D., Coimbra-Campos, L.M.C., Birbrair, A., Miglino, M.A.: Pericytes in the placenta: role in placental development and homeostasis. In: Birbrair, A. (ed.) Pericyte Biology in Different Organs. AEMB, vol. 1122, pp. 125–151. Springer, Cham (2019). https://doi.org/10.1007/978-3-030-11093-2_8
51. Bergers, G., Song, S.: The role of pericytes in blood-vessel formation and maintenance. Neuro Oncol. **7**(4), 452–464 (2005)
52. Grant-Jacob, J.A., et al.: A neural lens for super-resolution biological imaging. J. Phys. Commun. **3**(6), 065004 (2019)
53. Santosh, K.C., Roy, P.P.: Arrow detection in biomedical images using sequential classifier. Int. J. Mach. Learn. Cybern. **9**(6), 993–1006 (2016). https://doi.org/10.1007/s13042-016-0623-y

Estimating the False Positive Prediction Rate in Automated Volumetric Measurements of Malignant Pleural Mesothelioma

Owen Anderson[1,2(✉)], Andrew C. Kidd[3], Keith A. Goatman[1], Alexander J. Weir[1], Jeremy P. Voisey[1], Vismantas Dilys[1], Jan P. Siebert[2], and Kevin G. Blyth[3,4]

[1] Canon Medical Research Europe, 2 Anderson Place, Edinburgh, UK
owen.anderson@eu.medical.canon
[2] School of Computing Science, University of Glasgow, 18 Lilybank Gardens, Glasgow, UK
[3] Pleural Disease Unit, Queen Elizabeth University Hospital, 1345 Govan Road, Glasgow, UK
[4] Institute of Infection, Immunity and Inflammation, University of Glasgow, 120 University Place, Glasgow, UK

Abstract. Malignant Pleural Mesothelioma (MPM) is a rare cancer associated with exposure to asbestos fibres. It grows in the pleural space surrounding the lungs, exhibiting an irregular shape with high surface-to-volume ratio. Reliable measurements are important to assessing treatment efficacy, however these tumour characteristics make manual measurements time consuming, and prone to intra- and inter-observer variation. Previously we described a fully automatic Convolutional Neural Network (CNN) for volumetric measurement of MPM in CT images, trained and evaluated by seven-fold cross validation on 123 CT datasets with expert manual annotations. The mean difference between the manual and automatic volume measurements was not significantly different from zero ($27.2\,\text{cm}^3$; $p = 0.225$), the 95% limits of agreement were between -417 and $+363\,\text{cm}^3$, and the mean Dice coefficient was 0.64. Previous studies have focused on images with known MPM, sometimes even focusing on the lung with known MPM. In this paper, we investigate the false positive detection rate in a large image set with no known MPM. For this, a cohort of 14,965 subjects from the National Lung Screening Trial (NLST) were analysed. The mean volume of "MPM" found in these images by the automated detector was $3.6\,\text{cm}^3$ (compared with $547.2\,\text{cm}^3$ for MPM positive subjects). A qualitative examination of the one hundred subjects with the largest probable false detection volumes found that none of them were normal: the majority contain hyperdense pathology, large regions of pleural effusion, or evidence of pleural thickening. One false positive was caused by liver masses. The next step will be to evaluate the automated measurement accuracy on an independent, unseen, multi-centre data set.

X. Ye et al. (Eds.): BIOSTEC 2020, CCIS 1400, pp. 116–139, 2021.
https://doi.org/10.1007/978-3-030-72379-8_7

Keywords: Malignant Pleural Mesothelioma (MPM) · Deep learning (DL) · Convolutional Neural Network (CNN) · Computed tomography (CT) · Image segmentation

1 Introduction

Mesothelioma is the cancer associated with exposure to asbestos fibres. In around 90% of cases the cancer develops in the pleural space surrounding the lungs [4], where it is known as Malignant Pleural Mesothelioma (MPM). Many European countries have restricted the use of asbestos, however the delayed onset of the disease (in extreme cases more than 70 years after exposure [5]) means that the rate of cases has only recently begun to slow. In countries with no legislation preventing the use of asbestos, mortality rates from mesothelioma continue to increase [1].

Care for patients diagnosed with MPM is likely to be palliative—current treatments for the disease are often ineffective, and only around 7% of subjects survive five or more years beyond their initial diagnosis. The volume of the mesothelioma tumour is a key feature for determining response to treatment. However, it is extremely difficult to measure the tumour because of its shape and appearance.

An automated detector that is both fast and accurate could have a number of practical applications, including helping to assess the right treatment regime for each patient, or as a measure of efficacy in a clinical trial, or as an automated incidental finding integrated in a radiology reading system. However, to be effective, automated incidental findings require low false alarm rates, or they will distract and annoy, rather than support, the radiologist. In this paper we assess both measurement accuracy and false positive detection rates for the automated MPM detector.

1.1 Tumour Measurement

Although volume is the most representative tumour size measurement, it is common practice to use surrogate metrics which can be performed much faster. In contrast to mesothelioma, most tumours can be assumed to be roughly spherical. This allows a simple diameter measurement to be used to accurately track tumour volume over time. This is used by the RECIST (Response Evaluation Criteria in Solid Tumours) score [22], that is routinely used, for example, in the measurement of lung nodules.

MPM tumours, however, are not remotely spherical. They develop in the tight pleural space around the lungs, growing with an irregular shape having a high surface area-to-volume ratio. The routine surrogate metric for MPM measurement is the modified RECIST (or mRECIST) score [8]. It requires tumour thickness measurements at multiple locations, perpendicular to the lung wall. The sum of these thickness measurements taken at two time points are used to generate the mRECIST report, which categorises the tumours as either [11]:

- Complete Response (CR), indicating a disappearance of all known disease;
- Partial Response (PR), indicating a 30% or more decrease in the mRECIST score;
- Stable disease/No change, indicating that no new lesions have appeared, and the mRECIST score has not significantly changed;
- Progressive Disease (PD), indicating a 20% or more increase in the mRECIST score, or the appearance of new lesions.

The mRECIST score has poor intra- and inter-annotator agreement [27]. A major component of the variability arises from the choice of the line locations. However, Armato *et al.* [3] showed that even when multiple experts are given the coordinates for the line centres, significant variability in the mRECIST score remains due to variation in the choice of line angle. A further component of the measurement variability arises from interpretation of the images. Labby *et al.* [17] describe a 95% confidence interval between five observers spanning 311% and 111% for single time-point *area* measurements of baseline and response images respectively. The research suggests that CT images of MPM are inherently ambiguous.

Although tumour volume is the most representative measurement, such measurements are too time-consuming for routine care and the mRECIST measurement remains the *clinical* standard due to its feasibility.

1.2 Overview of Existing Measurement Tools

Several semi-automated approaches have been developed to decrease the time required to interpret CT images. Some target the measurement of pleural thickening, while others specifically target MPM tumour measurements. Pleural effusion is a common confounding feature when measuring MPM. In CT images, the MPM and effusion can have overlapping CT (Hounsfied Unit) values [20], making differentiation technically challenging. For any measurements of tumour volume progression, this distinction is necessary because any volume of fluid and tumour are unrelated.

Gudmundsson *et al.* [13] describe the use of deep CNNs to segment pleural thickening (which can include MPM tumour, pleural effusion, and pleural plaques) from CT images. The images are pre-processed to remove the patient couch and air. Images are then passed to one of two U-Nets, dependent on the laterality of the disease, which must be manually identified. Median area Dice coefficients ranging from 0.662 to 0.800 are achieved across two test sets (totalling 131 slices from 43 patients). The two test sets were manually annotated for MPM tumour (rather than pleural thickening) by 3 and 5 observers, providing inter-observer Dice coefficients ranging from 0.648 to 0.814, which are similar to those achieved by the automated method. As this approach does not aim to distinguish effusion from tumour, the authors describe that 7 out of 15 outlier slices where the method over-predicts tumour area contain pleural effusion. This is explored and addressed in their later publications [12,14], where they train the CNNs to exclude pleural effusion from the segmentation, and examine performance across two test sets—one of which selected to contain slices showing pleural effusion. Training the algorithm to distinguish pleural effusion improved average area Dice coefficients (0.499 to 0.690 in the pleural effusion test set).

Chen *et al.* [9] describe semi-automated measurement of tumour volume in CT images by a random walk segmentation. The random walk segmentation is initialised by 20–30 manually placed seed points per slice within the MPM tumour area. For each slice, this requires expert interaction lasting around 20–30 s. Across a test set of 15 subjects, a mean Dice coefficient of 0.825 is achieved.

Sensakovic *et al.* [23] semi-automate the measurement of a pleural volume. The method first segments the lung parenchyma and hemi-thoratic cavity. User input is required for segmentation around the liver boundary. Based on the segmentations, the pleural volume is derived. Evaluation of the method is at a CT slice level, where a median area Jaccard index of 0.484 is achieved over 31 patients (which is equivalent to a Dice coefficient of 0.652). The median Jaccard index for the same slices annotated by three observers is 0.517 (equivalent to a Dice coefficient of 0.682).

Brahim *et al.* [7] detect the thoracic cavity, and use texture analysis to locate regions of MPM tumour. They achieve a Dice coefficient of 0.88 across a test set of 10 CT images.

This manuscript builds on our previous work [2], which described the preliminary findings from an internal validation study of our fully automatic, deep learning-based volumetric segmentation tool, based on 123 CT scans and expert annotations (from 108 patients). This manuscript contributes an extended analysis of the specificity of the technique, using a large, independent dataset from the National Lung Screening Trial (NLST) study to examine the false positive detection rate in a dataset where true MPM is unlikely.

2 Method

An automated detector has been developed for the segmentation of MPM tumour from CT images as part of a retrospective cohort study funded by the Cancer Innovation Challenge (Scottish Health Council), which will conclude in 2020 following the analysis of 403 patients with MPM.

2.1 Data

123 volumetric CT datasets from 108/403 subjects recruited to the DIAPHRAGM and PRISM research studies were used to train and cross-validate the automated method, all of which had a confirmed histological diagnosis of MPM. A further subset of CT datasets from the NLST archive were utilised to test the automated detector.

PRISM. (Prediction of ResIstance to chemotherapy using Somatic copy number variation in Mesothelioma) [6] is a retrospective cohort study to determine a genomic classifier that predicts chemo-resistance in MPM. The study involves retrieval of tumour blocks pre- and post-chemotherapy from 380 subjects across five UK centres. 123 CT images from 85/380 PRISM subjects are included in this study (43 images acquired pre-treatment, and 80 images acquired post-treatment), from centres in Glasgow.

DIAPHRAGM. (Diagnostic and Prognostic Biomarkers in the Rational Assessment of Mesothelioma) [26] was a 3 year prospective observational study, which involved 747 patients from 23 UK sites. Subjects were recruited to the study upon first presentation of MPM. A suncohort of 23/747 subjects from Glasgow centres (who had both MRI and CT images) were selected. All the selected images were acquired pre-treatment. Contemporaneous MRI images are useful in disambiguating some confounding features in CT images.

NLST. (National Lung Screening Trial) [19] was a multicentre study which aimed to compare low-dose CT with chest radiography for lung cancer screening. The study targeted older (55–74 years) ex- and current smokers. 46,613 CT images from 14,965 subjects are used to test detector specificity.

The images from the DIAPHRAGM study were acquired earlier in development of MPM with respect to those from the PRISM study, and consequently the tumour volumes tend to be smaller and thinner in the DIAPHRAGM study. Slices from a PRISM and DIAPHRAGM dataset are compared in Fig. 1.

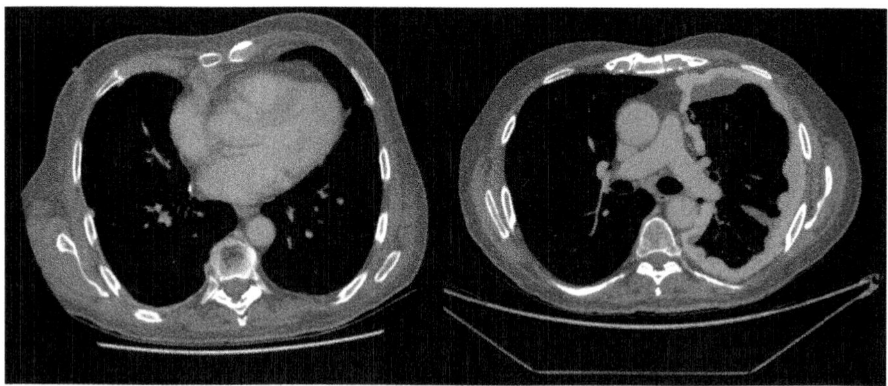

Fig. 1. Two axial CT slices from two subjects in the cohort, with manually derived MPM tumour segmentation shown in red. Top: A slice from a CT image taken in the DIAPHRAGM study. Bottom: A slice from a CT image taken in the PRISM study. The unsegmented areas (in grey) represent adjacent pleural fluid. Figure from [2]. (Color figure online)

Ground Truth Generation. A respiratory clinician with training in image analysis and mesothelioma identification manually segmented the MPM tumour in 123 CT images from the PRISM and DIAPHRAGM studies. Tumour segmentation was performed in the axial plane using Myrian software (Intrasense,

Paris). Segmentations were performed in all slices containing tumour for 80/123 images. For 43/123 images a more sparse annotation was performed where every fifth slice was annotated. Consecutive slices are highly correlated—both in appearance and in terms of the tumour characteristics. Annotating a subset of slices allowed a greater number of subjects to be included in the training set, increasing the diversity of this cohort. Although beneficial to training the algorithm, a sparser annotation resulted in datasets which could not be used to evaluate volume accuracy, and were not included in the evaluation of the algorithm.

Ground Truth Inter-slice Consistency Processing. The MPM tumour was manually segmented in the axial plane. A free-hand segmentation was required to capture the complex shape of the tumour, and inevitably this leads to some annotation inconsistencies between slices. These appear as a discontinuities of the tumour segmentation in the orthogonal, sagittal and coronal planes, contrasting with the continuous nature of the tumour viewed in the axial plane of annotation (Fig. 1). For many measurements inconsistencies of this nature are negligible, however for MPM measurement the between-slice inconsistency can have a significant effect on volumetric measurements. To improve between-slice consistency, a three-dimensional binary closing operation (Fig. 3) was performed using an $11 \times 11 \times 11$ voxel structuring element. A limitation of this approach is that any genuine holes in the tumour smaller than five voxels will be removed.

2.2 Cross-Validation

The algorithm was evaluated by k-fold cross validation, where a setting of $k = 7$ was found to provide robust group statistics for each test set, whilst maximising the amount of training data at each fold. As described in Sect. 2.1, 43/123 datasets were sparsely annotated, and could not be used to evaluate volumetric accuracy. These datasets were used in the training set for all seven folds. The 80/123 datasets with full annotation were randomly assigned to seven folds, to provide a validation set of 11 or 12 datasets per fold. The 68 or 69 remaining datasets are further sub-divided by a 30:70 split, where 30% is used to determine the best model and select an optimal model threshold (referred to as the internal validation set), and 70% is used as the training set, to which the 43 sparsely annotated datasets are added.

Neighbouring CT slices are highly correlated, and including all the slices from a CT images biased the algorithm towards maximising performance on the images with the greatest number of slices. To counter this, fully segmented CT images were also subsampled to 100 slices when training the algorithm.

Performance Metrics. Absolute volume correspondence and segmentation accuracy are used to evaluate agreement between the automated method and manual observer. Given only single time-point images were available in this preliminary evaluation, we were unable to evaluate volume *change* accuracy.

Bland-Altman analysis [18] is used to evaluate volumetric agreement between the automated and manual segmentations. This plots the difference of two measurements against the mean of the two measurements, together with the mean difference and the 95% limits of agreement. The following summarises the volumetric agreement statistics:

1. The mean difference (or bias) between the two measurement methods
2. A test for whether the mean difference between the two measurement methods is significantly different from zero, determined using a two-sided paired t-test (MATLAB statistics toolbox, Mathworks, Natick).
3. The 95% limits of agreement [18].
4. A test whether the difference between the measurement methods increases (or decreases) as the tumour volume increases. This was determined from the slope of a least squares regression fit to the points in the Bland-Altman plot. Specifically, it tests whether the slope is statistically different from a zero gradient, based on t-statistics (MATLAB statistics toolbox, Mathworks, Natick).

The Dice Score is used to measure region overlap between the manual and automated measurements. Although volumetric agreement is the primary property of interest, it does not show whether the same regions have been delineated, or whether the regions intersect. The Dice score provides a measure of these properties.

2.3 Algorithm

To automatically segment MPM tumour, a Convolutional Neural Network (CNN) was trained.

Architecture. The CNN was a U-Net architecture [21]—similar to the method used by Gudmundsson *et al.* [13,14]. Our network (Fig. 2) takes three axial slices at a time, and predicts a segmentation at the central of these slices. The encoder is pre-trained in a VGG classifier on the ImageNet challenge data [16]. For pre-training, the three-channel input was used to consume three-colour natural images.

All network activations are rectified linear units, aside from the ultimate layer of the network, which was a softmax activation. Dropout (with a rate of 0.2) [25] was used to prevent over-fitting and batch normalisation [15] was used at the locations illustrated in Fig. 2 to improve the training characteristics. The network was implemented and trained using the Keras framework [10].

Image Pre-processing: CT image intensities input to the network are clipped to [−1050, +1100] Hounsfield Units, and normalised to range [−1, +1]. The images are retained at their original resolution (which is typically within the range 0.71 mm to 1.34 mm).

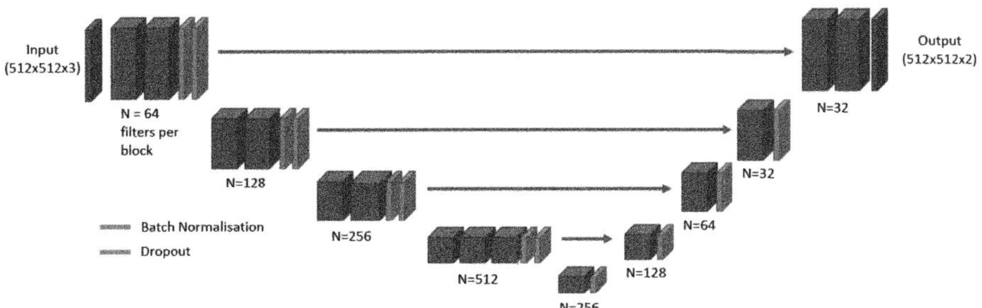

Fig. 2. A schematic of the U-Net model architecture. The blue boxes represent a stack of convolutional filters, with the number of filters per stack shown to the left of each box. All filters have a dimensionality of 3×3. Green and orange boxes represent dropout and batch normalisation layers respectively. The blue arrows represent skip connections by feature concatenation. Figure from [2]. (Color figure online)

Training. The network was trained for 30 epochs, after which the best performing model is selected across the epochs. This model was chosen based on highest average voxel-level accuracy for the internal validation set. For training, the Adam optimiser was used, with a cyclic learning rate [24], where the learning rate (lr) has been set to oscillate between $lr = 0.0001$ and $lr = 0.003$, with a full cycle duration of one epoch. A batch size of 8 slices (with context) per batch allowed the model (10,019,874 parameters) to train on the available GPU.

Despite MPM tumour segmentation being a binary classification task, categorical cross-entropy was used as the objective function. Therefore, the output of the network was two-channel: one for tumour segmentation, and one for background segmentation. This objective function was found to improve convergence with respect to binary cross-entropy. The slices during training were randomly ordered, and it was possible that the class balance in the first batch was highly unbalanced. When batches were predominantly tumour negative in the first few batches, weights near the decoder of the network were optimised to zero, and training stopped as errors could no longer back-propagated. Categorical cross-entropy was used to overcome this, a non-zero signal is always required in one of the two output channels, regardless of the class balance of the example slice/batch. This regularising effect of categorical cross-entropy increased experiment repeatability between runs and folds of analysis.

Binarisation. The output of the CNN was a probability map, showing the probability of MPM tumour at every voxel in the input CT slice. This output was binarised by applying a threshold. The optimal threshold for the CNN was chosen to maximise the mean Dice coefficient between the binarised prediction and manual annotations in the internal validation set. The optimal threshold varied slightly between models—different training datasets had varying levels of complexity, resulting in models which predicted in varying probability ranges.

The internal validation sets at each fold also contained different disease characteristics, which added variance to the optimal threshold between folds.

Tumour Volume. For validation, the algorithm was used to segment the MPM tumour in every slice of the input CT images. Tumour volume was then calculated [2]:

$$M(x,y,z) = \begin{cases} 1 & \forall P(x,y,z) > t \\ 0 & \forall P(x,y,z) \leq t \end{cases} \tag{1}$$

where M describes a segmentation image of same dimensionality as the input CT image, with each voxel assigned a binary value of one to indicate MPM tumour and zero elsewhere. M was calculated by evaluating the probability map $(P(x,y,z))$ with respect to the optimal threshold, t. This binary segmentation was then converted into a measurement of tumour volume (V) [2]:

$$V = S_x S_y S_z \sum_{x=0}^{X} \sum_{y=0}^{Y} \sum_{z=0}^{Z} M(x,y,z), \tag{2}$$

where S_x, S_y and S_z denote the image voxel sizes in x,y and z respectively.

2.4 False Positive Rate Estimation

NLST Study Data. The National Lung Screening Trial (NLST) study enrolled 53,454 persons at high risk for lung cancer between 2002 and 2004 from 33 centres in the United States. The study had two arms, comparing chest X-rays and CT imaging for detecting lung cancer. 26,722 participants were enrolled in the CT arm of the study. Of these, 14,965 subjects are used to provide a further testing set for the automated mesothelioma detector. The subset of NLST images was selected to include subjects with reported lung abnormalities and lung nodules. The NLST study was not focused on mesothelioma, and it is unlikely that many images in the study contain mesothelioma (it was not indicated as an incidental finding for any images in the study). Hence this dataset is used to analyse the specificity of the automated detector across a large and independent cohort. Since imaging alone cannot give a definite diagnosis of mesothelioma—the appearance of the tumour in CT images is similar to many other findings—biopsy is often the only definitive test. For this reason, it is possible that images acquired for the NLST study contain one or more subjects with mesothelioma.

Time-Points. The CT images acquired for the NLST study spanned three annual time-points. Participation was terminated upon either: a) completion of the third time point, b) subject drop out, or c) a significant finding impeding the ability to complete the study. In this analysis, images from all the available time points were included in the analysis.

Study Findings. As a part of the NLST study, a variety of findings of relevance were recorded. For the purposes of this analysis, hyperdense pathologies which have a bright appearance in CT images are of relevant—such findings are most likely to be confused with MPM by the automated detector. The specific NLST findings of interest are listed in Table 1. Note that since the NLST study recorded findings by *subject* rather than by image, not all of the images from a subject with a positive finding will necessarily contain evidence of the specific finding(s).

Table 1. List of NLST study findings considered positive in the false positive detection rate analysis.

NLST findings of interest
Pleural thickening or effusion
Non-calcified hilar/mediastinal adenopathy or mass
Chest wall abnormality
Consolidation
Emphysema

Reconstruction Kernel: The CT images acquired for the NLST study were reconstructed using "hard" (sharp) kernels, "soft" kernels. For some subjects images were reconstructed from the same acquisition data using both types of kernel. CT manufacturers offer a variety of different reconstruction kernels, described by their own naming conventions. Table 2 lists the kernels by CT manufacturer that were considered hard for the purposes of this study. In total, this resulted 20,139 hard image reconstructions and 26,474 soft image reconstructions.

2.5 Experiments

The convolutional neural network was trained seven times on seven folds of the training dataset, as described in Sect. 2.2. The seven resulting CNN models were combined into an ensemble to generate the final volume measurement result, by calculating the mean of the volumes from the seven models. The results obtained by this method were:

1. Compared with those obtained from the individual seven models for all subjects with histologically confirmed MPM (DIAPHRAM and PRISM),
2. Stratified by whether hyperdense pathology is present (NLST),
3. Stratified by hard/soft kernel reconstructions (NLST).

The 100 cases where the algorithm finds the largest volumes of tumour were qualitatively analysed.

Table 2. List of CT reconstruction kernels considered "hard" and "soft" in this study. Kernels names used to reconstruct two or more images are listed.

Manufacturer	Hard kernel names	Soft kernel names
GE	LUNG and BONE	STANDARD, BODY FILTER/STANDARD and BODY FILTER/BONE
Philips	D and B	A, C and EC
Siemens	B50f, B60f, B80f and B45f	B30f, B20f, B31f, B30s, B50s, B70f, B31s, B40f, B60s and B35f
Toshiba/Canon	FC51, FC53	FC01, FC30, FC50, FC02, FC10, FC82 and FC11

3 Results

Manual annotation time varied between subjects, taking approximately 2.5 h per image. Automated measurements required approximately 60 s per image, using an Nvidia 1080Ti graphics processing unit (GPU), 32 GB of RAM and a 12-core Intel Xeon CPU (3.40 GHz).

3.1 Inter-slice Consistency Processing

Three-dimensional binary closing was proposed to increase between-slice manual segmentation consistency (c.f. Sect. 2.1). This processing increased detected plural volume from 301.1 cm^3 (standard deviation 263.9 cm^3) to 514.7 cm^3 (standard deviation 336.1 cm^3) over the cohort. Figure 3 shows a typical binary closing result, and highlights the additional voxels added by the closing operation. Visually, the closed version appears more contiguous and physically plausible.

3.2 Volumetric Agreement

The cohort mean predicted volume was 547.2 cm^3 (standard deviation 290.9 cm^3) across seven-folds of analysis.

Raw Manual Annotations. The mean tumour volume in the raw manual segmentations is 405.1 cm^3 (standard deviation 271.5 cm^3), which is significantly lower than the automatically detected volume. The Bland-Altman plot in Fig. 4 shows a minor, though statistically significant, trend where the volume error increases slightly with tumour volume ($p < 0.001$). This indicates that on average, the algorithm over-segments the tumour compared with the raw ground truth (here the manual measurement is *without* the binary closing operation to increase consistency between slices).

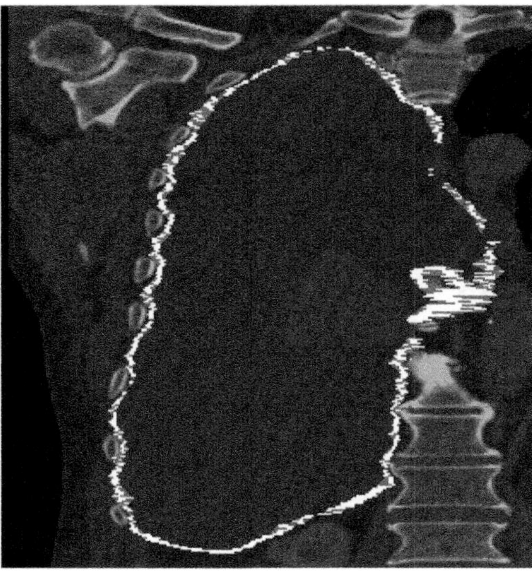

Fig. 3. A CT coronal view of a subject with MPM, showing the right lung. The white annotation indicates the location of tumour, as drawn by an expert annotator in the axial plane, which follows the bounds of the pleural cavity, surrounding a region of pleural effusion. Red shows the regions which are closed by a binary closing operation. Figure from [2]. (Color figure online)

Closed Manual Annotations. Binary closing increased the mean tumour volume of the manual segmentations to 574.4 cm^3 (standard deviation 327.1 cm^3). The Bland-Altman plot in Fig. 5 shows that using closed manual annotations gives a mean difference of $-27.2\,cm^3$, which is not significantly different from zero mean difference ($p = 0.225$). To facilitate comparison to other methods, the results are equivalent to 95% limits of agreement which span 129.2% of the total tumour volume.

Four measurement differences in Fig. 5 are outliers (outside of the 95% limits of agreement): three of these are where the algorithm predicts a higher volume of tumour than recorded by the observer. Inspection of these cases showed extremely narrow tumour in these images. The algorithm often identifies the bulk of the tumour mass (where it is thicker and more visible), but does not propagate the tumour into the rind-like surface which, although narrow, encloses a significant proportion of the lung surface area. This is potentially where the slice-based nature of the approach limits performance. A fully 3D CNN approach may offer higher accuracy in such cases. Inspection of the remaining outlier (under-segmentation by the algorithm) showed tumour which was unusually thick compared with the other images in the training cohort. For this case, it is likely the algorithm failed to generalise to this degree of tumour thickness, unseen during training.

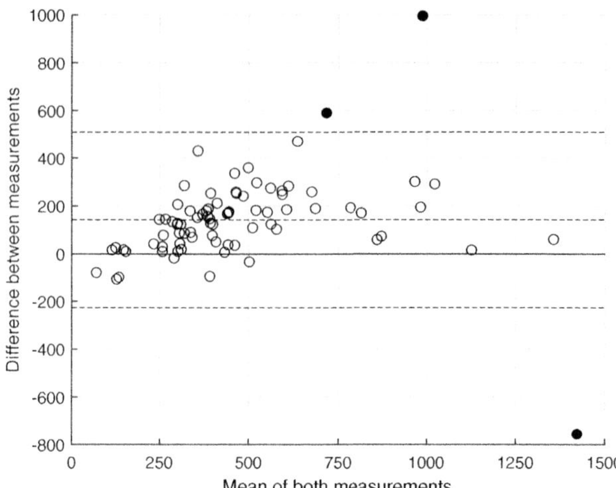

Fig. 4. Bland-Altman plot of the algorithm-annotator agreement for tumour volume measurements, across 80 subjects. The central dashed line indicates a mean difference of 142.2 cm^3 over-segmentation by the algorithm. Outer dashed lines indicate upper and lower 95% limits of agreement of [−224.1, +508.5] cm^3 respectively. Figure from [2].

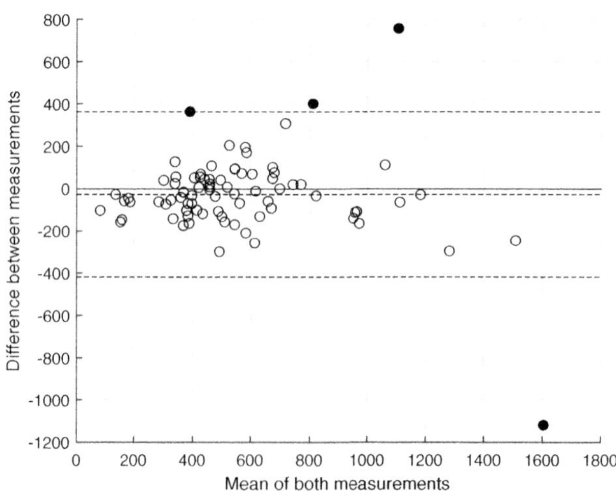

Fig. 5. Bland-Altman plot of the algorithm-annotator agreement for tumour volume measurements across 80 subjects, using cleaned ground truth. The central dashed line indicates a mean difference of −27.2 cm^3 under-segmentation by the algorithm. Outer dashed lines indicate upper and lower 95% limits of agreement of [−414.2, +360.5] cm^3 respectively. Figure from [2].

3.3 Region Overlap (Dice Score)

The mean overall Dice coefficient was 0.64 (standard deviation 0.12) using the binary closed ground truth. In comparison, the Dice score was 0.55 (standard deviation also 0.12) using the raw ground truth, confirming higher voxel-wise correspondence following binary closing to improve inter-slice consistency. Dice coefficients varied between subjects and between analysis folds. Due to the wide range of tumour shapes and volumes in this dataset (c.f. Sect. 2.1), some test sets simply contained more difficult cases. Figure 6 shows the ground truth and predicted tumour for a subject from the PRISM sub-cohort.

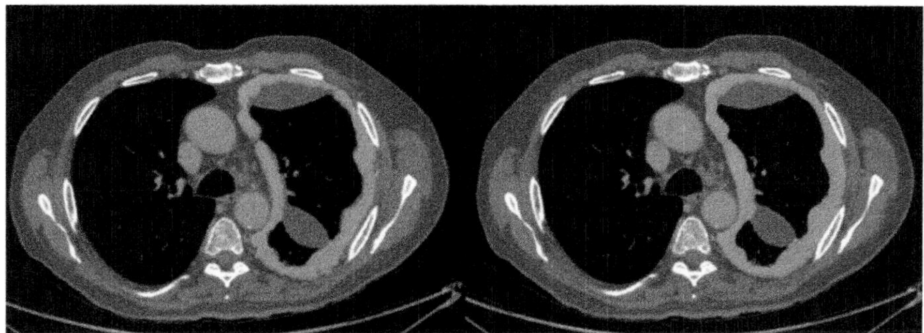

Fig. 6. A CT slice from a subject positive for MPM. Top: Image overlaid with the ground truth segmentation (in red). Bottom: The corresponding predicted segmentation from one of the seven-fold models. Figure from [2]. (Color figure online)

3.4 False Positive Rate Estimation

Using the ensembled algorithm, prediction time increased to around 120 s per image, using an Nvidia 1080Ti graphics processing unit (GPU), 32 GB of RAM and a 12-core Intel Xeon CPU (3.40 GHz).

Comparison to MPM Positive Images. For the NLST dataset, which should contain little or no mesothelioma, in the vast majority of images the automated detector segmented very little. Figure 7 shows the predicted volumes for the NLST hard kernel images, together with the mesothelioma positive volumes from the DIAPHRAM and PRISM studies. The average volume measurement from the hard kernel NLST images is 3.6 cm^3 (standard deviation 6.5 cm^3). In contrast the mean automated volume measurement in the DIAPHRAGM and PRISM datasets was 547.2 cm^3 (standard deviation 290.9 cm^3).

Stratification by NLST Finding. Of the hard kernel images, 11,157 were finding positive and 8,982 were finding negative (see Table 1 for details of the positive and negative groups).

Across the hard kernel image reconstructed images there was a small but significant ($p < 0.001$) difference between the algorithm predictions for finding positive and finding negative images. The mean segmented volume in finding negative images was 2.9 cm^3 (s.d. 3.4 cm^3, median 2.0 cm^3). For the finding positive images this increased to 4.1 cm^3 (s.d. 8.2 cm^3, median 2.2 cm^3). Given that the finding positive subjects may have up to two time-points where no pathology was present, as the pathology finding is per subject rather than per image, an overlap of the groups is to be expected. Figure 8a shows predicted volumes for the NLST datasets, stratified by whether the image was graded as finding negative or finding positive.

Effect of Reconstruction Kernel. Of the soft kernel images, 14,763 were finding positive and 11,711 were finding negative.

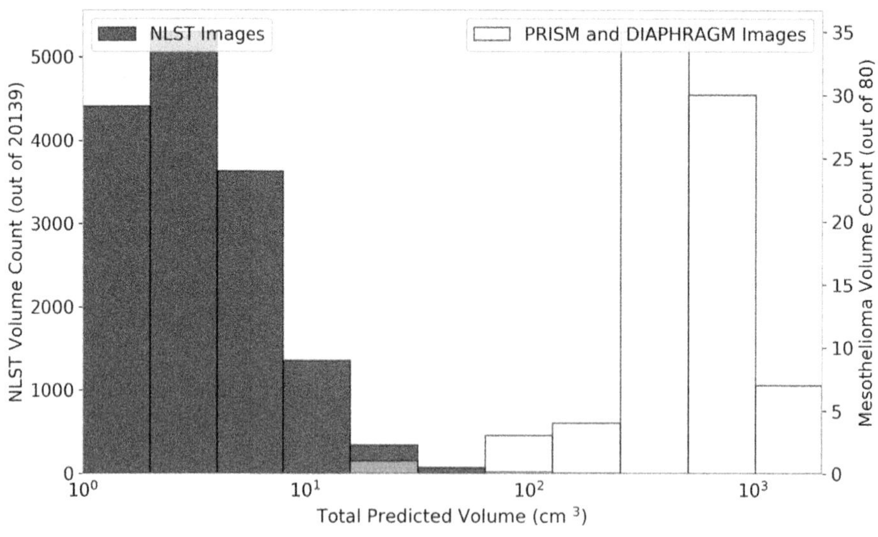

Fig. 7. A histogram of predicted MPM volumes across CT images from the NLST study with reference to the volume results from the multi-fold analysis across images from the PRISM and DIAPHRAM studies. The NLST images are reconstructed using hard kernels. For the volume measurements, a logarithmic scale is used.

For the soft kernel reconstructions the mean detected volume was 10.1 cm^3 (s.d. 13.8 cm^3), an increase compared with the mean volume of 3.6 cm^3 for the hard kernels. Figure 9 shows the distribution of detected volumes for all the images reconstructed with the soft and hard kernels. Figure 10 shows a direct comparison between the hard and soft kernel image segmentations, where the softer kernel results in a thicker segmentation. The figure also provides an example of how the appearance of the images may change between the reconstruction kernel used.

Using the soft kernel images, differentiation by bright pathology finding is less clear. The mean segmented volume in finding negative images was 9.0 cm^3 (s.d. 8.8 cm^3, median 6.5 cm^3). For the finding positive images this increased to 11.0 cm^3 (s.d. 16.7 cm^3, median 7.1 cm^3). Although remaining statistically significant ($p < 0.001$), this difference is less apparent than for hard kernel images (Fig. 8b).

In general across the images, a softer kernel results in a thicker segmentation. Due to the nature of the segmented regions, any volume measurements are extremely sensitive to this thickness change. In some cases (and as shown in Fig. 9), a difference in volume arises because new regions were segmented—sometimes regions which are segmented in hard kernel images extend further in the equivalent soft kernel images. This may be due to an increased ambiguity—areas which the algorithm could differentiate in hard kernel images may be less distinguishable in soft kernel images. This may also arise because of a minimum tumour thickness which the algorithm can segment (this is discussed further in Sect. 4.1).

Observation of Outliers. Using both hard and soft kernel reconstructed images, 94/100 upper outliers were for subjects reported to have a bright pathology finding. Many images show evidence of pleural thickening and considerable pleural effusion. Examples of 9/100 outliers are provided in Fig. 11. The training data only contains unilateral examples of MPM, however it is likely the algorithm has not fit to this aspect of the data. Several of the upper outliers in Fig. 11 show subjects with pathologies in both lungs which have been identified by the algorithm. By design, the algorithm had sufficient receptive field to encompass the entire image, and had the capability to use information in one lung to guide any tumour delineation in the other, however the unilateral nature of the disease in the training data appears not to have been learned. It is likely the algorithm would generalise to measurement of bilateral examples of MPM, although such cases are exceptionally rare. The remaining 6/100 images with no reported bright pathology finding associated were abnormal. For one, the automated method segmented volume in the liver. Generally, the algorithm segmented more around the diaphragm, and this region was where false positives were most frequent. This is a region where axial slices are particularly difficult to interpret, and where more extensive 3-D information could help disambiguate the images.

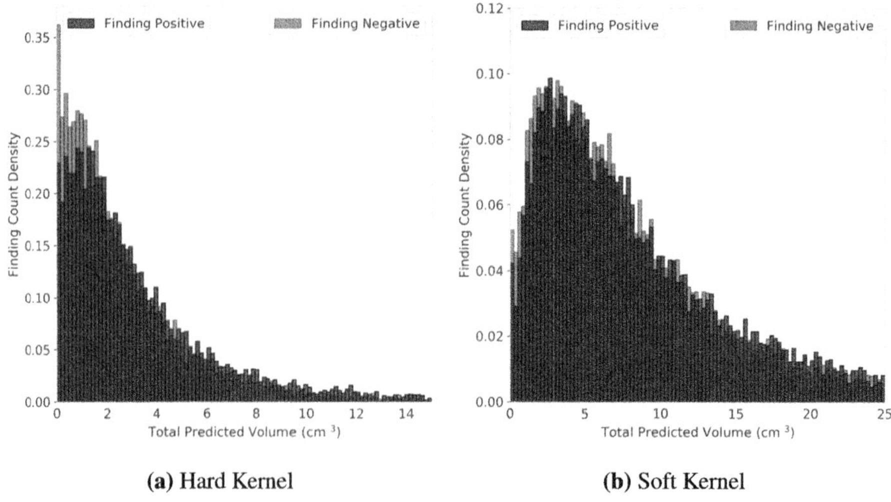

(a) Hard Kernel **(b)** Soft Kernel

Fig. 8. Comparison of predicted MPM volumes reconstructed by hard 8a and soft 8b kernels. Subjects are stratified into finding positive and finding negative. Note that different axis limits are used for the hard and soft kernel subplots.

4 Discussion

Although there is no curative treatment for MPM, tumour volume measurements would support clinicians to find the most effective care for each patient, and could enable more powerful clinical trials. Manual measurements of volume are too time-consuming to be routine, and still suffer from uncertainty. Some of this uncertainty arises from ambiguous features in the images—many structures appear very similar to MPM tumour in CT images. Manual measurements require significant clinical expertise to disambiguate the images, the expert uses an understanding of anatomy and experience of how the tumour develops. The distillation of such complex domain knowledge makes the application of traditional image analysis techniques complex. Such tasks, however, are where deep learning is readily applied.

Distilling expertise does not overcome the inherent uncertainty in annotating a tumour of this shape, with an unusually high surface-to-volume ratio. The large proportion of edge voxels means that any volume measurement is highly sensitive to the edge dilatation of the tumour segmentations - changing the boundary by half a voxel can change volume measurements by up to 60% (based on the analysis of tumour shapes from the DIAPHRAGM study). This poses many technical challenges—for the automated method, we have shown that in the regime of narrow segmented regions in MPM negative subjects, the choice of reconstruction kernel consistently impacts measurements.

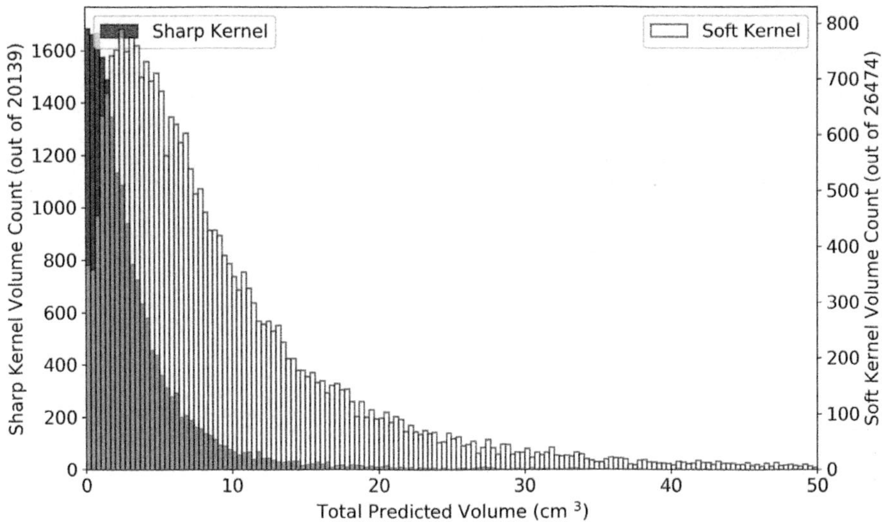

Fig. 9. A histogram of MPM volume predictions across the NLST dataset, stratified by hard or soft image reconstruction kernel.

4.1 Critical Analysis

Generally, the literature shows significant variability in MPM tumour measurements. Sensakovic *et al.* [23] found an inter-observer mean Dice coefficient of 0.68 across slices from 31 subjects. Gudmundsson *et al.* [14] achieve a mean Dice coefficient of 0.690 on slices which are selected to contain pleural effusion. This mean Dice coefficient increases to 0.780 on a second test set, containing different disease characteristics. Over full volume images from 15 subjects, Chen *et al.* [9] achieve a Dice score of 0.825. Our mean volumetric Dice coefficient of 0.64 is lower than that achieved by Chen *et al.* Some of the difference may arise from the semi-automated nature of their approach, however on some images we achieve similarly high Dice coefficients. Across our cohort, higher Dice scores were achieved for images where the tumour was thicker—these are images which are inherently easier to annotate, both manually and automatically, and a higher Dice coefficient is more easily achieved. Although these comparisons provide interesting context, we can only draw limited conclusions without a like-for-like comparison between methods on the same cohort.

Further large scale analysis across data from an independent study indicates that the algorithm is robust to the majority of negative cases. This is a one-sided analysis, and does not provide a measure of sensitivity, however analysis of outliers shows the algorithm is providing plausible output. Where the predicted volumes are highest, the algorithm confounds other bright pathologies with MPM tumour—most of the outliers are unhealthy, and many have images similar in appearance to those from MPM positive subjects. We would not expect

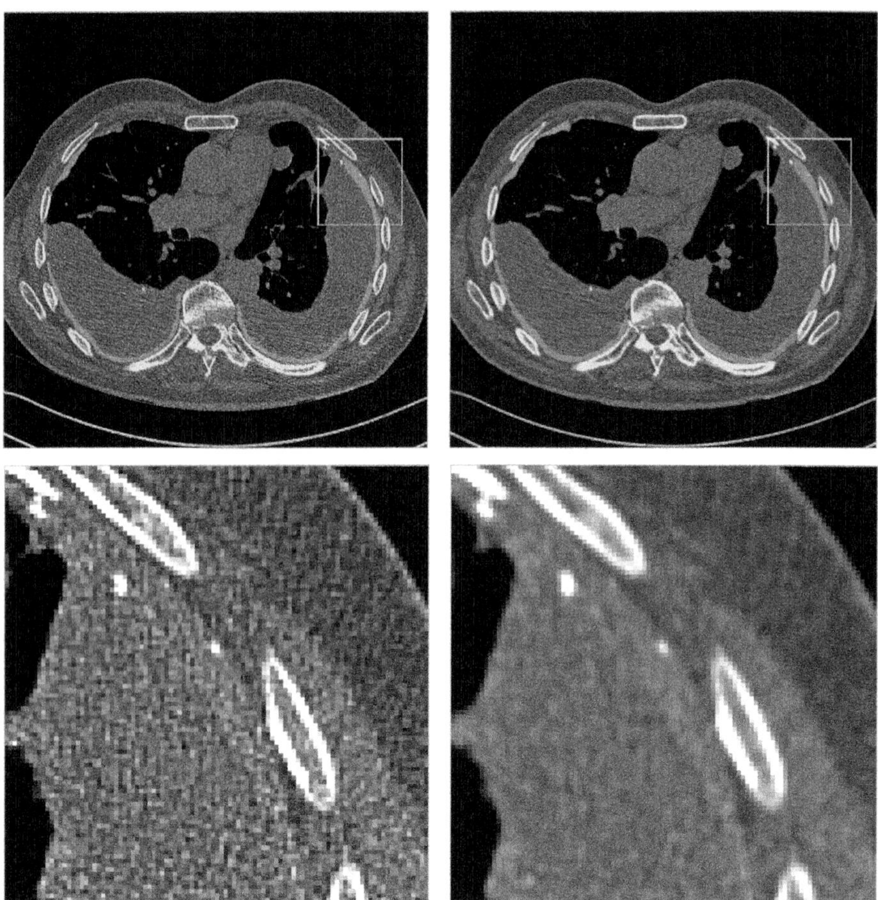

Fig. 10. Top row: a comparison of corresponding hard-kernel (left) and soft-kernel (right) reconstructed images from the NLST study, with an overlay the segmentation produced by one of the 7-fold models. Bottom row: A cropped region corresponding to the green box in the top row, showing the smoother appearance of the soft kernel reconstructed images. (Color figure online)

the algorithm to be capable of distinctions between many pathologies and MPM tumour based on the images alone.

The analysis suggests that the choice of CT reconstruction kernel is significant where there is little or no MPM present. Smoother images may increase the ambiguity in delineation at the edges of the tumour, and given the algorithm has only been trained on positive cases, it is likely to be biased towards inclusion of these ambiguous regions. As mentioned in Sect. 3.4, for some cases using a softer image reconstruction results in additional segmented areas, which could be due to an increased image ambiguity in these regions, or because a larger spatial extent is more likely to be detected by the algorithm. By its design, the

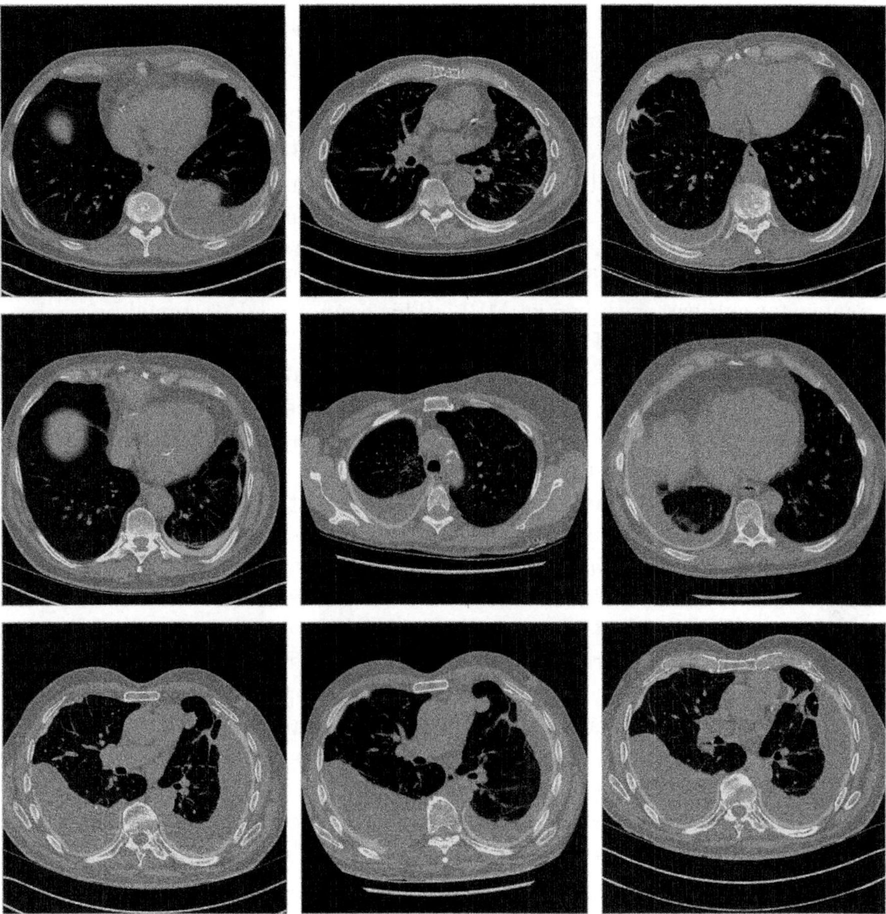

Fig. 11. A selection of images from the NLST study for which the algorithm predicted a relatively high volume of MPM tumour. The images are overlaid with segmentations by a random selection of the 7-fold models.

CNN outputs smooth and continuous probability maps. After thresholding, it is unlikely that segmented regions will be narrower than a few voxels. Generally, for measurements of MPM tumour this is not a problem, however for the NLST cohort images that show pleural thickening, it is possible that a thickened pleura is thinner than the algorithm can segment. In CT images, a healthy pleura is invisible, and a thickness of even one or two voxels may be significant. Expanding a region of bright pleural thickening (or other pathological regions) in the images by using a softer kernel may slightly increase the thickness of these regions, allowing them to be detected by the algorithm. We note that inspection of several outliers in the cross-validation on MPM positive subjects did show undetected, thin tumour regions (Sect. 3.2). It is possible that for these outliers, the choice of reconstruction kernel would also impact any automated measurements. To overcome this, an algorithm which segments the images at an increased resolution may be more appropriate.

Of the images from the PRISM and DIAPRAGM studies, 107/123 were reconstructed using soft kernels. This leaves 16/123 hard kernel images, and meaningful statistics could not be derived to measure how the manual annotations were impacted by reconstruction kernel. It may be that the algorithm is biased by reconstruction kernel imbalance in the training data—it is possible that segmenting greater volumes would be measured as higher segmentation performance for subjects with known MPM. This cannot be determined by analysis of cases with no known MPM.

For the task of MPM segmentation on histologically confirmed cases, where the disease characteristics can vary dramatically between subjects, as well as between time-points and observers, performance of an algorithm depends heavily on the training and testing cohort. An increased variance between subjects means that a large and diverse test set is required to truly establish whether any automated method can generalise to unseen cases. A potential limitation of this work is that we have demonstrated the performance of the algorithm on 80 subjects which have not undergone treatment for the disease, all from imaging centres based in Glasgow, all annotated by a single observer. Images from a further 14,965 subjects from 33 different centres have provided an insight into some aspects of algorithm performance on independent images. However, to truly understand performance, more images containing MPM tumour (with ground truth segmentations) are required. We have used an unusually large cohort with full volume annotation of MPM tumour, however a large, independent and varied test set by multiple observers is still necessary to truly determine the performance of this algorithm.

4.2 Future Work

Multi-fold analysis can only tell us so much about algorithm performance, given the data on which the analysis is based is not completely independent from what was used to develop the algorithm. An independent test set from a multiple institutions will provide a more unbiased indication of performance. Some aspects of performance on independent images have been measured using images from the NLST study, but other aspects of performance cannot be tested on images which contain no tumour. The algorithm is currently being evaluated on the remaining unseen evaluation datasets, which are histologically confirmed as MPM positive, acquired from multiple institutions (only 123/403 datasets were used in the internal validation). This will provide a more detailed, realistic and unbiased assessment of algorithm performance.

5 Conclusion

An internal validation to explore the utility of a deep leaning algorithm for volumetric segmentation of MPM in CT images has been performed. It was found that inter-slice consistency of manual annotations was improved by binary closing. There was no significant mean difference between the manual and automatic measurements following binary closing of the manual annotations. Images from an independent study with no known MPM were used as a further test set, and the majority of the volumes predicted to contain the highest volume of tumour by the algorithm are from subjects which were positive for other bright pathologies. To our knowledge, this is the first volumetric evaluation of a fully automated system to segment pleural volume. Future work will involve testing the method on the remaining evaluation set. The algorithm has potential application to routine care (for tumour assessment, to guide patient therapy), and the assessment of tumour development in clinical trials.

Acknowledgments. The authors thank the National Cancer Institute for access to NCI's data collected by the National Lung Screening Trial (NLST). The statements contained herein are solely those of the authors and do not represent or imply concurrence or endorsement by NCI.

References

1. Abdel-Rahman, O.: Global trends in mortality from malignant mesothelioma: analysis of WHO mortality database (1994–2013). Clin. Respir. J. (2018). https://doi.org/10.1111/crj.12778
2. Anderson, O., et al.: Fully automated volumetric measurement of malignant pleural mesothelioma from computed tomography images by deep learning: preliminary results of an internal validation. In: BIOIMAGING 2020–7th International Conference on Bioimaging, Proceedings; Part of 13th International Joint Conference on Biomedical Engineering Systems and Technologies, BIOSTEC 2020 (2020). https://doi.org/10.5220/0008976100640073
3. Armato, S.G., Nowak, A.K., Francis, R.J., Kocherginsky, M., Byrne, M.J.: Observer variability in mesothelioma tumor thickness measurements: defining minimally measurable lesions. J. Thoracic Oncol. (2014). https://doi.org/10.1097/JTO.0000000000000211
4. Attanoos, R.L., Gibbs, A.R.: Pathology of malignant mesothelioma. Histopathology **30**(5), 403–418 (1997). https://doi.org/10.1046/j.1365-2559.1997.5460776.x. https://onlinelibrary.wiley.com/doi/abs/10.1046/j.1365-2559.1997.5460776.x
5. Bianchi, C., Giarelli, L., Grandi, G., Brollo, A., Ramani, L., Zuch, C.: Latency periods in asbestos-related mesothelioma of the pleura. Eur. J. Cancer Prev. **6**, 162–166 (1997)
6. Blyth, K., et al.: An update regarding the Prediction of ResIstance to chemotherapy using Somatic copy number variation in Mesothelioma (PRISM) study. Lung Cancer (2018). https://doi.org/10.1016/s0169-5002(18)30090-4
7. Brahim, W., Mestiri, M., Betrouni, N., Hamrouni, K.: Malignant pleural mesothelioma segmentation for photodynamic therapy planning. Comput. Med. Imaging Graph. (2018). https://doi.org/10.1016/j.compmedimag.2017.05.006
8. Byrne, M.J., Nowak, A.K.: Modified RECIST criteria for assessment of response in malignant pleural mesothelioma. Ann. Oncol. (2004). https://doi.org/10.1093/annonc/mdh059

9. Chen, M., Helm, E., Joshi, N., Gleeson, F., Brady, M.: Computer-aided volumetric assessment of malignant pleural mesothelioma on CT using a random walk-based method. Int. J. Comput. Assist. Radiol. Surg. **12**(4), 529–538 (2016). https://doi.org/10.1007/s11548-016-1511-3
10. Chollet, F.: Keras (2015). https://keras.io/
11. Eisenhauer, E.A., et al.: New response evaluation criteria in solid tumours: revised RECIST guideline (version 1.1). Eur. J. Cancer (2009). https://doi.org/10.1016/j.ejca.2008.10.026
12. Gudmundsson, E., Straus, C., Li, F., Kindler, H., Armato, S.: P1.06-04 deep learning-based segmentation of mesothelioma on CT scans: application to patient scans exhibiting pleural effusion. J. Thoracic Oncol. (2019). https://doi.org/10.1016/j.jtho.2019.08.991
13. Gudmundsson, E., Straus, C.M., Armato, S.G.: Deep convolutional neural networks for the automated segmentation of malignant pleural mesothelioma on computed tomography scans. J. Med. Imaging (2018). https://doi.org/10.1117/1.jmi.5.3.034503
14. Gudmundsson, E., Straus, C.M., Li, F., Armato, S.G.: Deep learning-based segmentation of malignant pleural mesothelioma tumor on computed tomography scans: application to scans demonstrating pleural effusion. J. Med. Imaging (2020). https://doi.org/10.1117/1.jmi.7.1.012705
15. Ioffe, S., Szegedy, C.: Batch normalization: accelerating deep network training by reducing internal covariate shift. In: Proceedings of the International Conference on Machine Learning (ICML). Proceedings of Machine Learning Research, vol. 37, pp. 448–456 (2015). http://proceedings.mlr.press/v37/ioffe15.html
16. Deng, J., Dong, W., Socher, R., Li, L.-J., Li, K., Fei-Fei, L.: ImageNet: a large-scale hierarchical image database. In: 2009 IEEE Conference on Computer Vision and Pattern Recognition (2009). https://doi.org/10.1109/CVPRW.2009.5206848
17. Labby, Z.E., et al.: Variability of tumor area measurements for response assessment in malignant pleural mesothelioma. Med. Phys. (2013). https://doi.org/10.1118/1.4810940
18. Martin Bland, J., Altman, D.G.: Statistical methods for assessing agreement between two methods of clinical measurement. The Lancet (1986). https://doi.org/10.1016/S0140-6736(86)90837-8
19. National Lung Screening Trial Research Team: The national lung screening trial: overview and study design. Radiology (2011). https://doi.org/10.1148/radiol.10091808
20. Ng, C.S., Munden, R.F., Libshitz, H.I.: Malignant pleural mesothelioma: the spectrum of manifestations on CT in 70 cases. Clin. Radiol. (1999). https://doi.org/10.1016/S0009-9260(99)90824-3
21. Ronneberger, O., Fischer, P., Brox, T.: U-Net: convolutional networks for biomedical image segmentation. In: Medical Image Computing and Computer-Assisted Intervention (2015). https://doi.org/10.1007/978-3-319-24574-4_28. http://arxiv.org/abs/1505.04597
22. Schwartz, L.H., et al.: RECIST 1.1 - Update and clarification: from the RECIST committee. Eur. J. Cancer (2016). https://doi.org/10.1016/j.ejca.2016.03.081
23. Sensakovic, W.F., et al.: Computerized segmentation and measurement of malignant pleural mesothelioma. Med. Phys. (2011). https://doi.org/10.1118/1.3525836
24. Smith, L.N.: Cyclical learning rates for training neural networks. In: IEEE Winter Conference on Applications of Computer Vision (2017). https://doi.org/10.1109/WACV.2017.58

25. Srivastava, N., Hinton, G., Krizhevsky, A., Sutskever, I., Salakhutdinov, R.: Dropout: a simple way to prevent neural networks from overfitting. J. Mach. Learn. Res. **15**, 1929–1958 (2014). https://doi.org/10.1214/12-AOS1000
26. Tsim, S., et al.: Diagnostic and Prognostic Biomarkers in the Rational Assessment of Mesothelioma (DIAPHRAGM) study: Protocol of a prospective, multicentre, observational study. BMJ Open (2016). https://doi.org/10.1136/bmjopen-2016-013324
27. Yoon, S.H., Kim, K.W., Goo, J.M., Kim, D.W., Hahn, S.: Observer variability in RECIST-based tumour burden measurements: a meta-analysis. Eur. J. Cancer **53**, 5–15 (2016). https://doi.org/10.1016/j.ejca.2015.10.014

Combining Registration Errors and Supervoxel Classification for Unsupervised Brain Anomaly Detection

Samuel Botter Martins[1,2,3](✉), Alexandre Xavier Falcão[1], and Alexandru Cristian Telea[4]

[1] Laboratory of Image Data Science (LIDS), University of Campinas, Campinas, Brazil
{sbmmartins,afalcao}@ic.unicamp.br

[2] Bernoulli Institute, University of Groningen, Groningen, The Netherlands

[3] Federal Institute of São Paulo, Campinas, Brazil

[4] Department of Information and Computing Sciences, Utrecht University, Utrecht, The Netherlands
a.c.telea@uu.nl

Abstract. Automatic detection of brain anomalies in MR images is challenging and complex due to intensity similarity between lesions and healthy tissues as well as the large variability in shape, size, and location among different anomalies. Even though discriminative models (supervised learning) are commonly used for this task, they require quite high-quality annotated training images, which are absent for most medical image analysis problems. Inspired by groupwise shape analysis, we adapt a recent fully *unsupervised* supervoxel-based approach (SAAD)—designed for abnormal asymmetry detection of the hemispheres—to detect brain anomalies from registration errors. Our method, called BADRESC, extracts supervoxels inside the right and left hemispheres, cerebellum, and brainstem, models registration errors for each supervoxel, and treats outliers as anomalies. Experimental results on MR-T1 brain images of stroke patients show that BADRESC outperforms a convolutional-autoencoder-based method and attains similar detection rates for hemispheric lesions in comparison to SAAD with substantially fewer false positives. It also presents promising detection scores for lesions in the cerebellum and brainstem.

Keywords: Brain anomaly detection · Supervoxel segmentation · One-class classification · Registration errors · MRI

The authors thank CNPq (303808/2018-7), FAPESP (2014/12236-1) for the financial support, and NVIDIA for supporting a graphics card.

X. Ye et al. (Eds.): BIOSTEC 2020, CCIS 1400, pp. 140–164, 2021.
https://doi.org/10.1007/978-3-030-72379-8_8

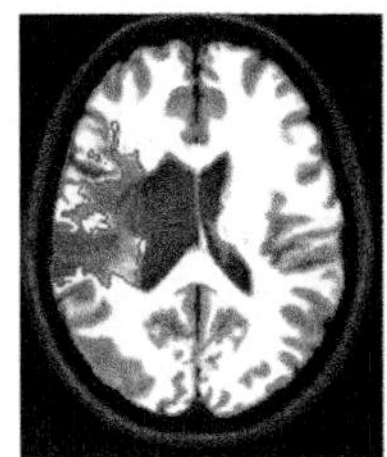
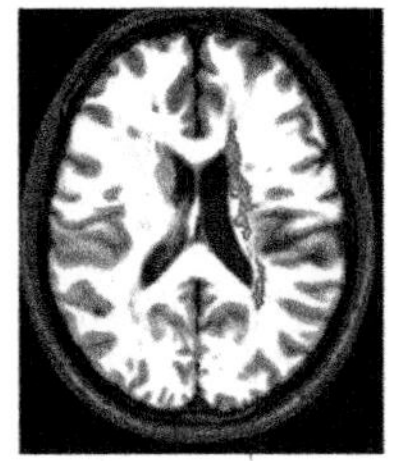
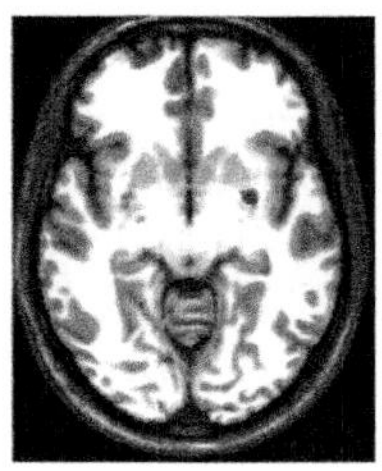

Fig. 1. Axial slices of three stroke patients from the ATLAS dataset [19] with lesions (ground-truth borders in red) that significantly differ in location, shape, and size. Figure referenced from [23]. (Color figure online)

1 Introduction

Quantitative analysis of MR brain images has been used extensively for the characterization of brain disorders, such as stroke, tumors, and multiple sclerosis. Such methods rely on delineating objects of interest—(sub)cortical structures or lesions to solve detection and segmentation simultaneously. Results are usually used for tasks such as quantitative lesion assessment (*e.g.,* volume), surgical planning, and overall anatomic understanding [7,17,35]. Note that *segmentation* corresponds to the exact delineation of the object of interest, whereas *detection* consists of finding the rough location of such objects (*e.g.,* by a bounding box around the object), in case they are present in the image.

The simplest strategy to detect brain anomalies consists of a visual slice-by-slice inspection by one or multiple specialists. This process is very laborious, time-consuming, easily prone to errors, and even impracticable when a large amount of data needs to be processed. Continuous efforts have been made for automatic anomaly detection that delineates anomalies with accuracy close to that of human experts. However, this goal is challenging and complex due to the large variability in shape, size, and location among different anomalies, even when the same disease causes these (see, *e.g.,* Fig. 1). These difficulties have motivated the research and development of automatic brain anomaly detection methods based on *machine learning* algorithms.

Most automatic methods in the literature rely on supervised machine learning to detect or segment brain anomalies. They train a classifier from training images—which must be previously labeled (*e.g.,* lesion segmentation masks) by experts—to delineate anomalies by classifying voxels or regions of the target image. Traditional image features (*e.g.,* edge detectors and texture features) and deep feature representations (*e.g.,* convolutional features) are commonly used [3,13,30,34,35]. Some works propose a groupwise shape analysis based on estimating the deformation field between a target image and a template (reference image) after image registration [13,34].

However, these methods commonly have three main limitations. First, they require a large number of high-quality annotated training images, which is absent for most medical image analysis problems [1,15,40]. Second, they are only designed for the lesions found in the training set. Third, some methods still require weight fine-tuning (retraining) when used for a new set of images due to image variability across scanners and acquisition protocols, limiting its application into clinical routine.

All the above limitations of supervised methods motivate research on *unsupervised* anomaly detection approaches [4,8,14,23–25,33]. From a training set with images of *healthy* subjects *only*, these methods encode general knowledge or assumptions (*priors*) from healthy tissues, so that an outlier who breaks such general priors is considered anomaly [14]. As unsupervised brain anomaly detection methods do not use labeled samples, they are less effective in detecting lesions from a specific disease than supervised approaches trained from labeled samples for the same disease. For the same reason, however, unsupervised methods are generic in detecting any lesions, *e.g.*, coming from multiple diseases, as long as these notably differ from healthy training samples.

Since many neurological diseases are associated with abnormal brain asymmetries [43], an *unsupervised* method called Supervoxel-based Abnormal Asymmetry Detection (SAAD) [24] was recently proposed to detect abnormal asymmetries in MR brain images. SAAD presents a mechanism for asymmetry detection that consists of three steps: (i) it registers all images to the same symmetric template and then computes asymmetries between the two hemispheres by using their mid-sagittal plane (MSP) as reference; (ii) a supervoxel segmentation method, named SymmISF, is used to extract pairs of symmetric supervoxels from the left and right hemispheres for each test image, guided by their asymmetries. Supervoxels define more significant volumes of interest for analysis than regular 3D patches; and (iii) each pair generates a local one-class classifier trained on control images to find supervoxels with abnormal asymmetries on the test image. SAAD was further extended to detect abnormal asymmetries in the own native image space of each test image [25].

Although SAAD claims to obtain higher detection accuracy even for small lesions compared to state-of-the-art detection methods, its analysis is limited to asymmetric anomalies in the brain hemispheres, ignoring lesions in the cerebellum and brainstem. Moreover, if the same lesion is localized in both hemispheres roughly in the same position (*e.g.*, some cases of multiple sclerosis), it is not detected due to the lack of asymmetries.

Inspired by groupwise shape analysis, in this work, we present BADRESC, an *unsupervised* method for Brain Anomaly Detection based on Registration Errors and Supervoxel Classification in 3T MR-T1 images of the brain. After registering a target image to a standard template with *only* healthy tissues by deformable registration, BADRESC assumes that registration errors for anomalies are considerably different from the registration errors for healthy tissues. Thus, BADRESC adapts the SAAD framework as follows. First, it replaces the asymmetry maps with registration errors. A robust preprocessing is considered to improve the quality of image registration. Second, it then analyses four macro-objects of interest—right and left hemispheres, cerebellum, and brainstem—by extracting supervoxels for each one *separately*. Finally, each supervoxel generates a local one-class classifier for healthy tissues to detect *outliers* as anomalies.

This work is an extension of a previous one presented in [23], which originally introduced BADRESC. While considering the same macro-objects of interest and datasets, our contributions include:

- a more detailed explanation of BADRESC's steps, especially supervoxel segmentation (Sect. 2 and Appendix A);
- an extended evaluation that considers another unsupervised baseline (like ours), which consists of a convolutional-autoencoder-based approach; and
- more evaluation metrics: Dice, mean recall, and three other false-positive metrics.

Experimental results on 3D MR-T1 brain images of stroke patients confirm the accuracy of BADRESC to detect hemispheric lesions with only a few false positives. Additionally, BADRESC presents promising results for the detection of lesions in the cerebellum and brainstem.

This paper is organized as follows. Section 2 introduces preliminary concepts on supervoxel segmentation and the considered framework used by BADRESC. Section 3 presents BADRESC. Section 4 presents experiments, while Sect. 5 reports and discusses results. Section 6 concludes the paper and discusses some possible future directions.

2 Iterative Spanning Forest (ISF)

One crucial step of our proposed method consists of extracting supervoxels inside each macro-object of interest for subsequent analysis. *Supervoxels* are groups of voxels with similar characteristics resulting from an oversegmentation of a 3D image or region of interest. We call *superpixels* for 2D images. They preserve intrinsic image information (*e.g.*, the borders of tissues and lesions) and are used as an alternative to patches to define more meaningful VOIs for computer-vision problems [37,45] and some medical image applications [35,44]. Supervoxels are a better alternative than 3D regular patches for our target problem, as (i) they better fit lesions and tissues, and (ii) their voxels contain minimum heterogeneous information.

In this work, we rely on the Iterative Spanning Forest (ISF) framework [42] for supervoxel segmentation. ISF is a recent approach for both superpixel and supervoxel segmentation that has shown higher effectiveness than several state-of-the-art counterparts, especially when used for 3D MR image segmentation of the brain [42]. ISF consists of three key steps: (i) seed sampling followed by multiple iterations of (ii) connected supervoxel delineation based on the image foresting transform (IFT) algorithm [11] (Appendix A), and (iii) seed recomputation to improve delineation. We next present the theoretical background for ISF as well as its algorithm.

2.1 Theoretical Background

Let the pair $\hat{I} = (D_I, \vec{I})$ be a d-dimensional multi-band image, where $D_I \subset Z^d$ is the *image domain*, and $\vec{I} : D_I \rightarrow \mathbb{R}^c$ is a mapping function that assigns a vector of c real-valued intensities $\vec{I}(p)$—one value for each band (channel) of the image—to each element $p \in D_I$. For simplicity, assume that the term *voxels* represents the d-dimensional-image elements.

An image can be interpreted as a graph $G_I = (D_I, \mathcal{A})$, whose *nodes* are the voxels, and the *arcs* are defined by an *adjacency relation* $\mathcal{A} \subset D_I \times D_I$, with $\mathcal{A}(p)$ being the *adjacent set* of a voxel p. In this work, we consider the 6-neighborhood adjacency for ISF. We refer to Appendix A for more details about image graphs, paths, and connectivity functions.

For a given *initial seed set* $\mathcal{S}$, labeled with consecutive integer numbers $\{1, 2, \cdots, |\mathcal{S}|\}$, and a *connectivity function* f, ISF computes each supervoxel as a *spanning tree* rooted at a *single* seed, such that seeds compete among themselves by offering lower-cost paths to conquer their most strongly connected voxels. We use the following connectivity function f given by

$$
\begin{aligned}
f(\langle q \rangle) &= \begin{cases} 0, & \text{if } q \in \mathcal{S}, \\ +\infty, & \text{otherwise}, \end{cases} \\
f(\pi_p \cdot \langle p, q \rangle) &= f(\pi_p) + \left[\alpha \cdot \|\vec{I}(q) - \vec{I}(R(p))\|\right]^\beta + \|q - p\|,
\end{aligned} \tag{1}
$$

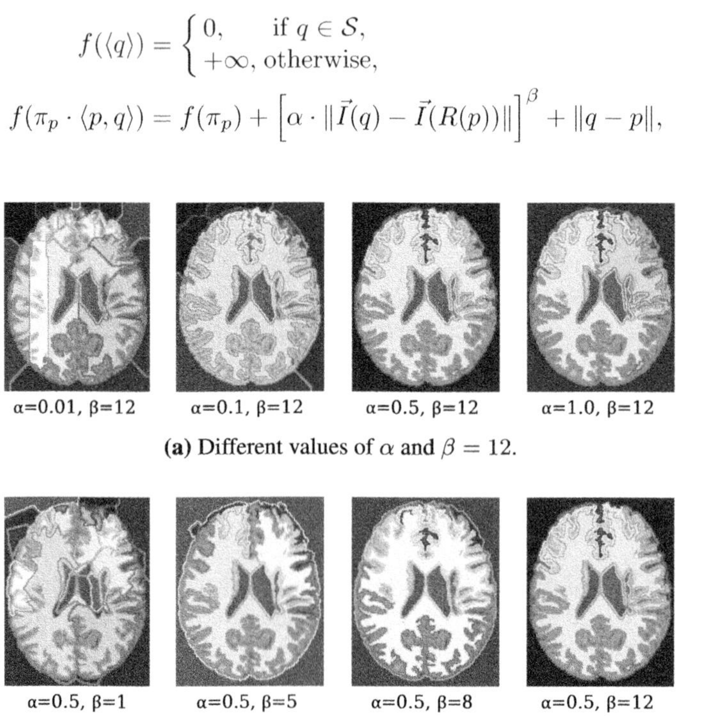

Fig. 2. The impact of the factors α and β for superpixel segmentation by ISF. Each superpixel is represented by a different color. For all cases, we performed ISF on the same 2D brain image with 10 iterations and identical 30 initial seeds selected by grid sampling. (Color figure online)

where $\|\vec{I}(t) - \vec{I}(R(p))\|$ is the Euclidean distance between the intensity vectors at voxels $R(p)$ and q, $\|q - p\|$ the Euclidean distance between the voxels p and q, $\langle q \rangle$ is a trivial path, $\pi_p \cdot \langle p, q \rangle$ the extension of a path π_p with terminus q by an arc $\langle p, q \rangle$, and $R(p)$ the starting node (seed) of π_p. The factors α and β serve to control a compromise between supervoxel boundary adherence and shape regularity. Although the authors of ISF have fixed $\alpha = 0.5$ and $\beta = 12$ during the experiments [42], such factors are problem-dependent and should be optimized to yield more accurate supervoxels. Figure 2 shows the impact of α and β for the superpixel segmentation of a 2D brain image.

2.2 The ISF Algorithm

Algorithm 1 presents a pseudo code for the Iterative Spanning Forest framework. At each iteration (Lines 2–4), ISF performs connected supervoxel delineation on the image I based on IFT (Line 3)—as described by Algorithm 2 (Appendix A)—from a given seed set $\mathcal{S}'$, adjacency relation $\mathcal{A}$, and the connectivity function f described by Eq. 1. The seed set at Iteration 1 is the initial seed set $\mathcal{S}$ (Line 1). Next, the seed set is recomputed by the function *SeedRecomputation* to improve delineation (Line 4). This process continues until reaching N iterations. The algorithm returns the optimum-path forest (predecessor map), root map, path-cost map, and the supervoxel label map. Figure 3 illustrates the execution of ISF.

Algorithm 1. Iterative Spanning Forest.

Input: Image $\hat{I} = (D_I, \vec{I})$, adjacency relation $\mathcal{A}$, connectivity function f, initial seed set $\mathcal{S} \subset D_I$, and the maximum number of iterations $N \geq 1$.
Output: Optimum-path forest P, root map R, path-cost map C, and supervoxel label map L.
Aux: Seed set $\mathcal{S}'$, and the variable i.

```
1 S' ← S
2 for i ← 0 to N − 1 do
3 |  (P, R, C, L) ← IFT(Î, A, f, S') /* see Alg. 2 */
4 |_ S' ← SeedRecomputation(Î, S', P, R, C)
5 return (P, R, C, L)
```

In this work, we adopted a seed-recomputation strategy proposed by Vargas-Muñoz *et al.* [42], as detailed next. At each iteration, we promote the *centroids* from the obtained supervoxels—*i.e.*, their geometric centers—to be the seeds of the next iteration. If a given centroid c_i is out of its supervoxel L_i—due to the non-convex shape of L_i—we select the voxel of L_i that is the closest to c_i. We refer to Vargas-Muñoz *et al.* [42] for more specific details.

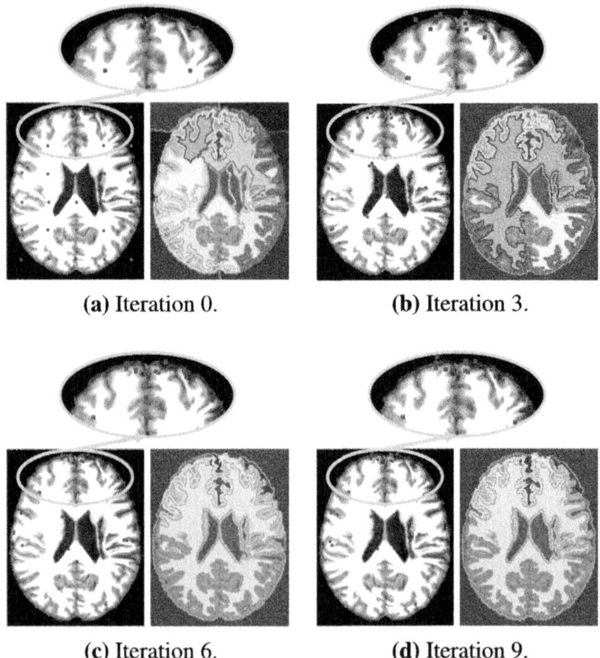

Fig. 3. Example of the ISF execution (10 iterations with $\alpha = 0.5$ and $\beta = 12$) on a 2D brain image. **(a)–(b)** Four iterations of ISF. For each iteration, we show its input seeds (red points) and the resulting obtained superpixels (each color represents a different superpixel). Iteration 0 shows the initial seed set obtained by grid sampling; the other seed sets are obtained by seed recomputation. As the insets show, most seeds do not change positions over iterations. (Color figure online)

A crucial step for the success of ISF consists of performing a robust *initial seed estimation*. This step, however, is problem-dependent, so that simple and general strategies—*e.g.*, a grid sampling in the input image—can provide unsatisfactory results (*e.g.*, undersegmentating a lesion). Section 3.3 details our strategy to select the initial seed for our problem.

3 Description of BADRESC

Figure 4 presents the pipeline of BADRESC which consists of five steps: 3D image preprocessing, image registration, registration error computation, supervoxel segmentation, and classification. We next describe all these steps to detect anomalies in the brain hemispheres, cerebellum, and brainstem.

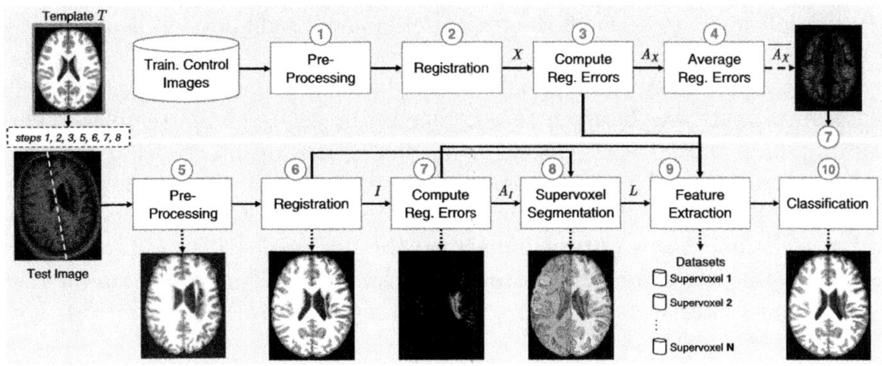

Fig. 4. Pipeline of BADRESC [23]. The upper blue part is computed offline. The bottom orange part is computed for each test image. The template (reference image) is used in both parts (Steps 1, 2, 3, 5, 6, 7, and 8). (Color figure online)

3.1 3D Image Preprocessing and Registration

MR images are affected by image acquisition issues such as noise and intensity heterogeneity. This makes their automated analysis very challenging since intensities of the same tissues vary across the image. To alleviate these and make images more similar to each other, we use typical preprocessing steps known in the literature [16,21,24], as shown in Fig. 5.

For each 3D image (Fig. 5a), we start performing noise reduction by median filtering, followed by MSP alignment, and bias field correction by N4 [41]. As voxels from irrelevant tissues/organs for the addressed problem (*e.g.*, neck and bones) can negatively impact the image registration and intensity normalization,

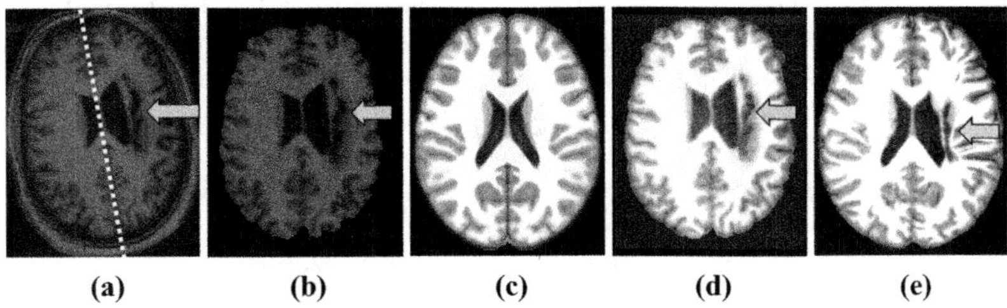

Fig. 5. 3D image preprocessing and registration steps. **(a)** Axial slice of a raw test 3D image. The dashed line shows its mid-sagittal plane (MSP) and the arrow indicates a stroke lesion. **(b)** Test image after noise filtering, MSP alignment, bias field correction, and brain segmentation. **(c)** Axial slice of the symmetric brain template (reference image). **(d)** Histogram matching between (b) and the template (intensity normalization). **(e)** Final preprocessed image after non-rigid registration and histogram matching with the template.

we use AdaPro [22] to segment the regions of interest: right and left hemispheres, cerebellum, and brainstem (Fig. 5b).

To attenuate differences in brightness and contrast among images, we apply a histogram matching between the segmented images and the template. This operation only considers the voxels inside the regions of interest (Fig. 5d). We then perform deformable registration to place all images in the coordinate space of the ICBM 2009c Nonlinear Symmetric template [12]. Since the image registration technique has a critical impact on the analysis, we use Elastix [18], a popular and accurate image registration method.[1] Finally, we perform another histogram matching between the registered images and the template (Fig. 5e).

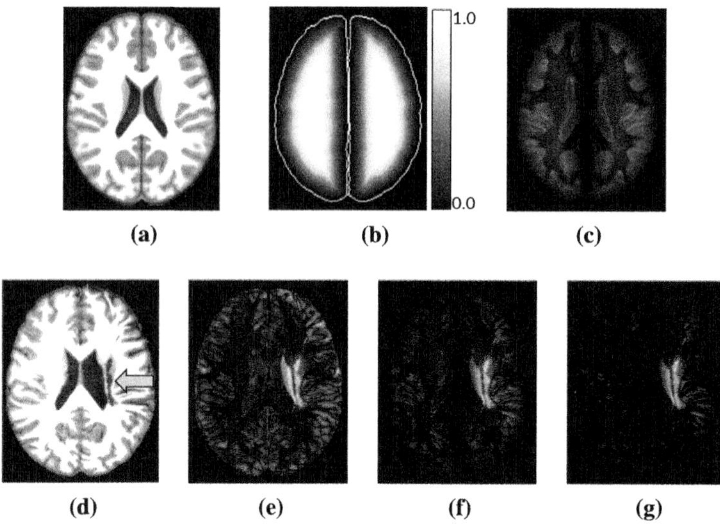

Fig. 6. Registration error computation. **(a)** Axial slice of the brain template. (b) Euclidean Distance Transform (EDT) normalized within $[0, 1]$ computed for the brain segmentation mask defined for the template. Brain borders are shown only for illustration purposes. **(c)** Common registration errors for control images. **(d)** Axial slice of a test stroke image after preprocessing and registration in (a). The arrow indicates the stroke lesion. **(e)** Registration errors. **(f)** Attenuation of **(e)** for the cortex based on the EDT. **(g)** Final registration errors for the test image: positive values of the subtraction between (f) and (c). Figure referenced from [23].

3.2 Registration Error Computation

When registering images to a standard template with *only* healthy tissues, we expect that registration errors (REs)—*i.e.*, voxel-wise absolute differences

[1] We used the *par0000* files available at http://elastix.bigr.nl/wiki/index.php.

between the registered image and the template—are lower and present a different pattern compared to anomalies (Fig. 6e). However, some healthy structures in the cortex, such as gyri and sulci, present high REs due to their complex shapes and very large variability between subjects—observe the cortex of the template and the registered image in Figs. 6a and d; note its resulting REs in Fig. 6e. As such, we need to apply some attenuation-process to avoid detecting false positives in this region.

Let T be the template (Fig. 6a) and M_T its predefined brain segmentation mask for the right hemisphere, left hemisphere, cerebellum, and brainstem (background voxels have label 0 and each object has a different label). Let $X = \{X_1, \cdots, X_k\}$ be the set of k registered training images (output of Step 2 in Fig. 4) and I the test image after preprocessing and registration (output of Step 6 in Fig. 4; see also Fig. 6d).

Firstly, we compute the Euclidean Distance Transform (EDT) for each object of M_T and normalize the distances within $[0, 1]$ to build the map E (Fig. 6b). Next, we obtain the set of registration errors R_X for all X by computing the voxel-wise absolute differences between X and T (Fig. 4, Step 3; see also Fig. 6e). For each training image $X_i \in X$, we attenuate REs in its cortex such that for each voxel $v \in X_i$,

$$\begin{aligned} f(v) &= 1 - (E(v) - 1)^{\lambda} \\ A_{X_i}(v) &= R_{X_i}(v) \cdot f(v), \end{aligned} \tag{2}$$

where $E(v)$ is the euclidean distance for the voxel v, $f(v)$ is its attenuation factor within $[0, 1]$, λ is the exponential factor of the function, and A_{X_i} is the map with the attenuated REs for X_i. In this work, we considered $\lambda = 4$. Thus, REs of voxels close to the brain borders are extremely attenuated, whereas those from voxels far from the borders are slightly impacted (Fig. 6f). A downside of this approach is that subtle lesions in the cortex tend to be missed due to the lack of REs.

In order to even ignore REs caused by noises or small intensity differences in regions/tissues far from the cortex, we create a *common registration error map* $\overline{A_X}$ by averaging the attenuated REs from A_X (output of Step 4 in Fig. 4; see also Fig. 6c). Finally, we repeat the same steps to compute the attenuated REs for the test image I and then subtract $\overline{A_X}$ from them. Resulting positive values form a final attenuated registration error map A_I for I (output of Step 7 in Fig. 4; see also Fig. 6g).

3.3 Supervoxel Segmentation

The direct comparison between the registered image and its template, or even between large 3D regular patches, is not useful as it will not tell us where *small-scale* REs occur—a similar parallel is done for asymmetries in [25]. Conversely, a voxel-wise comparison is risky, since individual voxels contain too little information to capture REs. These difficulties motivate the use of *supervoxels* as the unit of comparison (Step 8 in Fig. 4).

Inspired by the SymmISF method [24] used in SAAD for symmetrical supervoxel segmentation, we propose a new technique that extracts supervoxels in the brain guided by registration errors, as shown in Fig. 7. Our supervoxel segmentation is also based on the recent Iterative Spanning Forest (ISF) framework [42] for superpixel segmentation (Sect. 2) and has three steps: (i) seed estimation; (ii) connected supervoxel delineation (multiple iterations); and (iii) seed recomputation to improve delineation, as follows.

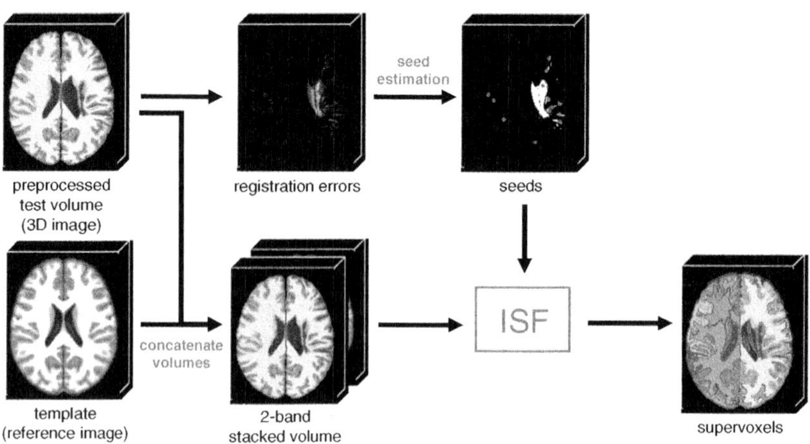

Fig. 7. Pipeline of the proposed supervoxel segmentation. The method stacks the input preprocessed test 3D image (segmented objects are colored) with the template to build a 2-band volume. An initial seed set is obtained from the registration errors of the test image. For each object of the segmentation brain mask, the ISF framework [42] estimates supervoxels inside the object from the initial seeds. Resulting supervoxels are combined and relabeled to form the final label map. (Color figure online)

Recall a template T, its predefined brain segmentation mask M_T (objects of interest), a preprocessed 3D test image I registered on T, and its attenuated registration error map A_I. Equivalently to SymmISF, we find initial seeds by selecting one seed per local maximum in A_I (see the seeds in Fig. 7). We compute the local maxima of the foreground of a binarized A_I at $\gamma \times \tau$, where τ is Otsu's threshold [28]. The higher the factor γ is, the lower is the number of components in the binarized A_I. We extend the seed set with a fixed number of seeds (*e.g.*, 100) by uniform grid sampling the regions with low REs of the binarized image, resulting in the final seed set $\mathcal{S}$.

By stacking I and T as the input 2-band volume (Fig. 7), we perform ISF inside each object of interest in M_T, *separately*, from the initial seeds. The results are label maps wherein each supervoxel is assigned to a distinct number/color. We then combine and relabel the resulting supervoxels to build the final supervoxel map L (output of Step 8 in Fig. 4).

3.4 Feature Extraction and Classification

Our feature extraction and classification steps are very similar to those of SAAD [24], as detailed next. BADRESC relies on an outlier detection approach that designs a set of *specialized* one-class classifiers (OCCs) specific for each test 3D image, as shown in Fig. 8. For each 3D test image, each supervoxel in L is used to create a *specialized* one-class classifier (OCC) using as feature vector the *normalized histogram* of the attenuated registration errors (REs) in A_I (Step 9 in Fig. 4). Classifiers are trained from *control images* only, thus locally modeling normal REs for the hemispheres, cerebellum, and brainstem. BADRESC uses the one-class linear Support Vector Machine (oc-SVM) for this task [20].

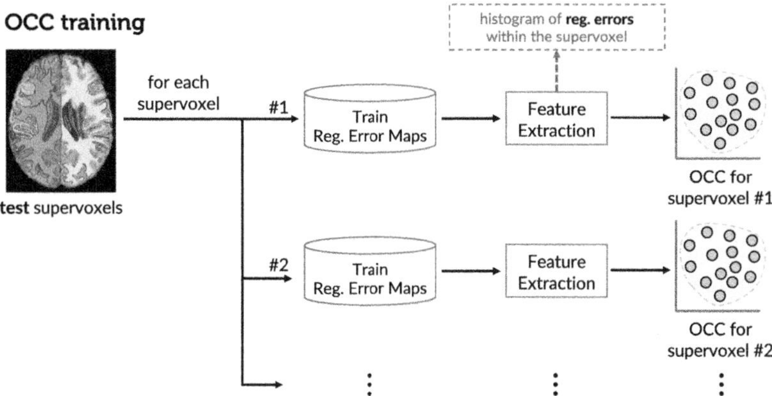

Fig. 8. One-class classifier (OCC) training to detect abnormal registration errors. For each supervoxel from a given test 3D image, BADRESC trains an OCC from the training normal registration errors previously computed.

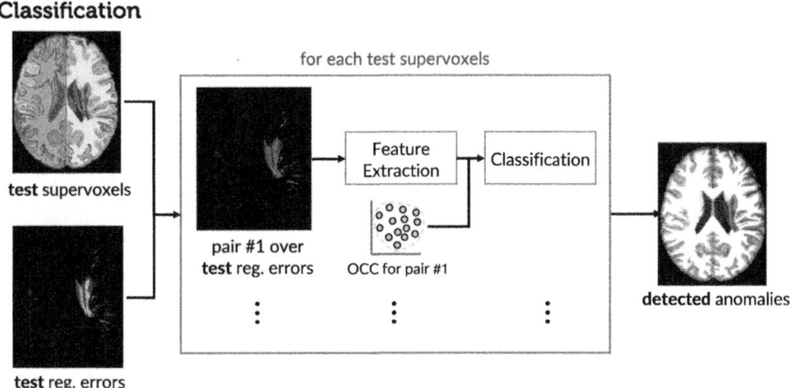

Fig. 9. Detection of abnormal registration errors of a test 3D image by supervoxel classification. For each supervoxel, BADRESC uses the corresponding OCC to classify the registration errors inside it.

Finally, BADRESC uses the trained OCCs to find supervoxels with abnormal REs in I (Step 10 in Fig. 4). Figure 9 illustrates the supervoxel classification.

When *dynamically* designing specialized one-class per-supervoxel classifiers for each test image, BADRESC implicitly considers the *position* of the supervoxels when deciding upon their registration errors. The central premise for this is that a *single* global classifier cannot to separate normal and anomalous tissues by only using texture features.

4 Experiments

To assess the performance of BADRESC, we conducted a set of experiments. This section describes the MR-T1 image datasets, baselines, and the evaluation protocol considered for the experiments. All computations were performed on the same Intel Core i7-7700 CPU 3.60 GHz with 64 GB of RAM.

4.1 Datasets

To evaluate BADRESC, we need datasets with *volumetric* MR-T1 brain images (i) from *healthy* subjects for training, and (ii) with lesions of different appearance (especially small ones) and their segmentation masks. First, we considered the CamCan dataset [39], which has 653 MR-T1 images of 3T from healthy men and women between 18 and 88 years. As far as we know, CamCan is the largest public dataset with 3D images of healthy subjects acquired from different scanners. To avoid noisy data in the training set, we removed some images with artifacts or bad acquisition after a visual inspection in all MR-T1 images, yielding 524 images.[2]

For testing, we chose the Anatomical Tracings of Lesions After Stroke (ATLAS) public dataset release 1.2 [19] in our experiments. ATLAS is a challenging dataset with a large variety of manually annotated lesions and images of 1.5T and 3T acquired from different scanners. It contains heterogeneous lesions that differ in size, shape, and location (see Fig. 1). All images only have a mask with the stroke region, ignoring other possible anomalies caused by those lesions. Current state-of-the-art segmentation results [31] for ATLAS from a *supervised* method based on U-Net are inaccurate yet (Dice score of 0.4867).

Since the considered training images have a 3T field strength, we selected all 3T images from ATLAS for analysis (total of 269 images). All images were registered into the coordinate space of ICBM 2009c Nonlinear Symmetric template [12] and preprocessed as outlined in Sect. 3.1.

4.2 Baselines

We compared BADRESC against two baselines: (i) the SAAD method proposed in [24], which in turn was also evaluated with the ATLAS dataset as reported

[2] A link to all these images will be added in the camera-ready paper.

in [24], and (ii) the convolutional-autoencoder-based approach (CAE) from Chen *et al.* [8], which is, as far as we know, the current state-of-the-art *unsupervised* method for the ATLAS dataset.

We considered the 2D axial slices of all preprocessed training images to train CAE, which has the following architecture: three 2D convolutional layers with 16, 8, and 8 filters of patch size 3×3, respectively, followed by $ReLU$ activation and 2D max-pooling in the *encoder*, and the corresponding operations in the *decoder*. The Nadam gradient optimizer [38] minimized the mean squared error between reconstructed and expected 2D axial slices during training. The method detects anomalies by thresholding the residual image of the input image *vs* its reconstruction to obtain a binary segmentation, similarly to Baur *et al.* [4] and Chen *et al.* [8]. We followed Baur *et al.* [4] by selecting two thresholds as the 90th and 95th percentile from the histogram of reconstruction errors on the considered training set, resulting in the brightness of 194 and 282, respectively. For simplicity, we call CAE-90 and CAE-95 for the versions with the 90th and 95th percentile, respectively.

For a fair comparison, we evaluated SAAD for all 3T images that only contain lesions in the hemispheres. Additionally, we evaluated BADRESC and CAE for all considered testing images, including the ones with stroke lesions in the cerebellum and brainstem. We used the following parameters for BADRESC, empirically obtained from the observation on a few training control images: $\alpha = 0.06$, $\beta = 5.0$, $\gamma = 3$, histograms of 128 bins, and $\nu = 0.01$ for the linear oc-SVM.

4.3 Quality Metrics

Although BADRESC detects anomalies regardless of their types or diseases, we can compute quantitative scores only over those lesions that are labeled in ATLAS, which are a subset of what BADRESC can detect. Thus, we propose a set of metrics to evaluate detection quality, as follows. We start computing the detection rate based on at least 15% overlap between supervoxels detected by the methods and lesions labeled in ATLAS (Tables 1 and 2, row 1). We then computed the *true positive rate* (recall) that measures the percentage of lesion voxels correctly classified as abnormal (Tables 1 and 2, row 2). Although our focus is on *detecting* abnormal asymmetries, we also measured the *Dice score* between lesions and the detected supervoxels to check BADRESC's potential as a *segmentation method* (Tables 1 and 2, row 3). However, observe that true anomalies detected by our method that are not annotated as lesions in the ground-truth masks will be incorrectly considered as false-positive and, thus, underestimating the Dice score. We could then consider only supervoxels overlapped with the annotated lesions to compute Dice scores, but this would be unfair to the considered baselines.

We provided false-positive (FP) scores in terms of both voxels and supervoxels regarding the ground-truth stroke lesions of ATLAS. Hence, some anomalies with no labeled masks in ATLAS are considered FP. This is the best we can do in the absence of labeled masks for all kinds of abnormalities in this dataset. We computed the *mean number of FP voxels*, *i.e.*, incorrectly classified as abnormal (Tables 1 and 2, row 4). We normalized this count with respect to all classified voxels (Tables 1 and 2, row 5), *i.e.*, the total number of voxels inside the right hemisphere for SAAD and all voxels from the hemispheres, cerebellum, and brainstem for BADRESC and CAE.

At the next level, we estimated FP supervoxels as those whose voxels overlap less than 15% with ground-truth lesion voxels. We computed the mean number of FP supervoxels and their proportions to the total number of supervoxels (Tables 1 and 2, rows 6 and 7). The first metric gives us an estimation of the visual-inspection user effort. The second metric checks how imprecise detection is regarding the total number of regions that the user has to analyze visually.

When visually analyzing FP supervoxels, it is harder to check many disconnected supervoxels spread across the brain than a few connected ones. Hence, we gauge visual analysis user-effort by evaluating the two metrics outlined above on the level of connected FP supervoxel components (Tables 1 and 2, rows 8 and 9). Finally, we also computed the mean processing times of each method (Tables 1 and 2, row 10) for preprocessed images, thus excluding the mean time of the preprocessing step (Sect. 3.1), which is 90 s on average.

5 Evaluation Results

Table 1 summarizes quantitative results of the baselines for stroke lesions in the hemispheres, while Fig. 10 presents some corresponding visual results. CAE-90 presents considerably higher detection scores (0.953) than SAAD (0.845) and BADRESC (0.82). However, these impressive results are misleading as CAE reports considerably more false-positive voxels than SAAD (about 6.75×), being drastically worse than BADRESC (about 48×)—compare rows 4 and 5 in Table 1. For instance, CAE-90 misclassifies 23.7% of the hemispheres as abnormal, which is far from being reasonable and hinders the visual analysis (we expect just a small portion of the brain, *e.g.*, 1%). These high FP rates explain the poor Dice scores for CAE in Table 1, which in turn are compatible with the ones reported in [8].

Additionally, CAE is speedy (running time about 2 s per image) and yields very noisy disconnected regions, especially in regions with transitions between white and gray matter (*e.g.*, the cortex), that hinder the subsequent visual inspection (see the results in Fig. 10). Even though the number of FP voxels decrease for a higher threshold, the detection score can be hugely impacted; for example, the threshold at the 95th percentile approximately halves both the detection score and FP voxels rates compared with the results for the 90th percentile in Table 1. CAE might present better results by using a considerable large training set and/or some additional post-processing, but this is not considered in [4,8]. CAE presents better results for other medical imaging modalities, such as CT and T2 [4,8].

SAAD reports a better detection rate and mean recall for hemispheric lesions than BADRESC, although the difference between such scores is not accentuate—*e.g.*, SAAD has a detection rate of 0.845 while BADRESC has 0.82. BADRESC,

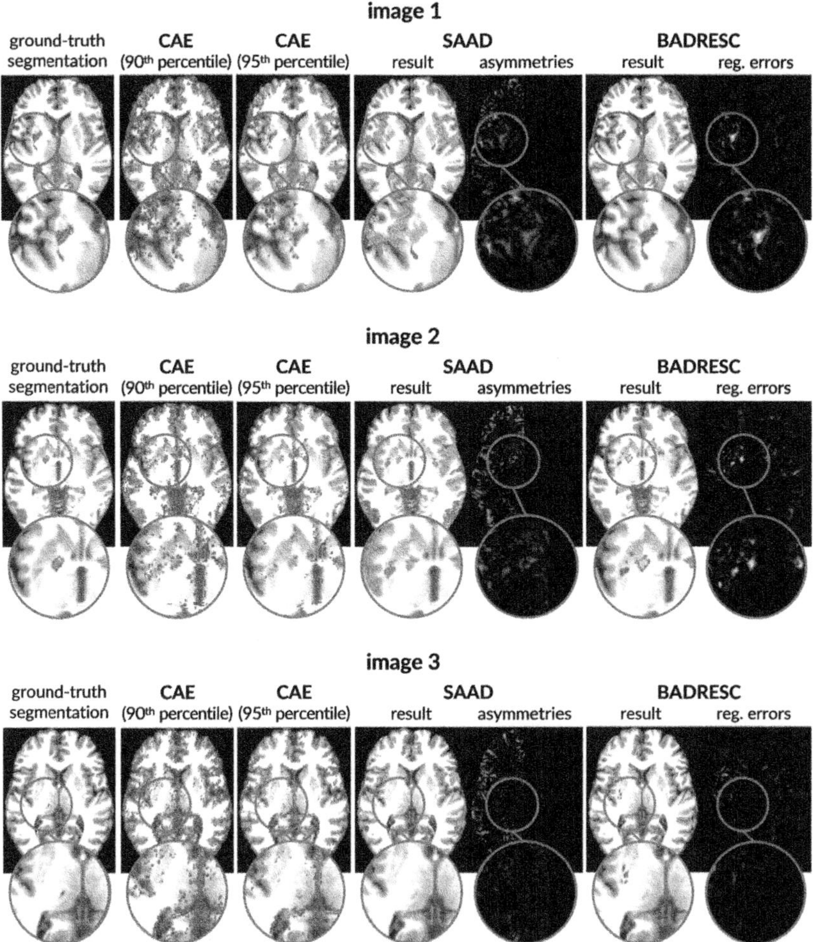

Fig. 10. Comparative results between the baselines for stroke lesions in the hemispheres. For each image (axial slice), we present an inset surrounding the lesion whose border color indicates if the lesion was detected (green) or missed (red). (Color figure online)

in turn, reports a better Dice score (0.17) than SAAD (0.12). However, as outlined in Sect. 4.3, this score is underestimated since real unlabeled anomalies detected by the methods are considered false-positive. If we considered only supervoxels overlapped with the annotated lesions, such a Dice score leverages to 0.42. While still low, this score is not far from state-of-the-art results (Dice score 0.4867) on the ATLAS dataset from a *supervised* method based on U-Net [31]. Interestingly, our method is noticeably superior to CAE, which is an *unsupervised* method (like ours), reporting Dice scores of 0.015.

Table 1. Quantitative comparison between the baselines for images from the ATLAS dataset with stroke lesions in the hemispheres. **Top part:** higher values mean better accuracies. **Bottom part:** lower values mean better accuracies. The abbreviation k denotes thousands.

		CAE-90	CAE-95	SAAD	BADRESC
1	Detection rate	**0.953**	0.567	0.845	0.82
2	True positive rate (mean recall)	0.34 ± 0.15	0.21 ± 0.13	$\mathbf{0.44 \pm 0.25}$	0.39 ± 0.26
3	Dice	0.015 ± 0.023	0.015 ± 0.024	0.12 ± 0.15	$\mathbf{0.17 \pm 0.15}$
4	# FP voxels	432k ± 186k	207k ± 45k	64k ± 37k	**9k ± 11k**
5	FP voxel rate	0.237 ± 0.102	0.113 ± 0.025	0.08 ± 0.05	$\mathbf{0.005 \pm 0.01}$
6	# FP supervoxels	method does not use supervoxels		58.87 ± 22.45	$\mathbf{21.46 \pm 13.86}$
7	FP supervoxel rate			0.2 ± 0.06	$\mathbf{0.1 \pm 0.07}$
8	# FP connected supervoxels			53 ± 17.31	$\mathbf{16.61 \pm 9.21}$
9	FP connected supervoxel rate			0.18 ± 0.05	$\mathbf{0.08 \pm 0.042}$
10	Mean processing time (in secs)	2.09 ± 0.08	2.04 ± 0.16	63.03 ± 6.73	54.17 ± 1.3

Table 2. Quantitative comparison between CAE and BADRESC for images from the ATLAS dataset with stroke lesions in the cerebellum and brainstem. **Top part:** higher values mean better accuracies. **Bottom part:** lower values mean better accuracies. The abbreviation k denotes thousands.

		CAE-90	CAE-95	BADRESC
1	Detection rate	**0.878**	0.365	0.683
2	True positive rate (mean recall)	$\mathbf{0.3 \pm 0.145}$	0.17 ± 0.14	0.26 ± 0.26
3	Dice	0.01 ± 0.02	0.01 ± 0.01	$\mathbf{0.1 \pm 0.15}$
4	# FP voxels	434k ± 68k	225k ± 67k	**8.7k ± 7.9k**
5	FP voxel rate	0.238 ± 0.038	0.124 ± 0.037	$\mathbf{0.005 \pm 0.004}$
6	# FP supervoxels	method does not use supervoxels		$\mathbf{23.43 \pm 15.25}$
7	FP supervoxel rate			$\mathbf{0.09 \pm 0.05}$
8	# FP connected supervoxels			$\mathbf{18.41 \pm 10.19}$
9	FP connected supervoxel rate			$\mathbf{0.08 \pm 0.03}$
10	Mean processing time (in secs)	2.09 ± 0.08	2.04 ± 0.16	54.17 ± 1.3

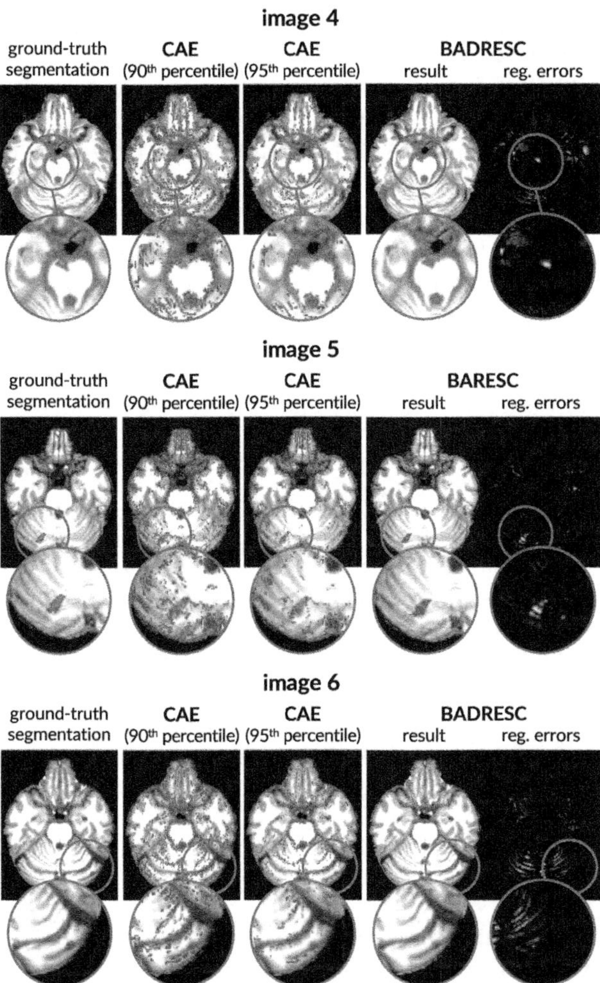

Fig. 11. Comparative results between CAE and BADRESC for stroke lesions in the cerebellum and brainstem. For each image (axial slice), we show an inset surrounding the lesion whose border color indicates if the lesion was detected (green) or missed (red). (Color figure online)

When analyzing supervoxels, both SAAD and BADRESC output more meaningful regions for visual analysis than CAE—compare the detected regions in Fig. 10. They can accurately detect small asymmetric lesions in the hemispheres (Fig. 10, Image 1) since asymmetries and registration errors successfully emphasize such lesions (see these for Image 1 in Fig. 10). SAAD cannot detect lesions with low asymmetries, while BADRESC does not have this limitation—compare the results, asymmetries, and registration errors for Image 2 in Fig. 10. However, both methods are ineffective in detecting tiny anomalies (Fig. 10, image 3) since asymmetries and registration errors cannot highlight such anomalies.

BADRESC is a bit faster and reports seven times fewer false-positive (FP) voxels than SAAD (Table 1, rows 4, 5, and 10): an average of 9000 FP voxels against approximately 64000, respectively. Concerning FP supervoxel scores, BADRESC is consistently better than SAAD (scores roughly three times higher)—compare rows 6–9 in Table 1. For instance, SAAD incorrectly classifies 58.87 supervoxels on average, which consists of 20% of all analyzed supervoxels and 8% of the analyzed voxels in the hemisphere respectively. BADRESC, in turn, reports an average of 21.46 FP supervoxels, which corresponds to 10% of analyzed supervoxels and only 0.5% of voxels in the whole brain. When grouping connected detected supervoxels, BADRESC reports only 16 FP supervoxels. Hence, a user will need far less effort and time to visually analyze results from BADRESC than from SAAD.

BADRESC is less accurate when detecting lesions in the cerebellum and brainstem (detection rate of 0.683) than in the hemispheres, as shown in Table 2 and Fig. 11. Some of these lesions are indeed challenging, especially in the cerebellum, whose appearances are similar to their surrounding tissues (Fig. 11, Image 6). BADRESC reports similar FP scores to those of hemispheric lesions, which confirms the stability of the method (compare rows 4–9 for BADRESC in Figs. 10 and 11). The considered registration-error attenuation (Eq. 2 with $\alpha = 4$) seems to be very strong for the cerebellum and brainstem, which impairs the representation of the lesions. However, as SAAD cannot detect lesions in the cerebellum and brainstem, BADRESC is a more interesting solution to be further investigated and improved, especially in such macro-objects of interest.

6 Conclusion

We presented a new *unsupervised* method for brain anomaly detection that combines registration errors and supervoxel classification. Our approach, named BADRESC, adapts a recent supervoxel-based approach (SAAD) to detect *outliers* as anomalies from registration errors in the hemispheres, cerebellum, and brainstem. This work is an extension of a previous one, which originally introduces BADRESC. Its main contributions include a more detailed explanation of the method, especially concerning supervoxel segmentation, and an extended evaluation (more baselines and evaluation metrics).

BADRESC was validated on 3T MR-T1 images of stroke patients with annotated lesions, outperforming a convolutional-autoencoder-based approach, and attaining similar detection accuracy to SAAD for lesions in the hemispheres and substantially fewer false positives. BADRESC also detects lesions in the cerebellum and brainstem with promising results.

For future work, we intend to improve BADRESC by optimizing its parameters and using additional visual analytics techniques to improve seeding and further investigate other anomaly features and classifiers to yield better detection rates, especially for the cerebellum and brainstem.

A Appendix

Image Foresting Transform

The *Image Foresting Transform (IFT)* is a methodology for the design of image operators based on optimum connectivity [11]. For a given connectivity function and a graph derived from an image, the IFT algorithm minimizes (maximizes) a connectivity map to partition the graph into an *optimum-path forest* rooted at the minima (maxima) of the resulting connectivity map. The image operation resumes to a post-processing of the forest attributes, such as the root labels, optimum paths, and connectivity values. IFT has been successfully applied in different domains, such as image filtering [10], segmentation [6,22,36], superpixel segmentation [5,24,42], pattern classification [2,29], and data clustering [27,32]. This appendix presents preliminary concepts and introduces the IFT algorithm.

Preliminary Concepts

Image Graphs. A *d-dimensional multi-band image* is defined as the pair $\hat{I} = (D_I, \vec{I})$, where $D_I \subset Z^d$ is the *image domain*—*i.e.*, a set of elements (pixels/voxels) in Z^d—and $\vec{I} : D_I \rightarrow \mathbb{R}^c$ is a mapping function that assigns a vector of c intensities $\vec{I}(p)$—one value for each band (channel) of the image—to each element $p \in D_I$. For example, for 2D RGB-color images: $d = 2$, $c = 3$; for 3D grayscale images (*e.g.*, MR images): $d = 3$, $c = 1$. We represent a *segmentation* of $\hat{I}$ by a label image $\hat{L} = (D_I, L)$, wherein the function $L : D_I \rightarrow \{0, 1, \cdots, M\}$ maps every voxel of $\hat{I}$ to either the background (label 0) or one of the M objects of interest.

Most images, like the ones used in this paper, typically represent their intensity values by *natural numbers* instead of *real numbers*. More specifically, $\vec{I} : D_I \rightarrow [0, 2^b - 1]$, where b is the *number of bits* (pixel/voxel depth) used to encode an intensity value.

An image can be interpreted as a graph $G_I = (D_I, \mathcal{A})$, whose *nodes* are the voxels and the *arcs* are defined by an *adjacency relation* $\mathcal{A} \subset D_I \times D_I$, with $\mathcal{A}(p)$ being the *adjacent set* of a voxel p. A *spherical adjacency relation* of radius $\gamma \geq 1$ is given by

$$\mathcal{A}_\gamma : \{(p, q) \in D_I \times D_I, \|q - p\| \leq \gamma\}. \tag{3}$$

The image operators considered in this paper use two types of adjacency relations: $\mathcal{A}_1$ (6-neighborhood) and $\mathcal{A}_{\sqrt{3}}$ (26-neighborhood), as illustrated in Fig. 12.

Paths. For a given image graph $G_I = (D_I, \mathcal{A})$, a *path* π_q with terminus q is a sequence of distinct nodes $\langle p_1, p_2, \cdots p_k \rangle$ with $\langle p_i, p_{i+1} \rangle \in \mathcal{A}$, $1 \leq i \leq k - 1$, and $p_k = q$. The path $\pi_q = \langle q \rangle$ is called *trivial path*. The concatenation of a path π_p and an arc $\langle p, q \rangle$ is denoted by $\pi_p \cdot \langle p, q \rangle$.

Connectivity Function. A *connectivity function* (path-cost function) assigns a value $f(\pi_q)$ to any path π_q in the image graph $G_I = (D_I, \mathcal{A})$. A path π_q^* ending

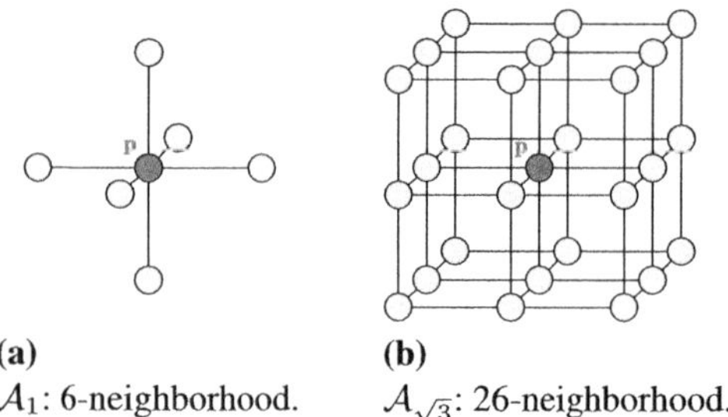

(a) $\mathcal{A}_1$: 6-neighborhood. (b) $\mathcal{A}_{\sqrt{3}}$: 26-neighborhood.

Fig. 12. Examples of adjacency relation for a given voxel p (red). (Color figure online)

at q is optimum if $f(\pi_q^*) \leq f(\tau_q)$ for every other path τ_q. In other words, a path ending at q is optimum if no other path ending at q has lower cost.

Connectivity functions may be defined in different ways. In some cases, they do not guarantee the optimum cost mapping conditions [9], but, in turn, can produce effective object delineation [26]. A common example of connectivity function is f_{max}, defined by

$$
\begin{aligned}
f_{max}(\langle q \rangle) &= \begin{cases} 0 & \text{if } q \in \mathcal{S}, \\ +\infty & \text{otherwise.} \end{cases} \\
f_{max}(\pi_p \cdot \langle p, q \rangle) &= \max\{f_{max}(\pi_p), w(p,q)\},
\end{aligned} \tag{4}
$$

where $w(p,q)$ is the arc weight of $\langle p, q \rangle$, usually estimated from $\hat{I}$, and $\mathcal{S}$ is the labeled seed set.

The General IFT Algorithm

For multi-object image segmentation, IFT requires a labeled seed set $\mathcal{S} = \mathcal{S}_0 \cup \mathcal{S}_1 \cup \cdots \mathcal{S}_M$ with seeds for object i in each set $\mathcal{S}_i$ and background seeds in $\mathcal{S}_0$, as

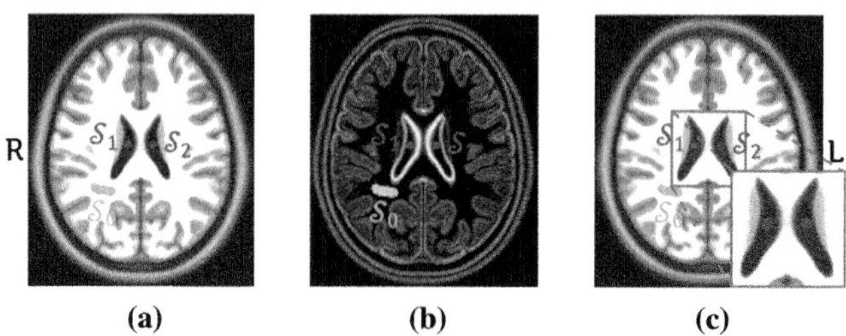

(a) **(b)** **(c)**

Fig. 13. Multi-object image segmentation by IFT. **(a)** Axial slice of a brain image with seeds $\mathcal{S}_0$ for the background (orange), $\mathcal{S}_1$ for the right ventricle (red), and $\mathcal{S}_2$ for the left ventricle (green). **(b)** Gradient image for (a) that defines the arc weights for seed competition. Arcs have high weights on object boundaries. **(c)** Resulting segmentation mask for the given seeds and arc weights. Red and green voxels represent object voxels, whereas the remaining ones are background. (Color figure online)

illustrated in Fig. 13. The algorithm then promotes an optimum seed competition so that each seed in $\mathcal{S}$ conquers its most closely connected voxels in the image domain. This competition considers a connectivity function f applied to any path π_q.

Defining Π_q as the set of all possible paths with terminus q in the image graph, the IFT algorithm minimizes a path cost map

$$C(q) = \min_{\forall \pi_q \in \Pi_q} \{f(\pi_q)\}, \tag{5}$$

by partitioning the graph into an optimum-path forest P rooted at $\mathcal{S}$. That is, the algorithm assigns to q the path π_q^* of minimum cost, such that each object i is defined by the union between the seed voxels of $\mathcal{S}_i$ and the voxels of D_I that are rooted in $\mathcal{S}_i$, *i.e.*, conquered by such object seeds.

Algorithm 2 presents the general IFT approach. Lines 1–7 initialize maps, and insert seeds into the priority queue Q. The state map U indicates by $U(q) =$

Algorithm 2. The General IFT Algorithm.

Input: Image $\hat{I} = (D_I, I)$, adjacency relation $\mathcal{A}$ connectivity function f, and seed set $\mathcal{S} \subset D_I$ labeled by λ.
Output: Optimum-path forest P, root map R, path-cost map C, and label map L.
Aux: Priority queue Q, state map U, and variable *tmp*.

```
1  foreach q ∈ D_I do
2      P(q) ← ∅, R(q) ← q
3      C(q) ← f(⟨q⟩), L(q) ← 0
4      U(q) ← White
5      if q ∈ S then
6          insert q into Q
7          L(q) ← λ(q), U(q) ← Gray
8  while Q ≠ ∅ do
9      Remove p from Q such that C(p) is minimum
10     U(p) ← Black
11     foreach q ∈ A(p) such that U(q) ≠ Black do
12         tmp ← f(π*_p · ⟨p, q⟩)
13         if tmp < C(q) then
14             P(q) ← p, R(q) ← R(p)
15             C(q) ← tmp, L(q) ← L(p)
16             if U(q) = Gray then
17                 update position of q in Q
18             else
19                 insert q into Q
20                 U(q) ← Gray
21 return (P, R, C, L)
```

White that the voxel q was never visited (never inserted into Q), by $U(q) = Gray$ that q has been visited and is still in Q, and by $U(q) = Black$ that q has been processed (removed from Q).

The main loop (Lines 8–20) performs the propagation process. First, it removes the voxel p that has *minimum path cost* in Q (Line 9). Ties are broken in Q using the first-in-first-out (FIFO) policy. The loop in Lines 11–20 then evaluates if a path with terminus p extended to its adjacent q is cheaper than the current path with terminus q and cost $C(q)$ (Line 13). If that is the case, p is assigned as the predecessor of q, and the root of p is assigned to the root of q (Line 14), whereas the path cost and the label of q are updated (Line 15). If q is in Q, its position is updated; otherwise, q is inserted into Q. The algorithm returns the optimum-path forest (predecessor map), root map, path-cost map, and the label map (object delineation mask).

References

1. Akkus, Z., et al.: Deep learning for brain MRI segmentation: state of the art and future directions. J. Digit. Imaging **30**(4), 449–459 (2017)
2. Amorim, W.P., Falcão, A.X., Papa, J.P., Carvalho, M.H.: Improving semi-supervised learning through optimum connectivity. Pattern Recogn. **60**, 72–85 (2016)
3. Aslani, S., et al.: Deep 2D encoder-decoder convolutional neural network for multiple sclerosis lesion segmentation in brain MRI. In: Medical Image Computing and Computer-Assisted Intervention (MICCAI), pp. 132–141 (2018)
4. Baur, C., Wiestler, B., Albarqouni, S., Navab, N.: Deep autoencoding models for unsupervised anomaly segmentation in brain MR images. In: International MICCAI Brainlesion Workshop, pp. 161–169 (2018)
5. Belém, F., Melo, L., Guimarães, S.J.F., Falcão, A.X.: The importance of object-based seed sampling for superpixel segmentation. In: Conference on Graphics, Patterns and Images (SIBGRAPI), pp. 108–115 (2019)
6. Bragantini, J., Martins, S.B., Castelo-Fernandez, C., Falcão, A.X.: Graph-based image segmentation using dynamic trees. In: Iberoamerican Congress on Pattern Recognition (CIARP), pp. 470–478 (2018)
7. Chen, H., et al.: VoxResNet: deep voxelwise residual networks for brain segmentation from 3D MR images. Neuroimage **170**, 446–455 (2018)
8. Chen, X., et al.: Deep generative models in the real-world: an open challenge from medical imaging. arXiv preprint arXiv:1806.05452 (2018)
9. Ciesielski, K.C., Falcão, A.X., Miranda, P.A.V.: Path-value functions for which Dijkstra's algorithm returns optimal mapping. J. Math. Imaging Vision **60**(7), 1025–1036 (2018)
10. Falcão, A.X., Cunha, B.S., Lotufo, R.A.: Design of connected operators using the image foresting transform. SPIE Med. Imaging **4322**, 468–479 (2001)
11. Falcão, A.X., Stolfi, J., de Alencar Lotufo, R.: The image foresting transform: theory, algorithms, and applications. IEEE Trans. Pattern Anal. **26**(1), 19–29 (2004)
12. Fonov, V.S., et al.: Unbiased nonlinear average age-appropriate brain templates from birth to adulthood. Neuroimage **47**, S102 (2009)
13. Gao, Y., Riklin-Raviv, T., Bouix, S.: Shape analysis, a field in need of careful validation. Hum. Brain Mapping **35**(10), 4965–4978 (2014)

14. Guo, D., et al.: Automated lesion detection on MRI scans using combined unsupervised and supervised methods. BMC Med. Imaging **15**(1), 50 (2015)
15. Havaei, M., et al.: Brain tumor segmentation with deep neural networks. Med. Image Anal. **35**, 18–31 (2017)
16. Juan-Albarracín, J., et al.: Automated glioblastoma segmentation based on a multiparametric structured unsupervised classification. PLoS One **10**(5), e0125143 (2015)
17. Kamnitsas, K., et al.: Efficient multi-scale 3D CNN with fully connected CRF for accurate brain lesion segmentation. Med. Image Anal. **36**, 61–78 (2017)
18. Klein, S., Staring, M., Murphy, K., Viergever, M.A., Pluim, J.P.W.: elastix: a toolbox for intensity-based medical image registration. IEEE Trans. Med. Imaging **29**(1), 196–205 (2010)
19. Liew, S.L., et al.: A large, open source dataset of stroke anatomical brain images and manual lesion segmentations. Sci. Data **5**, 180011 (2018)
20. Manevitz, L.M., Yousef, M.: One-class SVMs for document classification. J. Mach. Learn. Res. **2**(Dec), 139–154 (2001)
21. Manjón, J.V.: MRI preprocessing. In: Martí-Bonmatí, L., Alberich-Bayarri, A. (eds.) Imaging Biomarkers, pp. 53–63. Springer, Cham (2017). https://doi.org/10.1007/978-3-319-43504-6_5
22. Martins, S.B., Bragantini, J., Yasuda, C.L., Falcão, A.X.: An adaptive probabilistic atlas for anomalous brain segmentation in MR images. Med. Phys. **46**(11), 4940–4950 (2019)
23. Martins, S.B., Falcão, A.X., Telea, A.C.: BADRESC: brain anomaly detection based on registration errors and supervoxel classification. In: Biomedical Engineering Systems and Technologies: BIOIMAGING, pp. 74–81 (2020). Best student paper awards
24. Martins, S.B., Ruppert, G., Reis, F., Yasuda, C.L., Falcão, A.X.: A supervoxel-based approach for unsupervised abnormal asymmetry detection in MR images of the brain. In IEEE 16th International Symposium on Biomedical Imaging (ISBI), pp. 882–885 (2019)
25. Martins, S.B., Telea, A.C., Falcão, A.X.: Extending supervoxel-based abnormal brain asymmetry detection to the native image space. In: IEEE Engineering in Medicine and Biology Society (EMBC), pp. 450–453 (2019)
26. Miranda, P.A.V., Mansilla, L.A.C.: Oriented image foresting transform segmentation by seed competition. IEEE Trans. Image Process. **23**(1), 389–398 (2014)
27. Montero, A.E., Falcão, A.X.: A divide-and-conquer clustering approach based on optimum-path forest. In: Conference on Graphics, Patterns and Images (SIBGRAPI), pp. 416–423 (2018)
28. Otsu, N.: A threshold selection method from gray-level histograms. IEEE Trans. Syst. Man Cybern. **9**(1), 62–66 (1979)
29. Papa, J.P., Falcão, A.X., Suzuki, C.T.N.: Supervised pattern classification based on optimum-path forest. Int. J. Imaging Syst. Technol. **19**(2), 120–131 (2009)
30. Pinto, A., Pereira, S., Correia, H., Oliveira, J., Rasteiro, D.M., Silva, C.A.: Brain tumour segmentation based on extremely randomized forest with high-level features. In: IEEE Engineering in Medicine and Biology Society (EMBC), pp. 3037–3040 (2015)
31. Qi, K., et al.: X-net: brain stroke lesion segmentation based on depthwise separable convolution and long-range dependencies. In: Medical Image Computing and Computer-Assisted Intervention (MICCAI), pp. 247–255 (2019)

32. Rocha, L.M., Cappabianco, F.A.M., Falcão, A.X.: Data clustering as an optimum-path forest problem with applications in image analysis. Int. J. Imaging Syst. Technol. **19**(2), 50–68 (2009)
33. Sato, D., et al.: A primitive study on unsupervised anomaly detection with an autoencoder in emergency head CT volumes. In: SPIE Medical Imaging, p. 105751P (2018)
34. Shakeri, M., et al.: Statistical shape analysis of subcortical structures using spectral matching. Comput. Med. Imaging Graph. **52**, 58–71 (2016)
35. Soltaninejad, M., et al.: Automated brain tumour detection and segmentation using superpixel-based extremely randomized trees in FLAIR MRI. Int. J. Comput. Assist. Radiol. Surg. **12**(2), 183–203 (2016). https://doi.org/10.1007/s11548-016-1483-3
36. Sousa, A.M., Martins, S.B., Falcão, A.X., Reis, F., Bagatin, E., Irion, K.: ALTIS: a fast and automatic lung and trachea CT-image segmentation method. Med. Phys. **46**(11), 4970–4982 (2019)
37. Stutz, D., Hermans, A., Leibe, B.: Superpixels: an evaluation of the state-of-the-art. Comput. Vision Image Understand. **166**, 1–27 (2018)
38. Sutskever, I., Martens, J., Dahl, G., Hinton, G.: On the importance of initialization and momentum in deep learning. In: International Conference on Machine Learning (ICML), pp. 1139–1147 (2013)
39. Taylor, J.R., et al.: The Cambridge centre for ageing and neuroscience (Cam-CAN) data repository: structural and functional MRI, MEG, and cognitive data from a cross-sectional adult lifespan sample. Neuroimage **144**, 262–269 (2017)
40. Thyreau, B., Sato, K., Fukuda, H., Taki, Y.: Segmentation of the hippocampus by transferring algorithmic knowledge for large cohort processing. Med. Image Anal. **43**, 214–228 (2018)
41. Tustison, N.J., et al.: N4ITK: improved N3 bias correction. IEEE Trans. Med. Imaging **29**(6), 1310–1320 (2010)
42. Vargas-Muñoz, J.E., Chowdhury, A.S., Alexandre, E.B., Galvão, F.L., Miranda, P.A.V., Falcão, A.X.: An iterative spanning forest framework for superpixel segmentation. IEEE Trans. Image Process. **28**(7), 3477–3489 (2019)
43. Wang, L., Joshi, S.C., Miller, M.I., Csernansky, J.G.: Statistical analysis of hippocampal asymmetry in schizophrenia. Neuroimage **14**(3), 531–545 (2001)
44. Wu, W., Chen, A.Y.C., Zhao, L., Corso, J.J.: Brain tumor detection and segmentation in a CRF (conditional random fields) framework with pixel-pairwise affinity and superpixel-level features. Int. J. Comput. Assist. Radiol. Surg. **9**(2), 241–253 (2013). https://doi.org/10.1007/s11548-013-0922-7
45. Yan, J., Yu, Y., Zhu, X., Lei, Z., Li, S.Z.: Object detection by labeling superpixels. In: Conference on Computer Vision and Pattern Recognition (CVPR), pp. 5107–5116 (2015)

A Framework Based on Metabolic Networks and Biomedical Images Data to Discriminate Glioma Grades

Lucia Maddalena[1(✉)], Ilaria Granata[1], Ichcha Manipur[1], Mario Manzo[2], and Mario R. Guarracino[3]

[1] ICAR, National Research Council, Via P. Castellino 111, 80131 Naples, Italy
{lucia.maddalena,ilaria.granata,ichcha.manipur}@icar.cnr.it
[2] ITS, University of Naples "L'Orientale", Via Nuova Marina 59, 80132 Naples, Italy
mmanzo@unior.it
[3] University of Cassino and Southern Lazio, Cassino, Italy
mario.guarracino@unicas.it

Abstract. Collecting and integrating information from different data sources is a successful approach to investigate complex biological phenomena and to address tasks such as disease subtyping, biomarker prediction, target, and mechanisms identification. Here, we describe an integrative framework, based on the combination of transcriptomics data, metabolic networks, and magnetic resonance images, to classify different grades of glioma, one of the most common types of primary brain tumors arising from glial cells. The framework is composed of three main blocks for feature sorting, choosing the best number of sorted features, and classification model building. We investigate different methods for each of the blocks, highlighting those that lead to the best results. Our approach demonstrates how the integration of molecular and imaging data achieves better classification performance than using the individual data-sets, also comparing results with state-of-the-art competitors. The proposed framework can be considered as a starting point for a clinically relevant grading system, and the related software made available lays the foundations for future comparisons.

Keywords: Data integration · Glioma grade classification · Metabolic networks · Omics imaging · Transcriptomics

1 Introduction

Gliomas are a type of neuroepithelial tumors that originate from glial cells and are the most common primary tumors of the central nervous system. Recent technological advances allow us to identify and characterize, with an increasing level of detail, the risk factors and the molecular basis underlying this aggressive and invasive class of tumors. According to the WHO 2016 classification system, five glioma subtypes are recognized based on histological and molecular parameters and graded from I (low-grade LGG) to II-IV (high-grade HGG).

X. Ye et al. (Eds.): BIOSTEC 2020, CCIS 1400, pp. 165–189, 2021.
https://doi.org/10.1007/978-3-030-72379-8_9

Nonetheless, the different subtypes and grades still present high phenotype and survival variability [37]. As for all cancer types, the greatest scientific challenge concerns the discovery of specific risk factors and early diagnostic markers. Early and precise diagnosis also has a crucial role in terms of treatment planning.

Surgical resection with subsequent radiotherapy and chemotherapy is the main treatment strategy for HGGs, and the incorrect diagnosis of HGGs as LGGs would lead to less aggressive treatment decisions [47]. Glioblastoma Multiformae (GBM) is a grade IV glioma and is characterized by high aggressiveness and poor prognosis. Nowadays, treatment options are still quite limited in the case of GBM diagnosis with poor outcomes. The therapy failures are due to late symptom onset and consequent delay in diagnosis and treatment. In this context, an accurate diagnosis cannot prescind from quantitative estimations [24]. The last decade has seen *radiomics* [28,29], which involves the extraction of high-throughput quantitative features from clinical images, as a rapidly evolving field. It allows the non-invasive quantification of tumor phenotypes, providing clinically significant diagnostic and prognostic imaging biomarkers [10]. Glioma grade classification using radiomic features from Magnetic Resonance Imaging (MRI) or other biomedical imaging techniques have been investigated in several studies [9,10,14,26,30,47,50–52].

Advanced omics technologies have enabled high-throughput biomolecular data acquisition and characterization. This has also made way to a new interdisciplinary field dealing with the integrated analysis of features extracted from medical images and multi-omics data. This field has been named *imaging genomics* [22,23,31] or *radiogenomics* [1,18,42], while we refer to it as *omics imaging* [3], as it better captures the essence of the integrated study of a wide range of omics (genomics, transcriptomics, proteomics, other omics) and medical imaging (structural, functional, and molecular) data. This approach has the potential to get novel insights about tumor molecular-morphology relationship, decipher disease behavior, and also identify clinically important molecular/imaging biomarkers [39]. Omics imaging studies in recent years have examined the association between GBM imaging phenotypes and gene-expression patterns, [7,44] or the prediction of GBM patient survival (e.g., [13,17]). However, to the best of our knowledge, only our previous study [32] analyzed the problem of integrating omics and imaging data for glioma grade classification. We showed that a suitable combination of both these kinds of data could provide more accurate classification results than their separate use. In that classification framework, our implementation choices have been guided by the established literature, rather than by their specific suitability for the problem at hand.

Here, we investigate whether the adoption of different classifier models, feature sorting, or feature selection algorithms may lead to better results for integrating multimodal data for glioma grade classification. Specifically, the main contributions can be summarized as a set of extended investigations on

- three methods for sorting features based on their importance for classification;
- two optimization criteria for choosing the best number of sorted features through cross-validation;

– three classification methods for evaluating testing performance.

Moreover, average performance results obtained by repeated application of the proposed framework on random partitions of the input data are compared to those obtained with a single training/test set, so as to analyze punctual performance results and the significance of the extracted features. Finally, we make the software and extracted data publicly available so as to lay the foundations for future comparisons.

2 Evaluation Framework

Figure 1 shows the adopted framework for classification evaluation, in the following referred to as CEF. The input data (either O, I, or OI features) is partitioned into a training and a testing set; the partitioning is chosen randomly, taking care to have the same distribution of samples over classes, both in training and test set. The training set is used to sort the features according to their decreasing importance for classification (SortFeatures module). Then, the optimal number NoF of sorted features is estimated (SelectOptNum module), and the first NoF sorted features are used to train a classification model M (ClassModel module). Finally, the model M trained using the training dataset is used to classify the test set and to estimate the related performance (Eval module). The described classification and evaluation procedure is repeated a number $numIter$ of times (in the experiments, $numIter$ is set to 100), each time randomly permuting the data so as to obtain different train/test subdivisions. Overall performance values are obtained as the average of those obtained at each iteration (i.e., for each of the partitions).

The main modules of the evaluation framework are briefly described in the following.

2.1 Feature Sorting Methods

Feature selection is a dimensionality reduction technique, whose aim is to choose a small subset of the relevant features from the original features by removing irrelevant, redundant, or noisy features [36]. It usually leads to higher learning accuracy, lower computational cost, and better model interpretability. Based on the searching strategy, feature selection methods can be classified as wrapper methods, that require the application of a classifier to evaluate the quality of selected features, filter methods, that select the most discriminating features directly from data, wrapper methods, that use the intended learning algorithm itself to evaluate the features, and embedded methods, that perform feature selection in the process of model construction, while learning optimal parameters.

In [32], we adopted the recursive feature elimination (RFE) [20] using Support Vector Machines (SVM) [48], a wrapper method that provides a ranked list of features ordered according to their relevance. Here, we also consider two other methods for sorting features according to their decreasing relevance for classification.

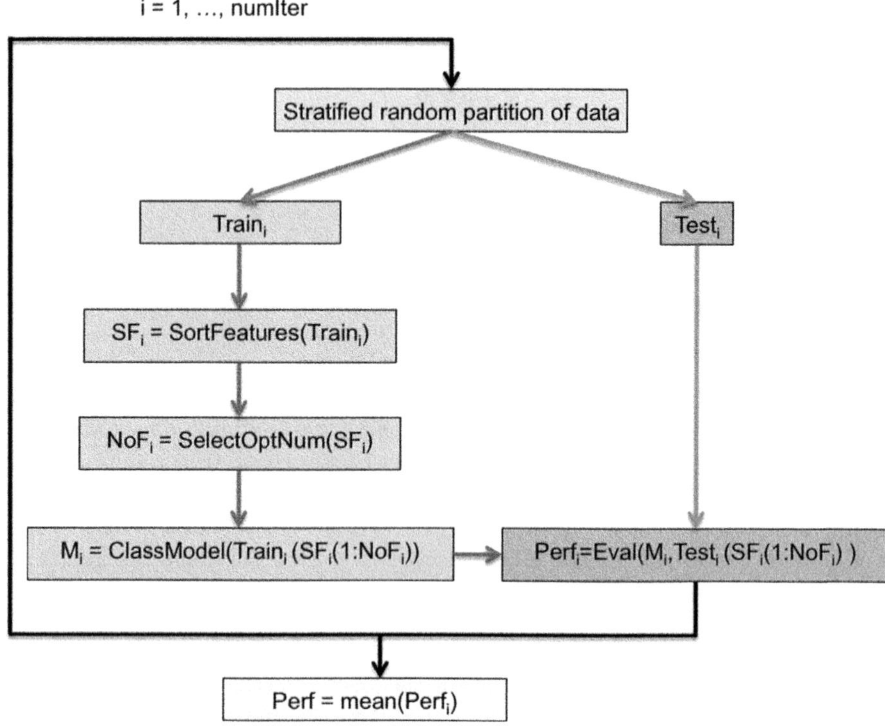

Fig. 1. CEF evaluation framework for classification.

Feature weighting using Neighborhood Component Analysis (NCA) [49] is a non-parametric and embedded method for selecting features with the goal of maximizing the prediction accuracy of a classification algorithm. Based on nearest neighbor feature weighting, it learns a feature weighting vector by maximizing, through a gradient ascent technique, the expected leave-one-out classification accuracy with a regularization term.

We further rank the features based on a class separability criterion based on entropy (ENTR), assessing the significance of every feature for separating two labeled groups. The relative entropy, also known as Kullback-Leibler distance or divergence, measures the distance between two probability distributions. Therefore it can be used to measure how different are the probability density functions of a feature in two classes.

2.2 Selection of the Optimal NoF

One of the usual means for deciding the number NoF of sorted features to be selected is to arbitrarily fix a threshold on the weight of the sorted features, taking only the first of them whose weight surpasses the threshold. Instead, in [32], the optimal NoF is automatically selected through k-fold cross-validation

(CV) of a classifier trained using the first NoF sorted features of the training data; the optimal value is chosen as the one that maximizes the AUC across the $numIter$ iterations of the process.

To better highlight the relationship between the classifier AUC value and error rate [12], here, we also consider the choice of NoF as the one that minimizes the loss across the iterations.

Both in [32] and here, to better handle class unbalancing of the considered dataset, oversampling in the training folds of the CV procedure is performed to balance the minority and majority classes. This is achieved using the adaptive synthetic sampling approach for imbalanced learning (ADASYN) method [21]. It adopts a weighted distribution for different minority class samples with reference to their level of difficulty. In this way, improvement during the learning procedure is twofold: first, a reduction of the bias introduced by the class imbalance, and, second, a shift of the classification decision boundary toward the more difficult samples.

2.3 Classifier Models

In [32], we adopted the k-Nearest Neighbor (kNN) [15] as a classification model trained on training data. Using kNN, each sample is classified by a majority vote of its neighbors, being assigned to the class most common amongst its k nearest neighbors measured by a distance function. In our case, $k = 1$, so that each sample is simply assigned to the class of its nearest neighbor.

Here, we consider two other classifiers. The first is a classification ensemble (in the following referred to as Ensemble), i.e., a predictive model composed of a weighted combination of multiple classification models. The Ensemble model is built by boosting classification trees via LogitBoost [16]. It includes a structural model for boosting, on the logistic scale, composed of different base learners providing additive components. An optimized set of learners works better than one. This configuration demonstrates that, in an empowerment situation where all basic learners are not equivalent, there is no unique optimal choice for all application contexts. This aspect explains many of the properties of boosting.

The second classifier (in the following referred to as Fitclinear) is a linear classifier. It trains linear classification models for binary class learning with high-dimensional, full or sparse predictor data. Moreover, it minimizes the objective function using techniques that reduce computing time (e.g., stochastic gradient descent). Here, we adopted a logistic regression model and the logit score transform function, $1/(1 + e^{-x})$.

3 Experimental Results

3.1 Data

RNA sequencing data was obtained from the NCI's Genomic Data Commons portal (https://portal.gdc.cancer.gov). This included FPKM (fragments per kilobase per million reads mapped) normalized gene counts from The Cancer Genome Atlas (TCGA) brain cancer projects TCGA-Glioblastoma Multiforme and TCGA-Low Grade Glioma (TCGA-GBM and TCGA-LGG). The TCGA-GBM contains 161 samples, and the TCGA-LGG contains 511 samples (refer to the TCGA column in Table 1). The brain tissue metabolic model [2] used in this study was downloaded from the Metabolic Atlas repository (https://metabolicatlas.org/). Sample-wise weighted and directed metabolic networks were constructed by combining the gene expression data and tissue-specific metabolic model, as in [19]. The nodes in the network represent the metabolites, while product-reactant metabolite pairs involved in the same reaction are connected by edges. These edges are weighted with the expression values of the enzymes corresponding to the reactions catalyzing the interacting metabolite couples. The simplification of the edges in the multigraphs is performed by taking the average of the enzyme expression of multiple edges connecting two nodes in the same reaction and then adding the means of different reactions. The resulting simple graphs contain 8458 edges, further reduced to 1375 by removing those edges with weights common to all samples, and are used in the experiments as omics features (O).

Table 1. Number of samples for each class (GBM and LGG) in the omics data (TCGA), the imaging data (TCIA1 publicly available, TCIA2 available on demand), their intersections (Set1 and Set2), and the union of these intersections (SetU).

	TCGA	TCIA1	TCIA2	Set1	Set2	SetU
GBM	161	102	33	21	9	30
LGG	511	65	43	63	41	104
Total	672	167	76	84	50	134

MRI pre-operative scans for a subset of patients from the TCGA-GBM and TGCA-LGG projects are available in The Cancer Imaging Archive (TCIA, cancerimagingarchive.net) [11]. Also available in the TCIA archive, are imaging features extracted from the TCGA-GBM and TGCA-LGG imaging collections by Bakas *et al.* [4–6] and are those used in our study (I). The authors selected a subset of radiological data that included pre-operative MRI baseline scans from the T1-weighted pre-contrast (T1), T1-weighted post-contrast (T1-Gd), T2, and T2- FLAIR (Fluid Attenuated Inversion Recovery) modalities. Pre-processing of MRI volumes and segmentation of glioma sub-regions was followed by volumetric feature extraction. This resulted in a panel of more than 700 features, with quantitative information regarding intensity, volumes, morphology, histogram-based, and textural parameters, as well as spatial information and parameters extracted from glioma growth models. The imaging features have been computed by the authors for 135 TCGA-GBM and 108 TGCA-LGG subjects. Among them, those for 102 GBM and 65 LGG samples (see column TCIA1 in Table 1) are publicly available through TCIA, while the remaining features (see column TCIA2 in

Table 2. Performance measures used in the experiments.

Name	Formula	Description
Accuracy	$\text{Acc} = \frac{\text{TP} + \text{TN}}{\text{TP} + \text{FN} + \text{FP} + \text{TN}}$	Percentage of correctly classified samples
Specificity	$\text{Spec} = \frac{\text{TN}}{\text{TN} + \text{FP}}$	Percentage of negative samples correctly identified
Sensitivity (or Recall or TPR)	$\text{Sens} = \frac{\text{TP}}{\text{TP} + \text{FN}}$	Percentage of positive samples correctly classified
Precision	$\text{Prec} = \frac{\text{TP}}{\text{TP} + \text{FP}}$	Percentage of positive samples correctly classified, considering the set of all the samples classified as positive
F-measure	$\text{F}_\beta = \frac{(1+\beta^2) \cdot \text{Prec} \cdot \text{Sens}}{(\beta^2 \cdot \text{Prec}) + \text{Sens}}$	Compromise between sensitivity and precision, weighted by $\beta \in \mathbb{R}^+$. In the experiments, $\beta = 1$
Adjusted F-measure	$\text{AGF} = \sqrt{F_2 \cdot InvF_{0.5}}$	Addresses imbalanced data, giving more weight to patterns correctly classified in the minority class [33]
G-mean	$\text{Gm} = \sqrt{\text{Sens} \cdot \text{Spec}}$	Geometric mean of the accuracy of both classes
Area Under the ROC Curve	$\text{AUC} = \int_0^1 \text{Sens}(x) dx,\ x = 1 - \text{Spec}$	Uses the ROC curve to exhibit the trade-off between the classifier's TP and FP rates

Table 1), are available only upon demand, as they have been used as test dataset for the MICCAI Brain Tumor Segmentation 2018 challenge (BraTS 2018)[1].

Matching the subject IDs of omics and imaging data, we obtained a total of 30 GBM and 104 LGG samples having both omics and imaging features (see SetU column in Table 1). This set is given by the union of the training set Set1 and the testing Set2, obtained by matching TCGA with TCIA1 and TCIA2 samples, respectively. In the following, we consider omics, imaging, and omics imaging features (denoted as O, I, and OI, respectively) for the matched samples belonging to sets Set1, Set2, and SetU.

3.2 Performance Measures

We consider the performance metrics summarized in Table 2, defined in terms of the number of true positives (TP), true negatives (TN), false positives (FP) and false negatives (FN). Here, the majority class (LGG) is assumed as the negative class, while the minority class (GBM) is assumed as the positive class.

For all the metrics, higher values indicate better performance results. While all of them contribute to investigating the performance results, in our analyses,

[1] https://www.med.upenn.edu/sbia/brats2018.html.

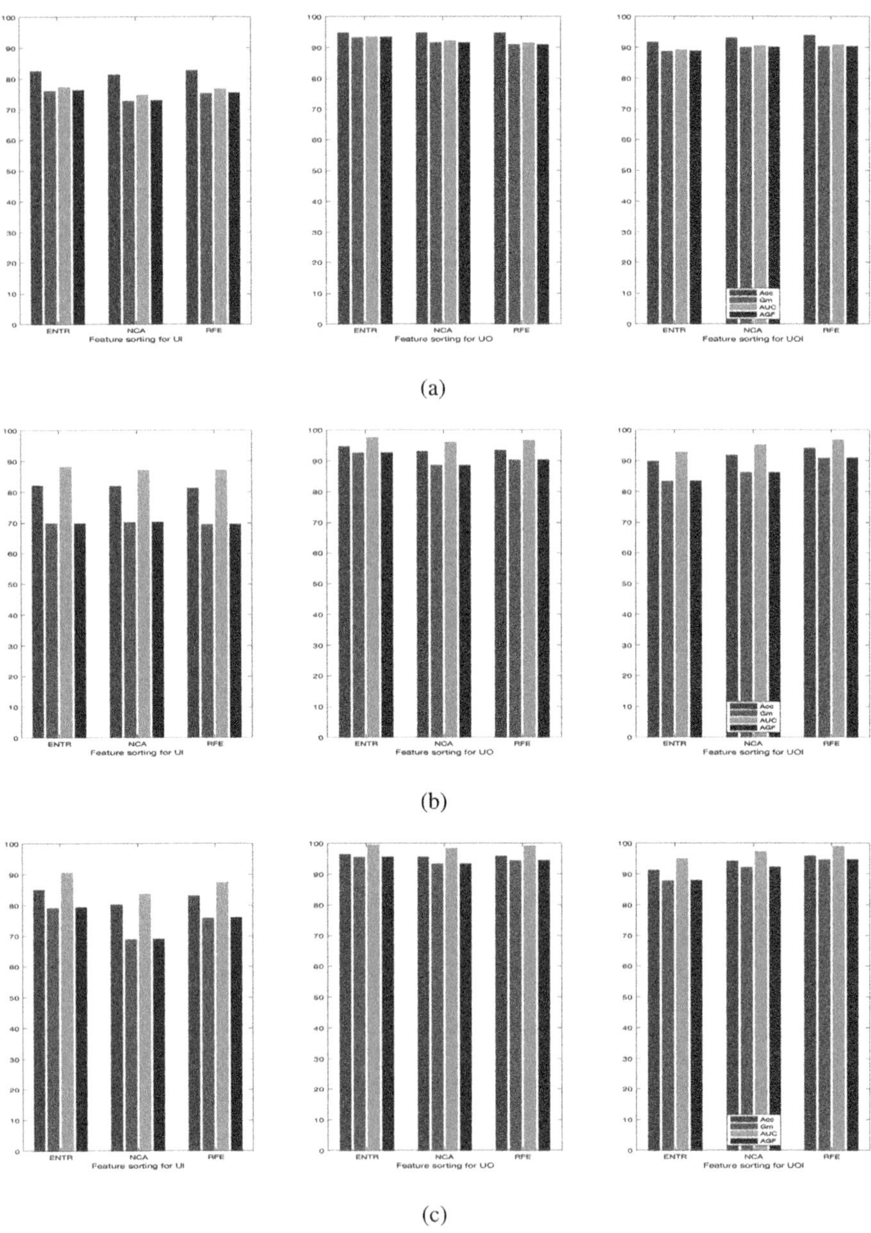

Fig. 2. Varying the feature sorting method: average performance on the I (left column), O (center column), and OI (right column) datasets using ENTR (left bars), NCA (center bars), and RFE (right bars) feature sorting and three classifiers (a) kNN, (b) Ensemble, (c) Fitclinear.

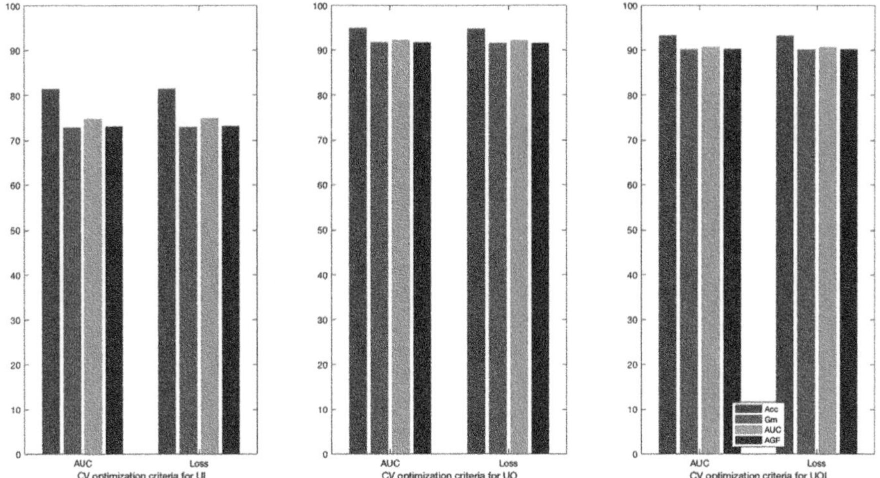

Fig. 3. Varying the optimization criterion for CV-based selection of NoF: average performance on the I (left column), O (center column), and OI (right column) datasets using AUC maximization (left bars) and Loss minimization (right bars).

we mainly refer to Acc, Gm, AUC, and AGF, as they better balance the contribution of the two unbalanced classes to the overall performance. Nonetheless, we provide values for all the metrics in our web pages, so as to make them available for future comparisons.

3.3 Performance Results in SetU

The CEF framework described in Sect. 2 has been evaluated on I, O, and OI features of SetU, varying the method for sorting features (Sect. 2.1), the criterion for computing the optimal number of features (Sect. 2.2), and the classifier model (Sect. 2.3).

The framework has been implemented in Matlab; all its scripts are made publicly available through our web pages. For feature sorting, we adopted the Matlab functions `fscnca` for NCA and `rankfeatures` for ENTR, while we used our implementation of RFE. The classifier models were built using the `fitcknn`, `fitcensemble`, and `fitclinear` Matlab functions and evaluated through the `predict` function. The number $numIter$ of iterations of the entire procedure was fixed to 100.

In Fig. 2, we report the average performance obtained by CEF varying the feature sorting method. Here, we observe that, generally, a) performance obtained using only I features is always lower than that achieved using O and OI features; b) best performances are obtained when sorting features based on ENTR in the case of I and O features and RFE in the case of OI features, and this holds whichever is the adopted classifier.

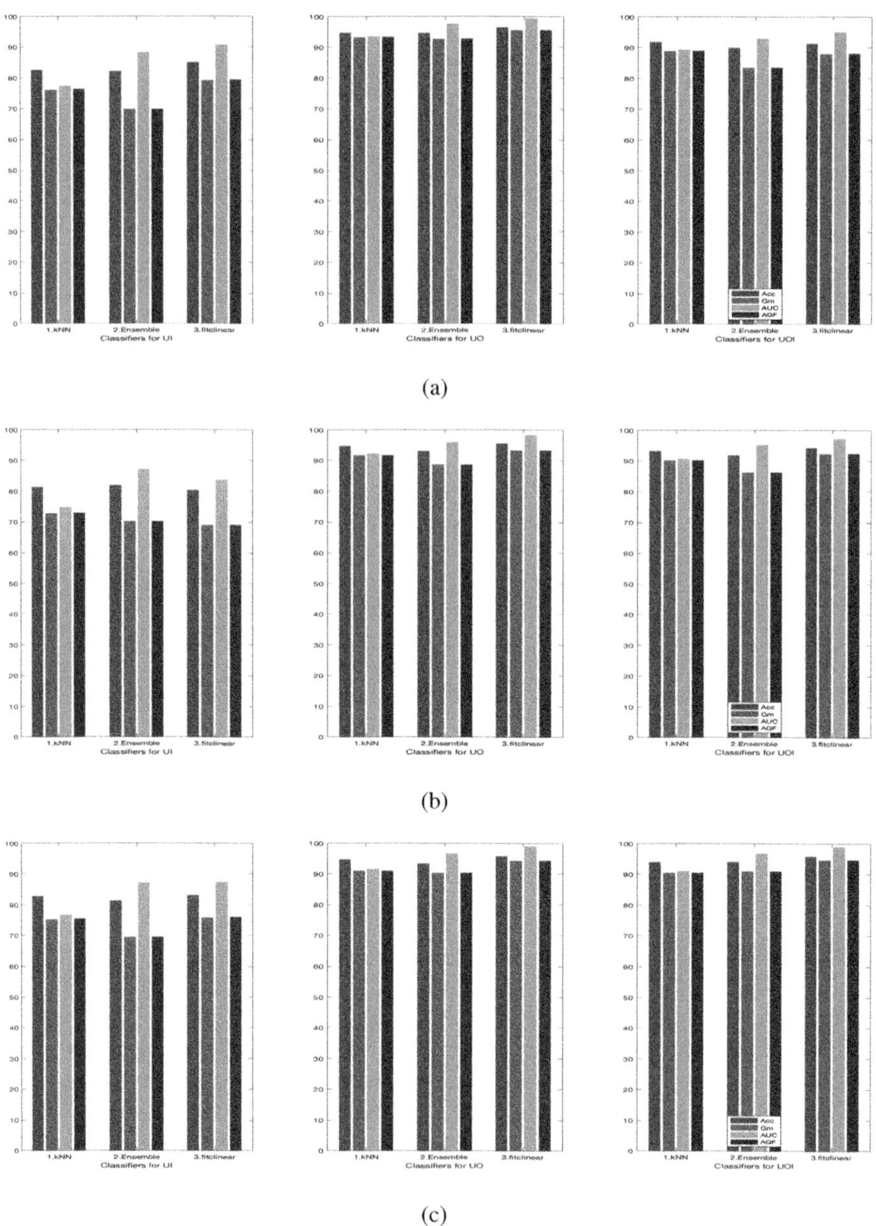

Fig. 4. Varying the classifier: average performance on the I (left column), O (center column), and OI (right column) datasets using the kNN (left bars), Ensemble (center bars), and Fitclinear (right bars) classifiers, with features sorted by (a) ENTR, (b) NCA, and (c) RFE.

Table 3. Summary of the compared methods for glioma grade classification.

1st author year [Ref]	# HGG	# LGG	Data & source	Method
Law, 2003 [30]	120	40	Perfusion MR, proton MR spectroscopy	Logistic regression and ROC analysis of relative cerebral blood volume (rCBV) and metabolite ratios (m.r.)
Zacharaki, 2009 [51]	52	22	MRI, perfusion MRI	SVM-RFE to select a subset from 161 imaging features + weighted SVM classifier
Ertosun, 2015 [14]	48	52	Digital pathology images (WSI) [27]	DL: Ensemble of CNNs
Togao, 2016 [47]	29	16	IntraVoxel Incoherent Motion (IVIM) MRI	ROC analysis to evaluate the diagnostic accuracy of various parameters (the best is the volume fraction within a voxel of water flowing in perfused capillars)
Chen, 2018 [9]	220	54	MRI [35]	Multiscale 3D CNN segmentation + SVM-RFE radiomics features selection + XGboost classifier
Cho, 2018 [10]	210	75	MRI [35]	MRMR algorithm to select 5 among 468 radiomics features, used to build 3 different classifier models
Khawaldeh, 2018 [26]	213	235	MRI [11,43]	DL: based on AlexNet, trained using single 2D MRI slices. Three class classification problem (including 139 healthy samples)
Yang, 2018 [50]	61	52	MRI ClinicalTrials.gov	DL: transfer learning from 2D GoogLeNet (manually specified ROIs)
Zhuge, 2020 [52]	210	105	MRI [6,35]	DL: 3D segmentation + 2D R-CNN on the slice with largest tumor area or 3DConvNet on the 3D segmentation

Figure 3 compares average performance results obtained using the two optimization criteria for choosing NoF, with NCA feature sorting and kNN classifier. It can be observed that no substantial difference can be found between results obtained by the two optimization criteria. This holds true also using other feature sorting methods and different classifiers (not shown here).

Average performance results obtained using the three different classifiers with features sorted by ENTR, NCA, and RFE methods are reported in Fig. 4. Here, it can be observed that Fitclinear leads to the best performance for all the types of data, regardless of the method adopted for sorting features.

3.4 Comparisons with Existing Classification Methods

Several methods have been proposed in the literature for the classification of glioma grades, exploiting various types of imaging sources. Some of them are summarized in Table 3, where we report bibliographic information (name of the

Table 4. Performance (%) of methods for glioma grade classification.

Method	Acc	Sens	Spec	AUC
Law *et al.* [30], only rCBV		95.0	57.5	
Law *et al.* [30], rCBV+m.r		93.3	60.0	
Zacharaki *et al.* [51]	87.8	84.6	95.5	89.6
Ertosun *et al.* [14]	96.0	98.0	94.0	
Togao *et al.* [47]		96.6	81.2	95.0
Chen *et al.* [9]	91.3	91.3		95.0
Cho *et al.* [10]	88.5	95.1	70.2	90.3
Khawaldeh *et al.* [26]	91.3	87.5	95.3	
Yang *et al.* [50]	94.5			96.8
Zhuge *et al.* [52], 2D R-CNN	96.3	93.5	97.2	
Zhuge *et al.* [52], 3DConvNet	97.1	94.7	96.8	
Maddalena *et al.* [32] I	80.5	69.5	83.7	76.6
Maddalena *et al.* [32] O	95.1	90.7	96.5	93.6
Maddalena *et al.* [32] OI	95.0	91.1	96.1	93.6
CEF I	85.1	71.4	89.1	90.6
CEF O	96.5	94.2	97.2	99.4
CEF OI	96.0	92.9	96.9	99.1

first author, year, and reference), the number of samples for the high-grade and low-grade glioma classes, the type of imaging data (eventually with reference to their source), and a very short description of the adopted method (here, DL stands for Deep Learning, one of the most recent, but now widespread, approaches).

In Table 4, we compare the performance of these methods (as reported by the authors themselves), bearing in mind that each has been validated by its authors on a different set of data. For direct comparison, we also report the best average performance results achieved for each of the data sources (I, O, and OI) in [32] and with CEF (Fitclinear classifier with ENTR feature sorting for I and O features and RFE feature sorting for OI features). Overall, we can conclude that the proposed approach based on using O and OI features shows average

Table 5. Best test performance on Set2.

	Acc	Sens	Spec	Prec	F_1	Gm	AUC	AGF
I	88.0	88.9	87.8	61.5	72.7	88.4	91.5	88.2
O	96.0	100.0	95.1	81.8	90.0	97.5	100.0	97.4
OI	98.0	100.0	97.6	90.0	94.7	98.8	100.0	98.7

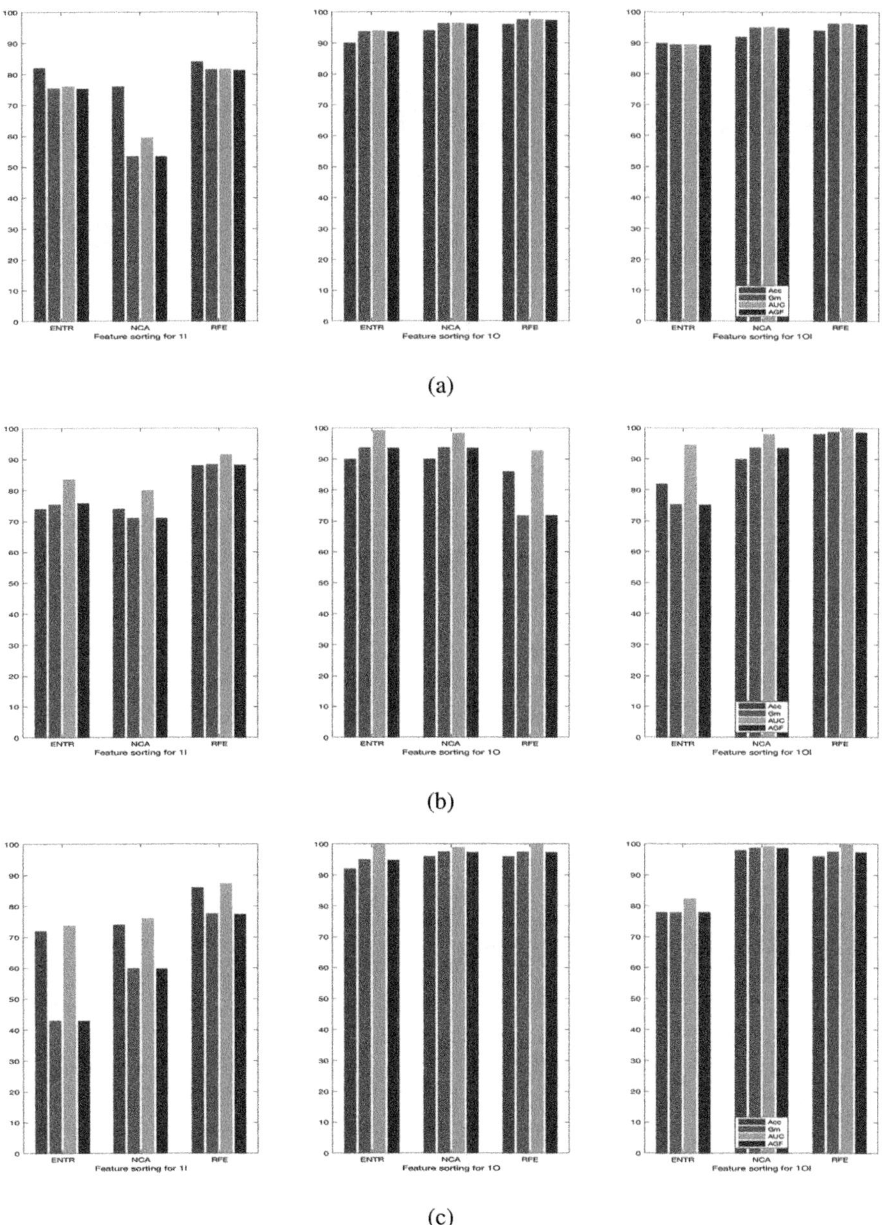

Fig. 5. Varying the feature sorting method on Set2: performance on the I (left column), O (center column), and OI (right column) datasets using ENTR (left bars), NCA (center bars), and RFE (right bars) feature sorting and three classifiers (a) kNN, (b) Ensemble, (c) Fitclinear.

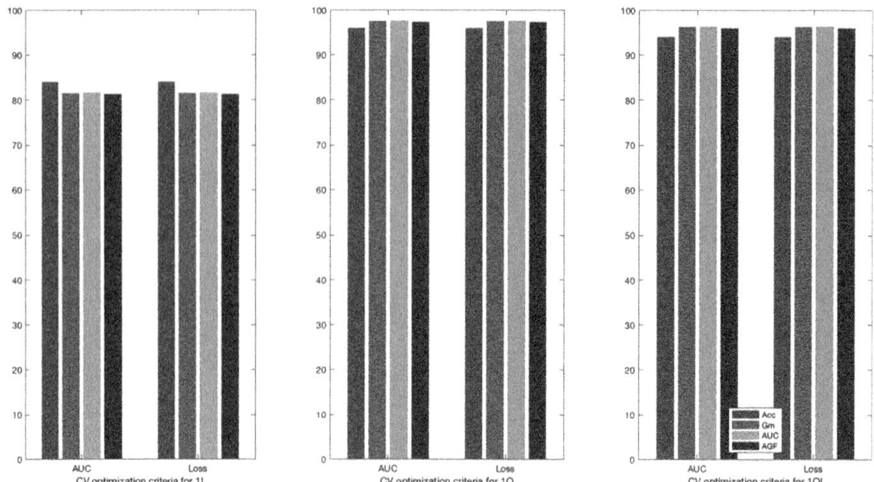

Fig. 6. Varying the optimization criterion for CV-based selection of NoF on Set2: performance on the I (left column), O (center column), and OI (right column) features using AUC maximization (left bars) and Loss minimization (right bars).

performance similar to or higher than most of the compared methods in terms of all the considered performance metrics. Moreover, the performance achieved with CEF surpasses that of the previous evaluation framework [32] in terms of all the metrics. However, contrary to our previous experience, it appears that, on average, omics features alone lead to better results than integrated omics and imaging features when using the best combination of feature sorting and classification methods. This point deserves further analysis, carried out in the following section.

3.5 Performance Results in Set2

Besides testing the performance in a generally agreed way, as an average over repeated training/test partitioning of the data (as done in Sects. 3.3 and 3.4), we want to verify the suitability of the adopted approach in a specific application, to better speculate in a real case scenario. Therefore, here, we consider a single iteration of our classification framework, where a classification model is learned solely on the Set1 training set and evaluated on the Set2 test set.

Figures 5, 6 and 7 report performance results on the I, O, and OI features of Set2, with training performed solely on Set1. As in Sect. 3.3, we vary the feature sorting method (Fig. 5), the optimization criterion for CV-based selection of NoF (Fig. 6), and the classification model (Fig. 7). Contrary to the average performance computed in the previous sections, best testing performances are obtained when sorting features based on RFE for most of the cases. ENTR and NCA are better suited for O data with the Ensemble classifier (Fig. 5-(b), center), while RFE leads to the best overall performance for OI data with the

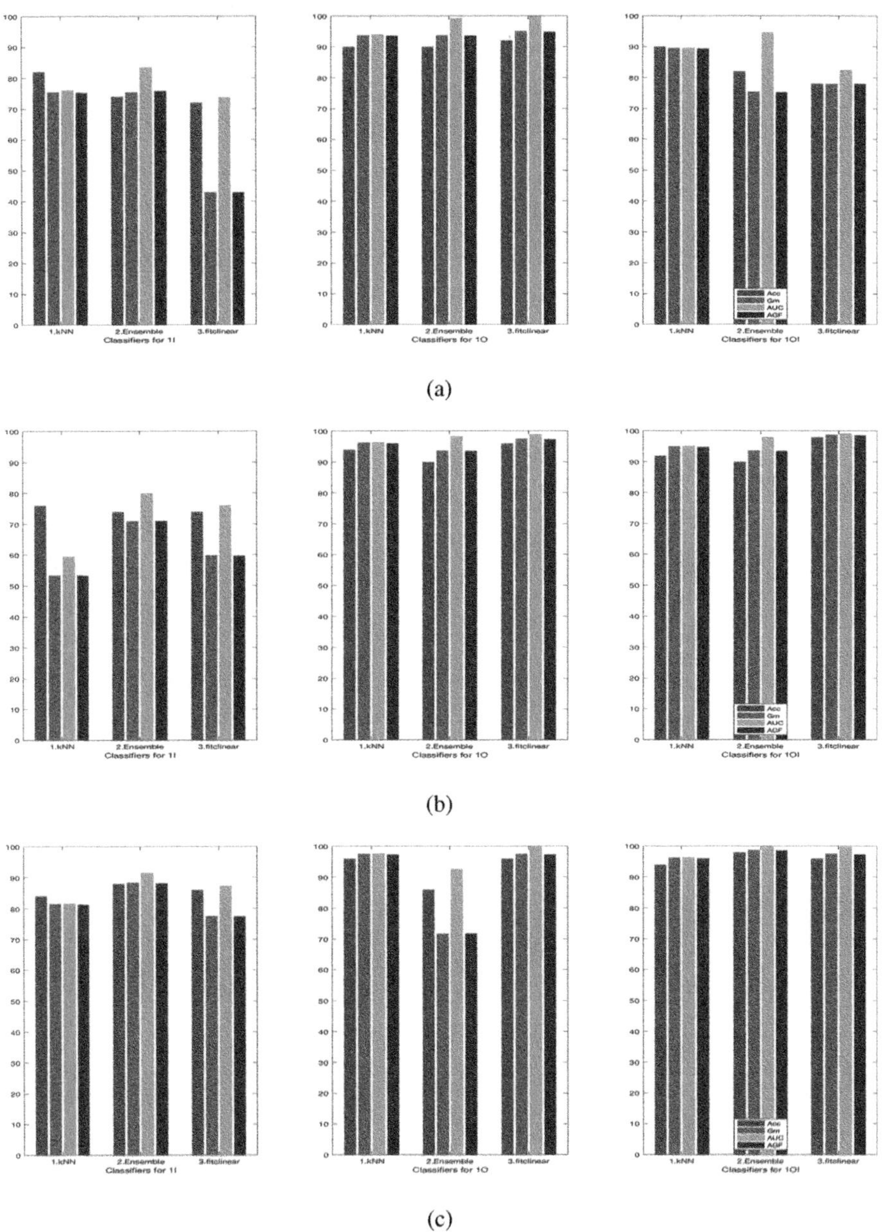

Fig. 7. Varying the classifier on Set2: performance on the I (left column), O (center column), and OI (right column) features using the kNN (left bars), Ensemble (center bars), and Fitclinear (right bars) classifier classifiers, with features sorted by (a) ENTR, (b) NCA, and (c) RFE.

Table 6. Omics features annotation.

Feature	Reaction	Enzymes symbol	Subsystem
m00247c_m00569c	HMR_4371	PGAM2, PGAM1, BPGM, PGAM4	Glycolysis
m01688c_m01680c	HMR_4570, HMR_6623, HMR_7851	NME family, TK1, SLC25A19	Purine, Pyrimidine, Transp. mitochondrial
m01306c_m00669c	HMR_3777	BCAT1	Valine, leucine, and isoleucine
m01694l_m01679l	HMR_8217	GLA	Sphingolipid
m01913s_m01910s	HMR_4416	GLA, GLB1, RPL36A	Galactose
m01734r_m01896r	HMR_7274	ALG3	N-glycan
m00826m_m02189m	HMR_3769 HMR_3770	IVD, ACADSB	Valine, leucine, and isoleucine; Glycine, serine and threonine
m02832r_m01230r	HMR_6650	RBP2, RBP1	Retinol
m01869g_m01870g	HMR_7329	MGAT4C	N-glycan
m01690c_m01939c	HMR_4391	TPI1, TPI1P2	Glycolysis
m02579c_2579s	HMR_5023	RHAG	Transp. extracellular
m01673c_m01755c	HMR_4641	TK1	Nucleotide
m01673c_m01680c	HMR_6623	TK1	Pyrimidine
m02845c_m02806c	HMR_4052	PRPS2, PRPS1	Pentose phosphate path.
m02870c_m02926c	HMR_4077	SMS, SRM	Arginine and proline
m01045c_m01700c	HMR_4644	TYMS	Pyrimidine
m02122m_m00053m	HMR_3156	ACADSB	β oxidation of even-chain FA (mitochondrial)
m01637m_m01642m	HMR_6612, HMR_6615, HMR_7854	DTYMK, NME family, SLC25A19	Pyrimidine, Transport mitochondrial
m01747m_m01642m	HMR_6612, HMR_7848	DTYMK, SLC25A19	Pyrimidine, Transport mitochondrial
m02344c_2344s	HMR_0190	CA family, NAE1, ABCA1, AP1G1	Transport extracellular
m00809c_m00968c	HMR_1500	HSD17B7	Cholesterol biosynthesis 1 (Bloch pathway)
m01939c_m00247c	HMR_4373	GAPDH, GAPDHS	Glycolysis
m00267l_m00266l	HMR_7916	GGH	Folate metabolism
m01427c_m02730c	HMR_0607	CDS2, CDS1	Glycerophospholipid
m01637m_m01752m	HMR_6612	DTYMK	Pyrimidine
m02008l_m01910l	HMR_0832	GLB1	Glycosphingolipid
m03108r_m03106r	HMR_7278, HMR_8248	ALG5, UGCG	N-glycan, Sphingolipid
m02583c_m00536c	HMR_7676	NNMT	Nicotinate and nicotinamide metabolism
m02139l_m01973l	HMR_7573	GUSB	Heparan sulfate degradation
m02870c_m01116c	HMR_4075	SRM	Arginine and proline
m01972l_m01430l	HMR_0787	GBA, SAPCD1	Glycosphingolipid
m01990c_m01992c	HMR_5397	GBE1	Starch and sucrose
m02133c_m02471c	HMR_3917 HMR_4699	MTR, BHMT2, BHMT	Cysteine, methionine; Glycine, serine, threonine
m02658c_m02812c	HMR_4212	ODC1	Arginine and proline
m01868g_m01869g	HMR_7328	MGAT5	N-glycan metabolism
m00240c_m02392c	HMR_0031	PLIN family, FITM1, BSCL2, CIDEA, FITM2	Pool reactions
m01965c_m01965g	HMR_7675	SLC2A1	Transp. Golgi
m01821s_m01822s	HMR_3991	CP, HSP3, FXN, FTH1, FTMT, FTH1P5	Porphyrin
m01307c_m02335c	HMR_5131	AARS1, AARS2	Aminoacyl-tRNA biosynthesis
m00351c_m00349c	HMR_8710	RDH5	Retinol
m00554c_m00555c	HMR_6587	PIK3C3	Inositol phosphate
m02026c_m02366c	HMR_1081	LTC4S	Leukotriene
m02409p_m02348p	HMR_3033 HMR_3034	SLC25A20, CROT, SLC25A29	Carnitine shuttle (peroxisomal)

Table 7. Selected features using ENTR for feature sorting on OI data.

Mode on SetU	On Set1
TEXTURE_GLRLM_ET_T1Gd_SRE	SPATIAL_Cere
TEXTURE_GLRLM_ET_T2_SRE	TEXTURE_GLSZM_NET_T1Gd_LZHGE
TEXTURE_GLSZM_NET_T1Gd_LZHGE	TEXTURE_GLCM_ET_T2_Energy
TEXTURE_GLRLM_ET_FLAIR_SRE	TEXTURE_GLCM_ET_T1Gd_Energy
TEXTURE_NGTDM_ET_T1Gd_Coarseness	TEXTURE_GLRLM_ET_T2_SRE
TEXTURE_GLSZM_ET_T1Gd_ZSV	TEXTURE_GLSZM_ET_FLAIR_GLV
TEXTURE_GLSZM_ET_FLAIR_GLV	TEXTURE_GLRLM_ET_T1Gd_SRE
TEXTURE_GLRLM_ET_T2_RP	TEXTURE_GLOBAL_ET_T1Gd_Kurtosis
TEXTURE_GLSZM_ET_T2_ZSV	TEXTURE_GLRLM_ET_FLAIR_SRE
TEXTURE_GLRLM_ET_T1_SRE	TEXTURE_GLSZM_ET_T2_GLV
TEXTURE_GLSZM_ET_T1_ZSV	TEXTURE_GLSZM_ET_T1Gd_ZSV
TEXTURE_GLSZM_ET_T2_GLV	TEXTURE_GLSZM_ET_T1_GLV
m02579c_2579s	TEXTURE_GLRLM_ET_T2_RP
TEXTURE_GLRLM_ET_T1Gd_RP	TEXTURE_GLSZM_ET_T1_ZSV
TEXTURE_NGTDM_ET_T1_Coarseness	TEXTURE_NGTDM_ET_T1Gd_Coarseness
TEXTURE_GLSZM_ET_T1_GLV	TEXTURE_GLRLM_ET_T1Gd_RP
TEXTURE_GLCM_ET_T1Gd_Energy	TEXTURE_GLCM_ET_FLAIR_Energy
TEXTURE_GLCM_ET_T2_Energy	TEXTURE_GLSZM_ET_T1Gd_GLV
TEXTURE_NGTDM_ET_T2_Coarseness	TEXTURE_GLRLM_ET_T1_SRE
TEXTURE_GLRLM_ET_FLAIR_RP	TEXTURE_GLSZM_NET_T1_LZHGE
TEXTURE_GLSZM_NET_T2_LZE	TEXTURE_GLSZM_NET_T2_LZLGE
TEXTURE_GLSZM_ET_T1Gd_GLV	TEXTURE_NGTDM_ET_T2_Coarseness
TEXTURE_GLSZM_NET_T2_LZLGE	TEXTURE_GLRLM_ET_FLAIR_RP
TEXTURE_GLCM_ET_FLAIR_Energy	TEXTURE_NGTDM_ET_T1_Coarseness
TEXTURE_GLOBAL_ET_T1Gd_Kurtosis	m02579c_2579s
TEXTURE_GLCM_ET_T2_Entropy	
TEXTURE_GLRLM_ET_T2_RLN	
TEXTURE_GLSZM_ET_FLAIR_ZSV	
TEXTURE_GLRLM_ET_T1Gd_RLN	
SPATIAL_Cere	

Ensemble classifier (Fig. 5-(b), right). Also NCA with the Fitclinear classifier leads to high performance for OI data (Fig. 5-(c), center).

As in the case of the whole SetU, no substantial difference can be perceived when varying the optimization criterion. This can be observed in Fig. 6, reporting performance results using RFE feature sorting and the kNN classifier.

Ensemble is the classifier model leading to the best performance in the case of I features (left column of Fig. 7), whichever sorted, while Fitclinear leads to the best performance for O features (center column of Fig. 7). In the case of OI data (right column of Fig. 7), each classifier leads to the highest performance with different feature sorting methods. The overall highest performance is achieved with RFE sorting on OI data using the Ensemble classifier (right plot of Fig. 7-(b)). The best test performance on Set2 for each type of feature is reported in Table 5. This is achieved using RFE for feature sorting and Ensemble (for I and OI features) or Fitclinear (for O features) classifiers.

Table 8. Selected features using NCA for feature sorting on OI data.

Mode on SetU	On Set1
m00247c_m00569c	m00247c_m00569c
m01688c_m01680c	m01688c_m01680c
VOLUME_ET_over_TC	m01306c_m00669c
VOLUME_NET_over_TC	VOLUME_ET_OVER_WT
m01694l_m01679l	m01694l_m01679l
m01913s_m01910s	m01734r_m01896r
m00826m_m02189m	m01913s_m01910s
m02832r_m01230r	m01869g_m01870g
m01690c_m01939c	m00826m_m02189m
m02579c_2579s	m01673c_m01755c
VOLUME_ET_OVER_WT	m01673c_m01680c
m02845c_m02806c	m02870c_m02926c
m01734r_m01896r	m01045c_m01700c
VOLUME_ET_OVER_BRAIN	m02122m_m00053m
m01637m_m01642m	m02832r_m01230r
m01747m_m01642m	TEXTURE_GLCM_ET_T2_Variance
m02344c_2344s	m00809c_m00968c
m01306c_m00669c	m01690c_m01939c
m01869g_m01870g	m01747m_m01642m
m01939c_m00247c	VOLUME_NET_over_TC
VOLUME_ET	VOLUME_ET_over_TC
m00267l_m00266l	m01427c_m02730c
m01673c_m01680c	m02845c_m02806c
m01673c_m01755c	m01637m_m01752m
m02008l_m01910l	m03108r_m03106r
m02583c_m00536c	TEXTURE_GLRLM_ET_T2_LRHGE
m02870c_m02926c	TEXTURE_GLCM_ET_T2_AutoCorrelation
VOLUME_ET_OVER_NET	m02139l_m01973l
TEXTURE_NGTDM_ET_T2_Busyness	m02870c_m01116c
m03108r_m03106r	m01939c_m00247c

Comparing performance results on Set2 with average results obtained on SetU (Sect. 3.3), we conclude that 1) the performance obtained using I features alone is always lower than that achieved using O and OI features; 2) for I features,

ENTR on average, but RFE in Set2, are the feature sorting methods of choice, regardless of the adopted classifier; 3) for O features, best results are obtained using ENTR on average, but RFE in Set2, except if used in conjunction with the Ensemble classifier (where ENTR and NCA provide better sorted features); 4) for OI features, RFE appears as the feature sorting method to choose, both on average and in Set2. In Set2, also NCA leads to effective sorted features when coupled with kNN and Fitclinear classifiers; 5) no substantial difference can be found between results obtained by the two optimization criteria for CV-based selection of the optimal number of sorted features, and this holds true regardless the feature sorting methods and classifier methods.

3.6 Analysis of the Selected Features

Table 7 reports the names of the features selected using the ENTR feature sorting method on OI data. Specifically, the left column reports the names of the thirty OI features most frequently selected in the training set of each of the 100 iterations of the CEF evaluation procedure on SetU. The right column reports the names of the NoF=25 OI features selected when training the classification model on the Set1 dataset (with NoF automatically computed by CV). Most of the compared features (96% of them) appear in both the columns. All the features, except one, belong to the imaging data and mainly deal with MRI image texture, as can be deduced by their names provided by the authors [5,6]. Only one of the selected features (m02579c_2579s, named according to the acronyms of the involved metabolites) belongs to the omics data. The integration of omics data into a metabolic model scaffold allowed us to build sample-specific networks from which to extract relevant biological information. The metabolites connection weighted by enzymes expression values, through the gene-protein-reaction relationship (GPR) annotations, represents the structure of the networks, as well as the features extracted by the different methods applied in this work. From the metabolites couple, various information can be recovered and exploited to furnish novel insights about candidate biomarkers and therapeutic targets. Indeed, the metabolic annotations can concern the compounds, the whole reaction with its related subsystem, and finally, the enzymes involved in catalyzing the reaction itself. For each extracted feature, the above-mentioned annotations are reported in Table 6.

In [32], we analyzed the first three most recurrent features obtained from omics and omics imaging over 50 iterations of the evaluation procedure (namely, m00247c_m00569c, m02579c_2579s, and m01972l_m01430l). They were exactly the same, confirming their strong discriminative power. The only omics feature selected in this case is one of the three, and its biological relevance associated with cellular growth, death, apoptosis has already been discussed in [32].

Analogously, Table 8 reports the names of the features selected using the NCA feature sorting method on OI data. Many of the compared features (66.67% of them) appear in both the columns. Here, only seven (left column) or six (right column) imaging features have been selected, related to imaging volumes and texture. Concerning omics features, in total, 17 metabolite couples are the same in both columns, out of 23 for the right one and out of 24 for the left one. The enzymes and reactions related to these common features are mostly involved in Glycolysis/Gluconeogenesis, Nucleotide, Branched-chain amino acid, and Sphingolipid metabolism. All these biological processes are known to be involved in cancer cell survival and invasion. Glycolysis, nucleotide, and amino acids metabolism are key factors for the higher energetic demand of cells aimed at incessantly proliferating. It is worth to cite PGAM1, the brain isoform of the phosphoglyceric acid mutase, which catalyzes the reaction 1,3-bisphospho-D-glycerate → 2,3-bisphospho-D-glycerate (m00247c_m00569c), since its abundance has been correlated to aggressiveness and poor prognosis of tumors [45]. Sphingolipids are highly abundant in the brain, as they are part of the myelin sheaths of nerve axons and are largely involved in cellular signaling triggered by external stimuli. Their metabolism represents, indeed, a novel resource for the treatment of GBM, as well as neurodegenerative disorders [41,46].

For the case of RFE feature sorting on OI data, Table 9 reports the names of the selected features. Many of the compared features (61.11% of them) appear in both the columns. Only three (left column) or four (right column) imaging features have been selected, related to imaging volumes, texture, histograms, and spatial properties. Intersecting the omics features of the left columns in Table 8 and Table 9, thirteen of them are commons, and again processes like Glycolysis, Amminoacids, and Nucleotides metabolism are enriched. The first metabolite couple (m00247c_m00569c), common to both the columns, is the same found using NCA feature sorting (see Table 8). The unique features extracted by the RFE sorting are also worth to be mentioned. In particular, iron regulation of the porphyrin metabolism, here charged by the reactions involving the metabolites couple m01821s_m01822s and the enzymes CP, HSP3, FXN, FTH1, FTMT, FTH1P5, is increasingly being associated with high tumor grade and poor survival in GBM [25,40]. The Leukotriene metabolism, here represented by the connection between Glutathione and Leukotriene C4 (m02026c_m02366c) from the reaction HMR_1081 (GSH[c] + leukotriene A4[c] → leukotriene C4[c]), has a role in the progression of several types of cancers as an inflammatory pathway and the expression of its products and related proteins is upregulated in glioma cells [38]. Cancer cells, moreover, exploit the fine carnitine system as a key resource for the metabolic plasticity, through the involvement of its carriers, such as SLC25A20, SLC25A29 and CROT, here catalyzing the reactions involving the link m02409p_m02348p [34]. In both NCA and RFE selection, features concerning the retinol metabolism are present. Gliomas show an imbalance in retinoid receptor expression that increases the endogenous production of retinoic acid (RA) in glia. Different types of alterations regarding the RA synthesis have been found in glioblastoma and, as novel insights from integrative approaches, may contribute to reconsider current RA treatment strategies [8]. Furthermore, the couple m02579c_2579s (found using ENTR feature sorting, see Table 7) is also here selected in both the columns.

Table 9. Selected features using RFE for feature sorting on OI data.

Mode on SetU	On Set1
m00247c_m00569c	m00247c_m00569c
m02579c_2579s	m01673c_m01755c
m01972l_m01430l	m02344c_2344s
m02344c_2344s	VOLUME_ET_OVER_BRAIN
m01688c_m01680c	m02026c_m02366c
m01690c_m01939c	m02870c_m02926c
m01990c_m01992c	m01972l_m01430l
m02133c_m02471c	m02658c_m02812c
VOLUME_ET_OVER_WT	m01990c_m01992c
m02658c_m02812c	VOLUME_ET
m01673c_m01755c	m02870c_m01116c
m01868g_m01869g	TEXTURE_GLSZM_NET_T2_SZLGE
m02845c_m02806c	m02579c_2579s
m01913s_m01910s	m01673c_m01680c
m00809c_m00968c	m00240c_m02392c
SPATIAL_Insula	m01673m_m01680m
m00240c_m02392c	m02409p_m02348p
m01965c_m01965g	HISTO_ED_T2_Bin3
m01939c_m00247c	
m00267l_m00266l	
VOLUME_ET	
m00826m_m02189m	
m01821s_m01822s	
VOLUME_ET_OVER_BRAIN	
m01673c_m01680c	
m02832r_m01230r	
VOLUME_ET_OVER_NET	
m01307c_m02335c	
m00351c_m00349c	
m00554c_m00555c	

4 Discussion and Conclusion

We investigated how the adoption of different classifier models or feature selection algorithms and the integration of imaging and omics data affect the performance results for the classification of glioma grades. Our analysis confirms that the performance obtained using only I features is always lower than that achieved using O and OI features. Moreover, it highlights that feature sorting methods should be chosen depending on the type of data (e.g., ENTR or RFE for I features, ENTR, RFE, or NCA for O features, RFE or NCA for OI features). This is not a limitation, as the choice can be performed automatically, based on cross-validated results on training data. Both the optimization criteria for CV-based selection of the optimal number of sorted features can be considered, as they lead to similar performance results. Finally, Fitclinear and Ensemble proved to be the preferred classifiers.

Performance results for a specific training/test setting allowed us to analyze punctual performance results and the significance of the extracted features, also from the biological point of view.

We are confident that making the software and the extracted data publicly available, as we did, can lay the foundations for future comparisons.

Availability

Matlab scripts are made available through our webpages. Extracted omics features for Set1 and Set2 are also made available. Imaging features for Set1 are already publicly available, while Set2 is available on demand.

Acknowledgments. The work was carried out also within the activities of all the authors as members of the ICAR-CNR INdAM Research Unit. M. Manzo acknowledges the guidance and supervision of Prof. Alfredo Petrosino during the years spent working together. The authors would like to thank G. Trerotola for technical support.

References

1. Acharya, U.R., Hagiwara, Y., Sudarshan, V.K., Chan, W.Y., Ng, K.H.: Towards precision medicine: from quantitative imaging to radiomics. J. Zhejiang Univ. Sci. B **19**, 6–24 (2018). https://doi.org/10.1631/jzus.B1700260
2. Agren, R., Bordel, S., Mardinoglu, A., et al.: Reconstruction of genome-scale active metabolic networks for 69 human cell types and 16 cancer types using INIT. PLoS Comput. Biol. **8**(5), e1002518 (2012)
3. Antonelli, L., Guarracino, M.R., Maddalena, L., et al.: Integrating imaging and omics data: a review. Biomed. Signal Process. Control **52**, 264–280 (2019). https://doi.org/10.1016/j.bspc.2019.04.032, http://www.sciencedirect.com/science/article/pii/S1746809419301326
4. Bakas, S., Akbari, H., Sotiras, A., et al.: Advancing the cancer genome atlas glioma MRI collections with expert segmentation labels and radiomic features. Sci. Data **4** (2017). https://doi.org/10.1038/sdata.2017.117
5. Bakas, S., Akbari, H., Sotiras, A., et al.: Segmentation labels and radiomic features for the pre-operative scans of the TCGA-GBM collection. Cancer Imaging Arch. (2017). https://doi.org/10.7937/K9/TCIA.2017.KLXWJJ1Q
6. Bakas, S., Akbari, H., Sotiras, A., et al.: Segmentation labels and radiomic features for the pre-operative scans of the TCGA-LGG collection. Cancer Imaging Arch. (2017). https://doi.org/10.7937/K9/TCIA.2017.GJQ7R0EF

7. Beig, N., et al.: Radiogenomic analysis of hypoxia pathway reveals computerized MRI descriptors predictive of overall survival in glioblastoma. In: Proceedings of SPIE, vol. 10134, pp. 101341U–101341U-10 (2017). https://doi.org/10.1117/12.2255694
8. Campos, B., et al.: Retinoid resistance and multifaceted impairment of retinoic acid synthesis in glioblastoma. Glia **63**(10), 1850–1859 (2015)
9. Chen, W., Liu, B., Peng, S., Sun, J., Qiao, X.: Computer-aided grading of gliomas combining automatic segmentation and radiomics. Int. J. Biomed. Imaging **2018**, 2512037:1–2512037:11 (2018). https://doi.org/10.1155/2018/2512037
10. Cho, H.H., Lee, S.H., Kim, J., et al.: Classification of the glioma grading using radiomics analysis. PeerJ **6** (2018). https://doi.org/10.7717/peerj.5982
11. Clark, K., et al.: The cancer imaging archive (TCIA): maintaining and operating a public information repository. J. Digit. Imaging **26**(6), 1045–1057 (2013). https://doi.org/10.1007/s10278-013-9622-7
12. Cortes, C., Mohri, M.: AUC optimization vs. error rate minimization. In: Advances in Neural Information Processing Systems. MIT Press (2004)
13. Diehn, M., et al.: Identification of noninvasive imaging surrogates for brain tumor gene-expression modules. Proc. Natl. Acad. Sci. U.S.A. **105**(13), 5213–5218 (2008). https://doi.org/10.1073/pnas.0801279105
14. Ertosun, M.G., Rubin, D.L.: Automated grading of gliomas using deep learning in digital pathology images: a modular approach with ensemble of convolutional neural networks. In: AMIA 2015 Annual Symposium Proceedings, pp. 1899–1908 (2015)
15. Fix, E., Hodges, J.: Discriminatory analysis, nonparametric discrimination: consistency properties. Technical report 4, USAF School of Aviation Medicine, Randolph Field, Texas (1951)
16. Friedman, J., Hastie, T., Tibshirani, R.: Additive logistic regression: a statistical view of boosting. Ann. Stat. **38**(2) (2000)
17. Gevaert, O., Mitchell, L., Achrol, A., et al.: Glioblastoma multiforme: exploratory radiogenomic analysis by using quantitative image features. Radiology **273**(1), 168–74 (2014). https://doi.org/10.1148/radiol.14131731
18. Gillies, R.J., Kinahan, P.E., Hricak, H.: Radiomics: images are more than pictures, they are data. Radiology **278**(2), 563–577 (2016). https://doi.org/10.1148/radiol.2015151169, pMID: 26579733
19. Granata, I., Guarracino, M.R., Kalyagin, V.A., et al.: Model simplification for supervised classification of metabolic networks. Ann. Math. Artif. Intell. **88**, 91–104 (2019). https://doi.org/10.1007/s10472-019-09640-y
20. Guyon, I., Weston, J., Barnhill, S., et al.: Gene selection for cancer classification using support vector machines. Mach. Learn. **46**(1), 389–422 (2002). https://doi.org/10.1023/A:1012487302797
21. He, H., Bai, Y., Garcia, E.A., et al.: ADASYN: adaptive synthetic sampling approach for imbalanced learning. In: 2008 IEEE International Joint Conference on Neural Networks (IEEE World Congress on Computational Intelligence), pp. 1322–1328, June 2008. https://doi.org/10.1109/IJCNN.2008.4633969
22. Hariri, A.R., Weinberger, D.R.: Imaging genomics. Br. Med. Bull. **65**(1), 259–270 (2003). https://doi.org/10.1093/bmb/65.1.259
23. Jaffe, C.C.: Imaging and genomics: is there a synergy? Radiology **264**(2), 329–331 (2012). https://doi.org/10.1148/radiol.12120871
24. Jakola, A.S., Reinertsen, I.: Radiological evaluation of low-grade glioma: time to embrace quantitative data? Acta Neurochir. **161**(3), 577–578 (2019). https://doi.org/10.1007/s00701-019-03816-5

25. Kaneko, S., Kaneko, S.: Fluorescence-guided resection of malignant glioma with 5-ala. Int. J. Biomed. Imaging **2016** (2016)
26. Khawaldeh, S., Pervaiz, U., Rafiq, A., et al.: Noninvasive grading of glioma tumor using magnetic resonance imaging with convolutional neural networks. Appl. Sci. **8**(1) (2018). https://doi.org/10.3390/app8010027, https://www.mdpi.com/2076-3417/8/1/27
27. Kong, J., Cooper, L., Moreno, C., et al.: In silico analysis of nuclei in glioblastoma using large-scale microscopy images improves prediction of treatment response. In: Proceedings of the IEEE Engineering in Medicine and Biology Society, pp. 87–90 (2011). https://doi.org/10.1109/IEMBS.2011.6089903
28. Kumar, V., et al.: Radiomics: the process and the challenges. Magn. Reson. Imaging **30**(9), 1234–1248 (2012). https://doi.org/10.1016/j.mri.2012.06.010. Quantitative Imaging in Cancer
29. Lambin, P., Rios-Velazquez, E., Leijenaar, R., et al.: Radiomics: extracting more information from medical images using advanced feature analysis. Eur. J. Cancer **48**(4), 441–446 (2012). https://doi.org/10.1016/j.ejca.2011.11.036
30. Law, M., Yang, S., Wang, H.A.: Glioma grading: sensitivity, specificity, and predictive values of perfusion MR imaging and proton MR spectroscopic imaging compared with conventional MR imaging. Am. J. Neuroradiol. **24**(10), 1989–1998 (2003). http://www.ajnr.org/content/24/10/1989
31. Lee, G., Lee, H.Y., Ko, E.S., et al.: Radiomics and imaging genomics in precision medicine. Precis. Future Med. **1**(1), 10–31 (2017). https://doi.org/10.23838/pfm.2017.00101
32. Maddalena, L., Granata, I., Manipur, I., Manzo, M., Guarracino, M.: Glioma grade classification via omics imaging. In: Proceedings of the 13th International Joint Conference on Biomedical Engineering Systems and Technologies - Volume 2 BIOIMAGING, pp. 82–92. INSTICC, SciTePress (2020). https://doi.org/10.5220/0009167700820092
33. Maratea, A., Petrosino, A., Manzo, M.: Adjusted f-measure and kernel scaling for imbalanced data learning. Inf. Sci. **257**, 331–341 (2014)
34. Melone, M.A.B., Valentino, A., Margarucci, S., Galderisi, U., Giordano, A., Peluso, G.: The carnitine system and cancer metabolic plasticity. Cell Death Dis. **9**(2), 1–12 (2018)
35. Menze, B.H., Jakab, A., Bauer, S., et al.: The multimodal brain tumor image segmentation benchmark (BRATS). IEEE Trans. Med. Imaging **34**(10), 1993–2024 (2015). https://doi.org/10.1109/TMI.2014.2377694
36. Miao, J., Niu, L.: A survey on feature selection. Procedia Comput. Sci. **91**, 919–926 (2016). https://doi.org/10.1016/j.procs.2016.07.111, http://www.sciencedirect.com/science/article/pii/S1877050916313047. Promoting Business Analytics and Quantitative Management of Technology: 4th International Conference on Information Technology and Quantitative Management (ITQM 2016)
37. Molinaro, A.M., Taylor, J.W., Wiencke, J.K., Wrensch, M.R.: Genetic and molecular epidemiology of adult diffuse glioma. Nat. Rev. Neurol. **15**(7), 405–417 (2019)
38. Piromkraipak, P., et al.: Cysteinyl leukotriene receptor antagonists inhibit migration, invasion, and expression of MMP-2/9 in human glioblastoma. Cell. Mol. Neurobiol. **38**(2), 559–573 (2018)
39. Ranjbar, S., Mitchell, J.R.: Chapter 8 - An introduction to radiomics: an evolving cornerstone of precision medicine. In: Depeursinge, A., Al-Kadi, O.S., Mitchell, J. (eds.) Biomedical Texture Analysis, pp. 223–245. Academic Press (2017). https://doi.org/10.1016/B978-0-12-812133-7.00008-9

40. Ravi, V., Madhankumar, A.B., Abraham, T., Slagle-Webb, B., Connor, J.R.: Liposomal delivery of ferritin heavy chain 1 (FTH1) siRNA in patient xenograft derived glioblastoma initiating cells suggests different sensitivities to radiation and distinct survival mechanisms. PloS One **14**(9), e0221952 (2019)
41. Russo, D., et al.: Glycosphingolipid metabolic reprogramming drives neural differentiation. EMBO J. **37**(7), e97674 (2018)
42. Sala, E., et al.: Unravelling tumour heterogeneity using next-generation imaging: Radiomics, radiogenomics, and habitat imaging. Clin. Radiol. **72**(1), 3–10 (2017)
43. Scarpace, L., Flanders, A., Jain, R., Mikkelsen, T., Andrews, D.: Data from REMBRANDT. Cancer Imaging Arch. **12** (2005). https://doi.org/10.7937/K9/TCIA.2015.588OZUZB
44. Smedley, N.F., Hsu, W.: Using deep neural networks for radiogenomic analysis. In: 2018 IEEE 15th International Symposium on Biomedical Imaging (ISBI 2018), pp. 1529–1533, April 2018. https://doi.org/10.1109/ISBI.2018.8363864
45. Sun, Q., et al.: Phosphoglyceric acid mutase-1 contributes to oncogenic mTOR-mediated tumor growth and confers non-small cell lung cancer patients with poor prognosis. Cell Death Differ. **25**(6), 1160 (2018)
46. Tea, M.N., Poonnoose, S.I., Pitson, S.M.: Targeting the sphingolipid system as a therapeutic direction for glioblastoma. Cancers **12**(1), 111 (2020)
47. Togao, O., Hiwatashi, A., Yamashita, K., et al.: Differentiation of high-grade and low-grade diffuse gliomas by intravoxel incoherent motion MR imaging. Neuro-Oncology **18**(1), 132–141 (2016). https://doi.org/10.1093/neuonc/nov147
48. Vapnik, V.: The Nature of Statistical Learning Theory. Springer, New York (1995). https://doi.org/10.1007/978-1-4757-2440-0
49. Yang, W., Wang, K., Zuo, W.: Neighborhood component feature selection for high-dimensional data. JCP **7**, 161–168 (2012)
50. Yang, Y., et al.: Glioma grading on conventional MR images: a deep learning study with transfer learning. Front. Neurosci. **12** (2018). https://doi.org/10.3389/fnins.2018.00804
51. Zacharaki, E.I., Wang, S., Chawla, S., et al.: Classification of brain tumor type and grade using MRI texture and shape in a machine learning scheme. Magn. Reson. Med. **62**, a609–1618 (2009). https://doi.org/10.1002/mrm.22147
52. Zhuge, Y., Ning, H., Mathen, P., et al.: Automated glioma grading on conventional MRI images using deep convolutional neural networks. Med. Phys. (2020). https://doi.org/10.1002/mp.14168

Bioinformatics Models, Methods and Algorithms

Efficient Algorithms for Co-folding of Multiple RNAs

Ronny Lorenz[1], Christoph Flamm[1], Ivo L. Hofacker[1,2], and Peter F. Stadler[1,3,4,5,6(✉)]

[1] Institute for Theoretical Chemistry, University of Vienna, Währingerstraße 17, 1090 Wien, Austria
{ronny,xtof,ivo,studla}@tbi.univie.ac.at
[2] Bioinformatics and Computational Biology, Faculty of Computer Science, University of Vienna, Währingerstraße 29, 1090 Wien, Austria
[3] Bioinformatics Group, Department of Computer Science, Interdisciplinary Center for Bioinformatics, and Competence Center for Scalable Data Services and Solutions Dresden/Leipzig, Universität Leipzig, Härtelstraße 16-18, 04107 Leipzig, Germany
studla@bioinf.uni-leipzig.de
[4] Max Planck Institute for Mathematics in the Sciences, Inselstraße 22, 04103 Leipzig, Germany
[5] Facultad de Ciencias, Universidad National de Colombia, Sede Bogotá, Colombia
[6] Santa Fe Institute, 1399 Hyde Park Road, Santa Fe, NM 87501, USA

Abstract. The simplest class of structures formed by $N \geq 2$ interacting RNAs consists of all crossing-free base pairs formed over linear arrangements of the constituent RNA sequences. For each permutation of the N strands the structure prediction problem is algorithmically very similar – but not identical – to folding of a single, contiguous RNA. The differences arise from two sources: First, "nicks", i.e., the transitions from one to the next piece of RNA, need to be treated with special care. Second, the connectedness of the structures needs to guaranteed. For the forward recursions, i.e., the computation of folding energies or partition functions, these modifications are rather straightforward and retain the cubic time complexity of the well-known folding algorithms. This is not the case for a straightforward implementation of the corresponding outside recursion, which becomes quartic. Cubic running times, however, can be restored by introducing linear-size auxiliary arrays. Asymptotically, the extra effort over the corresponding algorithms for a single RNA sequence of the same length is negligible in both time and space. An implementation within the framework of the `ViennaRNA` package conforms to the theoretical performance bounds and provides access to several algorithmic variants, include the handling of user-defined hard and soft constraints.

An earlier version of this contribution appeared in the Proceedings of the 13th International Joint Conference on Biomedical Engineering Systems and Technologies – Volume 3: Bioinformatics [26]. This work was supported in part by the German Federal Ministry of Education and Research (BMBF, project no. 031A538A, de.NBI-RBC, to PFS and project no. 031L0164C, RNAProNet, to PFS), and the Austrian science fund FWF (project no. I 2874 "Prediction of RNA-RNA interactions", project no. F 80 "RNAdeco" to ILH).

X. Ye et al. (Eds.): BIOSTEC 2020, CCIS 1400, pp. 193–214, 2021.
https://doi.org/10.1007/978-3-030-72379-8_10

Keywords: RNA folding · Interacting RNAs · Partition function · Outside recursion · Cubic-time algorithm

1 Introduction

RNA-RNA interactions play an important role in both eukaryotic [17] and procaryotic [14] gene regulation. In eukaryotes, RNA interference involves the binding of small RNAs from diverse sources to longer RNAs, usually leading to degradation. Post-transcriptional gene silencing by microRNAs is just one of the many variations on this theme. Both small interfering RNAs (siRNAs) and long non-coding RNAs (lncRNAs) are also involved in the regulation of splicing and the biogenesis of other RNAs, including microRNAs. RNA sponges, usually lncRNAs, sequester specific miRNAs to revert their silencing effects. The binding of lncRNAs such as *TINCR* to an mRNA can also contribute to the control of translation. In procaryotes, a large number of diverse and often lineage specific small RNAs (sRNAs) act as regulators of translation by binding to their target mRNAs inducing structural changes. In all these cases the RNAs interact by forming intermolecular base pairs. Such hetero-duplexes also form between spliceosomal RNAs during the assembly of the spliceosome and are crucial for the correct splicing. The maturation of ribosomal RNAs (rRNAs) and spliceosomal RNAs (snRNAs) requires chemical modifications, most of which are introduced by snoRNPs, which rely on the specific binding of small nucleolar RNAs (snoRNAs) with their rRNA or snRNA target.

An abundance of RNA-RNA interactions was recently reported by transcriptome-wide experiments [16]. This was not entirely unexpected as much earlier computations studies already found statistical evidence for extensive RNA-RNA interaction networks [38]. It is likely, therefore, that complexes composed of more than two RNAs may play important roles similar to the well-established protein complexes. In addition, higher order complexes have already be considered extensively in synthetic biology [8,21]. The prediction and analysis of multi-component RNA complexes thus has become an important task in computational biology, in particular in the context of strand displacement systems [3].

Many aspects of RNA structures, including their thermodynamic properties are well represented by their secondary structures, i.e., discrete base pairs. These already capture the dominating stabilizing and destabilizing contribution: the stacking of base pairs with in helical stem regions and the conformational entropy loss of unpaired regions relative to unconstrained RNA chains. These energetic contributions are compiled in the "loop-based" standard energy model [39]. Most computational studies of RNA structure exclude pseudoknots [31]. That is, secondary structures are not allowed to contain two base (i, j) and (k, l) such that $i < k < j < l$. This condition makes it possible to obtain efficient dynamic programming algorithms. Both the ground state structures [44] and the partition function of the equilibrium ensemble of secondary structures [28] can be computed in cubic time and quadratic space.

The formation of base pairs in a complex of two or more RNA molecules follows the same physical principles as the folding of a single, contiguous RNA chain. The same energy model (with a few simple extensions briefly discussed below) therefore applies to RNA-RNA interactions. However, complexes of multiple RNA strands fall into a class of structures that includes pseudoknot-like structures and thus is difficult to handle computationally. The pairwise case is captured well by the RIP model of [1]. Assuming that so-called tangle-structures do not occur, the RIP model is still amenable to dynamic programming solutions, although at the cost of $\mathcal{O}(n^6)$ time and $\mathcal{O}(n^4)$ space, for both ground-state structures and equilibrium base-pairing probabilities [9,20]. An extension to the multi-strand case was introduced in [29].

The full RIP model is computationally too demanding for most applications, hence approximations and simplifications are usually employed. Examples include a greedy, helix-based approach that allows essentially unrestricted matchings [6] and formalization as a constrained maximum weight clique problem [23]. An alternative is to assume a single, dominating interacting region, which is often – but not always – a plausible approximation, in particular if one of the partners is small as in the case miRNAs. In this scenario the energy of the interaction can decomposed into unfolding energies for the interaction sites on each partner and the hybridization energy of the exposed interaction regions [4,7,30]. A similar approach can be taken when interactions need to conform to specific patterns, is in the case of H/ACA snoRNAs binding to their targets [37].

In this contribution we consider a simplified model that excludes all pseudoknot-like structures. Conceputally, this amounts to computing a conventional, pseudoknot-free secondary on the concatenation of the interacting RNA strands, although with a suitably modified energy model (see below). Although some important types of interactions, in particular kissing-hairpins [13], cannot be modeled in this way, it is still a useful approximation in many situations. For $N = 2$ strands, this model has been analyzed in detail in [2,5,10]. For $N > 2$, the ground-state folding problem still remains essentially unchanged. The only necessary adaptation is a modification of the energy model to assign different energy contributions to substructures ("loops") that contain one or more *nicks*, as we shall the call the breakpoints between strands. Kinetic simulations of multistrand cofolding have been studied in [32]. For $N = 2$, the order of the strands does not matter. In fact, it is easy to see that every crossing-free set of base pairs on AB translates to a crossing-free set of pairs on the alternative order BA. This is no longer true for $N > 2$, however. We now have to consider the different permutations of the RNA strands. For connected structures, two permutations of the RNA strands either form the same set of crossing-free secondary structures (if one is a cyclic permutations of the other), or their sets of crossing-free secondary structures are disjoint [12]. As a consequence, it is necessary to compute the structures for all permutations (with a fixed first strand to exclude the equivalent cyclic permutations). Since the ensembles of (connected) structures are disjoint, one can perform these computations independently. An implementation for the general case is available in `NUPACK` [43].

The binding energies between strands in heteropolymeric structures are intrinsically concentration dependent because the number of particles changes when polymeric structures are formed [10]. Partition function computations therefore need to handle complexes separately that are composed of different combinations of strands. RNAcofold [5] initially ignores this issue and first computes a partition function Z_{AB} that includes both connected structures (in which the strands A and B are linked by at least one base pair) and conformation is which the monomers A and B form independent structures. The correct partition function is then obtained as $Z_{AB} - Z_A Z_B$. This approach seems to become tedious for higher-order interactions. NUPACK [12] instead considers only connected structures. It turns out that this leads only to a small modification of McCaskill's algorithm. While this avoids the complications arising from disconnected structures, it leads to more complicated outside recursions for computations of base pairing probabilities even though this step still follows the idea of McCaskill's outside recursions [28].

The key issue is that the computation of the probability of the base pair (k, l) needs to consider the case that (k, l) resides in a loop $\mathcal{L}$ with closing pair (i, j) that harbors *exactly* one nick. If the loop $\mathcal{L}$ were to contain two or more nicks, the structure would be disconnected, and hence excluded. Controlling the number nicks in the loop is conceptually simple. In practice, however, it is not trivial to handle without additional effort because all partition function variables computed in the inside recursions, outlined in Sect. 2, only cover connected substructures, and hence the cases with a nick in the exterior loop need to be handled separately. In Sect. 3 we show how this can be achieved efficiently. Section 5 briefly summarizes details and features of the implementation of RNAmultifold in the ViennaRNA package. Benchmarking data are provided in Sect. 6. Since RNA complex formation is inherently concentration dependent, Sect. 7 briefly describes how this issue is handled in RNAmultifold. Section 8 showcases the interactions between spliceosomal RNAs. Finally in Sect. 9 we address some questions and extensions that have been left open for future research and briefly discuss the limits of the approach taken in this contribution.

2 Inside Recursion

Our goal is to compute the partition function of an ensemble of connected, crossing-free secondary structures of $N \geq 1$ RNA strands with a total length n. We assume that the strands are given in a particular order π. Nucleotide positions are order consecutively from 1 to n is this order of strands. For fixed π, a structure is crossing-free if, given a base pair (i, j), another base pair with $i < k < j$ is allowed only if $i < l < j$. The set of crossing free structures remain the same under circular permutations and are disjoint for any other permutation of the strands [12]. The probability $p_{k,l}$ that (k, l) forms a base pair is therefore a weighted sum of of the base pairing probabilities $p_{k,l}[\pi]$ of all permutations π that fix the first strand. The contribution of each permutation π is proportional to its partition function $Q[\pi]$ [12], i.e., we have

$$p_{k,l} = \sum_{\pi} w(\pi) p_{k,l}[\pi] \quad \text{with} \quad w(\pi) = Q[\pi]/Q\,, \tag{1}$$

where $Q := \sum_{\pi} Q[\pi]$ is the total partition function of the complex. From an algorithmic point of view it therefore suffices to solve the folding problem for a fixed permutation π. We may therefore assume that the strands are indexed consecutively as $s = 1, \ldots, N$.

Complexes that contain the same RNA strand more than once imply symmetries that complicate the problem and need to considered at different levels [12]. Copies of the same RNA sequence are not distinguishable. In the general case, therefore, we have to interpret π not a permutation of the integers 1, 2, ..., N, but as the permutations of the letters in a word (with the first letter fixed), where letters correspond to strands accounting for the composition of the complex. We write $\Pi(\kappa)$ for the set of distinguishable non-cyclic permutations of the strands. For instance, we $\Pi('AAB') = \{AAB\}$ and $\Pi('ABAB') = \{AABB, ABAB\}$.

A related issue arises from secondary structures with r-fold rotational symmetry. Again, these are indistinguishable if they are formed over sequences with the same rotational symmetry. In the dynamic programming algorithm they cannot be separated from the non-symmetric structures. Algorithmically, therefore, they are over-counted by a factor of r, corresponding to an energy contribution of $-RT \ln r$. The same symmetry also reduces the distinguishable conformations by a factor of r, thus incurring an entropic penalty of $+RT \ln r$, exactly compensating the algorithmic overcounting [12]. As a consequence, the issue of rotational symmetry can be ignored in partition function calculations. We note that this not true for energy minimization. Since rotationally symmetric structures are destablized by the small – but not negligible – free energy contribution $RT \ln r$ that cannot be accounted for in the dynamic programming algorithm, the prediction of a symmetric ground state may be incorrect and the correct groundstate is the most stable non-symmetric structure, see [19] for details. Symmetries of the secondary structures also map nicks onto each other, r must be a divisor of N and in particular no symmetries are possible for $N = 1$, where the end of molecule is the only nick.

The standard energy model for RNA secondary structures [39] distinguishes three types of "loops": *Hairpin loops* contain no further interior base pairs. *Interior loops*, which contain stacked base pairs as the special case without intervening unpaired bases, contain exactly one interior base pair. *Multi-branch loops* (multi-loops for short) contain two more consecutive base pairs in their interior. Energy contributions for hairpin and interior loops are tabulated as function of closing (and interior) base pair and the sequence(s) of the unpaired stretches. In contrast, a linear approximation is used for multiloops to keep the number of parameters manageable and to ensure that the dynamic programming recursions can evaluated in cubic time and quadratic space.

McCaskill's original approach [28] to computing partition functions and the generalization to multi-strand problems considers *all* structures. Designed for single, contiguous sequences, of course all these structures are trivially connected. It is thus legitimate to re-interpret the variables appearing in McCaskill's algorithms as partition functions over *connected* structures only. As noted in [12] this implies that for $N > 1$ care has to be taken to enforce connectedness.

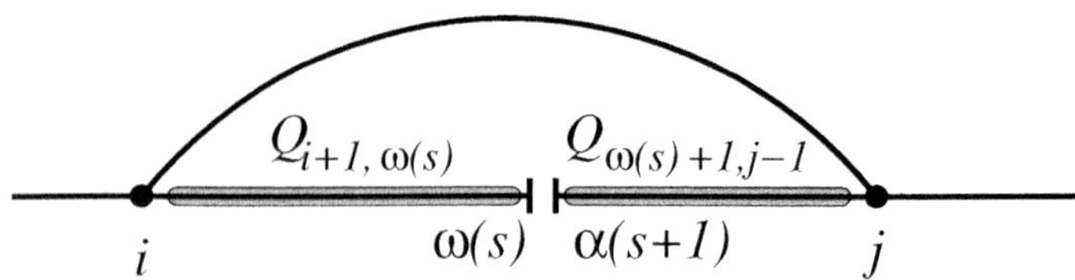

Fig. 1. Nicked loop case in the inside recursion. The RNA sequences are shown as horizontal line, base pairs as arcs. Here, the base pair (i, j) connects two connected components separated by a single nick between $\omega(s)$ and $\alpha(s+1) = \omega(s) + 1$. Nicked loops are exterior. The connected secondary structures on the intervals $[i+1, \omega(s)]$ and $[\alpha(s+1), j-1]$ therefore contribute independently. As limiting cases, the nick may be adjacent to i or j, in which case one of the two intervals $[i+1, \omega(s)] = [i+1, i]$ or $[\alpha(s+1), j-1] = [j, j-1]$ is empty. By definition it then contributes as factor of 1 to the partition function. Figure from [26].

The notation in the contribution follows previous presentations of the `ViennaRNA` package [18,25,27]. We write Q_{ij} for the partition function over all crossing-free connected structures on the interval $[i, j]$. The partition function over all crossing-free connected structures on the interval $[i, j]$ that are enclosed by the base-pair (i, j) are denoted by Q^B_{ij}. The additive approximation of multiloop energies implies that the partition function of a multiloop can be decomposed into multiplicative contributions, one for the its closing base pairs (i, j), a term $Q^M_{i+1,u}$ describing the left part of loop containing at least one stem, and a term $Q^1_{u+1,j-1}$ covering the rightmost component containing exactly one stem whose outer-most base pair starts a position $u+1$. For a detailed description we refer to [28].

In order to handle connectedness we first note that if a structure on $[i, j]$ to which the closing pair (i, j) is added is already connected, then the recursions are the same as in McCaskill's original algorithm. The difference for $N > 1$ thus comes from the situations in which (i, j) connects two distinct components. Since the variables Q_{ij}, Q^B_{ij}, $Q^M_{i+1,u}$, and $Q^1_{u+1,j-1}$ all refer to connected structures only, the latter case has to be included as additional alternative in the decomposition of Q^B_{ij} [12]. It pertains to "loops" enclosed by (i, j) in which exactly one nick is "exposed", i.e., not covered by another base pair. From an energetic point of view, such a loop is *external*, i.e., it does not incur the usual destabilizing entropic contributions. The situation is outlined in Fig. 1.

We will need a bit of notation. Denote by $\omega(s)$ the 3'-most nucleotide position of strand s. The contribution of "nicked loops" is then given by

$$Q^N_{ij} = \sum_{s:i\leq\omega(s)\leq j} \mathrm{e}^{-\varepsilon_{ij}/RT} Q_{i+1,\omega(s)} Q_{\omega(s)+1,j-1} \tag{2}$$

with the additional constraint that either both i and $i+1$ as well as $j-1$ and j must be on the same strand, or the nick is adjacent to the base (i, j), in which case either $i = \omega(s)$ and $j-1$ and j are on a common strand, or $j-1 = \omega(s)$ and

i and $i+1$ are on a common strand. The energy contribution ε_{ij} of the nicked loop comprises only the dangling end terms, see [39] for details.

3 Outside Recursion

In order to compute the base pairing probability $p_{k,l}[\pi]$ we need to evaluate the ensemble of secondary structures that contain the base pair (k, l). All such structures are combinations of a secondary structure on $[k, l]$ and a partial secondary structure outside on $[1, k] \cup [l, n]$. The non-crossing condition ensures that the inside and outside structures can be combined freely, with additive energies and thus multiplicative partition functions [28]. In fact, the "outside ensembles" can be constructed as complements of "inside ensembles" in a systematic manner [35]. A secondary structure containing (k, l) is connected if and only if both the substructures inside and outside of (k, l) are connected, where connectedness of the outside partial structure means that it is connected once the pair (k, l) is added. Denote by $\widehat{Q}_{k,l}[\pi]$ the partition function over all connected partial secondary structures outside of the base pair (k, l). The partition function over all connected structures that contain the pair (k, l) is then simply $\widehat{Q}_{k,l}[\pi]Q^B_{k,l}[\pi]$ and we obtain the base pairing probabilities for a given permutation of the strands as

$$p_{k,l}[\pi] = \widehat{Q}_{k,l}[\pi]Q^B_{k,l}[\pi]/Q[\pi] \tag{3}$$

where $Q[\pi] = Q_{1,n}[\pi]$ is the partition function over all connected secondary structures. The base pairing probabilities for a N-ary complex of interaction RNAs [12] therefore can be computed as

$$p_{k,l} = \sum_{\pi} w(\pi)p_{k,l}[\pi] = \frac{1}{Q}\sum_{\pi} \widehat{Q}_{k,l}[\pi]Q^B_{k,l}[\pi]\,. \tag{4}$$

The decomposition in Eq. (4) shows that we can compute the $p_{k,l}[\pi]$ independently for each permutation π. We therefore drop the reference to π in the following.

The ensemble of outside structures described by $\widehat{Q}_{k,l}$ consists of three mutually exclusive subsets of structures [28]: (1) structures in which (k, l) is not enclosed by any other base pair with partition function $\bar{Q}_{k,l}$ and (2) structures in which (k, l) is enclosed by another base pairs (i, j). The latter can be subdivided further depending on whether the loop enclosed by (i, j) contains (2a) no nick or (2b) exactly one nick. The corresponding partition functions are denoted by $\check{Q}_{k,l}$ and $\ddot{Q}_{k,l}$, respectively. Recall that two or more nicks in a loop imply that the secondary structure is not connected. The recursions for $\bar{Q}_{k,l}$ and $\check{Q}_{k,l}$ are identical to the ones developed in [28]. Since these recursions have been discussed repeatedly in the literature, we do not repeat the details here. It is worth noting, however, that a naïve implementation of the recursions for $\bar{Q}_{k,l}$ and $\check{Q}_{k,l}$ requires $\mathcal{O}(n^4)$ time. It is not difficult, however, to reduce the time complexity to cubic with the help of auxiliary arrays of size $\mathcal{O}(n)$ [25,28].

The focus of this contribution is the additional multi-strand case, i.e., the partition function $\ddot{Q}_{k,l}$. In order to avoid boundary cases we allow also terms of $Q_{i,i-1} = 1$ denoting denoting empty intervals [25]. Note, however $Q^B_{i,j} = 0$ unless $i < j$, and the terms also vanish if $|j - i| < 3$ unless there is a nick between i and j since a hairpin loop contains a minimum of three unpaired bases. Thus the minimum span of a base pair within a single RNA strand is $|j - i| = 4$. There is no distance constraint across nicks, however. We write $\alpha(s)$ and $\omega(s)$ to denote its 5'-most and 3'-most nucleotide position for strands s. Recall that strands are numbered consecutively w.r.t. the given order π. Thus $\alpha(s+1) = \omega(s) + 1$. Furthermore, we write $\sigma(i) = s$ if and only if $\alpha(s) \le i \le \omega(s)$, i.e., if position i occurs in strand s. Finally, we will need the *same-strand indicator function* defined by $\xi_i = 1$ if $\sigma(i) = \sigma(i+1)$ and $\xi_i = 0$ otherwise, as well as its complement $\bar{\xi}_i := 1 - \xi_i$.

To compute $\ddot{Q}_{k,l}$ we have to consider the relative position of focal base pair (k,l), the enclosing base pair (i,j) and the nick. There are two mutually exclusive cases: (1) the nick is located 3' (right) of (k,l), i.e., between l and j and (2) the nick is located 5' (left) of (k,l), i.e., between i and k. In either case the secondary structure enclosed by $[i,j]$ is divided into two independent parts by the nick, i.e., their partition functions can be computed separately, and we obtain

$$\ddot{Q}_{k,l} = \ddot{Q}^{3'}_{k,l} + \ddot{Q}^{5'}_{k,l} \qquad \text{with} \tag{5}$$

$$\ddot{Q}^{3'}_{k,l} = \sum_{\substack{1 \le i < k \\ l < j \le n}} \widehat{Q}_{i,j} Q_{i+1,k-1} \sum_{s | l < \alpha(s) \le j} Q_{l+1,\alpha(s)-1} Q_{\alpha(s),j-1} \tag{6}$$

$$\ddot{Q}^{5'}_{k,l} = \sum_{\substack{1 \le i < k \\ l < j \le n}} \widehat{Q}_{i,j} Q_{l+1,j-1} \sum_{s | i \le \omega(s) < k} Q_{i+1,\omega(s)} Q_{\omega(s)+1,k-1} \tag{7}$$

The evaluation of a single entry $\ddot{Q}_{k,l}$ according to Eqs. (6) or (7) requires $\mathcal{O}(n^2 N)$ operations for N strands with a total length n. The overall running time of $\mathcal{O}(n^4 N)$ by far exceeds the cubic time complexity of all other parts of the partition function algorithm. The additional factor nN is a serious practical burden. In the following section we show that time complexity can be reduced by rearranging these recursions in such a way that the recomputation of certain intermediate results can be avoided.

4 Computing $\ddot{Q}_{k,l}$ in Cubic Time

The key observation is that fixing the position l and computing the values of $\ddot{Q}_{k,l}$ consecutively for all k, we can pre-compute and store contributions that depend only on l and are required for all k. Again we have to consider nicks to the left and to right of (k,l) separately. Fixing the second index k in $\ddot{Q}^{5'}_{k,l}$, Eq. (7), only affects the number of choices for i and s. Moreover, for each strand s the choices of i are also fixed because i of the fixed upper bound $i \le \omega(s)$. This suggests to pre-compute parts of the outside contribution for every s with

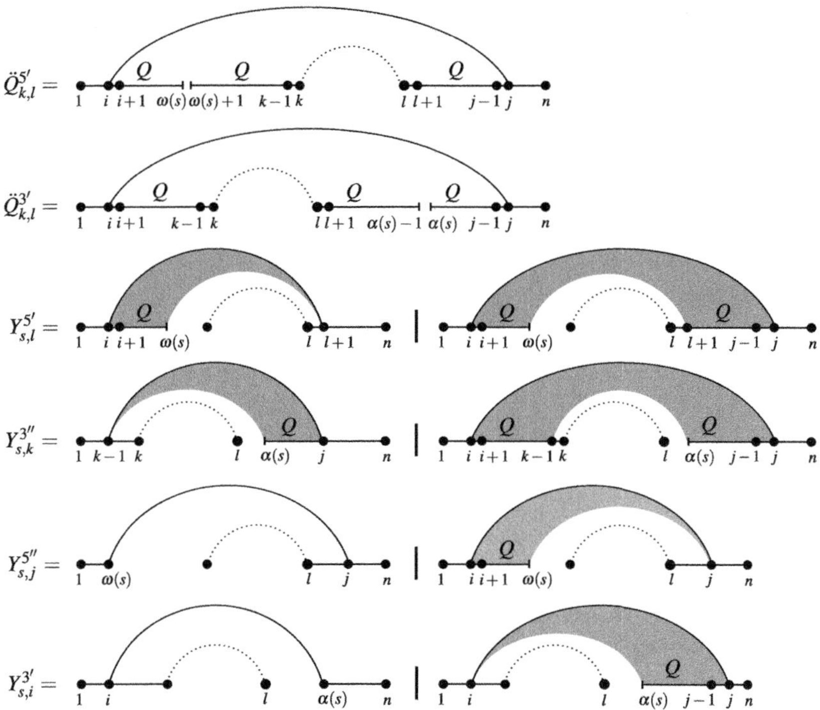

Fig. 2. Auxiliary arrays for computing base pair probabilities for the nicked-loop case. On top the two arrays $\ddot{Q}^{5'}_{k,l}$ and $\ddot{Q}^{3'}_{k,l}$ are sketched, showing the focal base pair (k, l), the enclosing pair (i, j), the position of the nick, and the partition function terms contributing to the loop. The two auxiliary arrays $Y^{5'}_{s,l}$ and $Y^{3''}_{s,k}$ (3rd and 4th line) collect contributions that are independent of the choice of i and j, thus reducing the effort to a sum over the strands s. Parts of these contributions are still re-computed repeatedly when iterating over the l and k. $Y^{5''}_{s,j}$ and $Y^{3'}_{s,i}$ (5th and 6th line) store these parts for reuse. Figure adapted from [26].

$\omega(s) < l$ and all possible choices of i and j. More precisely, we define, for each l, the auxiliary array

$$Y^{5'}_{s} = \xi_l \sum_{j>l} \xi_{j-1} Q_{l+1,j-1} \left(\widehat{Q}_{\omega(s),j} + \sum_{i<\omega(s)} \xi_i \cdot \widehat{Q}_{i,j} \cdot Q_{i+1,\omega(s)} \right). \tag{8}$$

A graphical representation of the contributions captured by $Y^{5'}_{s}$ is provided in Fig. 2. The auxiliary array (which can be overwritten as the outer loop progresses from value of l to the next, has size $\mathcal{O}(N)$ and each entry is computed in $\mathcal{O}(n^2)$ according to Eq. (8), resulting in a total effort of $\mathcal{O}(n^2 N)$. Equation (7) can now be rewritten as

$$\ddot{Q}^{5'}_{k,l} = \bar{\xi}_{k-1} Y^{5'}_{\sigma(k-1)} + \xi_{k-1} \sum_{s|\omega(s)<k} Q_{\omega(s)+1,k-1} Y^{5'}_{s}\,. \tag{9}$$

Each of the $\mathcal{O}(n^2)$ entries now requires $\mathcal{O}(nN)$ operations. Although we have achieved a reduction of the effort by a factor of n, the effort still exceeds the out goal of cubic time complexity.

A further improvement can be obtained by observing that parts of the sums required to compute $Y_s^{5'}$ for a given l can be re-used when $Y_s^{5'}$ is computed for $l-1$ because consecutive entries differ only by a single extra value of j. To make use of this observation we need to replace $Y_s^{5'}$ by $Y_{s,l}^{5'}$, i.e., an array of size $\mathcal{O}(nN)$ that retains the $Y_s^{5'}$ as l changes, together with an additional auxiliary array of the same size:

$$Y_{s,l}^{5'} = \xi_l \left(Y_{s,l+1}^{5''} + \sum_{j>l+1} Q_{l+1,j-1} \cdot Y_{s,j}^{5''} \right) \tag{10}$$

$$Y_{s,j}^{5''} = \xi_{j-1} \left(\widehat{Q}_{\omega(s),j} + \sum_{i<\omega(s)} \xi_i \widehat{Q}_{i,j} \cdot Q_{i+1,\omega(s)} \right). \tag{11}$$

Since $Y_{s,j}^{5''}$ is independent of l and k we can now re-use the stored contributions for every pair (k,l). Proper care has to be taken to properly interleave the computations of $Y_{s,j}^{5''}$ with the part of the computation that loops over variable l because $\widehat{Q}_{i,j}$ only become available for $l < j$. This does not affect the effort required to pre-fill the array $Y_{s,j}^{5''}$, which is still $\mathcal{O}(n^2N)$. Hence, the time complexity for the evaluation of one entry of $\ddot{Q}_{k,l}^{5'}$ reduces to $\mathcal{O}(n)$. The overall time complexity to compute (9) thus becomes $\mathcal{O}(n^2N)$ time and $\mathcal{O}(nN)$ space.

Let us now turn the second case, a nick located $3'$ of base pair (k,l). Conceptually, we can use the same re-arrangement and pre-computation as for 5' nicks; the details differ, however. We start by observing that fixing the value of the index k affects the possible choices of i only. The contributions to the left of the nick, however, do not contain a re-usable factor independent of k because the (i) recursion the involves the full contribution of $Q_{i+1,k-1}$ and (ii) the strand-changes we need to consider only depend on the current value of l. Instead, there are contributions on the right hand side that can be pre-computed. Define the auxiliary array

$$Y_{s,i}^{3'} = \xi_i \left(\widehat{Q}_{i,\alpha(s)} + \sum_{j>\alpha(s)} \xi_{j-1} \widehat{Q}_{i,j} Q_{\alpha(s),j-1} \right) \tag{12}$$

of size $\mathcal{O}(nN)$. We observe that $Y_{s,i}^{3'}$ is independent of both k and l and thus they can be pre-computed and then re-used for any pair (k,l). Substituting Eq. (12) into Eq. (6) yields

$$\ddot{Q}_{k,l}^{3'} = \xi_{k-1} \sum_{i<k} \xi_i Q_{i+1,k-1} \left(\bar{\xi}_l Y_{\sigma(l+1),i}^{3'} + \xi_l \sum_{s|\alpha(s)>l} Q_{l+1,\alpha(s)-1} Y_{s,i}^{3'} \right). \tag{13}$$

The $\mathcal{O}(n^2)$ values of $\ddot{Q}^{3'}_{k,l}$ therefore can be evaluated in total time $\mathcal{O}(n^3N)$ the expense of storing the nN auxiliary values $Y^{3'}_{s,i}$. This does not meet our goal of cubic time complexity, however. A further reduction can be achieved by observing that the order of summation in Eq. (13) can be changed to make the inner sum independent of l. This suggests to introduce the auxiliary array

$$Y^{3''}_{s,k} = \xi_{k-1} \sum_{i<k} \xi_i Q_{i+1,k-1} Y^{3'}_{s,i} \tag{14}$$

of size $\mathcal{O}(nN)$. Figure 2 gives a graphical representation of the class of structures contributing to $Y^{3''}_{s,k}$. The array can be computed from all positions k all strands s in $\mathcal{O}(n^2N)$ time. Substituting the auxiliary terms Eq. (14) into Eq. (6) yields a recursion similar to Eq. (9):

$$\ddot{Q}^{3'}_{k,l} = \bar{\xi}_l Y^{3''}_{\sigma(l+1),k} + \xi_l \sum_{s|\alpha(s)>l+1} Q_{l+1,\alpha(s)-1} Y^{3''}_{s,k}. \tag{15}$$

Assuming that the $\mathcal{O}(nN)$ values of $Y^{3''}_{s,k}$ are stored, it can be evaluated in $\mathcal{O}(n^2N)$ total time. As for the 5' nicks, proper interleaving into the recursion is necessary because $Y^{3'}_{s,i}$ depends on $\widehat{Q}_{i,j}$. To this end, we fill $Y^{3'}_{\sigma(l+1),i}$ for all i if $\xi_l = 1$ and subsequently re-compute $Y^{3''}_{s,k}$.

In order to achieve cubic running time we have introduced four auxiliary arrays of size $\mathcal{O}(nN)$, $Y^{5'}_{s,j}$, $Y^{5''}_{s,j}$, $Y^{3'}_{s,i}$, and $Y^{3''}_{s,i}$, each of which can be filled in total time $\mathcal{O}(n^2N)$. The matrix $\ddot{Q}^{3'}_{k,l}$ of course does not need to be stored. Instead, the value of $\ddot{Q}^{3'}_{k,l}$ can immediately be added to the other contributions of $\widehat{Q}_{k,l}$ and only the latter, or base pairing probabilities $p_{k,l}$, need to be committed to memory. The extra effort for the outside recursion thus matches the extra effort for the inside recursion of the multi-strand folding problem. The number of strands will be much smaller than the total sequence length, $N \ll n$, in any reasonable application scenario. The additional space and time resources required for the multi-strand version of McCaskill's partition function algorithms therefore are asymptotically negligible compared to the single-strand case.

5 Implementation

`RNAmultifold` is part of the `ViennaRNA` package [18,25], release `2.5.0a2`. It provides access to both minimum energy and partition function calculations for arbitrary numbers of strands N. The user can choose to either evaluate a single permutation of the given strands, all permutations corresponding to a given connected complex, or all connected complexes with up to N constituents. Figure 3 shows the base pairing probabilities of a toy example.

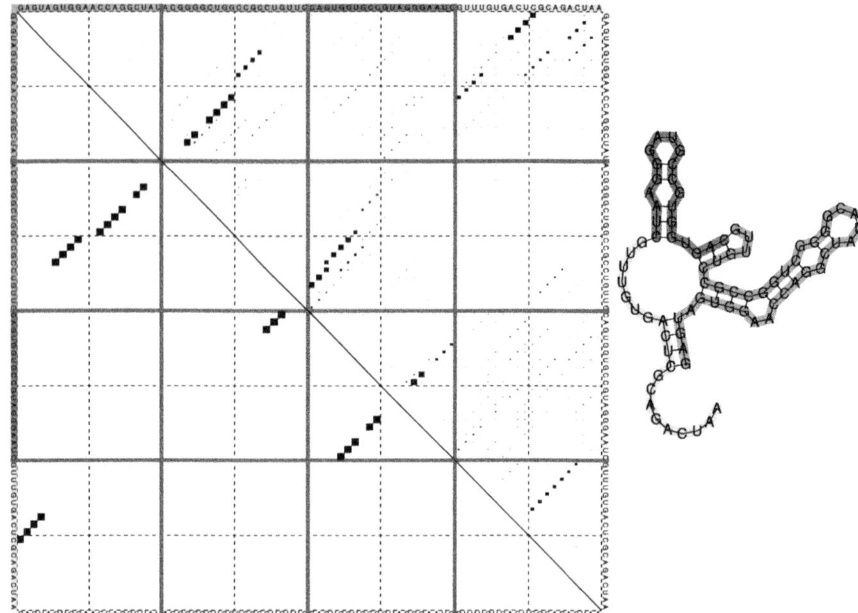

Fig. 3. Toy example with $N = 4$ strands (orange, cyan green and yellow) each of length 20, i.e., total length $n = 80$. The dot plot representation (left) shows the base pairing matrix for a fixed permutation π of the four strands in its upper right half. The lower left half shows the minimum free energy (MFE) structure for the same permutation. The area of each "dot" is proportional to $p_{ij}[\pi]$. Thick lines separate the four strand. The corresponding MFE structure is shown to the right.

A well-known practical issue for the implementations of partition function algorithms are overflow and underflow errors arising from the fact that partition functions consist of exponential terms that quickly grow beyond the range of floating point number as the system size n increases. The `ViennaRNA` package addresses this problem by working with rescaled terms of the form $q_{ij} := Q_{ij}/\zeta^{j-i+1}$. The scaling constant ζ is an estimate for the position-wise multiplicatice contribution to Q, i.e., $\sqrt[n]{Q} = \exp(-g/RT)$, where $g = G/n$ is an estimate for the free energy of folding per nucleotide position [18]. This approach is sufficient to keep q_{ij} and the corresponding restricted partition functions sufficiently close to 1 to avoid overflows for sequence length at least up to 10^4, which appears sufficient for practical applications. A very good estimate is to use the scaled ground state energy $g = E^*/n$. The value of E^* can be computed without numerical problem since the minimum energy computation is implemented using integer arithmetic [18].

The ViennaRNA package provides a flexible framework to handle constraints. It distinguishes *soft constraints*, which are implemented as additional pseudo-energy contributions associated with an unpaired base, a base pairs, or an loop, and *hard constraints* corresponding to forbidden or enforced base pairs [27]. A useful observation in this context is that hard constraints that enforce base pairs between strands can lead to forbidden permutations for $N > 2$: the observation that connected structures are crossing-free in only a single non-cyclic permutation also pertains to constraints. Three or more strands that are connected by hard constraints thus have feasible non-crossing structure only in a single permutation. All other permutations are excluded already during the preprocessing of the hard constraints. We note in passing that RNAmultifold also handles intra-strand G-quadruplexes in the same way as in a single RNA molecule [24]. Both RNA and DNA parameters can be used as in other components of the ViennaRNA package.

6 Benchmarking

We designed a benchmark data set aiming to minimize sequence-specific variations between instances with different numbers of strands. To this end we generated 10 random sequences for each length n and subdivided these into a different number N of separate strands. From the theoretical considerations in the Sect. 4 we expect that both memory consumption and running time should becomes independent of N for large values of the total sequence length n. Empirically, we found that the number of strands has a significant influence only for very short sequences with an average length of individual strands smaller than about 20 nt.

Figure 4 shows that RNAmultifold consistently outperforms NUPACK 3.2.2 [43]. For large sequences, the inside recursion of RNAmultifold is about 35× and the outside recursion is about 50–65× faster. The memory requirements of RNAmultifold are about 7× lower.

Both RNAfold and RNAcofold are contained in the ViennaRNA package and use identical energy parameters. The results of RNAmultifold and RNAfold ($N = 1$) as well as RNAcofold ($N = 2$) coincide within the expected numerical inaccuracies. These programs do not show significant differences in memory consumption. RNAfold is 10–15% faster than RNAmultifold. The outside recursion of RNAmultifold, however, is about two times faster than the corresponding part of RNAcofold. We do not show these small differences separately in Fig. 4.

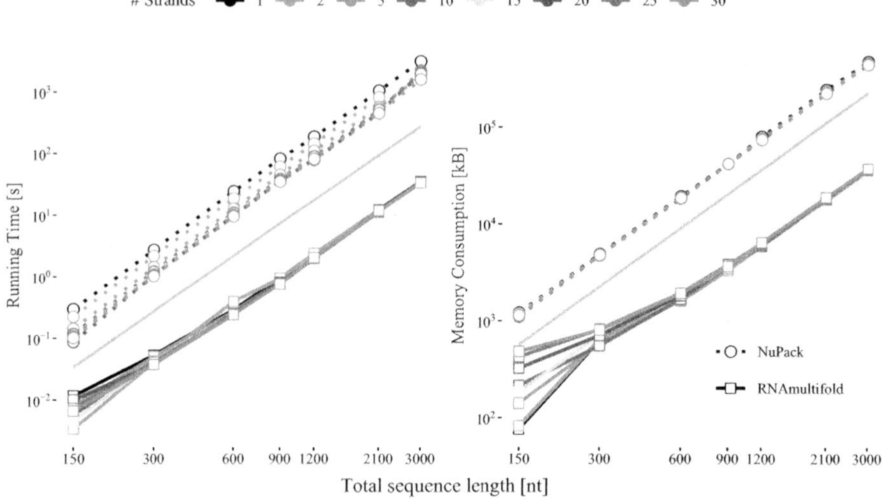

Fig. 4. Comparison of the performance measures for `NUPACK` (version 3.2.2) and `RNAmultifold` for different values of the total sequence length n and number N of strands. For each data point, 10 random instances were averaged. The theoretical asymptotic complexities $\mathcal{O}(n^3)$ for running time and $\mathcal{O}(n^2)$ for memory consumption are shown as thin gray lines. Figure adapted from [26].

7 Concentration Dependence

The formation of an RNA duplex is associated with an additional entropic contribution ε_0 for the initiation of helix formation. In the standard energy model, this term is already subsumed in the loop energies [33,39] and therefore does not appear for $N = 1$. In the case of RNA-RNA interactions, however, an initiation term must be associated with each nicked loop. Since a connected structure with N strands always has exactly $N - 1$ nicks, all connected structures in a complex with given composition are receive a contribution of $(N - 1)\varepsilon_0$, which cancels in Eq. (1) and thus can be ignored in the context of a fixed interaction complex. They do, however, play a role when complexes with a different number of constituents are compared. The partition function of the ensemble of connected structures of a complex κ composed of N (not necessarily distinct) RNA strands including the initiation correction is

$$Z_\kappa = \mathrm{e}^{-(N-1)\varepsilon_0/RT} \sum_{\pi \in \Pi(\kappa)} Q[\pi] \tag{16}$$

The stability of RNA-RNA complex is inherently concentration dependent. The easiest way to see this is to note that the association (and its reverse, the dissociation) of a complex

$$A_1A_2...A_k + B_1B_2...B_l \leftrightharpoons A_1A_2...A_kB_1B_2...B_l \tag{17}$$

changes the number of particles. The equilibrium constant for this reversible reaction is $K = Z_{A_1 A_2 \dots A_k B_1 B_2 \dots B_l} / Z_{A_1 A_2 \dots A_k} Z_{B_1 B_2 \dots B_l}$, see e.g. [5,10,12]. According to the law of mass action we can express the equilibrium constant for formation of κ from its constituent strands A_1, A_2,..., A_N as

$$K_\kappa = \frac{Z_\kappa}{Z_{A_1} Z_{A_2} \dots Z_{A_N}} = \frac{[\kappa]}{[A_1]\,[A_2] \cdots [A_N]}, \tag{18}$$

where [...], as usual in the chemical literature, denotes the concentration of a complex or individual strand.

We introduce the membership matrix $\mathbf{A}$ whose entries $\mathbf{A}_{\alpha,\kappa}$ count the number of strands of type α in complex κ. Assume that our systems contains the total concentration c_α of strand α. The concentration $[\alpha]$ of a strand α that is not contained in a complex is thus

$$[\alpha] = c_\alpha - \sum_\kappa \mathbf{A}_{\alpha,\kappa}[\kappa] \tag{19}$$

Since the system (17) of reversible reactions in particular can be endowed with mass action kinetics, there is a unique equilibrium point [34]. Alternatively, this can be proved starting from the partition function of the grand-canonical ensemble [12]. In the same contribution it is shown that the equilibrium concentrations can be computed by maximizing a function h [12, equ. (3.7)], which in our notation reads

$$h(\vec{\lambda}) = \sum_\alpha (\lambda_\alpha c_\alpha - Z_\alpha e^{\lambda_\alpha}) - \sum_\kappa Z_\kappa \exp\left(\sum_{\alpha'} \lambda_{\alpha'} \mathbf{A}_{\alpha',\kappa}\right) \tag{20}$$

Since the partition function for large molecules are in an “inconvenient” numerical range, we use the transformation $L_\alpha := \lambda_\alpha + \ln Z_\alpha$ to express the objective function in terms of the equilibrium constants and maximize:

$$h(\vec{L}) = \sum_\alpha (c_\alpha L_\alpha - e^{L_\alpha}) - \sum_\kappa K_\kappa \exp\left(\sum_{\alpha'} L_{\alpha'} \mathbf{A}_{\alpha',\kappa}\right), \tag{21}$$

where we have omitted the constant term $-\sum_\alpha c_\alpha \ln Z_\alpha$ since it does not affect the maximum. The equilibrium concentrations can then be obtained from [12, equ. (3.12)], which we can rewrite as

$$[\alpha] = e^{L_\alpha} \qquad\qquad [\kappa] = K_\kappa \prod_\alpha [\alpha]^{\mathbf{A}_{\alpha,\kappa}} \tag{22}$$

Note that the second equation recovers the law of mass action, Eq. (18). It is not difficult to obtain explicit expressions for the gradient and the Hessian of h (see Appendix). As suggested in [12], we use the Trust Region Method implemented as `find_min_trust_region()` in `dlib` [22]. Our implementation of $h(\vec{L})$ and its partial derivatives makes extensive use of the “log-sum-exp trick” to avoid overflow and underflow problems.

Writing $c = \sum_{\alpha} c_{\alpha}$ for the total concentration of RNA strands we can also compute the concentration-dependent probability of observing a base-pair between position i in strand α and position j in strand β by summing the $[\kappa]p_{ij}/c$ over all complexes κ (and strand α in case $\alpha = \beta$). If α and β appear more than once in a given complex, the base pairing probabilities need to be averaged over different combinations of interacting copies of α and β within each given complex.

8 Spliceosomale RNAs: A Showcase Applications

The spliceosome is highly dynamic, complex machinery comprising a multitude of proteins as well as the five spliceosomal snRNAs (U1, U2, U4, U5, U6). During the splicing reaction, its composition and internal structure, which also involves direct base pairing interactions between the snRNAs, is drastically rearranged [41]. Neglecting the mRNA target, the effect of RNA protein binding, and any chemical modifications of the snRNAs, we predict the formation of (parts of) the pre-catalytic spliceosome complex B, in particular its predecessor, the U4/U6.U5 tri-snRNP. To that end, we consecutively increased the concentrations of the individual snRNAs from an initial $0.05\mu M$ to $10\mu M$ in the order U6, U4, U5, and U2. Figure 5 shows the equilibrium concentrations of the snRNA complexes. We observe the formation of U4/U6 as soon as their constituents are available in sufficient concentrations. Upon adding U5, the U4/U6 complex becomes less favorable, instead the triplex U4/U6.U5 dominates the ensemble. Increasing the concentration of U2 afterwards, however, does not seem to affect the equilibrium concentration of U4/U6.U5 nor do we observe any appreciable increase in the concentration of the U4/U6.U5 + U2 tetraplex. Instead, U2 tends to form homo-tetramers. This discrepancy of the prediction with respect to the accepted model of splieceosomal complex formation might be attributed to our simplified model that omits the effect of chemical modifications of the snRNAs, and the impact of protein binding.

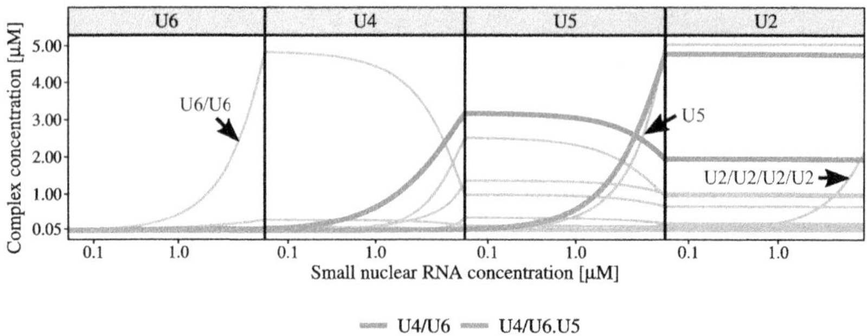

Fig. 5. Concentration dependence of the complexes formed by the human U6, U4, U5, and U2 spliceosomal snRNAs. The concentration of each snRNAs is increased from $0.05\mu M$ to $10\mu M$ in each sub-panel and then fixed at $10\mu M$ for the rest of the simulation. We observe the formation of the U4/U6 dimer complex and the U4/U6.U5 triplex. Increasing the concentration of U2 does not yield any noticable amounts of a U4/U6.U5 + U2 tetraplex. Instead, U2 tends to form homomultimers, possibly due to the lack of protein binding and chemical modifications of the snRNAs in our simplified model.

The base pairing probabilities $p_{k,l}$ can be used to obtain further derived quantities such as expected number N_{AB} of base pairs connecting any two strands A and B in a complex [12]. Since `RNAmultifold` provides access to the full framework for handling constraints in the `ViennaRNA` package [27], we easily can use hard constraints to exclude base pairs between certain strands. This provides a convenient thermodynamic estimate for the importance of a binary interaction in the complex. Denoting by Q the unconstrained partition function writing $Q_{A|B}$ for the partition function with the constraint that no base pairs can be formed between A and B. The contribution of the A-B interaction to the complex stability can then be measures by the partial opening energy

$$\Delta G_{A|B} = RT \ln Q - RT \ln Q_{A|B} \geq 0. \tag{23}$$

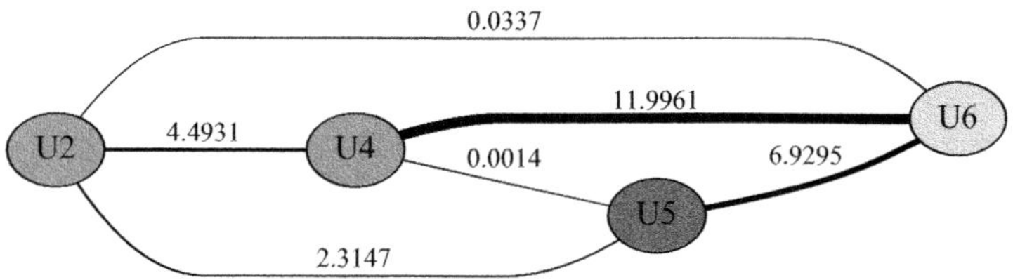

Fig. 6. Importance of binary interactions in the U2 + U4/U6.U5 snRNA complex expressed as $\Delta G_{A|B}$ in kcal/mol. The most stabilizing interactions are U4/U6 followed by U5/U6. Interactions of U2 with any snRNA other than U4 do not play an important role in the overall stability of the full tetraplex.

As an example, we again use the four snRNAs U2, U4, U5, and U6 and compute $\Delta G_{A|B}$ for each pair of interaction in the quaternary complex, see Fig. 6. The largest stabilizing contributions of any complex formed by the four snRNAs can be attributed to U4/U6 and U5/U6 interactions. While still noticable, the interaction between U2 and U4 only contributes a small amount to the overall energy of the complex. In particular, the interactions of U2 with any other snRNA appears energetically negligible.

9 Concluding Remarks and Future Challenges

`RNAmultifold` extends the `ViennaRNA` to handling the multi-strand RNA folding problem. For a fixed permutation π of the strands it computes the partition function (inside recursion) and the base pairing probabilities (outside recursion) in $\mathcal{O}(n^3)$ time and $\mathcal{O}(n^2)$. Our implementation has negligible overhead compared to `RNAfold` and `RNAcofold`. The performance compares favorably with `NUPACK`, at present the only competing software, saving nearly an order of magnitude in memory and about a factor of 50 in running time.

The ViennaRNA package provides access to multi-strand folding at three different levels of abstraction. First, computations can be conducted for fixed π as described at length in Sects. 2–6. The interface at the low level is useful in particular when large complexes are considered for which the set of permutations Π is too large to enumerate exhaustively. For smaller problems, functions are available that autonomously handle a complex with a given composition, returning e.g. aggregated base pairing probabilities, Eq. (1). At the top level, a mixture of strands and a list of allowed complexes can be defined to compute concentration-dependent observables.

Nevertheless, some issues remain open for future research. Some functionalities of the ViennaRNA are not yet available for multi-strand folding. Some of these features are straightforward extension of the partition function algorithms, and will become available with the next major release. This concerns in particular stochastic backtracking to sample individual structures with Boltzmann probabilities [11,36] and extensions of the RNA folding grammar necessary to handle multiple ligand binding sites [15] again making use of the constraints framework described in [27]. Since the symmetry effects compensate for partition functions, no symmetry corrections apply in the sampling process. The enumeration of suboptimal structures [42] is an extension of MFE folding algorithm [42]. Here we will have to take special care to properly treat the energy penalties associated with structures with symmetries that appear in particular in homo-dimers and -multimers [19].

A closer inspection of the folding recursions for different permutations π and π' reveals that parts of the arrays that need to be computed the forward recursions are identical. This suggests to avoid the recomputation to reduce the computational efforts. For larger numbers of strands and/or complexed composed of many strands it will be necessary to develop approximations that make it possible to decide without detailed computations which complexes and which permutations of strands within a complex need to be considered and which ones can be neglected.

RNAmultifold handles only pseudo-knot-free structures and thus excludes certain modes of RNA-RNA interactions such as kissing hairpins that are relevant both in biological and technological systems. While a large class of strand-displacement systems are pseudo-knot free, many of the sensor and signal amplification systems reviewed in [40] go beyond this paradigm. A simple extension of the approach taken here to pseudoknotted structures does not seem possible, however. Since there is no analog of the partitioning of connected structures into disjoint classes depending on the permutations of the strands, the entire "concatenation-like" paradigm becomes untenable. A possible alternative might be to used RNAup/intaRNA-like methods [4,7,30] to compute individual, localized interactions between entire complexes and to construct a network of exchange reactions between complexes. Such an approach, however, is very different from considering the full ensemble of all structures.

Availability

RNAmultifold can be downloaded as part of ViennaRNA Package 2.5.0a2 from www.tbi.univie.ac.at/RNA.

Appendix

Gradient and Hessian of *h*

Efficient optimization of h, Eq. (21), required the gradient and the Hessian of h, which we give here for convenience:

$$\begin{aligned}\frac{\partial h}{\partial L_\alpha} &= c_\alpha - \mathrm{e}^{L_\alpha} - \sum_\kappa \mathbf{A}_{\alpha,\kappa} K_\kappa \exp\left(\sum_{\alpha'} L_{\alpha'} \mathbf{A}_{\alpha',\kappa}\right) \\ \frac{\partial^2 h}{\partial L_\alpha \partial L_\beta} &= -\delta_{\alpha\beta}\mathrm{e}^{L_\alpha} - \sum_\kappa \mathbf{A}_{\alpha,\kappa}\mathbf{A}_{\beta,\kappa} K_\kappa \exp\left(\sum_{\alpha'} L_{\alpha'} \mathbf{A}_{\alpha',\kappa}\right)\end{aligned} \quad (24)$$

We note that the Hessian is negative definite since the sum can be written as $-\mathbf{M}\mathbf{M}^+$ with $\mathbf{M}_{\alpha,\kappa} = \mathbf{A}_{\alpha,\kappa}\sqrt{K_\kappa}\exp\left(\frac{1}{2}\sum_{\alpha'} L_{\alpha'}\mathbf{A}_{\alpha',\kappa}\right)$.

References

1. Alkan, C., Karakoç, E., Nadeau, J.H., Sahinalp, S.C., Zhang, K.Z.: RNA-RNA interaction prediction and antisense RNA target search. J. Comput. Biol. **13**, 267–282 (2006). https://doi.org/10.1089/cmb.2006.13.267
2. Andronescu, M., Zhang, Z.C., Condon, A.: Secondary structure prediction of interacting RNA molecules. J. Mol. Biol. **345**, 987–1001 (2005). https://doi.org/10.1016/j.jmb.2004.10.082
3. Badelt, S., Grun, C., Sarma, K.V., Wolfe, B., Shin, S.W., Winfree, E.: A domain-level DNA strand displacement reaction enumerator allowing arbitrary non-pseudoknotted secondary structures. J. R. Soc. Interface **17**, 20190866 (2020). https://doi.org/10.1098/rsif.2019.0866
4. Bernhart, S.H., Mückstein, U., Hofacker, I.L.: RNA accessibility in cubic time. Algorithms Mol. Biol. **6**, 3 (2011). https://doi.org/10.1186/1748-7188-6-3
5. Bernhart, S.H., Tafer, H., Mückstein, U., Flamm, C., Stadler, P.F., Hofacker, I.L.: Partition function and base pairing probabilities of RNA heterodimers. Algorithms Mol. Biol. **1**, 3 (2006). https://doi.org/10.1186/1748-7188-1-3
6. Bindewald, E., Afonin, K., Jaeger, L., Shapiro, B.A.: Multistrand RNA secondary structure prediction and nanostructure design including pseudoknots. ACS Nano **5**, 9542–9551 (2011). https://doi.org/10.1021/nn202666w
7. Busch, A., Richter, A., Backofen, R.: IntaRNA: efficient prediction of bacterial sRNA targets incorporating target site accessibility and seed regions. Bioinformatics **24**, 2849–2856 (2008). https://doi.org/10.1093/bioinformatics/btn544

8. Chappell, J., Watters, K.E., Takahashi, M.K., Lucks, J.B.: A renaissance in RNA synthetic biology: new mechanisms, applications and tools for the future. Curr. Opin. Chem. Biol. **28**, 47–56 (2015). https://doi.org/10.1016/j.cbpa.2015.05.018
9. Chitsaz, H., Salari, R., Sahinalp, S.C., Backofen, R.: A partition function algorithm for interacting nucleic acid strands. Bioinformatics **25**, i365–i373 (2009). https://doi.org/10.1093/bioinformatics/btp212
10. Dimitrov, R.A., Zuker, M.: Prediction of hybridization and melting for double-stranded nucleic acids. Biophys. J. **87**, 215–226 (2004). https://doi.org/10.1529/biophysj.103.020743
11. Ding, Y., Chan, C.Y., Lawrence, C.E.: Sfold web server for statistical folding and rational design of nucleic acids. Nucleic Acids Res. **32**, W135–W141 (2004). https://doi.org/10.1093/nar/gkh449
12. Dirks, R.M., Bois, J.S., Schaeffer, J.M., Winfree, E., Pierce, N.A.: Thermodynamic analysis of interacting nucleic acid strands. SIAM Rev. **49**, 65–88 (2007). https://doi.org/10.1137/060651100
13. Durand, G., et al.: A combinatorial approach to the repertoire of RNA kissing motifs; towards multiplex detection by switching hairpin aptamers. Nucleic Acids Res. **44**, 4450–4459 (2016). https://doi.org/10.1093/nar/gkw206
14. Dutta, T., Srivastava, S.: Small RNA-mediated regulation in bacteria: a growing palette of diverse mechanisms. Gene **656**, 60–72 (2018). https://doi.org/10.1016/j.gene.2018.02.068
15. Forties, R.A., Bundschuh, R.: Modeling the interplay of single stranded binding proteins and nucleic acid secondary structure. Bioinformatics **26**, 61–67 (2010). https://doi.org/10.1093/bioinformatics/btp627
16. Gong, J., Ju, Y., Shao, D., Zhang, Q.C.: Advances and challenges towards the study of RNA-RNA interactions in a transcriptome-wide scale. Quant. Biol. **6**(3), 239–252 (2018). https://doi.org/10.1007/s40484-018-0146-5
17. Guil, S., Esteller, M.: RNA-RNA interactions in gene regulation: the coding and noncoding players. Trends Biochem. Sci. **40**, 248–256 (2015). https://doi.org/10.1016/j.tibs.2015.03.001
18. Hofacker, I.L., Fontana, W., Stadler, P.F., Bonhoeffer, L.S., Tacker, M., Schuster, P.: Fast folding and comparison of RNA secondary structures. Monatshefte für Chemie **125**, 167–188 (1994). https://doi.org/10.1007/BF00818163
19. Hofacker, I.L., Reidys, C.M., Stadler, P.F.: Symmetric circular matchings and RNA folding. Discret. Math. **312**, 100–112 (2012). https://doi.org/10.1016/j.disc.2011.06.004
20. Huang, F.W.D., Qin, J., Reidys, C.M., Stadler, P.F.: Partition function and base pairing probabilities for RNA-RNA interaction prediction. Bioinformatics **25**, 2646–2654 (2009). https://doi.org/10.1093/bioinformatics/btp481
21. Isaacs, F.J., Dwyer, D.J., Collins, J.J.: RNA synthetic biology. Nat. Biotechnol. **24**, 545–554 (2006). https://doi.org/10.1038/nbt1208
22. King, D.E.: Dlib-ml: a machine learning toolkit. J. Mach. Learn. Res. **10**, 1755–1758 (2009). /http://dlib.net/
23. Legendre, A., Angel, E., Tahi, F.: RCPred: RNA complex prediction as a constrained maximum weight clique problem. BMC Bioinform. **20**, 128 (2019). https://doi.org/10.1186/s12859-019-2648-1
24. Lorenz, R., et al.: 2D meets 4G: G-quadruplexes in RNA secondary structure prediction. IEEE Trans. Comput. Biol. Bioinf. **10**, 832–844 (2013). https://doi.org/10.1109/TCBB.2013.7
25. Lorenz, R., et al.: ViennaRNA package 2.0. Algorithms Mol. Biol. **6**, 26 (2011). https://doi.org/10.1186/1748-7188-6-26

26. Lorenz, R., Flamm, C., Hofacker, I.L., Stadler, P.F.: Efficient computation of base-pairing probabilities in multi-strand RNA folding. In: de Maria, E., Fred, A., Gamboa, H. (eds.) Proceedings of the 13th International Joint Conference on Biomedical Engineering Systems and Technologies – Volume 3: Bioinformatics. pp. 23–31. Scitepress, Setúbal (2020)
27. Lorenz, R., Hofacker, I.L., Stadler, P.F.: RNA folding with hard and soft constraints. Algorithms Mol. Biol. **11**, 8 (2016). https://doi.org/10.1186/s13015-016-0070-z
28. McCaskill, J.S.: The equilibrium partition function and base pair binding probabilities for RNA secondary structure. Biopolymers **29**, 1105–1119 (1990). https://doi.org/10.1002/bip.360290621
29. Mneimneh, S., Ahmed, S.A.: Multiple RNA interaction: beyond two. IEEE Trans. Nanobiosci. **14**, 210–219 (2015). https://doi.org/10.1109/TNB.2015.2402591
30. Mückstein, U., et al.: Translational control by RNA-RNA interaction: improved computation of RNA-RNA binding thermodynamics. In: Elloumi, M., Küng, J., Linial, M., Murphy, R.F., Schneider, K., Toma, C. (eds.) BIRD 2008. CCIS, vol. 13, pp. 114–127. Springer, Heidelberg (2008). https://doi.org/10.1007/978-3-540-70600-7_9
31. Reidys, C.M.: Combinatorial Computational Biology of RNA. Springer, Heidelberg (2011). https://doi.org/10.1007/978-0-387-76731-4
32. Schaeffer, J.M., Thachuk, C., Winfree, E.: Stochastic simulation of the kinetics of multiple interacting nucleic acid strands. In: Phillips, A., Yin, P. (eds.) DNA 2015. LNCS, vol. 9211, pp. 194–211. Springer, Cham (2015). https://doi.org/10.1007/978-3-319-21999-8_13
33. Serra, M.J., Turner, D.H.: Predicting thermodynamic properties of RNA. Methods Enzymol. **259**, 242–261 (1995). https://doi.org/10.1016/0076-6879(95)59047-1
34. Shear, D.B.: Stability and uniqueness of the equilibrium point in chemical reaction systems. J. Chem. Phys. **48**, 4144–4147 (1968). https://doi.org/10.1063/1.1669753
35. Höner zu Siederdissen, C., Prohaska, S.J., Stadler, P.F.: Algebraic dynamic programming over general data structures. BMC Bioinform. **16**(19), S2 (2015). https://doi.org/10.1186/1471-2105-16-S19-S2
36. Tacker, M., Stadler, P.F., Bornberg-Bauer, E.G., Hofacker, I.L., Schuster, P.: Algorithm independent properties of RNA structure prediction. Eur. Biophys. J. **25**, 115–130 (1996). https://doi.org/10.1007/s002490050023
37. Tafer, H., Kehr, S., Hertel, J., Stadler, P.F.: `RNAsnoop`: efficient target prediction for box H/ACA snoRNAs. Bioinformatics **26**, 610–616 (2010). https://doi.org/10.1093/bioinformatics/btp680
38. Backofen, R., et al.: RNAs everywhere: genome-wide annotation of structured RNAs. J. Exp. Zool. B: Mol. Dev. Evol. **308**(B), 1–25 (2007). https://doi.org/10.1002/jez.b.21130. The Athanasius F. Bompfünewerer RNA Consortium
39. Turner, D.H., Mathews, D.H.: NNDB: the nearest neighbor parameter database for predicting stability of nucleic acid secondary structure. Nucleic Acids Res. **38**, D280–D282 (2010). https://doi.org/10.1093/nar/gkp892
40. Wang, F., Lu, C.H., Willner, I.: From cascaded catalytic nucleic acids to enzyme-DNA nanostructures: controlling reactivity, sensing, logic operations, and assembly of complex structures. Chem. Rev. **114**, 2881–2941 (2014). https://doi.org/10.1021/cr400354z
41. Will, C.L., Lührmann, R.: Spliceosome structure and function. Cold Spring Harb. Perspect. Biol. **3**, a003707 (2011). https://doi.org/10.1101/cshperspect.a003707

42. Wuchty, S., Fontana, W., Hofacker, I.L., Schuster, P.: Complete suboptimal folding of RNA and the stability of secondary structures. Biopolymers **49**, 145–165 (1999). https://doi.org/10.1002/(SICI)1097-0282(199902)49:2⟨145::AID-BIP4⟩3.0.CO;2-G
43. Zadeh, J.N., et al.: NUPACK: analysis and design of nucleic acid systems. J. Comput. Chem. **32**, 170–173 (2011). https://doi.org/10.1002/jcc.21596
44. Zuker, M., Stiegler, P.: Optimal computer folding of large RNA sequences using thermodynamics and auxiliary information. Nucleic Acids Res. **9**, 133–148 (1981). https://doi.org/10.1093/nar/9.1.133

Classification of Biochemical Pathway Robustness with Neural Networks for Graphs

Marco Podda, Pasquale Bove, Alessio Micheli, and Paolo Milazzo(✉)

Department of Computer Science, University of Pisa,
Largo B. Pontecorvo, 3, 56127 Pisa, Italy
{marco.podda,bovepas,micheli,milazzo}@di.unipi.it

Abstract. Dynamical properties of biochemical pathways are often assessed by performing numerical (ODE-based) or stochastic simulations. These methods are often computationally very expensive and require reliable quantitative parameters, such as kinetic constants and initial concentrations, to be available. Biochemical pathways are often represented as graphs, in which nodes and edges give a qualitative description of the modeled reactions, while node and edge labels provide quantitative details such as kinetic and stoichiometric parameters.

In this paper we propose the use of a neural network for graphs to predict dynamical properties of biochemical pathways by relying only on the structure of their graph representation (expressed in terms of Petri nets). We test our new methodology on a dataset of 706 pathways downloaded from the BioModels database, focusing on the dynamical property of concentration robustness. The proposed model allows us to predict robustness directly from the pathway structure, by avoiding the burden of performing numerical or stochastic simulations. Moreover, once trained, the model could be applied to predicting robustness properties for pathways in which quantitative parameters are not available.

Keywords: Systems biology · Deep graph networks · Pathway modelling · Robustness · Deep learning

1 Introduction

Biochemical pathways (or networks) are complex dynamical systems in which molecules interact with each other through chemical reactions. In these reactions, molecules can take different roles: reactant, product, promoter or inhibitor. Chemical kinetics laws, such as the law of mass action, allow describing and analysing the dynamics of a pathway through Ordinary Differential Equations

This work is supported by the Universitá di Pisa under the "PRA – Progetti di Ricerca di Ateneo" (Institutional Research Grants) - Project no. PRA_2020-2021_26 "Metodi Informatici Integrati per la Biomedica".

X. Ye et al. (Eds.): BIOSTEC 2020, CCIS 1400, pp. 215–239, 2021.
https://doi.org/10.1007/978-3-030-72379-8_11

(ODEs). Moreover, stochastic modelling and simulation approaches, based on Gillespie's simulation algorithm [9] or one of its many variants, are often adopted in the case of pathways involving molecules available in small concentrations, which make the dynamics of reactions sensitive to random events.

A common way of representing biochemical pathway is through graphs. Most graphical notations for pathways (see, e.g., [20,27,34]) represent molecules as nodes and reactions as multi-edges or as additional nodes. These notations enable network and structural analysis methods to be applied to the investigation of properties of the pathway as a whole. Moreover, they usually allow ODEs or stochastic models to be automatically generated in order to apply standard numerical simulation techniques.

The dynamics of a biochemical pathway is given by the variation over time of the concentrations of its molecules. Dynamical properties of interest usually concern the reachability of steady states, the occurrence of oscillatory behaviors, causalities between species, and robustness. The assessment of these properties often requires the execution of several numerical or stochastic simulations.

This article investigates the applicability of Machine Learning (ML) to the prediction of dynamical properties of biochemical pathways. In particular, we assume that some dynamical properties of pathways could be correlated with topological properties of the graphs by which such pathways are modeled. Thus, we study the use of neural networks for graphs (belonging to the broader class of Deep Learning [11] methods) to automatically infer those topological properties in a dataset of pathway graphs. Each graph is annotated with the desired property, calculated through numerical simulations based on ODE models of the associated pathways. Finally, we use the inferred topological properties to predict the dynamical property of interest on unseen pathway graphs.

If the initial assumption of the structure-dynamics correlation is correct, the obtained ML model could be able to predict whether the studied dynamical property holds, thus reducing the need of performing expensive numerical or stochastic simulations. Moreover, once trained the ML model could be applied to predicting dynamical properties of pathways for which quantitative parameters are not available, that is, pathways that cannot be analyzed by applying numerical or stochastic simulation methods.

To our knowledge, our approach is the first that addresses the open challenge of predicting dynamical properties from the pathway structure in a general way. Many approaches in literature applying inference methods to pathway models mainly focus on parameter estimation or on assessing relationships between the species involved in the pathway. Our methodology, instead, moves a step towards a paradigmatic shift for the assessment of dynamical properties, and it could be in principle applied to any dynamical property.

In order to test our approach, we focus on the assessment of the dynamical property of robustness [23] on the basis of a graph representation of biochemical pathways in terms of Petri nets [34]. Robustness is the ability of a pathway to preserve its dynamics despite the perturbation of some parameters or initial conditions. Its assessment usually requires a huge number of simulations in order to extensively explore the parameter space. We start from the creation of a dataset of Petri nets obtained from curated pathway models in SBML format downloaded from the BioModels[1] database [28]. Robustness indicators of these pathways (to be used as labels in the dataset) have been computed by performing ODE-based simulations using the `libRoadRunner` Python library [39]. In particular, given a pathway model and a pair of molecular species (called input and output species), the computed robustness value measures how much the concentration of the output species at the steady state is influenced by perturbations of the initial concentration of the input species. This is a notion of *concentration robustness* [37] which is to some extent correlated with the notion of global sensitivity [42].

The predictive task this study addresses is to classify whether an output species is robust to perturbations in the initial concentration on the input or not, for a given pathway network. To do so, we first create a dataset of pathway subgraphs, where each subgraph contains the input and output nodes, as well as all the other nodes in the original pathway that influence the reaction dynamics. Each subgraph is labeled by a binary indicator obtained by thresholding the actual robustness value associated to the input/output pair, as calculated via numerical simulations. We use this dataset to train a neural network for graphs composed of two modules: a Deep Graph Network (DGN) [1] to automatically extract structural information correlated with the robustness in the form of a vector; and a Multi-Layer Perceptron predictor [15] which takes as input the vectorial representation inferred by the DGN, and classifies the example as robust or not. In our experiments, we assess the predictive ability of the model under various performance metrics, showing that the model is able to predict robustness with reasonable accuracy.

This paper is a revised and extended version of [3]. With respect to [3], we have tested our methodology on a dataset with significantly larger graphs: we passed from a limit size of 40 nodes to 100. This is an important improvement that allows us to evaluate the scalability of the approach to complex pathway models whose dynamics is in often difficult to predict. Moreover, we have deepened the analysis of the performance of the neural network for graphs by considering additional performance metrics. We also widened the range of the neural network hyper-parameter selection, increasing the number of configurations explored by 50% with respect to the original work. Lastly, we have added a case study of pathway model taken from the BioModels database in order to illustrate the methodology and test it on a real example.

The paper is structured as follows. Section 2 contains background notions about Petri nets modeling of pathways, robustness properties, and Deep Graph Networks. In Sect. 3 we describe our methodology, defining the predictive task and providing details of the Deep Graph Network model. Section 4 describes the experimental setup. In Sect. 4.3 we discuss the results of our experiments. Finally, in Sect. 5 we draw our conclusions and discuss future work.

[1] BioModels: https://www.ebi.ac.uk/biomodels/.

2 Background

Before describing our methodology, we provide in this section some necessary background notions about the modeling of biochemical pathways with Petri nets, the dynamical property of concentration robustness and the class of Neural Networks for graphs (Deep Graph Networks) that we will use.

2.1 Petri Nets Modeling of Biochemical Pathways

Biochemical pathways are essentially sets of chemical reactions of the form

$$\ell_1 S_1 + \ldots + \ell_\rho S_\rho \xrightarrow{k} \ell'_1 P_1 + \ldots + \ell'_\gamma P_\gamma$$

where S_i, P_i are molecules (*reactants* and *products*, respectively), $\ell_i, \ell'_i \in \mathbb{N}$ are *stoichiometric coefficients* expressing the multiplicities of reactants and products involved in the reaction, and $k \in \mathbb{R}_{\geq 0}$ is the *kinetic constant*, used to compute the reaction rate according to standard chemical kinetic laws such as the law of mass action.

Moreover, in biochemical pathways reactions often include in their description some molecules, called *modifiers* that, although not consumed nor produced by the reaction, act either as *promoter* (increase the reaction rate) or as *inhibitor* (decrease the reaction rate). These molecules are hence not listed among reactants and products, but have a role in the kinetic formula (that in this case could no longer follow the mass action principle). Modifiers are used, for instance, also in the SBML language [16], a standard XML-based modeling language for biochemical pathways.

In Fig. 1a we show a table describing a biochemical pathway as a set of reactions (first column), some of which include a modifier (second column), namely A for the third reaction and F for the sixth. Each reaction is associated with its kinetic formula (third column), that, for simplicity, we be referenced in the

Reaction	Modifiers	Kinetics
$A + B \to 2B$		$r1 = k_1 AB$
$B \to A$		$r2 = k_2 B$
$C + D \to E$	A	$r3 = k_3 CDA$
$E \to F$		$r4 = k_4 E$
$F \to E$		$r5 = k_5 F$
$G \to H$	F	$r6 = \frac{k_6 G}{1+2F}$
$H \to G$		$r7 = k_7 H$

(a) Reactions

$$\begin{aligned}
\frac{dA}{dt} &= -k_1 AB + k_2 B \\
\frac{dB}{dt} &= k_1 AB - k_2 B \\
\frac{dC}{dt} &= -k_3 CDA \\
\frac{dD}{dt} &= -k_3 CDA \\
\frac{dE}{dt} &= k_3 CDA - k_4 E + k_5 F \\
\frac{dF}{dt} &= k_4 E - k_5 F \\
\frac{dG}{dt} &= -\frac{k_6 G}{1+2F} + k_7 H \\
\frac{dH}{dt} &= \frac{k_6 G}{1+2F} - k_7 H
\end{aligned}$$

(b) ODEs

Fig. 1. Example of biochemical pathway: list of reactions with information on modifiers and kinetic formulas and corresponding ODE model.

following through an alias of the form ri (reported in the table). From the kinetic formulas of the two reactions with modifiers, it is clear that A acts as a promoter (the rate is proportional to the concentration of A) and that F acts as inhibitor (the rate is inversely proportional to the concentration of F). Kinetic formulas can then be used to construct a system of Ordinary Differential Equations (ODEs) as shown in Fig. 1b.

A graphical representation of biochemical pathways can be given in terms of Petri nets [8,34]. Petri nets have been originally proposed as a formalism of the description and analysis of concurrent systems [33], but later have been adopted for the modeling of other kinds of systems, such as biological ones. Several variants of Petri nets exist. For the aim of this work we consider a version of *continuous* Petri nets [8] with promotion and inhibition arcs and general kinetic functions. We call this variant *pathway Petri nets*.

A pathway Petri net is essentially a bipartite graph with different types of arcs and with labels in both edges and arcs. According to standard Petri nets terminology, the two types of edges are called *places* and *transitions*. The dynamics (or semantics) of a Petri net in a continuous setting is described by a system of ODEs with one equation for each place. In the case of pathways, such a system of ODEs corresponds exactly to the one that can be obtained from the modeled chemical reactions (as in Fig. 1b). A state of a pathway Petri net (called *marking*) is then an assignment of positive real values to the variables of the ODEs. We denote with M the set of all possible markings.

A *pathway Petri net* can be defined as a tuple $N = (P, T, f, p, h, v, m_0)$ where:

- P and T are finite, non empty, disjoint sets of *places* and *transitions*, respectively;
- $f : ((P \times T) \cup (T \times P)) \rightarrow \mathbb{N}^{\geq 0}$ defines the set of *directed arcs*, weighted by non-negative integer values;
- $p, h \subseteq (P \times T)$ are the sets of *promotion* and *inhibition* arcs;
- $v : T \rightarrow \Psi$, with $\Psi = M \rightarrow \mathbb{R}^{\geq 0}$, is a function that assigns to each transition a function corresponding to the computation of a kinetic formula to every possible marking $m \in M$;
- $m_0 \in M$ is the initial marking.

The visual representation of a pathway Petri net is shown in Fig. 2, that is the net corresponding to the pathway in Fig. 1a. Places P and transitions T of a pathway Petri net represent molecules and reactants, and are depicted as circles and rectangles, respectively. In the figure, places contain the name of the corresponding molecule. Directed arcs f, depicted as standard arrows, connect reactants to reactions and reactions to products. The weight of such arcs (omitted if 1) correspond to the stoichiometric coefficient of the connected reactant/product. If 0 the whole arc is omitted. Promotion and inhibition arcs, p and h, connect molecules to the reactions they promote or inhibit, respectively, and they are depicted as arrows ended by a filled dot or a T. Kinetic formulas of reactions (for simplicity, their aliases defined in Fig. 1a) are depicted inside the rectangles of the corresponding Petri net transitions. We assume molecules connected through promotion arcs to give a positive contribution to the value of the kinetic formula, while molecules connected through inhibition arcs to give a negative (inversely proportional) contribution. Finally, the initial marking m_0 is not depicted in the figure: it has to be described separately.

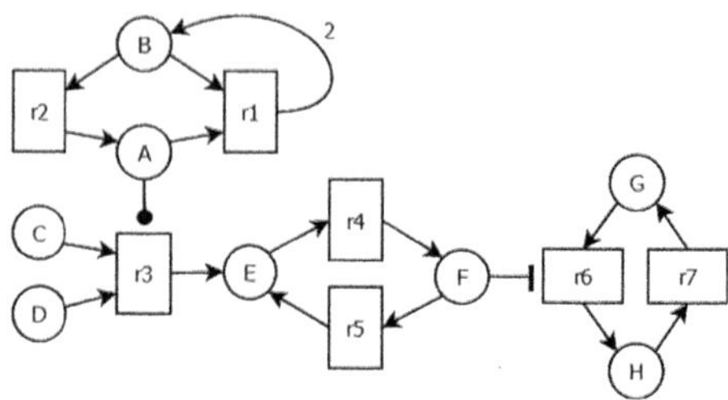

Fig. 2. Pathway Petri net corresponding to reactions in Fig. 1a.

2.2 Concentration Robustness

Robustness is the ability of a system to maintain its functionalities again external and internal perturbations [23]. It is a property observed in many biological systems. A general formalization of the notion of robustness has been proposed by Kitano in [24]. Such a formalization focuses on a specific functionality of the system and on a notion of *viability* of such a functionality measuring of the ability of the systems (e.g. a cell) to carry it out. This could be expressed, for instance, in terms of the synthesis/degradation rate or concentration level of some target substance, in terms of cell growth rate, or in terms of any other suitable quantitative indicator. Kitano's notion of robustness R of a system s with regard to a specific functionality a and against a set of perturbations P is then defined as:

$$R^s_{a,P} = \int_P \psi(p) D^s_a(p) dp$$

In this definition, $\psi(p)$ is the probability for perturbation p to take place, and $D_a(p)$ is a relative evaluation function for functionality a under perturbation p. More precisely, function $D_a(p)$ gives the viability of a under perturbation p relative to the viability of the same functionality in normal conditions. By assuming that in the absence of perturbations functionality a is carried out in an optimal way, we have $D_a(p) = 0$ for perturbations causing the system to fail in a, $D_a(p) = 1$ in the cases of no or irrelevant perturbations (i.e. having no influence), and $0 < D_a(p) < 1$ in the case of relevant perturbations.

Kitano's formulation of robustness has been improved in [35], where functionalities to be maintained are described as linear temporal logic (LTL) formulas and the impact of perturbations is measured through a notion of *violation degree* measuring the distance between the dynamics of the perturbed system and the LTL formula. Many more specific definitions exist, which differ either in the class of biological systems they apply to, or in the way the functionality to be maintained is expressed [25].

In the case of biochemical pathways, a common formulation of robustness, that can be reduced to the more general formulations in [24] and [35], can be expressed in terms of maintenance of the concentration levels of some species. In particular, the notion of *absolute concentration robustness* proposed in [37], compares the concentration level of given species at the steady state against perturbations in the kinetic parameters or in the initial concentration of some other species.

A generalization of absolute concentration robustness, called *α-robustness*, has been proposed in [31], where concentration intervals are considered both for the perturbed molecules (input species) and for the molecules whose concentration is maintained (output species). Roughly speaking, a biochemical pathway is α-robust with respect to a given set of initial concentration intervals if the concentration of a chosen output molecule at the steady state varies within an interval of values $[k-\alpha/2, k+\alpha/2]$ for some $k \in \mathbb{R}$. A relative version of α-robustness can be obtained simply by dividing α by k. The notion of α-robustness is related with the notion of global sensitivity [42] which typically measures the average effect of a set of perturbations.

Assessment of robustness properties is usually obtained by performing exhaustive (in the parameter space) numerical simulations [18,35]. In some particular cases there exist sufficient conditions on the biological network structure that can avoid simulations to be performed [37]. Moreover, the assessment of monotonicity properties in the dynamics of the network may allow the number of simulations to be significantly reduced [12].

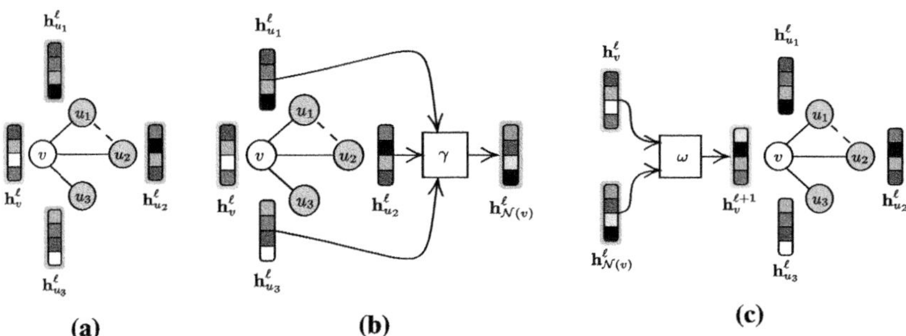

Fig. 3. The steps by which a Deep Graph Network layer is applied to a generic graph node. In a), an example graph is shown, with the embedding of the processed node v shaded in green, and its neighbor embeddings shaded in blue. In b), the three embeddings of the neighbors of v are passed to a function γ, which aggregates them into a neighborhood embedding (shaded in blue). In c), the current node embedding and the neighborhood embedding are combined by a function ω to produce the updated node embedding (in orange). In this last step, we omit the multiplication of the embedding with a weight matrix and the application of an activation function for simplicity. The letter ℓ is used to index the layers. (Color figure online)

2.3 Deep Graph Networks

Graphs allow the encoding of relational information in an expressive and concise way. However, the processing of graphs in ML requires to address several challenges, due to their nature. In fact, graphs have a discrete structure, and their size is variable. As such, to be exploited by many classes of ML models such as neural networks, graphs need to be transformed into real-valued vectors. Of course, this transformation cannot simply be arbitrary: given an associated predictive task, the mapping needs to be meaningful and functional to solving it. Deep Graph Networks (DGNs) [1] are neural network architectures able to learn the required graph-to-vector transformations adaptively from data.

The studies on the adaptive processing of graphs with neural networks originate from the seminal works on Recursive Neural Networks (RecNNs) in the nineties (see e.g. [2,6,40] and the references therein), which found application in the treatment of trees and, later, were extended to more complex structures such as directed acyclic graphs [13,30]. RecNNs, however, can be applied only to a restricted set of classes of graphs, since they cannot handle graph cycles in general. The first two models that allow the treatment of cycles were the Graph Neural Network (GNN) model [36] and the Neural Network for Graphs (NN4G) model [29]. While the former uses a state transition system to handle cycles, the latter breaks down the mutual dependencies introduced by cycles using a layering architecture. Below, we review how a DGN works from the perspective introduced by the NN4G, which was recently rediscovered (see e.g. [4,22,32]), and is currently the main modeling paradigm for learning in graph domains.

The core idea of DGNs is to associate a *state* vector $\mathbf{h}$ to all the nodes of the graph. These state vectors are usually called *node embeddings*. The values of a node embedding are updated according to the graph structure; more specifically, the update is calculated as a function of the current node embedding and the embeddings of the node neighbors. In DGN literature, this operation is referred to as applying a DGN *layer* to the node[2]. This process can be iterated arbitrarily many times by composing ("stacking") a series of DGN layers; at each new layer, the current node state is given by its embedding computed at the previous layer.

We shall now describe how a DGN layer is applied to a node in detail with the help of Fig. 3. Let us assume a graph such as in Fig. 3a. Furthermore, let us assume that we have already applied ℓ DGN layers to node v (our focus node), as well as to the neighbors of v: u_1, u_2 and u_3. To apply the $\ell + 1$ layer to v, its embedding needs to be updated according to the graph structure. This is accomplished in two step:

- *aggregation* (Fig. 3b): a *neighborhood function* $\mathcal{N}(v)$ selects the neighbors of v according to some criteria. The set of selected neighbor embeddings is then

[2] This definition of layer is adapted from the Deep Learning literature, where a layer is a parameterized function applied to an input, whose parameters are learned from data [11].

passed through a permutation-invariant function[3] γ. The end result is a neighborhood vector $\mathbf{h}^{\ell}_{\mathcal{N}(v)}$, which represents the aggregated state of the neighboring nodes of v;
- *combination* (Fig. 3c): in this phase, the embedding $\mathbf{h}^{\ell}_{v}$ of the current node, and the neighborhood vector $\mathbf{h}^{\ell}_{\mathcal{N}(v)}$ are combined together by a function ω to update the node embedding.

Altogether, the application of a DGN layer to the node is summarized by:

$$\mathbf{h}^{\ell+1}_{v} = \sigma(\mathbf{w}^{\ell+1} \cdot \omega(\mathbf{h}^{\ell}_{v}, \mathbf{h}^{\ell}_{\mathcal{N}(v)})),$$

where σ is a (possibly non-linear) function called *unit activation function*, and $\mathbf{w}$ is a vector of weights, whose values are optimized (usually trained with gradient descent) to best approximate the relationship between the input graph and the target property. Notice that each new layer reuses the embedding updated by the previous layer as its input. The process is bootstrapped by setting the initial embedding $\mathbf{h}^{0}_{v}$ as a vector of node descriptors (*features*). The layering mechanism effectively allows to pass information across the graph following its structure. In fact, as the number of layers increases, node embeddings acquire information coming from nodes farther away through their neighbors. In particular, in the ℓ-th layer, nodes can access information pertaining to nodes up to ℓ hops[4] (for a formal treatment, see [29]).

Conveniently, a DGN layer can be applied simultaneously to all the nodes in the graph. This corresponds to visiting each graph node in any order. Once a layer is applied, the information contained in the node embeddings is aggregated to produce a single embedding representing the entire graph. Specifically, one can compute $\mathbf{h}^{\ell}_{G}$, the graph embedding associated to the ℓ-th DGN layer, as:

$$\mathbf{h}^{\ell}_{G} = \tau(\{\mathbf{h}^{\ell}_{v} \mid v \in V_G\}).$$

Here, τ is another permutation-invariant function called *readout*, this time applied to the node set of the graph. Ultimately, stacking L DGN layers produces L different graph embeddings; each of them summarizes the information obtained from a progressively "broader" view of the graph. These layer-wise graph embeddings are then usually concatenated and fed to common ML algorithms, to be used for downstream tasks such as regression or classification. Note that by choosing different γ, ω and τ, different DGN variants are obtained. For example, γ and τ can be vector sum, while ω can be simple vector concatenation, or a more complex function approximated by a neural network. Details specific to our implementation are discussed in Sect. 4.1.

3 Methods

In this section we describe our methodology by starting from graph preprocessing and dataset construction, and by giving the model definition.

[3] A function f on an input set x is invariant with respect to a permutation π iff $f(x) = f(\pi(x))$. Note that, in the case of DGNs, the input set x is a set of node embeddings.

[4] A hop is defined as the shortest unweighted path between two nodes.

3.1 Graph Preprocessing

Pathway Petri nets representations of biochemical pathways are the basis for the creation of a dataset of graphs, which will be the input of our neural network for graphs. In order to let the ML method focus on the topological properties of the graphs, we made some *critical choices*. In particular, we decided to *omit* the following information from the Petri nets:

- kinetic formulas;
- multiplicities of reactants and products (i.e. arc labels);
- the initial marking m_0.

Consequently, by considering again the biochemical pathway presented in Fig. 1 we have that, by removing the mentioned information from its Petri net, we obtain the result shown in Fig. 4.

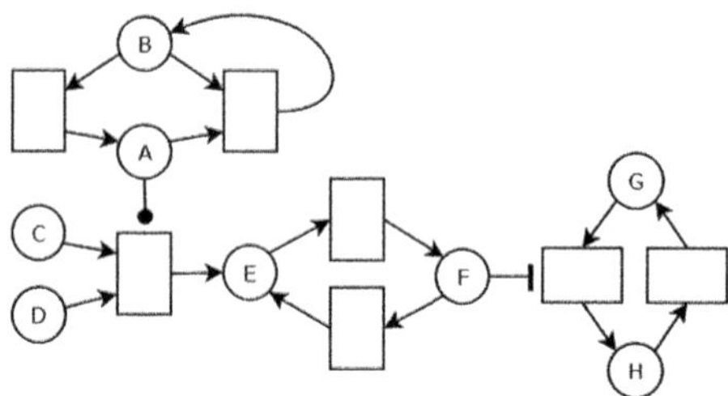

Fig. 4. Pathway Petri net obtained by omitting kinetic formulas and arc labels from the one in Fig. 2.

In order to be used by the neural network for graphs, we reformulate the "cleaned" Petri nets models of pathways into standard graphs. Hence, we represent a biochemical pathway as a directed graph $G = \langle V_G, E_G \rangle$, where $V_G = \{v_1, v_2, \ldots, v_n\}$ is a set of nodes, and $E_G = \{\langle u, v \rangle \mid u, v \in V\}$ is a set of edges. Furthermore, we define the neighborhood function of a node v as $\mathcal{N}(u) = \{v \mid (u, v) \in E_G\}$ for each node $u \in V_G$. Nodes can be of two types: *molecules*, denoted V^G_{mol}, and *reactions*, denoted V^G_{react}, with $V_G = V^G_{mol} \cup V^G_{react}$ and $V^G_{mol} \cap V^G_{react} = \emptyset$. Edges can be of three types: *standard*, denoted E^G_{std}, *promoters*, denoted E^G_{pro}, and *inhibitors*, denoted E^G_{inh}. Again, $E_G = E^G_{std} \cup E^G_{pro} \cup E^G_{inh}$ and $E^G_{std} \cap E^G_{pro} \cap E^G_{inh} = \emptyset$.

Given a pathway Petri net $N = (P, T, f, p, h, v, m_0)$ the corresponding graph G can be obtained by setting $V^G_{mol} = P$, $V^G_{react} = T$, $E^G_{std} = \{\langle u, v \rangle \in (P \times T) \cup (T \times P) \mid f(\langle u, v \rangle) > 0\}$, $E^G_{pro} = p$, $E^G_{inh} = h$. By construction, the obtained graph turns out to be bipartite. For graphs obtained in this way we adopt the same visual representation that we introduced for pathway Petri nets without kinetic formulas and arc multiplicities (see Fig. 4).

Let us define G', an *enriched* version of G, as follows: initially, $V_{G'} = V_G$, $E_{G'} = E_G$. Then, if $\langle u, v \rangle \in E^G_{std}$ is a standard edge connecting a molecule to a reaction, we augment $E_{G'}$ adding the same edge but with reversed direction. Formally, we define $E^{G'}_{std} = E^{G}_{std} \cup \{\langle v, u \rangle \mid \langle u, v \rangle \in E^{G}_{std}, u \in V^{G}_{mol}, v \in V^{G}_{react}\}$. Note that we do not reverse neither standard edges from reactions to molecules, nor promotion and inhibition edges.

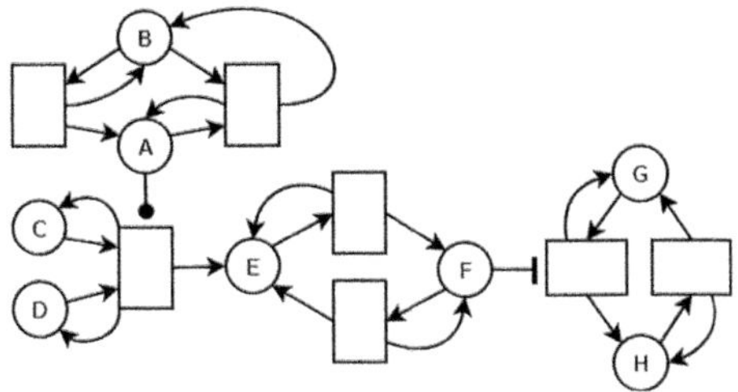

Fig. 5. Enriched version of the graph in Fig. 4.

Figure 5 shows the enriched version G' of the graph G obtained from the Petri net in Fig. 4. It now represents influence relationships between molecules and reactions. There is an edge (of any type) from a molecule to a reaction if and only if a perturbation in the concentration of the molecule determines a change in the reaction rate (that should be computed from the omitted kinetic formula). Similarly, there is an edge from a reaction to a molecule if and only if a perturbation in the reaction rate determines a change in the dynamics of the concentration of that molecule. This is intuitive for edges connecting reactions to products: the dynamics of the product accumulation is determined by the reaction rate. As regards the reversed edges we added in the enriched graph, they are motivated by the fact that a perturbation in the reaction rates determines a variation in the reactants consumption. The enriched graph essentially corresponds to the *influence graph* that could be computed from the Jacobian matrix containing the partial derivatives of the system of ODEs of the modelled pathway [5].

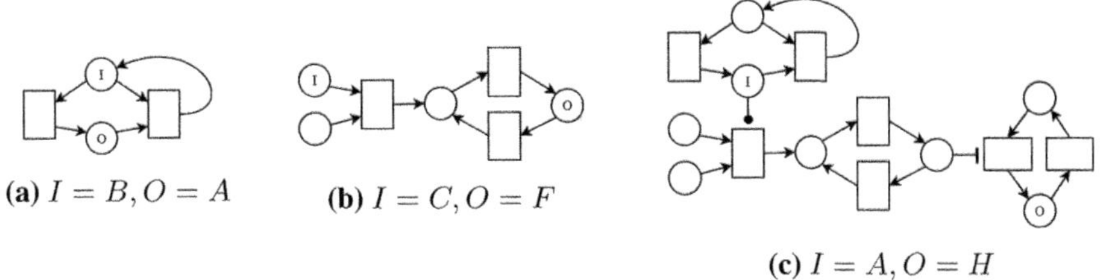

(a) $I = B, O = A$ **(b)** $I = C, O = F$ **(c)** $I = A, O = H$

Fig. 6. Examples of subgraphs of the graph in Fig. 4 induced by different input/output node pairs $(u, v) = (I, O)$.

Since we want to assess a property, concentration robustness, which expresses a relationship between an input and an output molecules of a given pathway, we can, through the enriched graph G', determine which portion of the graph modelling the pathway is relevant for the assessment of the property. Given a graph G, and a pair of nodes u and v, we define $S_{uv} = \langle V_{S_{uv}}, E_{S_{uv}} \rangle$, the *subgraph of G induced by the input/output node pair (u,v)*, informally as follows: S_{uv} is the smallest subgraph of G whose node set contains u, v, as well as nodes in every possible oriented path from u to v in G'. We remark that S_{uv} is a subgraph of G, although it is computed on the basis of the paths in G'. Figure 6 shows some examples of induced subgraphs extracted from the graph in Fig. 4. Induced subgraphs will allow us to apply the ML approach only on the portions of the graph relevant for the property, by getting rid of unnecessary nodes and edges.

3.2 Data Set

Our dataset originates from 706 SBML models of biochemical pathways downloaded from the BioModels database [26]. They correspond to the complete set of manually curated models present in the database at the time we started the construction of the dataset[5]. From these models, we built the associated Petri nets representations, which were saved as graphs in DOT format[6]. For the translation of the SMBL models into (pathway) Petri nets we developed a Python script that, for each reaction in the SMBL model extracts reactants, products and modifiers. It also checks the kinetic formula in order to determine whether each modifier is either promoter or an inhibitor. Subsequently, empty graphs (not containing any node) and duplicates were discarded. After this phase, the final graph dataset consisted of 484 pathway Petri networks. These were translated into graphs compliant with the notation described in Sect. 3.1, and the corresponding induced subgraphs for each input/output combination of interest were extracted. With respect to our previous work, we increased the maximum allowed size of the extracted induced subgraphs from 40 to 100 nodes. As a consequence, the dataset size changed from 7013 induced subgraphs in the original study to 44928 in this one, accounting for an approximate six-fold increase.

The robustness values to be used as labels of the induced subgraphs have been computed by following the relative α-robustness approach. The dynamics of each biochemical pathway has been simulated by applying a numerical solver (the `libRoadRunner` Python library) to its ODEs representation. Reference initial concentrations of involved molecules have been obtained from the original SBML model of each pathway. Moreover, 100 simulations have been performed for each molecule of the pathway by perturbing its initial concentration in the range $[-20\%, +20\%]$. The termination of each simulation has been set to the achievement of the steady state, with a timeout of 250 simulated time units.[7] For each couple of input/output molecules, we computed the width α of the

[5] May 2019.

[6] The DOT graph description language specification, available at: https://graphviz.gitlab.io/_pages/doc/info/lang.html.

[7] The concentration values obtained at the end of the simulation are considered as steady state values also in the cases in which the timeout has been reached.

range of concentrations reached by the output molecules by varying the input (α-robustness). A relative robustness $\overline{\alpha}$ has then been obtained by dividing α by the concentration reached by the output when the initial concentration of the input is the reference one (no perturbation). Finally, a robustness value $r \in [0, 1]$ to be used in the dataset has been computed by comparing $\overline{\alpha}$ (a relative representation of the output range) with 0.4 (a relative representation of the initial input range, that is 40%). Formally:

$$r = 1 - min(1, \frac{\overline{\alpha}}{0.4})$$

3.3 Model

Before training the ML model, a series of steps are needed in order to transform the available data in a way that allows them to be consumed by a neural network for graphs classifier. After the processing described in Sect. 3.1, we are given a set of graphs $\mathcal{G} = \{G_1, G_2, \ldots, G_N\}$, one for every pathway Petri network available. Each graph $G \in \mathcal{G}$ is associated to a set of tuples of the form

$$\{(S_{uv}, r) \mid u, v \in V^G_{mol}, r \in [0, 1] \subseteq \mathbb{R}\}.$$

Here, u and v are graph nodes, S_{uv} is the subgraph induced by input node u and output node v, and r is the associated concentration robustness calculated as explained in Sect. 3.2. For the purposes of this work, we seek to predict whether the output species is robust to perturbations of the input species or not. This corresponds to attaching a binary label to each subgraph S_{uv}: 1 if v is robust to perturbations on u, or 0 otherwise. To obtain such labels, we discretize the robustness values into binary indicators as follows:

$$y = \begin{cases} 1 & \text{if } r > 0.5 \\ 0 & \text{otherwise.} \end{cases}$$

As additional notation, we refer to the label 1 as the "positive class", and to the label 0 as the "negative class". After the discretization step, each graph $G \in \mathcal{G}$ is now associated to the following set of tuples:

$$\mathcal{T}_G = \{(S_{uv}, y) \mid u, v \in V^G_{mol}, y \in \{0, 1\}\}.$$

We construct our final dataset $\mathcal{D}$, on which the neural network for graphs is trained, as the union of all the tuple sets for each original graph of $\mathcal{G}$:

$$\mathcal{D} = \bigcup_{G \in \mathcal{G}} \mathcal{T}_G.$$

We can now formulate the predictive task informally as follows: given a previously unseen induced subgraph, we would like to predict its associated robustness indicator with reasonable accuracy. More specifically, we want to learn a function $f(S_{uv}) = \hat{y}$ that given an induced graph S_{uv}, predicts a robustness value

$\hat{y} \in [0, 1]$, which ideally is as close as possible to the ground truth robustness indicator y. In ML terms, this is achieved by training our model to minimize the following binary cross-entropy [19] (BCE) objective function:

$$\text{BCE}(\mathcal{D}) = -\frac{1}{|\mathcal{D}|} \sum_{(S_{uv}, y) \in \mathcal{D}} y \log(\hat{y}) + (1 - y) \log(1 - \hat{y}),$$

In this work, we propose to approximate f using a Deep Neural Network composed of two modules. The first module is a DGN with L layers, that receives an induced subgraph S_{uv} as input, and produces L graph embeddings $\mathbf{h}^{\ell}_{S_{uv}}$, with $\ell = 1, \dots, L$ as output. The second module is an MLP classifier, which takes as input the concatenation of the L graph embeddings, and outputs values $\hat{y} \in (0, 1)$, representing the probability of v being robust to perturbations in u in the induced subgraph S_{uv}. The corresponding predicted indicator can be obtained simply rounding this probability to the nearest integer. More formally, we implement f as:

$$f(S_{uv}) = \text{MLP}(\mathbf{h}^{1}_{S_{uv}}; \dots; \mathbf{h}^{L}_{S_{uv}}),$$

where $\mathbf{h}^{\ell}_{S_{uv}}$ are graph embeddings produced by the ℓ-th DGN layer, and the symbol ";" denotes vector concatenation. The weights of the model are learned through gradient descent. Figure 7 shows a high-level overview of our model.

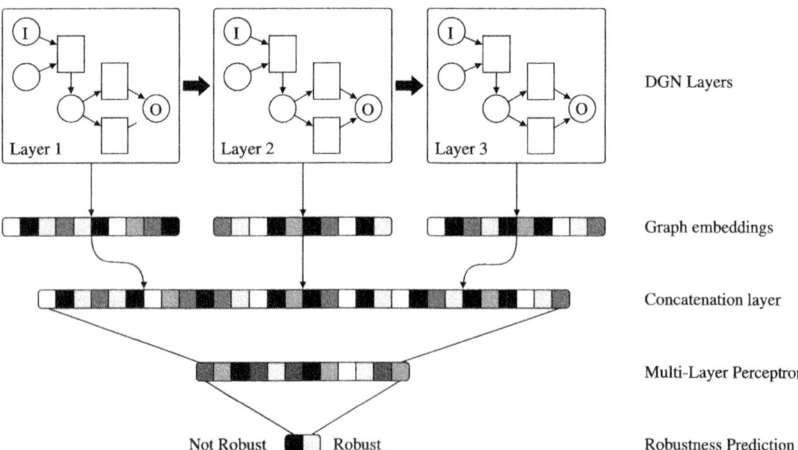

Fig. 7. A high-level overview of our model to predict robustness. For ease of visualization, we limit ourselves to the case where $L = 3$, and the MLP has only one hidden layer. The big black arrow connecting the layers indicates that the node embeddings computed at layer ℓ are reused as initial states in the subsequent layer $\ell + 1$. Note how each layer computes its own different graph embedding (where color intensity is used as a proxy for value magnitude).

4 Experiments

In this section, we provide all the necessary details concerning our experimental procedures. In particular, in Sect. 4.1, we describe the architecture of the Deep Neural Network in detail, while in Sect. 4.2, we discuss the assessment protocol by which we evaluated the proposed model on the predictive task. Finally, in Sect. 4.3, we report and comment on the experimental results.

4.1 Deep Neural Network Implementation

Before training the model, we set the initial node embeddings $\mathbf{h}^0$ to binary feature vector of size three. For each node, the three positions encode:

- whether the node is a molecule species (1) or a reaction (0);
- whether the node is an input species (1) or not (0);
- whether the node is an output species (1) or not (0).

As regards the DGN, we use element-wise mean as the aggregation function γ, and vector sum as the combining function ω, according to the formulation in [22,29]. To account for the different edge types representing the interactions between species and reactions, we used the following DGN layer:

$$\mathbf{h}_v^{\ell+1} = \sigma(\sum_{e \in \mathcal{E}} \mathbf{w}_e^\ell \cdot \omega(\mathbf{h}_v^\ell, \mathbf{h}_{\mathcal{N}(v,e)}^\ell)),$$

In the above formula, $\mathcal{E} = \{standard, promoter, inhibitor\}$ is the set of possible edge types, while $\mathcal{N}(v, e)$ is an edge-aware neighborhood function that selects only nodes connected to v by an edge of type $e \in \mathcal{E}$. This is equivalent to performing neighborhood aggregation separately for each edge type; the corresponding results are multiplied by a specific edge-type weight matrix and summed together before being passed to the activation function. This way, the network learns the contribution of the different edge types separately. We used Rectified Linear Units [10] (ReLU) as activation function σ, followed by a batch normalization layer [17].

As regards the MLP used for the downstream classification, it is composed of two hidden layers: the first has 128 units, while the second layer has 64. As activation function we choose ReLU for the hidden layers, while for the output layer we used a sigmoid function that maps its input to the $(0, 1)$ range. To prevent overfitting, the hidden layers are also regularized via Dropout [41], with drop probability of 0.1.

To train the network, we used the Adam optimizer [21] with an initial learning rate of 0.001, annealed every 50 epochs by a factor of 0.6. We trained with a batch size of 512 for a maximum of 1000 epochs, stopping training whenever 100 epochs passed without improvement on the validation accuracy. Other relevant network hyper-parameters such as the number of DGN layers and the dimension of the node embeddings were chosen via model selection, which we describe in detail in the following section.

The model has been implemented in Python, using the `PyTorch Geometric` library. All experiments were conducted on a single Tesla M40 GPU machine.

4.2 Performance Evaluation

To assess the performance of the proposed model, we use an evaluation framework based on 5-fold Cross-Validation (CV). Initially, we divide the dataset in five partitions of equal size. One of them is used as test set, and the other four are used as outer training set. The outer training set is split further into inner training set (80% of partition size) and validation set (20% of partition size) with the purpose of selecting, out of a set of candidates, the configuration of hyper-parameters that will best generalize on unseen data. Each candidate hyper-parameter configuration is trained on the inner training set, and its performance is assessed on the validation set. After all the candidates have been trained, the configuration with the best accuracy on the validation set is selected. This configuration is used to train a model on the outer training set (holding out another 10% of partition size for validation purposes), whose performance is assessed on the test set. The whole process is repeated five times, each time using a different combination of test and outer training folds. Finally, the five different test accuracies are averaged together to produce an estimate of the out-of-sample performance of the model. Note that, with this schema, the test data is never used for training purposes; thus, the resulting estimator is unbiased. In Fig. 8, we provide a high-level sketch of the evaluation procedure.

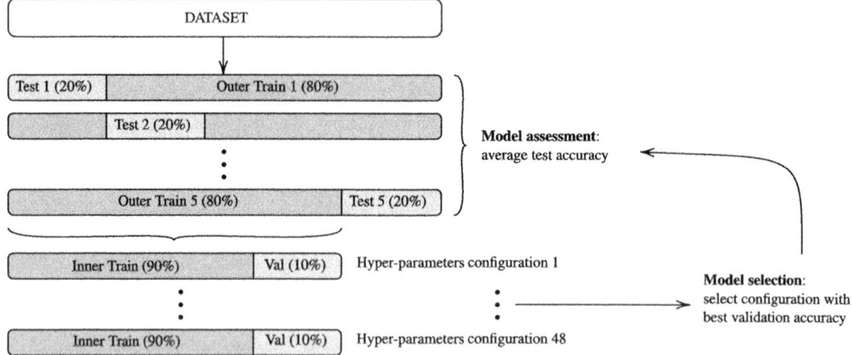

Fig. 8. The schematics of the evaluation framework. The dataset is divided in 5 non-overlapping folds of equal size. One of them is used as test set, the other four are used as outer training set. The outer training set is further divided into inner training set and validation set. This inner dataset is used to train all the candidate hyper-parameter configuration, selecting the one that achieves the best accuracy on the validation set. The winning configuration is ultimately trained on the outer training set and tested on the test set. At the end of the process, the five test accuracies are averaged to obtain the final model assessment. (Color figure online)

We optimized the following hyper-parameters: the number of units, i.e. the dimension of the node embeddings (choosing among 64 and 128), the number L of DGN layers (choosing in the set $\{1, \dots, 12\}$), and the type of readout function τ (choosing among element-wise sum, max and mean). In comparison with our original work [3], the size of the possible hyper-parameter configuration candidates has been increased by 50% (from 48 to 72 candidate configurations). Similarly, the total number of single experiments (model training) needed to carry on the model selection has increased from 240 to 360.

We assess the performances of the proposed model under various metrics. As usual for classification tasks, we use accuracy to measure the predictive performance of the proposed neural network. However, in our case, accuracy is affected by class imbalance (83% of the subgraphs belong to the positive class). Therefore, we also report five additional performance metrics to take this issue into account. These metrics are based on the notions of True Positives (TP), which indicate the ground truth examples correctly predicted by the classifier, and False Positives (FPs), which are negative examples wrongly predicted as positives by the classifier. True Negatives (TN) and False Negatives (FN) have symmetrical semantics. The reported metrics are thus the following:

- *Sensitivity*, defined as $TP/(TP + FN)$;
- *Specificity*, defined as $TN/(TN + FP)$.

All these metrics have been weighted by weighted by class proportions. Finally, we also compute the Area Under the Receiver Operating Characteristics (AU-ROC) curve [14], which quantifies the ability of the classifier to discriminate between negative and positive examples.

Table 1. Results of the 5-fold CV evaluation on the performance metrics of choice (weighted by class frequency). We report the global results as well as the results stratified by number of nodes per subgraph. For each stratification, we also report the related support (i.e. the average number of graphs in the strata).

Strata	Support	Accuracy	Sensitivity	Specificity	AU-ROC
1–10	243 ± 19	0.729 ± 0.020	0.851 ± 0.073	0.526 ± 0.113	0.820 ± 0.034
11–20	711 ± 30	0.843 ± 0.006	0.919 ± 0.021	0.629 ± 0.050	0.892 ± 0.008
21–30	526 ± 19	0.921 ± 0.008	0.969 ± 0.010	0.740 ± 0.052	0.954 ± 0.015
31–40	967 ± 27	0.889 ± 0.012	0.937 ± 0.005	0.757 ± 0.040	0.950 ± 0.009
41–50	1512 ± 21	0.928 ± 0.004	0.970 ± 0.008	0.635 ± 0.064	0.944 ± 0.011
51–60	1679 ± 28	0.921 ± 0.004	0.971 ± 0.006	0.588 ± 0.038	0.950 ± 0.005
61–70	1439 ± 23	0.947 ± 0.005	0.982 ± 0.006	0.644 ± 0.058	0.967 ± 0.005
71–80	1159 ± 28	0.941 ± 0.006	0.980 ± 0.010	0.712 ± 0.087	0.972 ± 0.007
81–90	372 ± 20	0.957 ± 0.008	0.998 ± 0.002	0.037 ± 0.075	0.925 ± 0.010
91–100	378 ± 14	0.850 ± 0.017	0.964 ± 0.024	0.536 ± 0.061	0.888 ± 0.026
Overall	$\mathbf{8985} \pm 1$	$\mathbf{0.913} \pm 0.003$	$\mathbf{0.965} \pm 0.006$	$\mathbf{0.646} \pm 0.042$	$\mathbf{0.948} \pm 0.004$

4.3 Results

The results of our experiments are reported in Table 1, where we average the metrics across the 5 test folds. In our analysis, we also stratify the performances by number of nodes, in order to understand how model performances vary in relation to the size of the input graph. It can be seen how our model accurately predicts robustness: in particular, we report an overall accuracy of 0.913 ± 0.003, as well as an AU-ROC of 0.948 ± 0.004. The model shows very high sensitivity (0.965 ± 0.006) but a lower specificity (0.646 ± 0.042); this is a consequence of class misproportion between negative (less frequent) and positive examples, indicating that it is "harder" for the model to predict input/output pairs that are not robust. Notice the very narrow standard deviations in all measurements, which indicate stable predictions across the different folds. To corroborate this finding, in Fig. 10 we show the ROC curves obtained on the test sets, where performances remain again consistent on all the five fold.

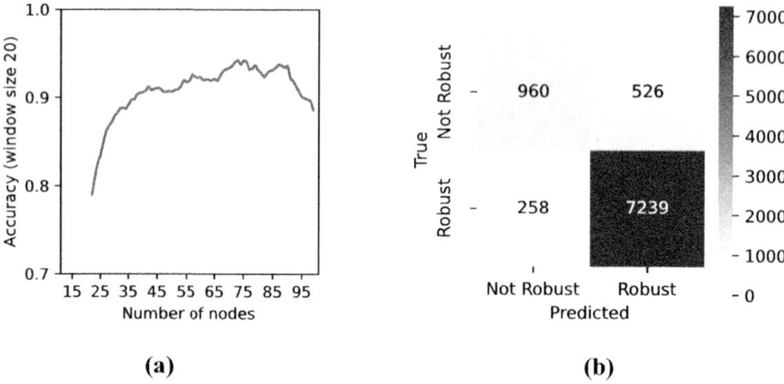

Fig. 9. a) Rolling mean accuracy showing increase in performance as the number of graph nodes grows, using a window of size twenty. b) Confusion matrix. The entries are computed as the mean of the five test folds. (Color figure online)

In Fig. 9b, we show the confusion matrix averaged over the five test folds. The results also highlight that the model performs well under all the considered data stratification. In particular, it performs better when dealing with graphs with at least 20 nodes. To visualize this trend, in Fig. 9a we show how the accuracy improves as the number of nodes of the considered graphs increases, by plotting the rolling accuracy on a window size of 20.

4.4 Case Studies

The lower prediction accuracy in the case of small graphs (1–10 nodes) can be explained by observing that we trained the model on a dataset of graphs in which kinetic, stoichiometric and initial concentration parameters have been omitted.

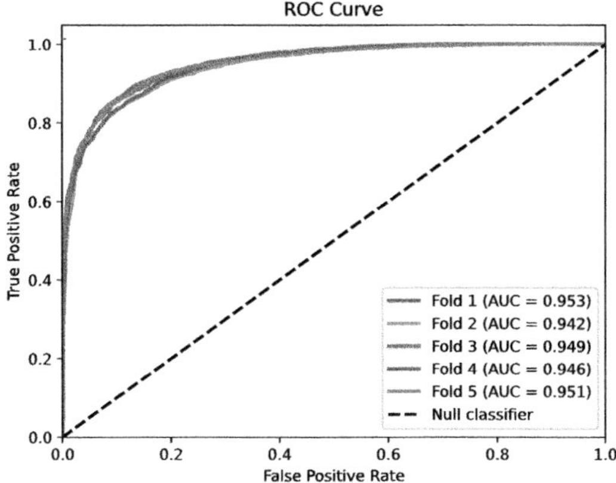

Fig. 10. ROC curves for each of the five test folds. The black dashed line shows the performance of a null classifier that always predicts one class. (Color figure online)

The smaller is the graph, the higher is, in general, the influence on its dynamics of these parameters.

For example, let us consider, as a first case study, the biochemical pathway introduced in Fig. 1 and the corresponding graph depicted in Fig. 4. Moreover, let us consider the following kinetic and initial concentration (marking) parameters:

$$k1 = 1.0 \quad k3 = 0.01 \quad k5 = 0.01 \quad k7 = 0.3 \quad k2 = 5.0 \quad k4 = 0.1 \quad k6 = 5.0$$
$$m_0(A) = 50 \quad m_0(B) = 50 \quad m_0(C) = 100 \quad m_0(D) = 100$$
$$m_0(E) = 0 \quad m_0(F) = 0 \quad m_0(G) = 100 \quad m_0(H) = 0$$

Table 2. Robustness values computed by numerical simulation of the ODEs in Fig. 1b. Input molecules with initial concentration equal to 0 are omitted. Output molecules with identical robustness values are merged.

Input	Output				
	A	B	C/D	E/F	G/H
A	1.0	0.73	0.99	1.0	1.0
B	1.0	0.73	0.99	1.0	1.0
C	1.0	1.0	0.0	0.99	0.99
D	1.0	1.0	0.0	0.99	0.99
G	1.0	1.0	1.0	1.0	0.5

On the basis of numerical simulations of the ODEs in Fig. 1b we obtained, by varying the initial concentration of each molecule in the interval $[-20\%, +20\%]$

Table 3. Probabilities of robustness obtained from the model for some relevant input/output combinations.

Input	Output	Probability
B	A	0.3798 ± 0.1249
A	F	0.7254 ± 0.1802
A	H	0.8835 ± 0.0499
C	F	0.0793 ± 0.1084
G	H	0.2351 ± 0.0054

the robustness values presented in Table 2. In Table 3, we list the average and standard deviations of the 5 different models evaluated in Sect. 4.2, when tasked to predict the robustness probabilities of some relevant input/output combinations. We remark that values in the two tables are not directly comparable: those in Table 2 are exact robustness values of this specific example while those in Table 3 are probabilities of the robustness values to be greater than 0.5 (averaged across 5 models). In this specific case, the prediction turns out to be accurate in the case of input/output pairs corresponding to big induced subgraphs. This happens in the cases of input A with output F or H. The prediction seems not correct in the case of input C and output F: the models gives a small probability while ODEs simulations give 0.99. We notice that the robustness value of this input/output combination is actually sensitive to the perturbation of parameters that have been omitted in the dataset. In particular, if the initial concentration of C, which was omitted in the dataset, was 80 instead of 100, the robustness value with input C and output F would become 0.5 rather than 0.99. The prediction turns out to be wrong also in the case of input B and output A. The probability is under 0.5, when numerical simulations say that robustness computed with this combination of input and output is 1. Also in this case the robustness is influenced by parameters that are not taken into account in the dataset, such as kinetic formulas and the label of the arc entering in node B. Finally, in the case of input G and output H the prediction gives a small probability of robustness and indeed the actual measured value is borderline (0.5). More in general, we observe a slight decrease in performance with respect to our previous work [3], where the predictions on this specific example of pathway were more accurate. Due to the higher heterogeneity of the extended dataset, it is possible that the model has learned to be more accurate on larger graphs, at the expense of performances of smaller ones.

As a second case study, let us consider the SBML model of the EGF pathway proposed by Sivakumar et al. in [38]. Such an SBML model is available in the BioModels database, where it is referenced as `BIOMD0000000394`. A graphical representation of the pathway automatically generated by the CellDesigner tool [7] is depicted in Fig. 11. This representation of the pathway can be trivially translated into a Pathway Petri net. We choose to adopt this representation for this case study for the sake of readability.

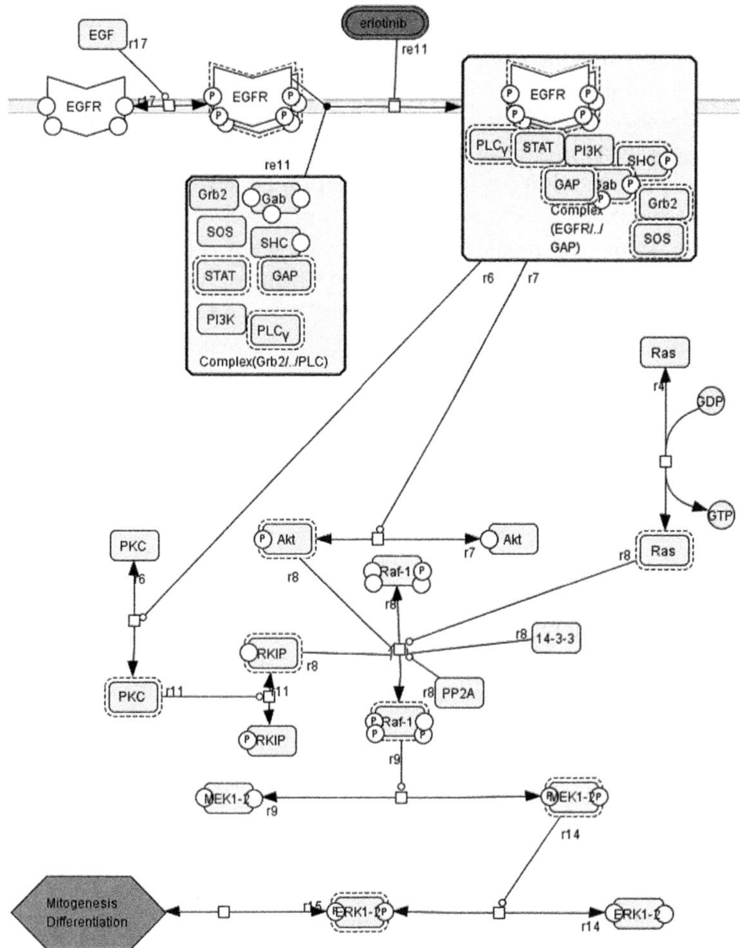

Fig. 11. Sivakumar et al. [38] model of the EGF pathway. Image generated form the SMBL file in the BioModels database using the CellDesigner tool. (Color figure online)

This pathway model describes, in a simplified way, the transduction of the EGF signal, and the consequent activation of the mitogenesis and cell differentiation processes (modelled as an abstract species in the pathway). The EGF signal protein, if available in the cell environment, can be perceived by the receptor protein EGFR, which then initiates a cascade of reactions inside the cell, ultimately leading to the activation of mitogenesis and differentiation. The first steps of the pathway are presented by the formation of a rather big complex involving an activated EGFR dimer and a number of other proteins (depicted as a big box in the upper-left corner of Fig. 11). The formation of such a complex is described in a very simplified way in this pathway model, by concentrating everything in only two reactions. The big complex then promotes a cascade of reactions inside the cell, this time modelled more in detail.

Numerical simulations say that the robustness of the mitogenesis and differentiation (abstract) species, considered as output, with respect to EGF and EGFR, considered as input, turns out to be very high (>0.995) in both cases. This is actually expected in a signal transduction pathway, since it behaves as an amplifier that must be able to activate the target cell process despite of perturbations in the signal and receptor concentrations. On the other hand, if we look at the robustness of the first portion of the pathway up to the creation of the big complex, we can then observe a different behavior. By considering the big complex as output, we still obtain a very high robustness (>0.999) with respect to input EGF, but a robustness value of only 0.19 when the input is EGFR. Again, this is not surprising, since EGF is actually in this pathway is modelled as a promoter of the first reaction (i.e., it is not consumed) while EGFR is a reactant a it will be included in the big complex.

In this case, the model correctly captured the different roles of EGF and EGFR. Indeed, in the case of EGF as input and the big complex as output, the model gives 0.9474 ± 0.014 as probability of robustness, whereas it gives 0.145 ± 0.121 with EGFR as input species. The model captured also the robustness in the whole model, namely when either EGF or EGFR are considered as input, and the abstract mitogenesis and differentiation as output. It gives probability 0.973 ± 0.005 with EGF as input and 0.970 ± 0.008 with EGFR as input.

5 Conclusions

The experimental results we obtained show that our model can infer topological properties of graphs which correlate with dynamical properties of the corresponding biochemical pathways. Such results are promising and let us believe that the approach deserves further investigation. Indeed, the assessment of new connections between structural and dynamical properties of biochemical pathways, and the development of automatic methods for their inference, could lead to new and more efficient ways of studying the functioning of living cells.

In our opinion, the proposed approach has two potentially impacting factors. First, predicting dynamical properties using neural networks for graphs is usually faster than performing numerical simulations. Once the model is trained, the network can be tested on novel subgraphs in milliseconds. In contrast, the numerical simulations we performed took times in the order of minutes, up to dozens of minutes or hours for the larger pathways. While it is true that the training process is time-consuming, it has to be performed only once. Hence, the cost of training is easily amortized as the size of the dataset grows, both in terms of number of pathways involved, and their size. Second, our approach is purposely based on relying on a restricted set of pathway features; the pathway structure, the input/output species, and the type of nodes and arcs in the related graph. Other features, like arc multiplicity, are not considered in our approach; this allows its applicability in cases where this minimal set of features is the only known information about the pathway.

The efficiency of our approach is based on the aim of replacing numerical simulations with the assessment of structural properties of pathways. Such an assessment is performed by the neural network for graphs. It is difficult to imagine how the same assessment could be done through an algorithm on graphs since the structural properties to be assessed are not known in advance, but inferred.

One important aspect to research in future works concerns model explainability. While being reliable as predictors, neural networks for graphs require additional effort in understanding the underlying function (from pathway structure to prediction) that they approximate. To this aim, generative models of pathways are a promising direction of research we intend to explore, as they can be helpful to study properties of the model and to provide explanations to the decisions taken by it.

Furthermore, we will consider enriching the dataset with information we have omitted in the present study. In particular, we may include arc labels (multiplicities of reactants/products) in order to evaluate their significance. Moreover, we may include something about kinetic formulas, such as their parameters (properly normalized). The latter addition could, in principle, improve the accuracy of the model on small subgraphs, but its effect on the accuracy of big ones has to be carefully evaluated.

Lastly, we plan to apply the approach to the assessment of other dynamical properties such as other notions of robustness as well as, for example, monotonicity, oscillatory and bistability properties.

References

1. Bacciu, D., Errica, F., Micheli, A., Podda, M.: A gentle introduction to deep learning for graphs. Neural Netw. **129**, 203–221 (2020). https://doi.org/10.1016/j.neunet.2020.06.006
2. Bianucci, A., Micheli, A., Sperduti, A., Starita, A.: Application of cascade correlation networks for structures to chemistry. Appl. Intell. **12**, 117–147 (2000). https://doi.org/10.1023/A:1008368105614
3. Bove, P., Micheli, A., Milazzo, P., Podda, M.: Prediction of dynamical properties of biochemical pathways with graph neural networks. In: Proceedings of the 13th International Joint Conference on Biomedical Engineering Systems and Technologies - Volume 3 BIOINFORMATICS, pp. 32–43. INSTICC, SciTePress (2020). https://doi.org/10.5220/0008964700320043
4. Duvenaud, D.K., et al.: Convolutional networks on graphs for learning molecular fingerprints. Adv. Neural. Inf. Process. Syst. **28**, 2224–2232 (2015)
5. Fages, F., Soliman, S.: From reaction models to influence graphs and back: a theorem. In: Fisher, J. (ed.) FMSB 2008. LNCS, vol. 5054, pp. 90–102. Springer, Heidelberg (2008). https://doi.org/10.1007/978-3-540-68413-8_7
6. Frasconi, P., Gori, M., Sperduti, A.: A general framework for adaptive processing of data structures. IEEE Trans. Neural Netw. **9**(5), 768–86 (1998). A publication of the IEEE Neural Networks Council
7. Funahashi, A., Morohashi, M., Kitano, H., Tanimura, N.: CellDesigner: a process diagram editor for gene-regulatory and biochemical networks. Biosilico **1**(5), 159–162 (2003)

8. Gilbert, D., Heiner, M., Lehrack, S.: A unifying framework for modelling and analysing biochemical pathways using Petri nets. In: Calder, M., Gilmore, S. (eds.) CMSB 2007. LNCS, vol. 4695, pp. 200–216. Springer, Heidelberg (2007). https://doi.org/10.1007/978-3-540-75140-3_14
9. Gillespie, D.T.: Exact stochastic simulation of coupled chemical reactions. J. Phys. Chem. **81**(25), 2340–2361 (1977)
10. Glorot, X., Bordes, A., Bengio, Y.: Deep sparse rectifier neural networks. In: Proceedings of the Fourteenth International Conference on Artificial Intelligence and Statistics, pp. 315–323 (2011)
11. Goodfellow, I., Bengio, Y., Courville, A.: Deep Learning. The MIT Press, Cambridge (2016)
12. Gori, R., Milazzo, P., Nasti, L.: Towards an efficient verification method for monotonicity properties of chemical reaction networks. In: Proceedings of the 12th International Joint Conference on Biomedical Engineering Systems and Technologies - Volume 3: BIOINFORMATICS, pp. 250–257. INSTICC, SciTePress (2019). https://doi.org/10.5220/0007522002500257
13. Hammer, B., Micheli, A., Sperduti, A.: Universal approximation capability of cascade correlation for structures. Neural Comput. **17**(5), 1109–1159 (2005)
14. Hastie, T., Tibshirani, R., Friedman, J.: The Elements of Statistical Learning. Springer, New York (2001). https://doi.org/10.1007/978-0-387-21606-5
15. Haykin, S.S.: Neural Networks and Learning Machines, 3rd edn. Pearson Education, London (2009)
16. Hucka, M., et al.: The systems biology markup language (SBML): language specification for level 3 version 2 core. J. Integr. Bioinform. **15**(1) (2018). https://doi.org/10.1515/jib-2017-0081. Article no. 20170081
17. Ioffe, S., Szegedy, C.: Batch normalization: accelerating deep network training by reducing internal covariate shift. In: Proceedings of the 32nd International Conference on International Conference on Machine Learning, ICML 2015, vol. 37, pp. 448–456. JMLR.org (2015)
18. Iooss, B., Lemaître, P.: A review on global sensitivity analysis methods. In: Dellino, G., Meloni, C. (eds.) Uncertainty Management in Simulation-Optimization of Complex Systems. ORSIS, vol. 59, pp. 101–122. Springer, Boston, MA (2015). https://doi.org/10.1007/978-1-4899-7547-8_5
19. Janocha, K., Czarnecki, W.: On loss functions for deep neural networks in classification. Schedae Informaticae **25**, 49–59 (2017)
20. Karp, P.D., Paley, S.M.: Representations of metabolic knowledge: pathways. In: ISMB, vol. 2, pp. 203–211 (1994)
21. Kingma, D.P., Ba, J.: Adam: a method for stochastic optimization. In: Proceedings of the 3rd International Conference on Learning Representations, ICLR (2015)
22. Kipf, T.N., Welling, M.: Semi-supervised classification with graph convolutional networks. In: 5th International Conference on Learning Representations, ICLR (2017)
23. Kitano, H.: Biological robustness. Nat. Rev. Genet. **5**(11), 826 (2004)
24. Kitano, H.: Towards a theory of biological robustness. Mol. Syst. Biol. **3**(1), 137 (2007)
25. Larhlimi, A., Blachon, S., Selbig, J., Nikoloski, Z.: Robustness of metabolic networks: a review of existing definitions. Biosystems **106**(1), 1–8 (2011)
26. Le Novere, N., et al.: BioModels database: a free, centralized database of curated, published, quantitative kinetic models of biochemical and cellular systems. Nucleic Acids Res. **34**(suppl_1), D689–D691 (2006)

27. Le Novere, N., et al.: The systems biology graphical notation. Nat. Biotechnol. **27**(8), 735 (2009)
28. Li, C., et al.: BioModels database: an enhanced, curated and annotated resource for published quantitative kinetic models. BMC Syst. Biol. **4** (2010). https://doi.org/10.1186/1752-0509-4-92. Article no. 92
29. Micheli, A.: Neural network for graphs: a contextual constructive approach. IEEE Trans. Neural Netw. **20**(3), 498–511 (2009)
30. Micheli, A., Sona, D., Sperduti, A.: Contextual processing of structured data by recursive cascade correlation. IEEE Trans. Neural Netw. **15**, 1396–1410 (2004)
31. Nasti, L., Gori, R., Milazzo, P.: Formalizing a notion of concentration robustness for biochemical networks. In: Mazzara, M., Ober, I., Salaün, G. (eds.) STAF 2018. LNCS, vol. 11176, pp. 81–97. Springer, Cham (2018). https://doi.org/10.1007/978-3-030-04771-9_8
32. Niepert, M., Ahmed, M., Kutzkov, K.: Learning convolutional neural networks for graphs. In: Proceedings of the 33rd International Conference on Machine Learning, vol. 48, pp. 2014–2023 (2016)
33. Peterson, J.L.: Petri nets. ACM Comput. Surv. (CSUR) **9**(3), 223–252 (1977)
34. Reddy, V.N., Mavrovouniotis, M.L., Liebman, M.N., et al.: Petri net representations in metabolic pathways. In: ISMB, vol. 93, pp. 328–336 (1993)
35. Rizk, A., Batt, G., Fages, F., Soliman, S.: A general computational method for robustness analysis with applications to synthetic gene networks. Bioinformatics **25**(12), i169–i178 (2009)
36. Scarselli, F., Gori, M., Tsoi, A.C., Hagenbuchner, M., Monfardini, G.: The graph neural network model. IEEE Trans. Neural Netw. **20**(1), 61–80 (2009)
37. Shinar, G., Feinberg, M.: Structural sources of robustness in biochemical reaction networks. Science **327**(5971), 1389–1391 (2010)
38. Sivakumar, K.C., Dhanesh, S.B., Shobana, S., James, J., Mundayoor, S.: A systems biology approach to model neural stem cell regulation by Notch, Shh, Wnt, and EGF signaling pathways. Omics: J. Integr. Biol. **15**(10), 729–737 (2011)
39. Somogyi, E.T., et al.: libRoadRunner: a high performance SBML simulation and analysis library. Bioinformatics **31**(20), 3315–3321 (2015)
40. Sperduti, A., Starita, A.: Supervised neural networks for the classification of structures. IEEE Trans. Neural Netw. **8**(3), 714–735 (1997)
41. Srivastava, N., Hinton, G., Krizhevsky, A., Sutskever, I., Salakhutdinov, R.: Dropout: a simple way to prevent neural networks from overfitting. J. Mach. Learn. Res. **15**, 1929–1958 (2014)
42. Zi, Z.: Sensitivity analysis approaches applied to systems biology models. IET Syst. Biol. **5**(6), 336–346 (2011)

Bio-inspired Systems and Signal Processing

The Extended i-NSS: An Intelligent EEG Tool for Diagnosing and Managing Epilepsy

Nadeem Ahmad Khan(✉), Gul Hameed Khan, Malik Anas Ahmad, M. Awais bin Altaf, and M. Osama Tarar

School of Science and Engineering,
Lahore University of Management Sciences (LUMS), Lahore, Pakistan
nkhan@lums.edu.pk

Abstract. The importance of Neurologists support system for EEG-based diagnosis of epilepsy as well as maintenance of EEG records of epileptic patients has risen with the passing time as the data from the patients and their numbers have increased. Requirements from such a system dealing with epileptic patient EEG files include accuracy in localization of epileptic events, customization of the system according to neurologists style of diagnosis, summarization of important events, less storage space, good fidelity of stored signal for later use, computational efficiency and finally a user friendly system interface. This work presents the extended i-NSS system with new experimental results on a combined scheme for classification and compression of EEG data. The same wavelet-transformed data used for classification is lossy encoded using either Huffman and Arithmetic coding techniques. This synergy not only decreases the overall computational effort, but also allows maintaining the classification fidelity of reconstructed signal greater than 99% with the classification results obtained on the original data. The proposed summarization and data reduction modes also allow selective archiving and retrieval of data. The classifier output apart from providing labelled EEG data also allows intelligent reduction of data and adaptive compression of EEG signal epochs according to its event labelling. The latter option can maintain low distortion levels (5–6% average PRD) for epileptic events at high overall compression ratios between 4–5. Results are presented on CHBMIT scalp EEG database.

Keywords: Neurologists support system · EEG tool · Epilepsy · Intelligent signal processing

---

Supported by the Higher Education Commission (HEC), Pakistan grant number 7978/Punjab/NRPU/R&D/HEC/2017 in addition to LUMS.

X. Ye et al. (Eds.): BIOSTEC 2020, CCIS 1400, pp. 243–262, 2021.
https://doi.org/10.1007/978-3-030-72379-8_12

1 Introduction

Electroencephalography (EEG) is extensively used for diagnosis of common neurological disorders like Epilepsy and Sleep disorders. Epilepsy is a recurring neurological disorder, which is characterized by excessive neural activity yield in the brain. Almost 1% of the human population suffers from epilepsy [1]. Epileptic seizures are accompanied by unique patterns in EEG, and therefore EEG is widely used to detect and locate the epileptic seizure and zone. It also helps to characterize the type of epilepsy. EEG signals are non-stationary. Usually the spectral content of the EEG is used for diagnosis which is considered in various frequency bands [10]: δ (0.4–4 Hz), θ (4–8 Hz), α (8–12 Hz) and β (12–30 Hz). δ (delta) are more prominent during deep sleep, θ (theta) waves are prominent during drowsiness, and α (alpha) waves are more prominent when a person is relaxed and closes his eyes, β (beta) waves are dominant during active thinking. Clinical findings of many disorders and seizures are indicated in terms of changes in these frequency bands of EEG [2].

Diagnostic procedures for epileptic patients may involve generating a huge amount of EEG data for inspection by a neurologist. Diagnosis at a clinic or hospital may typically involve several sessions of EEG recordings of duration 40 min to an hour. If these shorter recordings fail to capture a seizure, prolonged EEG up to 72 h can be conducted [3]. Recently portable, wearable and implantable EEG devices with wireless transmission capabilities are also being employed for advanced diagnosis, patient monitoring and treatment of epilepsy [4]. Unaided manual analysis is thus becoming a daunting task for a neurologist [6] given the increase in availability of data and the patient load. Prior manual marking of EEG by the technicians makes the busy clinician heavily dependent on the expertise of the technicians.

Computer-aided EEG analysis assists the Neurologists in two ways: Firstly, it provides an effective and user-friendly interface to examine and mark the multi-channel EEG data. Simultaneous examination of multiple channels also helps the clinicians to diagnose whether the epilepsy is generalized or focal. Secondly, it may automatically highlight the candidate EEG signal intervals depicting the epileptic patterns. If done accurately, it significantly reduces the data to be analyzed and lessen the fatigue upon the Neurologists. Currently available commercial tools for epilepsy are not user-friendly and if flexible require a prior understanding of signal processing techniques for utilizing its full functionalities. This brings their configuration into the hands of the technicians [5] rather than the clinician himself [6–10]. The results are, therefore, prone to misinterpretation and over-interpretation making the Neurologists inclined not to use these automatic tools. Last but not the least, these tools are generally not customizable as per clinician's approach and style of analysis.

The increasing availability of EEG data also calls for developing efficient means of storage and retrieval. For this purpose intelligent reduction and compression has gained significance. It applies to transmission of EEG data also where reduction in bandwidth and energy can result. However, the reduction and compression should preserve the most important events in good detail and introduce no significant artifacts leading to mistake in diagnosis.

Traditionally, the researchers have treated the task of EEG classification and that of reduction and compressions separately and many approaches to these ends have been proposed. However, this does not optimize overall computational efficiency and also does not minimizes the possibility that the introduced distortion and compression artifacts of the reconstructed signal will adversely affect the original classification results of EEG data. A synergy in the two approaches is, therefore, desirable. Some work like [13] and [14] have performed data reduction based on classification. These approaches employ very simple and less powerful methods of classification and compression, respectively, and the resulting encoded format does not allow any choices.

Based on all such considerations, one such initiative has been undertaken in our group under the Intelligent Neurologist Support System (*i*-NSS) project in which we have developed a joint intelligent compression and data reduction methodology. We have exploited wavelet transform and have shown its efficacy simultaneously for both tasks: Classification and compression (along with reduction). This paper updates about the recent extensions in *i*-NSS with new experiments and results. The rest of the paper is organized as follows: Sect. 2 briefly reviews the on going *i*-NSS project. Section 3 discusses the architecture of the *i*-NSS along with the recent extensions; Sect. 4 presents our experimental paradigm and our recent results. Section 5 holds discussion on the future prospects of our *i*-NSS project. Section 6 concludes the work.

2 The *i*-NSS Project

The initial scope of *i*-NSS project has been to develop a support system for Neurologists for reviewing EEG of epilepsy patients suffering from absence seizure and to provide automatic markings of potential epileptic events corresponding to Absence Seizures comprising 3 Hz Spike-and-Wave patterns. The system provides personalization to a Neurologist style and assessment through re-marking and re-training by the neurologist on the corrected events.

The progress made in the project has been covered in various papers published from time to time. [6] provides the overview of the technical approach, its user-interface and the support available to the neurologists. [16] presents its extension as an adaptive system that can be re-trained by the neurologists using corrective markings. In this context it discussed the potential of three classifiers that include Quadratic Discriminant Analysis (QDA), Artificial Neural Network (ANN) and Support Vector Machine (SVM) and shown the superiority of the latter. A recent paper [17] discusses its further extension how the patient data can be summarized, reduced and efficiently compressed maintaining excellent fidelity of the signal allowing its later use after decompression for the purpose of automatic classification or manual inspection by the neurologist.

In [17] we reported our key extension of a compression branch in the *i*-NSS system and demonstrated the usefulness of synergy between the process of compression and classification. The achieved compression performance is still equivalent to the state-of-the art methods though the synergy has led to efficient processing. The presented methodology first uses the classifier of the *i*-NSS system explained in [6] to automatically label the epileptic and non-epileptic epochs. This labeled EEG data is then efficiently compressed for storage or transmission in one of the multiple modes. The archiving is possible at different compression rates versus distortion levels depending on the requirement. System also allows data reduction and archiving of just the labeled epileptic seizures events that are of main interest to the neurologist. Non-epileptic epochs in the *i*-NSS classified data may be either be left out entirely or included at a coarser resolution as per neurologist's requirements.

In this work we first provide an overview of the extended system and report new performance results based on extensive testing on original and reconstructed data. Our earlier paper [16] discussed the classification performance of three types of classifiers: SVM, QDA, and ANN. SVM was chosen as a working classifier because of its best performance. In this work we have also experimented with more classifiers k Nearest Neighbor (KNN), Linear Discriminant Analysis (LDA), Decision Tree (DT) and shown that recognition performance of SVM is still superior. We have also conducted experiments with reconstructed signal and shown that reconstructed signal accuracy of classification is not dependent on classifier choice and remains equally good to the original data. Compared to [17], the reported results also cover the utilization of separate classifiers for each channel. The dataset used is also larger than [17]. The paper also covers more details of *i*-NSS project and discusses its future prospects.

3 Architectural Overview of the Extended *i*-NSS

Figure 1 shows the complete architecture of the proposed extended *i*-NSS system. After a common initial processing of data, the processing is divided in classification and compression branches. Processing at each step is explained as follows:

The process starts with selection of the EEG data file and a specific channel to process as the proposed algorithm works channel-wise. The next step is to extract a one second epoch. The epoch used are non-overlapping and contiguous. Classification and Compression is based on this unit of EEG sampled-data present in a epoch. Discrete Wavelet Transform (DWT) coefficients are calculated for each epoch in the next step. For every epoch, we applied multi-level DWT upto level 8 as the spectral content we re interested in lies between 0–30 Hz [12]. Daubechies-4 (db4) is used as mother wavelet. The detailed coefficients levels of the DWT are determined with respect to sampling frequency. The detailed levels are adjusted on the run according to the sampling frequency such as that we may get if not exact then at least the closest separate frequency bands i.e. Delta (δ: 0.4–4 Hz), Theta (θ: 4–8 Hz), Alpha (α: 8–12 Hz) and Beta (β: 12–30 Hz) component of the signal. Any detailed coefficients that does not contain frequency component from a frequency range of 0–30 Hz were discarded [16]. So, considering the fact of this frequency range, we are left with 5 DWT levels (3–7) of the data.

After calculating the DWT coefficients for each epoch, the proposed algorithm now divides into two branches which are explained separately as follows:

3.1 Classification Branch

This branch is dedicated for classifying the EEG data as epileptic or non-epileptic. The first step of this process is to calculate the statistical features. Instead of using all the detailed coefficients obtained from the DWT, we calculate the Mean, Standard Deviation and Power of every epoch for 5 selected DWT levels as suggested by [16]. Calculating Power, Mean absolute values and Standard deviations of 5 DWT levels (3–7), we obtain 15 features. Taking Ratio of Means of consecutive DWT levels (2–8) provide 6 features. So we have total 21 features. In order to normalize the whole data to one single level, Z-score normalization is used on these 21 statistical features in the next step [16].

In order to improve the performance of classifier, we applied Principal Component Analysis (PCA) technique that first reduces the dimensionality of the feature space for classification. The algorithm works on the principle of maintaining the data having maximum variance. So as a result we only contain the feature components which projected 93% of the total variance. So the 21 statistical features obtained from the previous step are now reduced to only 9 features.

These 9 features are now used for classifying the signal epoch as epileptic or non-epileptic. We have applied multiple classification algorithms to categorize the data as epileptic or non-epileptic. The list includes SVM, KNN, LDA and DT. Performance of these classifiers with parameter details is discussed in next section.

3.2 Compression Branch

This branch is devoted for compressing the EEG data. The first step in data compression process is the Data Selection stage. The same DWT coefficients computed for epochs for classification now labeled as epileptic or non-epileptic is utilized. They are selected or discarded for compression according to the test cases of data reduction and compression involved. For complete EEG compression case or adaptive compression all coefficients are utilized. For summarization and compression case, unwanted coefficients (like that of non-eplipetic intervals) are to be discarded.

The next step allows Quantization and Thresholding of these coefficients. The selected DWT coefficients are first thresholded using a single specified value or in case of adaptive mode using two (or more) threshold levels. Values below the used threshold are set to zero. By varying the level of threshold to be set, we can increase or decrease the number of wavelet coefficients being discarded. This controls the compression and also as consequence the accuracy of the reconstructed signal. For adaptive case, the classification labels are also utilized to select the right level of threshold for that interval. This is discussed further

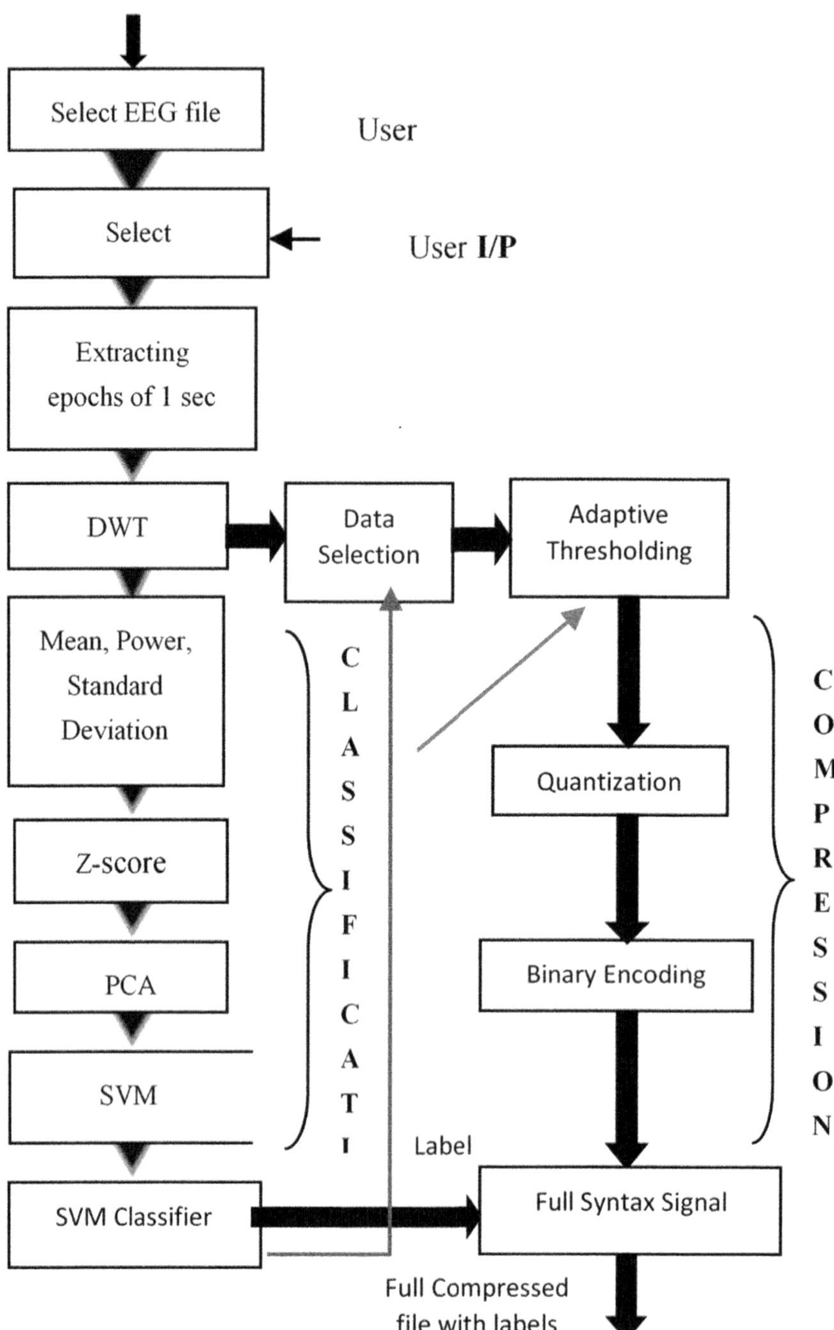

Fig. 1. Work flow architecture of the proposed algorithm [17].

in a later sections. The thresholded coefficients are then quantized for binary encoding.

Binary Encoding is the last stage of the process. We used both the Huffman and Arithmetic encoders separately. The binary coding was done using the standard built in functions of MATLAB library.

4 Results and Discussions

4.1 Dataset

In order to evaluate the performance of the proposed algorithm and to explore the merit of relation between compression and classification of EEG signals, the EEG data from Children's Hospital Boston dataset (CHBMIT) is used. The dataset consist of EEG recordings from paediatric subjects with unmanageable seizures. These recordings of 23 cases were gather round from 22 subjects (5 males, ages 3–22; and 17 females, ages 15–19). The EEG recordings were sampled 256 Hz. The International 10–20 electrode placement was used for recording EEG using 23 channels. The datasets is about generalized absence seizure categorized by 3 Hz spike and wave epileptic pattern in for every channel [16]. So the performance evaluation of the proposed algorithm in terms of classifying the epileptic and non-epileptic data corresponds to only one category of epilepsy which is absence seizure.

4.2 Performance Metrics

In this paper, we are using multiple metrics to evaluate the effectiveness of the proposed classification and compression methodologies. Performance evaluation in terms of classifying the EEG data as epileptic or non-epileptic, we are using the classification Accuracy, Specificity and Sensitivity. Accuracy, Specificity and sensitivity of the classifier are defined as (1), (2), and (3), respectively.

$$Accuracy = \frac{Number\ of\ true\ Labels}{Total\ number\ of\ Labels} \tag{1}$$

$$Specificity = \frac{TN}{TN + FP} \tag{2}$$

$$Sensitivity = \frac{TP}{TP + FN} \tag{3}$$

Where TN corresponds to True negative, FP is False positive, TP is True positive and FN is False negative. The performance measures for compression algorithms are Compression Ratio (CR), Percentage Root Mean Square Distortion (PRD). CR is defined as the ratio of the size of original data to that of the compressed data.

$$CR = \frac{LO}{LC} \tag{4}$$

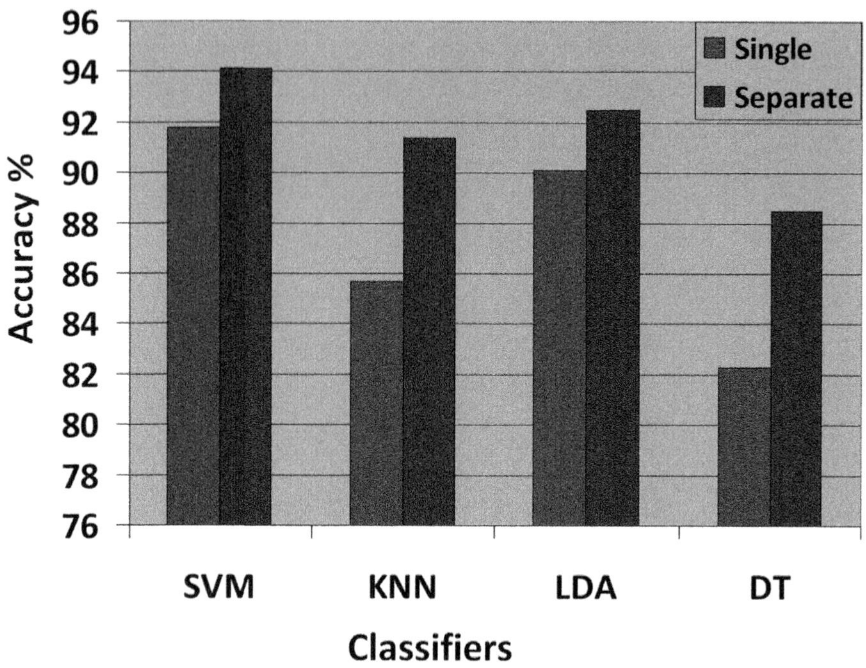

Fig. 2. Classification accuracy of single and separate classifiers.

where LO and LC corresponds to the size of EEG signal in bytes before and after compression, respectively. PRD is the standard measure to determine distortion between two signals, defined as

$$PRD = \sqrt{\frac{\sum_{n=1}^{N}(x[n] - x'[n])^2}{\sum_{n=1}^{N}(x[n])^2}} \tag{5}$$

Here $x[n]$ presents the original EEG signal whereas $x'[n]$ corresponds to the compressed EEG signal. N is the numbers of samples. Finally, the Similarity Index (SI) between original and decompressed EEG is calculated by dividing the number of classification labels of decompressed signal similar to the labels obtained for original EEG data by total number of classification labels given as

$$SI = \frac{Number\ of\ similar\ Labels}{Total\ number\ of\ Labels} \tag{6}$$

Another performance evaluation metric is the Data Reduction (DR), which is used for the case where we are summarizing the epileptic events by discarding non-epileptic epochs and compressing epileptic epochs. DR is measured as (Fig. 2):

$$DR = \frac{Number\ of\ original\ epochs}{Number\ of\ remaining\ epochs} \tag{7}$$

4.3 Experiments on Classification

In this work on extended i-NSS we present experimental results for classification using two training approaches and three new classifiers i.e. KNN, LDA and DT in addition to our original choice of SVM from our previous work. In the first approach a single shared classifier is used for all channels trained with EEG data from all channels. In the second approach we have separate classifiers for each channel.

For our current experiments we have used a portion of the CHBMIT dataset. The CHBMIT dataset is very biased towards non-epileptic events as compared to epileptic ones. Many EEG files are without any seizure event. To experiment with data balancing technique, we selected all the files of dataset that contained at least one epileptic seizure event. Within these files, the 1-sec epochs were randomly selected with non-epileptic and eplipetic epochs balanced in ratio of 67% to 33% respectively. Although we have applied some data balancing but still the ratio of non-epileptic events is higher. As a result, we have a total 30,165 epochs for classification. We used 10-fold cross validation scheme for performance evaluation of the proposed classification algorithm. We divided the data into ten parts out of which nine are used for training and one part is used for testing the classifier predictions. The process is repeated 10 times and after every iteration, testing data part is replaced with the new one. Purpose of using 10-fold cross validation is to reduce bias in the data. So using this method provides the advantage that each data points will be tested only once but processed in the training for 9 times.

We used MATLAB Classification Toolbox for classifiers. The choices of classifier configuration parameters are as follows: The Kernel function for SVM is linear with box-constraint of 0.75. The solver parameter is Sequential Minimal Optimization (SMO). In case of KNN, the Nearest-neighbors search method is 'kdtree' and number of nearest neighbors is one. The distance weighting function is 'equal' which assign equal weight to each neighbor. For LDA classifier, we are using 'IterationLimit' value of 100 for maximum number of iterations for batch processing and Solver for optimization is CGS (Collapsed Gibbs Sampling). Verbose is enabled with value 1. Hyperparameters to optimize DT are 'auto' and the predictor selection parameter is 'allsplits'.

Figure 1 shows the results obtained by these two approaches for SVM, KNN, LDA and DT. A significant increase in classification accuracy of all the listed classifiers can be seen in Fig. 1 on employing separate classifier approach. This is in line with our earlier reported results.

Table 1 shows the Average Accuracy, Sensitivity and Specificity of the proposed algorithm for different classifiers. The highest performance among all the utilized classifiers is achieved by SVM that is followed by LDA. Also channel-wise classification accuracy for SVM classifier is presented in Table 2. In this table accuracy obtained by using a single shared classifier for all the channels is compared when separate classifiers for each channel are utilized. As expected the performances in the second case is superior. Table 3, Table 4 and Table 5 presents both of these cases for KNN, LDA and DT respectively.

Table 1. Average accuracy, sensitivity and specificity of classifiers with separate classifier for every channel.

Classifier	Average accuracy (%)	Average sensitivity (%)	Average specificity (%)
SVM	94.1	87.2	96.1
KNN	91.4	79.3	89.3
LDA	92.5	83.9	94.3
DT	88.5	81.8	92.2

4.4 Experiments on Compression and Summarization

This section discusses our experiments on compression and summarization and explains how co-operation in classification can lead to intelligent compression. Though Neurologists requirement may vary, we will discuss three typical modes. We used EEG data from the same dataset for compression that we used for classification part.

Table 2. Channel wise classification accuracy of SVM.

Channel	Accuracy (%) using single classifier	Accuracy (%) using separate classifier
FP1F7	87.5	88.6
F7T7	89.9	92.4
T7P7	94.2	94.6
P7O1	92.8	96.3
FP1F3	91.6	92.6
F3C3	92.8	97.6
C3P3	90.9	93.1
FP2F4	88.4	88.6
F4C4	91.2	96.4
C4P4	92.5	94.7
P4O2	89.9	93.9
FP2F8	93.7	95.6
F8T8	92.6	97.8
T8P8	94.7	95.4
P8O2	90.1	96.2
FZCZ	91.8	93.9
CZPZ	89.9	90.1
P7T7	93.3	91.7
T7FT9	95.7	93.9
FT9FT10	92.8	96.8
FT10T8	94.8	97.2
T8P8	91.8	94.8
Average	91.8	94.1

Table 3. Channel wise classification accuracy of KNN.

Channel	Accuracy (%) using single classifier	Accuracy (%) using separate classifier
FP1F7	83.2	87.8
F7T7	87.6	88.3
T7P7	89.4	90.7
P7O1	86.8	89.3
FP1F3	91.7	94.8
F3C3	79.3	89.5
C3P3	74.8	82.1
FP2F4	83.0	91.2
F4C4	87.6	96.8
C4P4	89.3	90.9
P4O2	90.8	92.5
FP2F8	81.6	93.4
F8T8	75.8	87.9
T8P8	79.5	92.8
P8O2	92.9	93.1
FZCZ	85.4	89.9
CZPZ	89.1	94.5
P7T7	74.2	90.2
T7FT9	91.4	97.1
FT9FT10	87.3	90.8
FT10T8	93.7	95.5
T8P8	91.8	91.8
Average	85.7	91.4

Compression of Raw EEG Data. This is the simplest mode of compression where all unlabeled EEG data is compressed indiscriminately. Level 8 DWT coefficients are calculated prior to thresholding.

Figure 3 shows an epoch of a single channel non-epileptic EEG for raw and decompressed EEG data. The EEG epoch is taken from the first file of 'Patient 1' of the dataset. The channel is 'FP1F7' and the epoch is the first one. The decompressed epoch here is obtained by Arithmetic compression scheme with threshold levels 0 (PRD = 2.55), 2 (PRD = 5.06) and 4 (PRD = 6.87). We can see from the figure that both the raw and decompressed waveforms are quite similar perceptually. This is important so that the Neurologists assessment should not change on reconstructed data. Figure 3 shows the same scenario for an epileptic epoch with threshold levels 0 (PRD = 2.43), 2 (PRD = 4.32) and 4 (PRD = 5.56). This epileptic epoch corresponds to the third file of Patient 1. Epoch number is 3000 and the channel is 'FP1F7'.

Table 6 presents average CR and PRD of Arithmetic compression for multiple threshold levels. Table 6 witnesses the fact that increasing the threshold level

Table 4. Channel wise classification accuracy of LDA.

Channel	Accuracy (%) using single classifier	Accuracy (%) using separate classifier
FP1F7	89.2	89.7
F7T7	88.5	89.3
T7P7	90.0	91.6
P7O1	92.8	93.4
FP1F3	87.2	91.2
F3C3	91.7	92.1
C3P3	87.9	94.6
FP2F4	86.6	88.9
F4C4	91.9	91.9
C4P4	92.0	94.6
P4O2	89.3	95.8
FP2F8	91.9	93.5
F8T8	84.2	86.9
T8P8	89.8	93.9
P8O2	94.3	95.8
FZCZ	85.9	87.7
CZPZ	91.8	95.3
P7T7	86.6	90.1
T7FT9	93.3	93.8
FT9FT10	90.1	92.6
FT10T8	91.4	96.7
T8P8	94.9	94.9
Average	90.1	92.5

increases the CR but also the PRD. This implies that for a higher value of CR, distortion in the signal also increases so that we have to tradeoff between CR and PRD. Ratio of CR and PRD is also provided in the table. Here we can see that for a higher value of CR, PRD is also high but the ratio between these two metrics decreases for higher values of CR. This means the tradeoff is better for lower threshold values. Table 7 presents the same results as in Table 6 but for Huffman encoding scheme. Comparing the results shown in both the tables, we conclude that Arithmetic encoding scheme achieved better results in terms of CR versus PRD for lower threshold values but this preference recedes to equivalence on choice of higher thresholds for more compression. In Table 11 we have presented CR and PRD of a few existing EEG compression techniques. The comparison shows that the performance of our compression scheme is towards the better side.

Table 8 shows results of SI (Similarity Index) in percentage between the classification results of original EEG data and the decompressed data using Arithmetic compression scheme for different classifiers. All the results presented in this

Table 5. Channel wise classification accuracy of DT.

Channel	Accuracy (%) using single classifier	Accuracy (%) using separate classifier
FP1F7	87.6	88.5
F7T7	85.1	91.7
T7P7	85.8	89.3
P7O1	82.0	86.9
FP1F3	80.9	83.4
F3C3	84.8	91.5
C3P3	78.6	83.1
FP2F4	76.0	90.6
F4C4	77.6	85.8
C4P4	79.3	91.3
P4O2	80.2	89.1
FP2F8	80.4	94.2
F8T8	82.0	84.2
T8P8	83.3	86.3
P8O2	86.7	93.9
FZCZ	80.8	87.4
CZPZ	77.0	82.6
P7T7	77.1	86.5
T7FT9	85.8	91.1
FT9FT10	84.0	87.3
FT10T8	88.5	93.9
T8P8	88.5	88.5
Average	82.3	88.5

table are obtained by using threshold level zero. SVM achieved highest similarity for Arithmetic coding among all the listed classifiers followed by LDA having quite similar results as SVM. Table 9 discusses the same results as Table 8 but for Huffman encoding scheme. Similarity for SVM, KNN and LDA are comparable in both encoding modes and for DT it is somewhat higher using Huffman coding. Overall we see that similarity in classification for original and reconstructed remains close to 100% (very few changes in decisions) irrespective of classifier type.

Table 10 presents the SI of SVM classifier with different threshold levels. Though SI decreased somewhat with increase in threshold level it. Still hovers around 100% (Fig. 4).

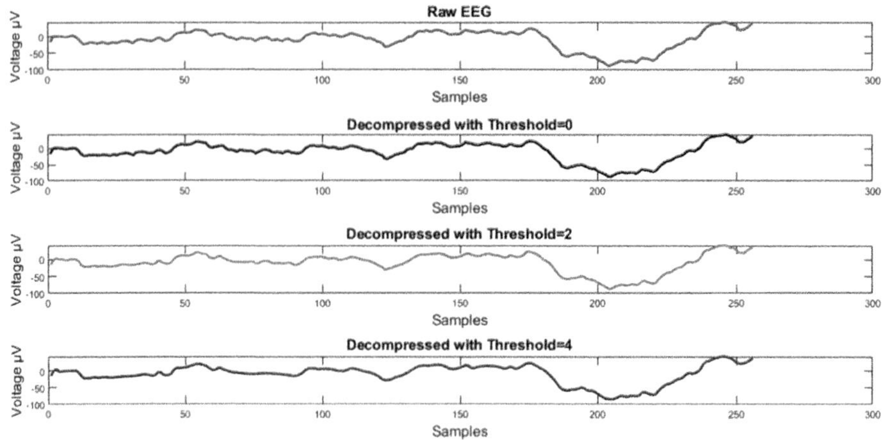

Fig. 3. Raw and decompressed EEG of a single channel for non-epileptic epoch.

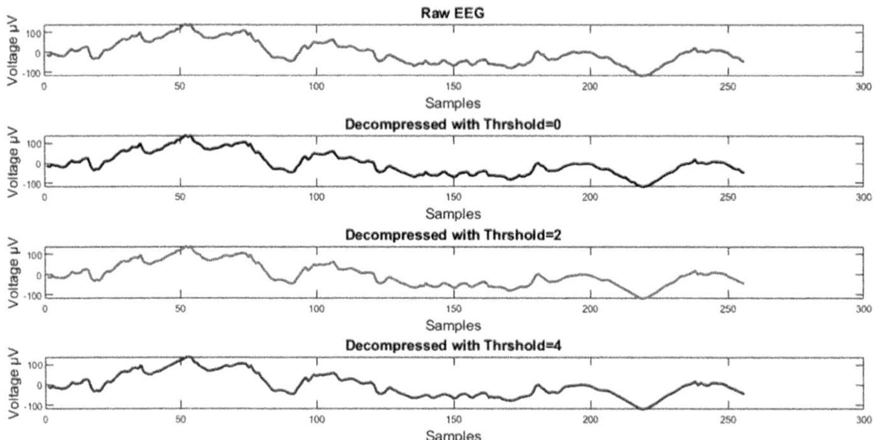

Fig. 4. Raw and Decompressed EEG of a single channel for epileptic epoch.

Adaptive Compression of EEG on Prepared Summary. In this case different EEG intervals undergo compression at different rates. We cover one option here but different variants of adaptive compression are possible. After, the classification branch categorizes the epochs as epileptic or non-epileptic, the idea is to compress the epileptic epochs at the lowest threshold of 0 for maintaining highest quality. Furthermore, the non-epileptic epochs are compressed at the highest threshold level of 4 to provide more compression. The main goal is to make the quality of signal indifferent intervals adaptive to the importance of the signal and minimizes the chances of any adverse effect on the neurologist's decision. Tables 12 and 13 present the results obtained for Huffman and Arithmetic compression schemes applied on EEG data. The epileptic epochs are still

Table 6. CR and PRD of Huffman compression for SVM with different threshold levels.

Serial No	Threshold level	Average CR	Average PRD (%)	CR/PRD
1	0	3.65	4.31	0.84
2	1	4.06	5.83	0.69
3	2	4.86	7.80	0.62
4	3	5.06	9.11	0.55
5	4	5.34	10.68	0.50

Table 7. CR and PRD of Arithmetic compression for SVM with different threshold levels.

Serial no	Threshold level	Average CR	Average PRD (%)	CR/PRD
1	0	3.72	3.81	0.97
2	1	4.29	5.36	0.80
3	2	4.67	7.26	0.64
4	3	5.38	8.08	0.66
5	4	6.18	12.05	0.49

Table 8. Similarity index of Arithmetic compression for classifiers with threshold level 0.

Classifier	Average similarity%	Max similarity%
SVM	99.1	99.8
KNN	98.2	99.3
LDA	99.0	99.6
DT	96.7	99.1

Table 9. Similarity index of Huffman compression for classifiers with threshold level 0.

Classifier	Average similarity%	Max similarity%
SVM	99.2	99.7
KNN	97.8	99.8
LDA	99.4	99.9
DT	98.2	99.7

maintained at an acceptable PRD though the overall average compression ratio is maintained high (see Table 6 for reference). For this mode it is advisable to train the classifier for higher sensitivity (so that no true positive undergoes a high distortion despite increase of false positives). The neurologists on inspection can successfully eliminate a false positive stored with low distortion [5].

Table 10. Similarity index of SVM with different threshold levels for Arithmetic compression.

No	Threshold	Average similarity%	Max similarity%
1	0	99.1	99.8
2	1	99.1	99.9
3	2	98.9	99.8
4	3	98.8	99.5
5	4	98.4	99.3

Table 11. Comparison of compression and distortion results with existing approaches [17].

Ref	Technique	CR	PRD (%)
[15]	JPEG 2000	5	10
[19]	JPEG 2000 arithmetic code	5	7
[20]	Biorthogonal 4.4 DWT; SPIHT	5	7
[21]	SPIHT	6	7
[22]	Biorthogonal 4.4 DWT; SPIHT	7	10
[23]	CDF 9/7 DWT	8	10
[25]	DWT with adaptive arithmetic coding	11	10
[26]	Channel Clustering	1.89	–

Table 12. Adaptive compression results using Huffman scheme[17].

	Mean	Max	Min
CR	5.042	5.842	3.953
PRD (%)	10.72	19.92	6.256
PRD epileptic epochs only (%)	5.6054	7.8447	3.4437
PRD non-epileptic epochs only (%)	11.3604	19.2689	6.7594

Table 12 presents the achieved CRs and PRDs in this mode in terms of Mean, Max and Min values for Huffman compression scheme. Table 13 shows the same results for Arithmetic compression scheme. Though as per Table 10, automatic classification decisions on reconstructed signal are not likely to change at the used distortion levels still maintaining the low PRD for epileptic events keeps the fidelity of signal high enough for no perceivable difference during manual inspection thus reassuring the correctness of earlier classification results.

Summarization and Compression. A summary of EEG is very useful for Neurologists for quick review of epileptic events and their statistics. This mode allows saving of all the epochs labeled as epileptic events and discarding the non-

Table 13. Adaptive compression results using Arithmetic scheme[17].

	Mean	Max	Min
CR	5.208	6.123	4.072
PRD (%)	10.77	19.93	6.256
PRD epileptic epochs only (%)	5.63	7.84	3.44
PRD non-epileptic epochs only (%)	11.33	19.26	94.69

Table 14. Data reduction ratio[17].

Serial Noe	
1	6.2
2	6.5
3	7.1
4	7.6

epileptic epochs. Rest of the data is then compressed. The compression versus distortion performance is nearly the same as in Table 1 and Table 2. Compression after selective data reduction effectively reduces the overall file size as compared to the raw EEG compression file. Table 14 shows the data reduction ration (DR) for different threshold levels. Experiment with re-classification of decompressed data generated singular all epileptic classification labels as expected.

5 Discussion and Future Prospects

i-NSS is an ongoing alive project with the expectation to report more developments in future. The performance results both for classification and compression has been reported in our earlier publications [6,16,17] and the current one that has been shown to be state-of-the-art. The system was initially deployed as an analysis tool for Punjab Institute of Mental Health (PIMH) and our earlier publication [6,16] also presented results on PIMH database. We would be going for more extensive clinical feedback in near future. The key focus in this regard would be to formalize a new EEG summarization and compression format that can be used to store the compressed data, classification information along with clinical annotations for storage and later retrieval according to various cases discussed in this paper. One of non-trivial work would be the incorporation of the artefact reduction and filtering tool in the EEG signal before the actual analysis processing. For further performance improvement of our system, we intend to try out other wavelet families for analysis and Deep Learning approaches for classification. On the compression side we like to exploit lossless methods as well that keep the PRD still below 10%.

The expectation with automatic and semi-automatic support system is now increasing towards the requirement of supporting the neurologist in diagnosis of the epilepsy type and identifying specific epileptic patterns appearing in the EEG. There are almost ten types of epileptic patterns as mentioned by Noachtar et al. patterns like spikes, sharp wave, benign epileptic discharges of childhood, spike-wave complexes, slow spike-wave complexes, 3-Hz spike-wave complexes, polyspikes, hypsarrhythmia, seizure pattern, status pattern are considered as epileptic [6]. One challenge to move in this direction is that no open dataset is available to support this research and would require simultaneous effort of building a pre-marked data to this effect. Long-term prospects of this tool lay in extending the system for other neurological disorders. This especially include EEG analysis in diagnosis of Sleep Apnea, which is also a common Neurological disorder encountered by the Neurologists. In recent years, research regarding the development and utilization of biomarkers for diagnosis and even early diagnosis of Alzheimer/Parkinson disease is picking up while some work on EEG analysis for Autism can also be found in literature [4]. As databases are still rare for these diseases, the tool can aid neurologists to gather and build databases of potential biomarkers for research in this area.

6 Conclusion

In this paper we have provided a comprehensive view for our ongoing *i*-NSS project and updated the progress made in this regard. We also discussed the future prospects of this on going work to extend it as a general clinician and a research tool for the neurologists. The recently extended *i*-NSS system not only can be used to support Neurlogists regarding initial diagnosis of commonly occurring epilepsy type, Absence Seizure, but is also being extended for supporting Neurologists in management of data of epileptic patients. In this regard cases have been experimented with to summarize EEG file events, reduce data and store it in a lossless compressed form.

For this extended system, we have explored the synergy between classification and compression of epileptic EEG data. This is meant to make the processing efficient and maintain the fidelity of the signal with original classification and visual validation by the Neurologists. It successfully eliminates the need of taking DWT twice on the same data as would be required for separate compression and classification task. The *i*-NSS incorporated in our framework performed dual task. Firstly, it helped in intelligent compression of data by providing classification labels for epileptic and non-epileptic data. We have used Arithmetic and Huffman for encoding purpose and have achieved comparable compression and reconstruction quality results. However, we have observed that optimal efficiency may require a mix use of both approaches depending on the desired CR (Compression ratio) and PRD (Percentage Root Mean Square Distortion). Moreover, classification performed on decompressed signals yield nearly same results as of the classification of raw EEG signals. The classification fidelity achieved is greater than 99% based on this synergy between classification and compression. This implies that artefacts produced in the signal due to compression do not affect signal quality. It was found that by using the labels for classification from

i-NSS we may improve our compression results. For example, in adaptive mode, when we used the labels for epochs and compressed the epileptic epochs at low and non-epileptic epochs at high threshold, we observed that we can maintain low PRD of 5–6% for epileptic events at high overall compression ratios between 4–5. Firstly, this means that we can efficiently use the classification results to reduce and compress the data. Secondly, it can also provide us with classified data for storage of selective data that is deemed significant by the user. The novel shared scheme employed, in which classification and compression of EEG data simultaneously takes place, results in decrease in computational complexity and increase in efficacy of the system.

In the coming future we are planning deployment of our system with the clinicians for extensive field-testing. For that we intend to first complete the development work on the format of compressed EEG data files supporting the aforementioned cases. Another challenge will be incorporation of pre-processing for effective filtering or suppressing the real-life EEG artifacts.

References

1. Neligan, A., Sander, L.: The incidence and prevalence of epilepsy (2001)
2. Subasi, A., Gursoy, M.I.: EEG signal classification using PCA, ICA, LDA and support vector machines. Expert Syst. Appl. **37**(12), 8659–8666 (2010)
3. Higgins, G., et al.: The effects of lossy compression on diagnostically relevant seizure information in EEG signals. IEEE J. Biomed. Health Inform. **17**(1), 121–127 (2013)
4. Aslam, A., et al.: A10. 13uJ/classification 2-channel deep neural network-based SoC for emotion detection of autistic children. In: IEEE Custom Integrated Circuits Conference (CICC), pp. 1–4, March 2020
5. Benbadis, S.R., Tatum, W.O.: Overinterpretation of EEGs and misdiagnosis of epilepsy. J. Clin. Neurophysiol. **20**, 42–44 (2003)
6. Ahmad, M.A., Majeed, W., Khan, N.A.: Advancements in computer aided methods for EEG-based epileptic detection. In: Proceedings of the 7th International Conference on Bio-inspired Systems and Signal Processing (BIOSIGNALS), Eseo, Angers, Lorie Valley, France (2014)
7. Brain Products GmbH/Products and Applications/Analyzer 2. http://www.brainproducts.com/productdetails.php?id=17. Accessed 17 May 2013
8. Neuralynx Spike Sort 3D Software. http://neuralynx.com/research_software/spike_sort_3d. Accessed 20 May 2013
9. NeuroExplorer Home. http://www.neuroexplorer.com/. Accessed 5 May 2013
10. Noachtar, S., Rémi, J.: The role of EEG in epilepsy: a critical review. Epilepsy Behav. **15**, 22–33 (2009)
11. Goldberger, A.L., et al.: PhysioBank, PhysioToolkit, and PhysioNet: components of a new research resource for complex physiologic signals. Circulation **101**(23), e215–e220 (2000). Circulation Electronic Pages http://circ.ahajournals.org/cgi/content/full/101/23/e215
12. Mahmood, A., Zainab, R., Ahmad, R.A., Saeed, M., Kamboh, A.M.: Classification of multi-class motor imagery EEG using four band common spatial pattern. In: 39th Annual International Conference of the IEEE Engineering in Medicine and Biology Society (EMBC), pp. 1034–1037 (2017)

13. Casson, A.J., Villegas, E.R.: Toward online data reduction for portable electroencephalography systems in epilepsy. IEEE Trans. Biomed. Eng. **56**(12), 2816–2825 (2009)
14. Chiang, J., Ward, R.: Data reduction for wireless seizure detection systems. In: 6th Annual International IEEE EMBS Conference on Neural Engineering, San Diego, California, 6–8 November (2013)
15. Higgins, G., et al.: EEG compression using JPEG2000: how much loss is too much? In: Annual International Conference of the IEEE Engineering in Medicine and Biology Society (EMBC), pp. 614–617 (2010)
16. Ahmad, M.A., et al.: Comparative analysis of classifiers for developing an adaptive computer-assisted EEG analysis system for diagnosing epilepsy. BioMed. Res. Int. 14, Article ID 638036 (2015)
17. Basir, R., Khan, N.A.: Exploring the merit of collaboration in classification and compression of epilepsy EEG signal. Biosignals (2020)
18. Khan, Z.A., Mansoor, S.B., Ahmad, M.A., Malik, M.M.: Input devices for virtual surgical simulations: a comparative study. In: Proceedings of the 16th International Multi Topic Conference (INMIC), Lahore (2013)
19. Higgins, G., McGinley, B., Jones, E., Glavin, M.: Efficient EEG compression using JPEG2000 with coefficient thresholding. In: Signals and Systems Conference (ISSC 2010), IET Irish, pp. 59–64 (2010)
20. Daou, H., Labeau, F.: Pre-Processing of multi-channel EEG for improved compression performance using SPIHT. In: Annual International Conference of the IEEE Engineering in Medicine and Biology Society (EMBC), pp. 2232–2235 (2012)
21. Higgins, G.H., McGinley, B., Jones, E., Glavin, M.: An evaluation of the effects of wavelet coefficient quantisation in transform based EEG compression. Comput. Biol. Med. **43**, 661 (2013)
22. Hoda, D., Labeau, F.: Dynamic dictionary for combined EEG compression and seizure detection. IEEE J. Biomed. Health Inform. **18**, 247–256 (2014)
23. Higgins, G., McGinley, B., Glavin, M., Jones, E.: Low power compression of EEG signals using JPEG2000. In: Pervasive Health 2010, pp. 1–4 (2010)
24. NeuroExplorer Home. http://www.explorer.com/. Accessed 5 May 2013
25. Nguyen, B., Nguyen, D., Ma, W., Tran, D.: Wavelet transform and adaptive arithmetic coding techniques for EEG lossy compression. In: 2017 International Joint Conference on Neural Networks (IJCNN), Anchorage, AK, pp. 3153–3160 (2017). https://doi.org/10.1109/IJCNN.2017.7966249
26. Hejrati, B., Fathi, A., Abdali-Mohammadi, F.: Efficient lossless multi-channel EEG compression based on channel clustering. Biomed. Signal Process. Control **31**, 295–300 (2017)

Idle State Detection with an Autoregressive Multiple Model Probabilistic Framework in SSVEP-Based Brain-Computer Interfaces

Rosanne Zerafa[1(✉)], Tracey Camilleri[1], Owen Falzon[2], and Kenneth P. Camilleri[1,2]

[1] Department of Systems and Control Engineering, Faculty of Engineering, University of Malta, Msida, Malta
rosanne.zerafa@um.edu.mt
[2] Centre for Biomedical Cybernetics, University of Malta, Msida, Malta

Abstract. The detection of the idle state is a key feature in developing asynchronous steady-state visual evoked potential (SSVEP)-based brain-computer interfaces (BCIs). Despite the large number of successful SSVEP detection methods, only a few studies have explicitly included the detection of the idle state. This work demonstrates the feasibility of a novel autoregressive multiple model (AR-MM) probabilistic framework for the detection of SSVEPs and the idle state. In a MM framework an SSVEP is identified by selecting one of the candidate models, each representing a particular SSVEP class, that best represents the dynamics of the data. An average classification accuracy of 78.94 ± 10.28% and an information transfer rate (ITR) of 28.85 ± 9.39 bpm are obtained for the 6-class SSVEP dataset in a longitudinal study. Furthermore, this work quantifies the performance of the AR-MM framework, that provides a measure of probability, for idle state detection. An average area under curve (AUC) of 0.83 is achieved with different threshold settings for idle state detection. The idle state could be detected with 81% average accuracy when considering maximum idle state and non-idle state detection rates. The results, obtained from a single-channel analysis, validate that the AR-MM framework is a good candidate for SSVEP detection and also for the idle state detection when compared with two multivariate methods, the canonical correlation analysis (CCA) and its extension, the filter bank canonical correlation analysis (FBCCA). With only a pair of electrodes required for the AR-MM approach, this is more practical for daily use of BCI applications, where a minimal amount of channels are desirable.

Keywords: Steady-state visually evoked potential · Asynchronous BCI · Self-paced BCI · No control state · Work state · Rest state · Single-channel · Univariate · Multiple modelling · AR models · Brain machine interface

X. Ye et al. (Eds.): BIOSTEC 2020, CCIS 1400, pp. 263–288, 2021.
https://doi.org/10.1007/978-3-030-72379-8_13

1 Introduction

Steady-state visually evoked potentials (SSVEPs) are electrical potentials evoked in the brain in response to a repetitive visual stimulus that is flickering at a specific frequency [54]. This neural response consists of oscillatory activity at the fundamental frequency and harmonics of the visual stimulus, and is prominent in the occipital region of the brain. SSVEPs have been used in non-invasive electroencephalogram (EEG)-based brain-computer interfaces (BCIs) by uniquely associating the brain patterns, generated in response to the flickering visual stimuli, to specific commands to control an application [5,31,34,56].

An SSVEP-based BCI may be asynchronous (self-paced), giving the user the flexibility of voluntarily issuing a command at any time instant independently of any cues, unlike synchronous (cue-based) BCIs [8]. This requires more complex SSVEP detection techniques because the BCI must be able to distinguish between an SSVEP response and background or noise EEG. The former refers to an intentional control (IC) state [16], also referred to as the work state [41], where the user requests control of the system by attending to a stimulus. The latter refers to a non-intentional control (NC) state [57], also typically referred to as the idle state [45], no control state [8] or rest state [19], which occurs while the user is not attending to any of the stimuli. Compared to the vast number of SSVEP detection methods developed, there are a limited number of studies that are focused on the detection of the idle state in SSVEP-based BCIs. The two main idle state detection techniques are the threshold-based approach for rejecting/confirming idle states, and alternatively the training of a supervised classifier with control and idle states [19]. The determination of an idle state has also been addressed by the use of an on/off BCI switch, or by setting a time threshold that limits the execution of a control state until this is validated. A detailed review of the different idle state detection methods applied to asynchronous SSVEP-based BCIs found in the literature is given in Sect. 2.

This work investigates multiple models (MMs) as an alternative approach to current SSVEP detection methods. The concept of MMs in adaptive control was primarily introduced to efficiently deal with large and abrupt time-varying parameters of control systems [28,32]. Some control systems may have various behaviours suited for different environments. These systems should be able to recognize the specific environment and adapt in a rapid and efficient manner to these time-varying environments [40]. The basic assumption of MMs techniques is that a system may be represented by a finite number of models known a priori. However, at a particular time instant only one model or a mixture of the models is expected to provide a correct representation of the system. The problem of state estimation is reduced to the search of which model from the set of known models best represents the actual system at any given time [17]. The same concept has been applied as a classification technique to time series data and particularly of interest to biosignal data [6,13,42,44,47,50,65]. An SSVEP response consists of an oscillatory activity at a specific frequency that is well defined and distinct from background EEG activity. In an SSVEP-based BCI, as a user attends to different flickering stimuli, the EEG data recorded is expected to change from

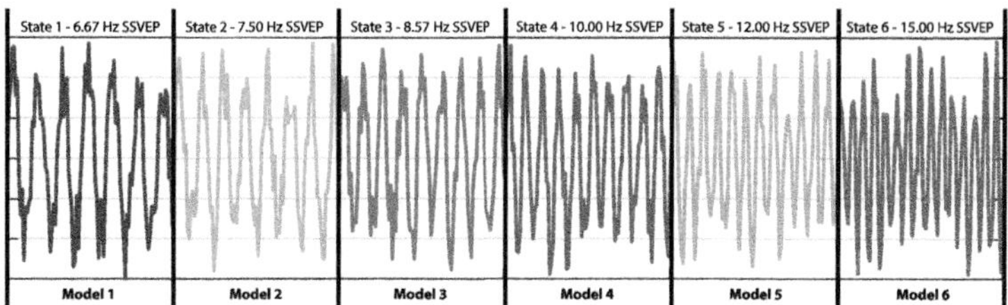

Fig. 1. Expert models each representing different SSVEP classes.

one state to another, representing distinct oscillatory activities in response to the different flickering visual stimuli. In this work it is shown that a MM framework is able to capture the different states of the EEG data.

In a MM approach different models may be trained to represent the different states of the data, each referred to as an expert model [25]. For an SSVEP-based BCI, each expert model would represent an SSVEP class that is attributed to a specific flickering stimulus, as shown in Fig. 1. This means that an SSVEP class can be identified by selecting one of the candidate models that best represents the current state of the data. In this work, each expert model is represented as a linear Gaussian state space model [20] with an autoregressive process. The use of parametric models, particularly autoregressive (AR) models and its variants, have been successfully applied to the analysis of EEG signals. For example, AR models have been used in spectral estimation [10,27,46,52], artifact/noise rejection [1,9,18,21,22,24,55] and for the estimation of the cortical functional connectivity [3]. In BCI related literature AR features are also commonly used directly for classification [26,48,51,66], however in this work AR models are used for prediction. The residual between the actual and predicted data is used to determine which model best represents the data. This residual is incorporated within a probabilistic framework in order to provide a probabilistic decision for classification [6].

A novel autoregressive multiple model (AR-MM) probabilistic framework has been presented for the detection of SSVEPs in BCIs in our previous work [62]. The proposed framework was compared to a number of other SSVEP detection techniques using a 12-class SSVEP dataset from 10 subjects [36]. The results obtained revealed that the univariate AR-MM probabilistic approach can yield a significant improvement in performance compared to power spectral density analysis (PSDA), a standard single-channel SSVEP detection method. The method was also compared to two state-of-the-art multivariate methods, specifically the canonical correlation analysis (CCA) and its extension, the filter bank canonical correlation analysis (FBCCA) methods. The results showed only a slightly lower performance compared to the CCA and FBCCA methods, specifically of 2.29% and 3.73%, respectively, with the advantage of requiring only a single-channel for SSVEP detection.

In this study, an extension of the investigation on the proposed AR-MM framework is presented, with the following goals:

(i) To demonstrate the feasibility of the AR-MM probabilistic framework for SSVEP detection on a larger dataset, which includes 6 SSVEP classes and an idle class, with data recorded from 10 subjects and repeated over three different days, such that the variation in performance is also investigated longitudinally.
(ii) To quantify the performance of the AR-MM framework with the inclusion of idle state detection, specifically demonstrating that the framework provides a measure of probability for each SSVEP class, which can be used as a measure of certainty in the decision making process of idle state detection.
(iii) To compare the performance of the single channel AR-MM framework for idle state detection with the performance of two standard multi-channel SSVEP detection techniques, specifically CCA and FBCCA, thus extending our previous work by demonstrating that even when incorporating the idle state detection the performance of the AR-MM framework remains comparable to the multi-channel methods while being more practical for real world BCI applications due to the lower number of required channels.

This article is organised as follows. A literature review on the different idle state detection techniques found in SSVEP-based BCI literature is given in the next section. Section 3 then gives a detailed mathematical description of the proposed AR-MM probabilistic framework for SSVEP detection which is followed by an overview of the reference SSVEP detection methods used for comparison in this study. The dataset containing both SSVEP and idle state classes is presented in Sect. 4 and the results obtained with the AR-MM probabilistic framework are presented in Sect. 5 and compared to the performance of the reference methods. Classification is initially based on SSVEP classes only and then the detection of the idle state class is also introduced. The results are then evaluated and discussed in Sect. 6.

2 Literature Review on Idle State Detection in SSVEP-based BCIs

The detection of the idle state is an essential feature for asynchronous BCIs. A literature review of the idle state detection methods applied in SSVEP-based BCIs has been conducted and the methods have been grouped into four categories as defined below:

- The threshold-based approach is the most common method for idle state identification in SSVEP-based BCIs [8,19,45]. This is a two-step process in which a standard SSVEP detection technique is primarily used to extract SSVEP features from an unlabelled trial. In the second step the features extracted are used to determine if the EEG data corresponds to an actual SSVEP trial or an idle state trial. Generally the feature with the largest value is associated with the target SSVEP class and this value is typically significantly larger than the values of the features associated with the rest of the non-target SSVEP classes. It is therefore assumed that in the case of an idle state trial, (i) the largest feature value obtained is relatively less than that typically obtained by a target SSVEP trial and (ii) that all the features obtained have equally low values. Based on these two assumptions, a threshold is set to distinguish between an SSVEP class and an idle state class. In some works this is done by fixing a threshold on the maximum feature value, which specifies if this is large enough to be considered as an SSVEP class or otherwise [8,67]. In other works a threshold on the difference among all the feature values is set to determine the confidence level of selecting a target SSVEP class [2,35,57,64]. The features obtained in the first step may be projected into a probability space before a threshold is set on the original features [8,33]. The selection of the thresholds may be fixed [8], subject-specific [64] or adaptive [2]. These thresholds vary significantly the level of sensitivity and specificity of the BCI system. Depending on the application, different rate of false positives with respect to false negatives may be preferred [45,67].

- Another idle state identification approach is that of a BCI with a trained classifier that is able to distinguish an idle state class from SSVEP classes [19]. This means that labelled idle state data and SSVEP state data are used for training. In case of an unlabelled trial, SSVEP features are first extracted using a standard SSVEP detection technique and then these features are fed to a supervised classifier. Binary classifiers such as the support vector machine (SVM) [53,63], k-means cluster analysis [49], and linear discriminant analysis (LDA) [41] trained to discriminate between idle state class and one SSVEP class have been implemented. In the case of multiple SSVEP classes, a second classification criteria is taken after results are obtained from the multiple binary classifiers. Alternatively, multiclass classifiers have also been applied in which case the classifier is specifically trained to discriminate the idle class from several other SSVEP classes [1,16,58,60].
- A different approach that has been used involves the introduction of an on/off switch, sometimes also referred to as a brain switch, that switches the BCI system on and off. A dedicated SSVEP flickering stimulus may be used to control the on/off state of the BCI, that is the start/stopping of the rest of the flickering stimuli corresponding to the different BCI commands [14, 29,45]. In this way, the idle state identification problem is only encountered when starting the BCI, during which only one stimulus corresponding to the BCI switch is flickering. Once the system is activated it works only in synchronous mode. Alternatively, hybrid BCI switches that combine SSVEPs with an additional physiological signal have also been developed [7,23], in which case the idle state detection is completely avoided.
- Another indirect approach to tackle non-intentional control states is achieved by the setting of a time threshold that limits the issuing of a control state. In this way a control signal is executed only if the identification of the same SSVEP class is maintained for a determined period of time. Otherwise the

system remains in a no control state. This technique has been used to reduce false negatives [15,43] or to adjust the individual SSVEP detection time in a dynamic stopping approach [39].

In this work a threshold-based approach is taken to distinguish the idle state from the SSVEP classes in the AR-MM probabilistic framework. The separability between idle state and non-idle state features is first evaluated using the area under the receiver operating characteristics (AUROC) curve and this is compared to the separability obtained using the CCA and FBCCA methods. This gives an overall indication of the measure of separability between features without the subjective selection of a threshold value. The detection of the idle state was then evaluated in terms of classification accuracy where different thresholds were chosen to find the best compromise between the idle state and non-idle state detection rates.

3 Methodology

3.1 Autoregressive Multiple Modelling (AR-MM) Probabilistic Framework

In this section, a mathematical description of the AR-MM probabilistic framework specifically applied to detect SSVEPs from a single channel of EEG data is presented. In this multiple model approach, different expert models, which are assumed to be autoregressive, represent different SSVEP classes. An unknown SSVEP class is then identified by selecting one of the candidate models that best represents the dynamics of the EEG data.

Let $\boldsymbol{Y}^T = y_1, ..., y_T$ be a sequence of EEG data having dynamics that depend upon the sequence of p-dimensional latent state variables $\boldsymbol{X}^T = \boldsymbol{x}_1, ..., \boldsymbol{x}_T$. Thus the joint distribution between $\boldsymbol{X}^T$ and $\boldsymbol{Y}^T$ of a linear Gaussian state space model that follows a Bayesian network is given by [20]:

$$p(\boldsymbol{X}^T, \boldsymbol{Y}^T) = p(\boldsymbol{x}_1) \prod_{t=2}^{T} p(\boldsymbol{x}_t|\boldsymbol{x}_{t-1}) \prod_{t=1}^{T} p(y_t|\boldsymbol{x}_t) \tag{1}$$

where $p(\cdot)$ denotes the probability density function and $\boldsymbol{x}_t$ is assumed to be a continuous real-valued hidden state variable. Assuming linearity and Gaussianity, the state space model is represented by the following state and measurement equations:

$$\boldsymbol{x}_t = \boldsymbol{\Phi} \boldsymbol{x}_{t-1} + \boldsymbol{w}_t \tag{2}$$

$$y_t = \boldsymbol{H}_t \boldsymbol{x}_t + v_t \tag{3}$$

where y_t is the observed EEG data from a single channel at time t, $\boldsymbol{x}_t = [-a_1, ..., -a_p]^\top$ is the hidden state vector made up of p autoregressive parameters, $\boldsymbol{H}_t = [y_{t-1}, ..., y_{t-p}]$ is the observation vector made up of p past EEG data samples, $\boldsymbol{\Phi}$ represents the state transition matrix, and $\boldsymbol{w}_t$ and v_t are two independent Gaussian noise processes assumed to have zero mean and covariance $\boldsymbol{Q}$

and variance R, respectively. In this work, $\boldsymbol{H}_t$ is taken to consist of the past p narrow band pass filtered EEG data, specifically filtered around the first H harmonic frequency components corresponding to the SSVEP class being modelled by that state space model, and y_t is made up of unfiltered EEG data at time t. Apart from the unknown AR parameters $\boldsymbol{x}_t$, the unknown parameters that characterise the model are collectively represented by $\boldsymbol{\Theta} = [R, \boldsymbol{Q}, \boldsymbol{\Phi}, \boldsymbol{\mu}, \boldsymbol{\Sigma}]$, where $\boldsymbol{\mu}$ represents the initial hidden state vector and $\boldsymbol{\Sigma}$ its corresponding covariance.

In a MM system, a set of N expert models each represented by unique state space Eqs. (2) and (3) and having system parameters $\boldsymbol{\Theta}^i$ for $i = 1, ..., N$, need to be trained. The training process to learn these system parameters $\boldsymbol{\Theta}$ is described in the next section. Once the different models are trained to represent each of the classes in the system, a probabilistic approach may be used to identify which of the candidate models best represents the data.

Under this framework, the posterior probability for each model M^i given $\boldsymbol{Y}^t$, which represents the observed EEG data up till time t, is given by Bayes' rule as follows [17]:

$$Pr(M^i|\boldsymbol{Y}^t) = Pr(M^i|y_t, \boldsymbol{Y}^{t-1}) = \frac{p(y_t|M^i, \boldsymbol{Y}^{t-1})Pr(M^i|\boldsymbol{Y}^{t-1})}{\sum_{j=1}^{N} p(y_t|M^j, \boldsymbol{Y}^{t-1})Pr(M^j|\boldsymbol{Y}^{t-1})} \tag{4}$$

where $Pr(M^i|\boldsymbol{Y}^{t-1})$ is the prior probability and $p(y_t|M^i, \boldsymbol{Y}^{t-1})$ is the likelihood function. The likelihood function for each MM is assumed to be Gaussian with mean $\hat{\boldsymbol{y}}_t^i$ and covariance $\boldsymbol{C}_t^i$ is estimated as follows:

$$p(y_t|M^i, \boldsymbol{Y}^{t-1}) = -\frac{1}{(2\pi)^{\frac{1}{2}}|\boldsymbol{C}_t^i|^{\frac{1}{2}}} \exp^{-\frac{1}{2}(y_t - \hat{y}_t^i)'(C_t^i)^{-1}(y_t - \hat{y}_t^i)} \tag{5}$$

In Eq. (5), $(y_t - \hat{y}_t^i)$ represents the difference between the observation y_t and its mean estimate $\hat{y}_t^i$, referred to as the residual. The mean estimate of the observation $\hat{y}_t^i$ is given by:

$$\hat{y}_t^i = \boldsymbol{H}_t^i \hat{\boldsymbol{x}}_{t|t-1}^i \tag{6}$$

where $\hat{\boldsymbol{x}}_{t|t-1}^i$ denotes the conditional expectation of state $\boldsymbol{x}_t$. In Eq. (5), $\boldsymbol{C}_t^i$ is the variance of $\hat{y}_t^i$ estimated as follows:

$$\boldsymbol{C}_t^i = \boldsymbol{H}_t^i \boldsymbol{P}_{t|t-1}^i \boldsymbol{H}_t^{i^{\top}} + R^i \tag{7}$$

where $\boldsymbol{P}_{t|t-1}^i$ denotes the corresponding state estimation error covariance.

When evaluating the posterior probability $Pr(M^i|\boldsymbol{Y}^t)$ in Eq. (4), the prior probability of the model $Pr(M^i|\boldsymbol{Y}^{t-1})$ is taken into consideration. The prior probabilities are here set to be uniformly distributed, that is, each model has equal chance of modelling new data. This was done by setting all prior probabilities equal to $1/N$, where N represents the number of models.

Given the assumption of stationarity within a fixed time window, a non-adaptive approach is considered, where the hidden state vector and its covariance are not updated but remain constant over time. Therefore, the initial state vector

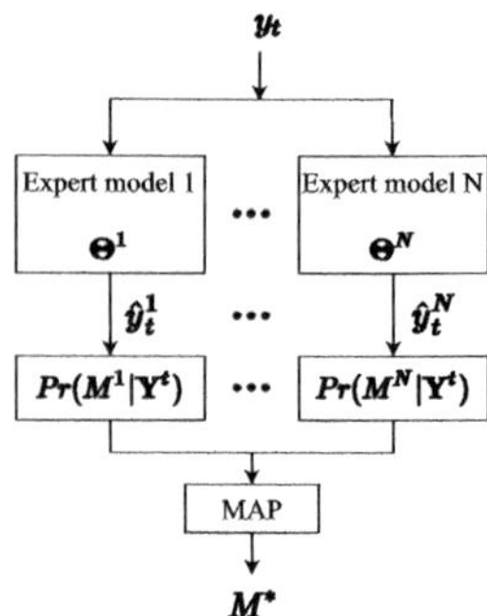

Fig. 2. AR-MM probabilistic framework with N expert models acting as candidates to model the observed sequence y_t. The model M^* that has the highest posterior probability is considered as the model that best represents the data [62].

and its corresponding covariance remain the same $\boldsymbol{\mu} = \boldsymbol{x}_t$ and $\boldsymbol{\Sigma} = \boldsymbol{Q}$. Consequently in Eqs. (6) and (7), the initial state vector and corresponding covariance are used to calculate the posterior probability, $\hat{\boldsymbol{x}}^i_{t|t-1} = \boldsymbol{\mu}^i$ and $\boldsymbol{P}^i_{t|t-1} = \boldsymbol{\Sigma}^i$ for all t. It follows that $\boldsymbol{\Phi} = I$ in Eq. (2).

Under this framework, N probabilities corresponding to the N models are obtained at each time instance with Eq. (4). The model M^* that has the maximum a posteriori (MAP) probability is then considered as the model that best represents the incoming data from the set of available models. Figure 2 shows a block diagram of the AR-MM probabilistic framework.

Training for the Probabilistic AR-MM Framework. The process of learning the AR parameters $\boldsymbol{x}^i_t$ and system parameters $\boldsymbol{\Theta}^i$ in a multiple modelling framework requires SSVEP training data for each class. Let z^i be a vector of a single channel SSVEP EEG data, with $i = 1, ..., N_f$ representing the number of target stimulus frequencies. This data is then narrow band pass filtered around the fundamental frequency f and the first H harmonic components corresponding to the SSVEP class i and is represented here by z^i_f. The estimation of parameters $\boldsymbol{x}^i_t$ and $\boldsymbol{\Theta}^i$ is then being carried out as follows [62]:

- The AR parameters $\boldsymbol{x}^i_t$ for the expert model M^i are found using the filtered training data z^i_f. AR parameters are estimated using Burg's method and the length of $\boldsymbol{x}^i_t$ represents the AR model of order p which was here set to 20.
- The unknown variance R is estimated from Eq. (3), where the observation vector y_t is replaced with training data z_t, i.e. $v_t = z_t - \boldsymbol{H}_t\boldsymbol{x}_t$. In this case $\boldsymbol{H}_t$ represents p past narrow bandpass filtered training data, i.e. $\boldsymbol{H}_t = [z_{f_{t-1}}, ..., z_{f_{t-p}}]$. The variance σ^i_l of the resulting v_t is obtained from each training trial of all the classes $i = 1, ..., N_f$, where $l = 1, ..., L$ represents the number of training trials. The mean variance across all the training trials gives R, i.e. $R = 1/(N_f L)\sum_{i=1}^{N_f}\sum_{l=1}^{L}\sigma^i_l$.
- The unknown covariance $\boldsymbol{Q}^i$ for model M^i is estimated from Eq. (2), where for the non-adaptive approach $\boldsymbol{x}^i_t = \boldsymbol{x}^i_{t-1} + \boldsymbol{w}_t$. Therefore, the covariance of

$\boldsymbol{x}_t^i \in \mathbb{R}^p$ obtained from AR parameters across different training trials gives $\boldsymbol{Q}^i \in \mathbb{R}^{p \times p}$.

- As discussed earlier, following the non-adaptive approach, the rest of the unknown system parameters are defined as $\boldsymbol{\mu} = \boldsymbol{x}_t$, $\boldsymbol{\Sigma} = \boldsymbol{Q}$ and $\boldsymbol{\Phi} = I$.

3.2 Comparative Methods

The performance of the proposed AR-MM method is compared to a single-channel PSDA method, as well as the CCA and FBCCA multi-channel methods. In our previous study [62] the results obtained for the single-channel AR-MM probabilistic framework showed significant improvement over the single-channel PSDA method. Even more promising, the classification accuracies obtained were only slightly lower compared to the multichannel methods, CCA and FBCCA, for most time windows. As an extension of the previous work [62], a threshold-based idle detection method is used for AR-MM, CCA and FBCCA and their relative performances is compared using a new SSVEP dataset which also includes the idle state. A brief mathematical description of CCA and FBCCA is presented below.

Canonical Correlation Analysis (CCA). In the literature, CCA is one of the most frequently used methods to detect SSVEPs and is generally used as a reference method with respect to which new SSVEP methods are compared [61]. In CCA the underlying correlation between two sets of multidimensional variables is determined. In this case the correlation between multi-channel EEG signals and a set of sine-cosine reference signals that model the SSVEPs evoked by each stimulus frequency [30].

Let $\boldsymbol{Y}$ and $\boldsymbol{X}_f$ be two multidimensional variables representing the multi-channel EEG signals of length T and a set of SSVEP reference signals of the same length as $\boldsymbol{Y}$, respectively. The sine-cosine reference signals $\boldsymbol{X}_f$ for the target stimulus frequency f are defined by [4]:

$$\boldsymbol{X}_f = \begin{pmatrix} \sin(2\pi f \frac{t}{F_s}) \\ \cos(2\pi f \frac{t}{F_s}) \\ \vdots \\ sin(2\pi H f \frac{t}{F_s}) \\ \cos(2\pi H f \frac{t}{F_s}) \end{pmatrix}^{\top}, \qquad t = 1, \ldots, T \tag{8}$$

where F_s is the sampling frequency, T is the number of samples and H is the number of harmonics. In this work the number of harmonic frequency components was set to $H = 3$.

CCA finds the linear combinations $y = \boldsymbol{Y}^{\top} \boldsymbol{W}_y$ and $x_f = \boldsymbol{X}_f^{\top} \boldsymbol{W}_{x_f}$, such that the correlation between the two canonical variants y and x_f is maximized [30]. The weight vectors $\boldsymbol{W}_y$ and $\boldsymbol{W}_{x_f}$ are found by solving the following optimization problem [38]:

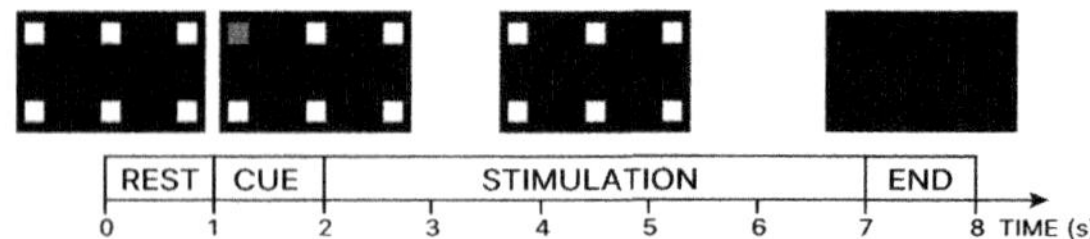

Fig. 3. Representation of the experimental protocol. Each trial consisted of an initial 1 s interval during which all 6 stimuli were static. A visual cue then instructed the user to direct their attention to one target stimulus highlighted in red for a stimulus trial or to the centre of the screen for an idle trial. After this 1 s cue, all the 6 stimuli flickered for 5 s at their respective frequency. Subjects directed their attention either at the target stimulus, or at the centre of the screen for a stimulus or an idle trial, respectively. This stimulus period was followed by a blank screen which indicated the end of the trial [59]. (Color figure online)

$$\max_{\boldsymbol{W}_y, \boldsymbol{W}_{x_f}} \rho_f(y, x_f) = \frac{\mathrm{E}[y^\top x_f]}{\sqrt{\mathrm{E}[y^\top y]\mathrm{E}[x_f^\top x_f]}} = \frac{\mathrm{E}[\boldsymbol{W}_y^\top \boldsymbol{Y} \boldsymbol{X}_f{}^\top \boldsymbol{W}_{x_f}]}{\sqrt{\mathrm{E}[\boldsymbol{W}_y^\top \boldsymbol{Y}\boldsymbol{Y}^\top \boldsymbol{W}_y]\mathrm{E}[\boldsymbol{W}_{x_f}^\top \boldsymbol{X}_f \boldsymbol{X}_f{}^\top \boldsymbol{W}_{x_f}]}} \tag{9}$$

For each reference signal, a maximum canonical correlation ρ_f is obtained and used as an SSVEP feature. The hypothesis is that the reference signal with the largest correlation contains SSVEP at the same frequency as the stimulus signal.

Filter Bank Canonical Correlation Analysis (FBCCA). Various CCA extensions have been developed in the literature [61]. The FBCCA method is one of the CCA variants that has been shown to improve the frequency detection of SSVEPs [11]. This filter bank has also been applied to different SSVEP detection methods as a pre-processing step before feature extraction [12,37]. The FBCCA method decomposes SSVEPs into multiple sub-band components and performs separate CCAs between each of the sub-band components and sine-cosine reference signal to obtain a weighted sum of the canonical correlation coefficients from each band.

The filter bank designed consists of K sub-bands covering multiple harmonic frequency bands [11]. In this work the lower and upper cut-off frequencies of the kth sub-band were set to $k \times 6.67$ Hz 80 Hz respectively, and the number of sub-bands was set to $K = 4$. The correlation values between the sub-band components $\boldsymbol{Y}_{SB_k}, k = 1, ..., K$ from the original EEG signals $\boldsymbol{Y}$ and the reference signals $\boldsymbol{X}_f$ corresponding to all stimulation frequencies f are estimated to form a correlation vector $\boldsymbol{\rho}_f = [\rho_f^1, \ldots, \rho_f^K]^\top$.

A weighted sum of squares of the correlation values corresponding to all sub-band components is then calculated as the feature for SSVEP detection as follows [11]:

$$\tilde{\rho}_f = \sum_{k=1}^{K} \boldsymbol{w}(k) \cdot (\rho_f^k)^2 \tag{10}$$

where $\boldsymbol{w}(k)$ are the weights of the sub-band components. These weights are set by the observation that the signal to noise ratio (SNR) of SSVEP harmonics decreases as the response frequency increases [11]:

$$\boldsymbol{w}(k) = k^{-a} + b, \quad k = 1, ..., K \tag{11}$$

where a and b are constants that maximize the classification performance and were fixed to 1.25 and 0.25 respectively, based on the findings in [11]. The frequency of the reference signals having the maximum correlation $\tilde{\rho}_f$ is then considered to be the target stimulus.

4 Materials

The dataset used in this study was originally used in our previous work in a comparative study to analyse the effect of distractors in SSVEP-based BCIs [59]. The segment of data with no external distractors is used for this work. Ten healthy subjects participated in this study, which was approved by the University Research Ethics Committee at the University of Malta. All volunteers had normal or corrected-to-normal vision and were free from any medication known to affect EEG recordings. Subjects went through a screening process and were excluded from the study if they had known neurological conditions, a history of epilepsy, seizure, or any adverse reaction to light or pattern stimulation. Two of the subjects had previous experience with EEG recordings, however only one of the subjects had experience with SSVEP setups.

Each subject participated in three recording sessions, with approximately three weeks between each session. Experiments were conducted in a quiet research laboratory where subjects were seated approximately 1 m away from a 15.4" LCD screen. During the experiments, subjects were instructed to direct their attention towards one of the six flickering stimuli presented as white squares on a black background, following the protocol shown in Fig. 3. The six stimuli presented were 6.67 Hz, 7.50 Hz, 8.57 Hz, 10.00 Hz, 12.00 Hz and 15.00 Hz, chosen as divisors of the display refresh rate 60 Hz. In addition to the SSVEP data, an idle state was recorded during which the subjects were instructed to focus at a fixation cross at the centre of the screen and ignore all the flickering stimuli. Each stimulation frequency and idle state was presented for 10 repetitions in a randomized order.

EEG data from eight active electrodes positioned over the occipital and parietal regions at locations O1, Oz, O2, PO7, P03, POz, PO4 and PO8, with a common ground at AFz and reference electrode at A2 were used in this analysis. g.tec g.ACTIVE electrodes and two g.USBamp biosignal amplifiers with a sampling rate 256 Hz were used to acquire the EEG data. The data was digitally bandpass filtered between 6–80 Hz and a latency delay in the visual system of 135 ms was considered after each stimulus onset. No artifact removal was carried out.

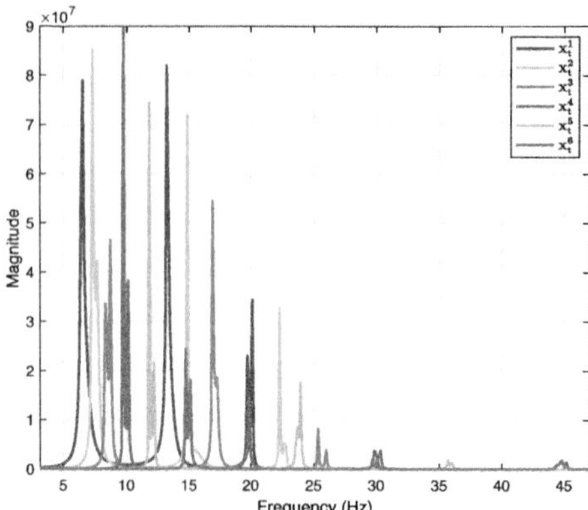

Fig. 4. An example of the spectra of a set of trained AR models representing the six SSVEP classes.

5 Results

AR Models. Six AR models were trained, one for each of the 6 SSVEP classes in the dataset. The training data was narrow band pass filtered around the first three harmonic frequency components $H = 3$ corresponding to the actual SSVEP response such that background activity not corresponding to the SSVEP response is filtered out and hence not modelled. An AR model of order 20 was then fit to the data. Given the narrow band filtering done at the pre-processing stage, this model order was found to give a good representation of the data irrespective of the stimulus class. A set of AR parameters $\boldsymbol{x}_t^i = \{-a_1, ..., -a_p\}$, for each model $i = 1, .., N_f$ was then obtained using Burg's method, where $N_f = 6$ is the number of stimuli classes. Figure 4 shows the spectra of 6 trained AR models, as an example. Each trained AR model, having parameter vectors $\boldsymbol{x}_t^i$, was then used to estimate $\hat{y}_t$, the predicted value of y_t using Eq. (6).

SSVEP Classification Results of the AR-MM Probabilistic Framework. As a first step, the classification between the SSVEP classes only is considered and then the identification of the idle state is included in the next section. In order to compare the performance of the AR-MM probabilistic approach with that of the CCA and FBCCA methods, batch mode classification is considered in which each trial is first segmented and then passed through the AR-MM probabilistic process. Labelling of one trial is done by finding:

$$\arg\max_{M} \sum_{t=1}^{T} Pr(M^i|\boldsymbol{Y}^t) \tag{12}$$

where T is the time window considered. Different window lengths for SSVEP detection are evaluated in this analysis. The classification accuracy was estimated

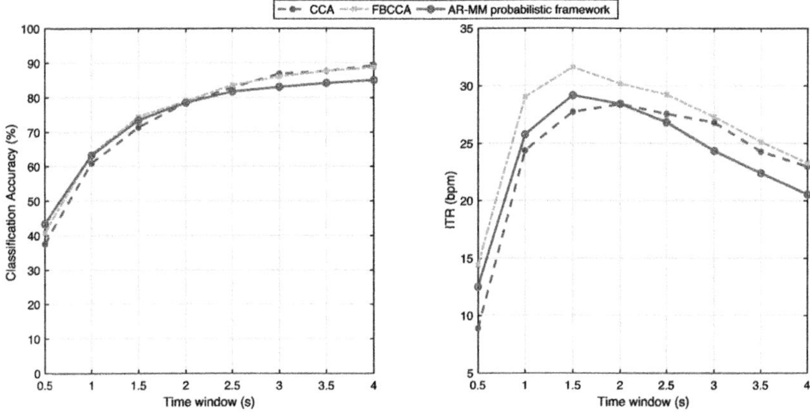

Fig. 5. Performance comparison of the AR-MM probabilistic framework, CCA and FBCCA methods. (a) Average classification accuracy (%) and (b) ITR (bpm) across all subjects for different time windows (s).

by considering 2 trials per class as training data to generate the AR parameters $\boldsymbol{x}_t$ of the 6 AR models, together with the noise covariances R and $\boldsymbol{Q}$, and the remaining 8 trials were used for testing. A minimum of 2 training trials were necessary to estimate the covariance $\boldsymbol{Q}$ of the state vector. Cross validation was then carried out by repeating the process five times such that all of the 10 trials per class were considered once for training, and then an average classification accuracy was computed. The information transfer rate (ITR) in bits per minute (bpm) [56] is also presented as a performance measure and was calculated as:

$$ITR = \frac{60}{T}\left(\log_2 N_f + P\log_2 P + (1-P)\log_2\left(\frac{1-P}{N_f-1}\right)\right) \tag{13}$$

where P is the classification accuracy, and T is the average time for selection in seconds. An additional gaze shifting time of 1 s was included in the estimation of the ITR.

Figure 5 shows the average classification accuracy (%) and ITR (bpm) obtained with the AR-MM probabilistic framework across all subjects and sessions for different data lengths from 0.5 s to 4 s, in steps of 0.5 s. The performance of the AR-MM probabilistic approach is compared with that of the CCA and FBCCA methods. In the case of the AR-MM probabilistic approach, the performance for each bipolar channel combination was computed and the highest performance associated with the best bipolar channel (BBC) was reported. On the other hand, all 8 channels were used in the estimation of the CCA and FBCCA multivariate methods.

To compare the performance of the proposed AR-MM probabilistic framework with the reference SSVEP detection methods, two-way repeated measures ANOVA were performed on the classification accuracies obtained across all the time windows. This indicated no significant ($p > 0.05$) differences between the

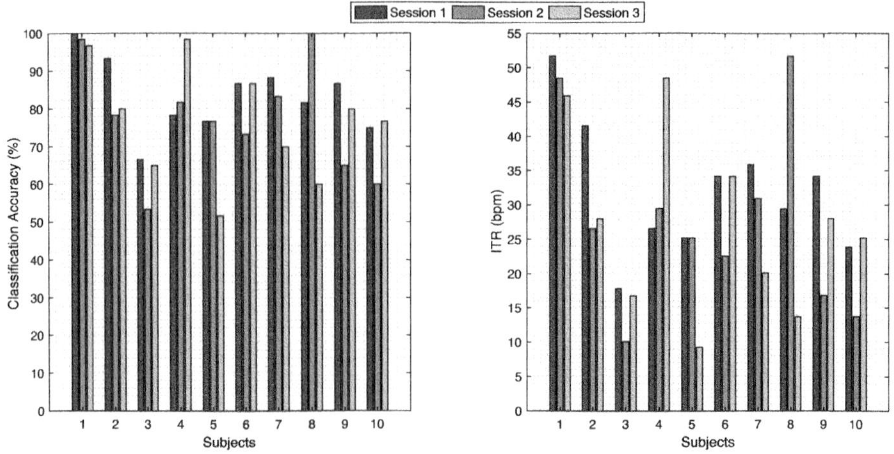

Fig. 6. (a) Classification accuracy (%) and (b) ITR (bmp) of the 10 subjects obtained in the 3 sessions with the AR-MM probabilistic framework for a 2 s time window.

classification accuracies obtained by the single channel AR-MM probabilistic framework compared to both multichannel methods, the CCA and the FBCCA methods, for all time windows. There was also no significant ($p > 0.05$) differences between the classification accuracies of the CCA and the FBCCA methods.

Figure 6 provides insight on individual subjects' performance across the 3 sessions recorded on different days with the AR-MM probabilistic framework for a time window of 2 s. The results obtained demonstrate that there is a large variation in performance between sessions of the same subject. In fact there is no particular trend in which performance varied across sessions for each subject. For example, Subject 1 obtained a consistent overall SSVEP classification accuracy between the 3 sessions while Subject 8 had a considerable difference in the classification accuracy for the 3 sessions.

Since the results obtained in consecutive sessions did not show consistent performance, the data from all 3 sessions of each subject were grouped to depict an overall individual subject performance. Table 1 shows the average results of each subject obtained with the AR-MM probabilistic framework for a 2 s time window. The performance varied significantly between subjects, from a maximum classification accuracy of 98.33% and ITR of 48.70 bpm for Subject 1, to a minimum classification accuracy of 61.67% and ITR of 14.90 bpm for Subject 3. In fact the classification accuracy was above 80% for 6 subjects, between 70% and 80% for 2 subjects, and between 60% and 70% for the remaining 2 subjects.

Idle State Detection. In this part of the analysis the idle state trials were added to the SSVEP trials. The same features described in Sect. 3 were obtained for each trial, including the idle state trials. Figure 7 shows the features obtained by each method for each SSVEP and idle state trials.

Table 1. AR-MM results for the 10 subjects averaged over the 3 sessions with a 2 s window and 1 s gaze shift.

Subject	Accuracy (%)	ITR (bpm)
1	98.33	48.70
2	83.89	32.02
3	61.67	14.90
4	86.11	34.83
5	68.34	19.88
6	82.22	30.31
7	80.55	29.00
8	80.56	31.61
9	77.22	26.30
10	70.56	20.92
Mean ± STD	**78.94 ± 10.28**	**28.85 ± 9.39**

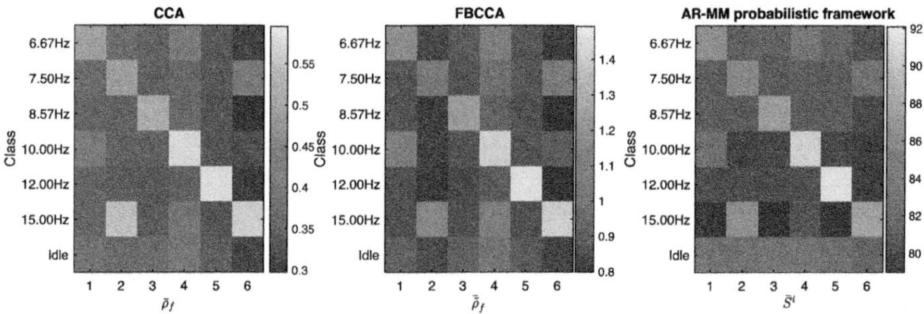

Fig. 7. Average SSVEP features of the (a) CCA, (b) FBCCA, and (c) AR-MM methods obtained per class with a 2 s window.

In the case of the CCA method, a maximum canonical correlation ρ_f was obtained for each class and used as a feature. Similarly, a weighted sum of squares of the correlation values corresponding to all sub-band components $\tilde{\rho}_f$ were used as features in the FBCCA method. Figure 7(a) and (b) show $\bar{\rho}_f$ and $\bar{\tilde{\rho}}_f$ that represent the CCA and FBCCA features respectively averaged across all trials and sessions. The features obtained with the AR-MM probabilistic framework for each trial were $S^i = \sum_{t=1}^{T} Pr(M^i|\boldsymbol{Y}^t)$, where T is the time window considered. Figure 7(c) shows the mean of these features over all sessions, cross validations and trials, i.e. $\bar{S}^i = \frac{1}{30\times5\times8}\sum_{N_s=1}^{30}\sum_{N_{cv}=1}^{5}\sum_{N_{trial}=1}^{8} S^i$, where N_s is the number of sessions, N_{cv} is the number of cross validations, and N_{trial} is the number of testing trials per class.

In the case of the AR-MM probabilistic framework, the model that has the MAP probability at each sample is considered as the model which best represents

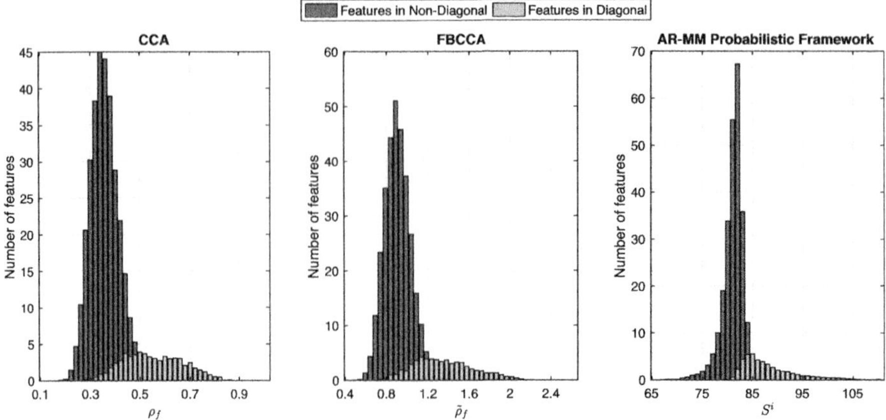

Fig. 8. Average histograms presenting the distributions of diagonal vs. non-diagonal features shown in Fig. 7 of the (a) CCA method, (b) FBCCA method, and (c) AR-MM probabilistic framework.

the SSVEP data. The probabilities of the other five models are expected to have a lower probability of representing the data.

Figure 7(c) shows this clearly whereby the sum of probabilities S^i for each trial are larger along the diagonals of the first six rows, corresponding to the six SSVEP classes, then on the non-diagonals. For the idle class however, which is represented by the 7th row in Fig. 7(c), all S^i values are relatively low, meaning that none of the trained AR models on SSVEP data may adequately represent the idle state data. A similar trend can be observed for both the CCA and FBCCA reference methods, in which case the correlation coefficients are considered as features. It was also observed in these figures that some features which are not along the diagonal also had relatively high values. In these occurrences the SSVEP classes have harmonics that coincide with those of other stimulating frequencies. For example, the 7.50 Hz SSVEP trials have the second harmonic which corresponds with the first harmonic of the 15.00 Hz SSVEP trials. As a consequence the 6th feature of the 7.50 Hz SSVEP trials and the 2nd feature of the 15.00 Hz SSVEP trials are relatively large. Likewise the 6.67 Hz SSVEP trials have the third harmonic conflicting with the second harmonic of the 10.00 Hz SSVEP trials.

To analyse the distribution of the diagonal and non-diagonal feature values shown in Fig. 7, histograms were obtained for each session. Figure 8 represents the average of 30 histograms obtained across all subjects, with each of the SSVEP detection method, from each session. To eliminate the effect of coinciding harmonics, these particular features in the non-diagonals were not considered in these histograms. For each method, the two distributions can be clearly identified and distinguished, where the features in the diagonal, corresponding to SSVEP classes, all have larger features than those found in the non-diagonal. Based on these distributions one can choose a threshold to distinguish the low

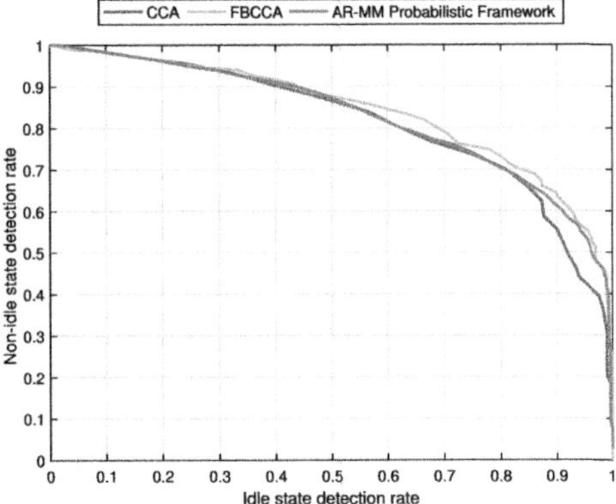

Fig. 9. Average ROC curves of the AR-MM probabilistic framework, CCA and FBCCA methods obtained with varying threshold values to distinguish between SSVEP classes and idle state classes for a 2 s time window.

feature values from the high feature values, which clearly indicate an idle state class or an SSVEP class respectively. The selection and optimization of this threshold value varies the performance of the idle state detection significantly.

In order to classify the idle class, the largest feature value of each unlabelled trial was evaluated with different threshold settings. If this was larger than the threshold set, the trial was considered as an SSVEP class, else rejected as an idle state class. A receiver operating characteristic (ROC) curve was obtained with each method in Fig. 9, where every point on the curve represents the non-idle state detection rate and the idle state detection rate obtained with different threshold values. The ROC curves are averaged across all 30 sessions. In the case of the AR-MM method these are also averaged across all cross validated sets. After observing the feature distributions in Fig. 8, the thresholds on the largest feature value, that is $\max S$ for the AR-MM method, were varied between 70 and 105 in steps of 0.1. The thresholds on the $\max \rho$ and $\max \tilde{\rho}$ were varied in steps of 0.01 between 0.2 and 0.9, and between 0.5 to 2.4, for the CCA and FBCCA respectively.

The area under the ROC curve (AUC) is then used as an overall indication and comparison of the performance of the different methods in identifying the idle state from the SSVEP classes without a subjective selection of thresholds for each method. The average AUCs obtained are 0.83, 0.81 and 0.84 for the AR-MM, CCA and FBCCA methods respectively. Paired t-tests were conducted to analyse the difference in performance between the AR-MM approach and the two reference methods across all the sessions. These indicated that no significant ($p > 0.05$) difference was found between the AUCs of the AR-MM probabilistic framework and the CCA method, and likewise between the AUCs of the AR-MM probabilistic framework and the FBCCA method. These results also revealed that the AUC obtained with FBCCA method was significantly ($p < 0.05$) larger than the AUC of the CCA method.

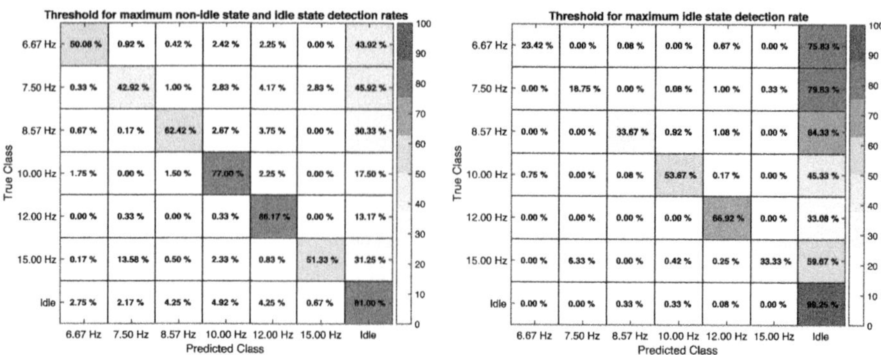

Fig. 10. Confusion matrices showing average classification accuracies (%) for the six SSVEP classes and idle state class with the AR-MM method for a 2 s time window obtained with (a) a threshold that obtains the maximum non-idle and idle state detection rates and (b) a threshold that obtains maximum idle state detection rate.

The ROC curve of Fig. 9 shows the relationship between the idle state-detection rate, showing the percentage of correctly classified idle state, with respect to the non-idle state detection rate, showing the percentage of SSVEP classes classified as an SSVEP class. To get the best compromise between the two rates, the threshold value closest to the point (1,1) on the ROC curve was found using the Euclidean distance. For the AR-MM framework, this is equivalent to a threshold value of 84.7 which corresponds to a non-idle state detection rate of 0.7 and an idle state detection rate of 0.8. Fig. 10(a) then presents the confusion matrix associated with this threshold value, showing that the six SSVEP classes can be classified with an average accuracy of 61.65% whereas the idle state can be detected with 81.00% accuracy. This confusion matrix highlights the fact that most misclassifications of the SSVEP classes were in fact misclassified as an idle class. This is better than having the SSVEP class misclassified to another SSVEP class as in practice a misclassification to an idle class implies that the BCI will take no action and the user has to initiate another control signal.

Since in practice a delayed response may be preferred to an incorrect SSVEP class label, one may opt to choose a threshold which corresponds to an idle state detection rate close to 100%. Specifically, for the AR-MM framework, a threshold value of 87.8 will give an idle state detection rate close to 1 and a non-idle state detection rate of 0.4. Figure 10(b) shows the confusion matrix for this condition where the idle state detection accuracy is now at 99.25%, at the expense of a low SSVEP class detection accuracy. Most significant however, is the fact that the incorrectly classified SSVEP classes have reduced to almost zero, which may be ideal for a practical BCI.

6 Discussion

The results obtained in the previous section demonstrate the potential of using the proposed AR-MM probabilistic framework for the detection of SSVEPs as well as the idle state in BCIs.

In our previous work [62] it was shown that AR models provide a good fit for the EEG data by capturing the dynamics of the underlying SSVEP signal. Therefore these were used as a model structure in the proposed probabilistic multiple modelling framework. The standard approach of using AR models in EEG analysis is to find AR parameters for incoming EEG data to form features which can then be used for classification. In this work however, AR expert models were trained for each SSVEP class, each of which has a distinct frequency, and then used for prediction on new EEG data. The residual between the true and the reconstructed signals was used to calculate the likelihood function in the MM framework. A probability measure for each model in representing incoming data was then obtained at each time instance and this result was then evaluated to find which model gave the best representation within a fixed time window, allowing batch mode classification as done with other state-of-the-art techniques.

The performance of the AR-MM probabilistic framework in detecting SSVEPs was compared to the multivariate CCA and FBCCA methods. It must be highlighted that multichannel SSVEP detection methods are known to benefit from an optimized combination of multiple signals. In fact it has been shown that this results in a greater robustness against noise and hence improved performance compared to single channel methods [4,18]. The results obtained with the single-channel AR-MM probabilistic framework, however, show that comparable classification performance to the two considered multi-channel methods could be obtained. Specifically, for the 6-class SSVEP data a classification accuracy of $78.94 \pm 10.28\%$ and an ITR of 28.85 ± 9.39 bpm averaged over 30 sessions with a 2 s time window was obtained, which was found to be comparable to the performance obtained with the multi-channel CCA and FBCCA methods. In all three cases, the SSVEP classification may have suffered because the dataset had some stimulation frequencies with coinciding harmonics. This could be rectified by the selection of different stimulation frequencies.

Since the same experiments were repeated by each subject on three different days, we also analysed how the SSVEP performance with the AR-MM framework varied longitudinally to mimic the use of a BCI system in real life. Although the results varied significantly between subjects, a significant above-chance level performance for the six class BCI system could be obtained with all the subjects in all the sessions. No particular trend in performance could however be seen as the sessions progressed, with some subjects showing consistent results across the three sessions while the performance of other subjects varied considerably between sessions.

Furthermore, we analysed the detection of idle state in SSVEP data using the AR-MM probabilistic framework and compared it to the multichannel reference methods. The features obtained for the idle state class were clearly distinct from the SSVEP classes as observed from the feature distributions of the three methods. Having obtained these features, a simple threshold-based approach was adopted to identify the idle state from the SSVEP classes. This was also done to obtain a measure of performance which could be used as a comparative measure between the three methods. The averaged ROC curves obtained in Fig. 9 illustrate the performance of the AR-MM framework at various thresholds compared with the reference methods. The AUC was used to compare the degree of separability between the detection rates of the idle state and non-idle state obtained without selection of a particular threshold. The AR-MM framework obtained an average AUC of 0.83, which revealed a good measure of separability between idle state and non-idle state. In addition, based on the AUC, the AR-MM framework gave comparable results to the AUCs of 0.81 and 0.84 for the CCA and FBCCA methods respectively, when trying to distinguish between an idle state and non-idle state class.

This result can also be compared to results found in the literature that similarly used the AUC to show the general performance of idle state detection algorithms. Du et al. [16] obtained an average AUC of 0.89 and Zhang et al. [63] obtained an average AUC of 0.94 to identify control versus no control states. Notably in these two particular studies, supervised classifiers were used to distinguish between the two states. In the present study the features obtained could similarly be fed to a supervised classifier, such as an LDA or SVM, and trained specifically to distinguish between various stimuli and idle state classes. This could potentially improve the performance of idle state detection with the drawback of requiring further user training, which may effect the practicality of the system.

The ROC curve obtained with the AR-MM method was also used to show the performance of the idle state detection that is dependent on the selection of the threshold value. The average classification accuracy for idle state detection with a threshold that gave the best compromise between idle and non-idle state detection rates was of 81.00%, while with a threshold that maximized the idle state detection rate, the classification accuracy was of 99.25%. The choice of this threshold value depends on the particular BCI application. In some situations, for example a BCI game, a shorter response time is beneficial at the expense of some SSVEPs being misclassified. In other situations, such as in a brain-controlled wheelchair, any incorrectly classified SSVEP classes may be dangerous [45] and hence a slower BCI response time may be preferred.

An alternative to the proposed idle state detection method could be to specifically train an additional model to represent the idle state class. In future work this would involve the investigation of which model would best fit idle state data. Once an expert model is trained for idle state this would be one of the candidate models that may represent the EEG data in the multiple model framework.

7 Conclusion

A univariate autoregressive multiple model (AR-MM) probabilistic framework for the detection of SSVEPs in BCIs was presented. The success of this technique to detect SSVEPs has been demonstrated in this work by its implementation on a dataset in a longitudinal study. More importantly, we focus on the detection of the idle state, which is a necessary feature in asynchronous BCIs. The motivation behind this analysis was that despite the large number of successful SSVEP detection methods that have been developed, few studies have been specifically focused on the detection of the idle state in SSVEP-based BCIs.

The proposed framework provides a measure of probability for each SSVEP class and this was used as a measure of selectivity between an idle state class and an SSVEP class. Compared to popular multi-channel techniques, specifically the CCA method and FBCCA method, the results revealed that the proposed single-channel approach could similarly discriminate reliably idle state classes from SSVEP classes. This further highlights the practicality of this single channel AR-MM probabilistic framework, which can also be used in real-world asynchronous BCIs where a minimal amount of channels are advantageous.

Acknowledgements. This work was partially supported by the project BrainApp, financed by the Malta Council for Science & Technology through FUSION: The R&I Technology Development Programme 2016.

References

1. Abu-Alqumsan, M., Peer, A.: Advancing the detection of steady-state visual evoked potentials in brain-computer interfaces. J. Neural Eng. **13**(3), 036005 (2016). https://doi.org/10.1088/1741-2560/13/3/036005
2. Ajami, S., Mahnam, A., Abootalebi, V.: An adaptive SSVEP-based brain-computer interface to compensate fatigue-induced decline of performance in practical application. IEEE Trans. Neural Syst. Rehabil. Eng. **26**(11), 2200–2209 (2018). https://doi.org/10.1109/TNSRE.2018.2874975
3. Babiloni, F., et al.: Estimation of the cortical functional connectivity with the multimodal integration of high-resolution EEG and fMRI data by directed transfer function. Neuroimage **24**(1), 118–131 (2005). https://doi.org/10.1016/j.neuroimage.2004.09.036
4. Bin, G., Gao, X., Yan, Z., Hong, B., Gao, S.: An online multi-channel SSVEP-based brain-computer interface using a canonical correlation analysis method. J. Neural Eng. **6**(4), 046002 (2009). https://doi.org/10.1088/1741-2560/6/4/046002
5. Blankertz, B., et al.: The Berlin brain–computer interface: non-medical uses of BCI technology. Front. Neurosci. **4**(198), 1–17 (2010). https://doi.org/10.3389/fnins.2010.00198. http://journal.frontiersin.org/article/10.3389/fnins.2010.00198/abstract
6. Camilleri, T.A., Camilleri, K.P., Fabri, S.G.: Automatic detection of spindles and K-complexes in sleep EEG using switching multiple models. Biomed. Signal Process. Control **10**, 117–127 (2014). https://doi.org/10.1016/j.bspc.2014.01.010. https://linkinghub.elsevier.com/retrieve/pii/S1746809414000111
7. Cao, L., Li, J., Ji, H., Jiang, C.: A hybrid brain computer interface system based on the neurophysiological protocol and brain-actuated switch for wheelchair control. J. Neurosci. Methods **229**, 33–43 (2014). https://doi.org/10.1016/j.jneumeth.2014.03.011

8. Cecotti, H.: A self-paced and calibration-less SSVEP-based brain-computer interface speller. IEEE Trans. Neural Syst. Rehabil. Eng. **18**(2), 127–133 (2010). https://doi.org/10.1109/TNSRE.2009.2039594. http://ieeexplore.ieee.org/document/5378643/
9. Cerutti, S., Chiarenza, G., Liberati, D., Mascellani, P., Pavesi, G.: A parametric method of identification of single-trial event-related potentials in the brain. IEEE Trans. Biomed. Eng. **35**(9), 701–711 (1988). https://doi.org/10.1109/10.7271
10. Chen, L.L., Madhavan, R., Rapoport, B.I., Anderson, W.S.: Real-time brain oscillation detection and phase-locked stimulation using autoregressive spectral estimation and time-series forward prediction. IEEE Trans. Biomed. Eng. **60**(3), 753–762 (2013). https://doi.org/10.1109/TBME.2011.2109715
11. Chen, X., Wang, Y., Gao, S., Jung, T.P., Gao, X.: Filter bank canonical correlation analysis for implementing a high-speed SSVEP-based brain-computer interface. J. Neural Eng. **12**(4), 046008 (2015). https://doi.org/10.1088/1741-2560/12/4/046008
12. Chen, X., Wang, Y., Nakanishi, M., Gao, X., Jung, T.P., Gao, S.: High-speed spelling with a noninvasive brain-computer interface. Proc. Natl. Acad. Sci. **112**(44), E6058–E6067 (2015). https://doi.org/10.1073/pnas.1508080112
13. Chen, Z. (ed.): Advanced State Space Methods for Neural and Clinical Data. Cambridge University Press, Cambridge (2015). https://doi.org/10.1017/CBO9781139941433
14. Cheng, M., Gao, X., Gao, S., Xu, D.: Design and implementation of a brain-computer interface with high transfer rates. IEEE Trans. Biomed. Eng. **49**(10), 1181–1186 (2002). https://doi.org/10.1109/TBME.2002.803536
15. Diez, P.F., Mut, V.A., Avila Perona, E.M., Laciar Leber, E.: Asynchronous BCI control using high-frequency SSVEP. J. Neuroeng. Rehabil. **8**(39), 1–8 (2011). https://doi.org/10.1186/1743-0003-8-39
16. Du, J., et al.: A two-step idle-state detection method for SSVEP BCI. In: 2019 41st Annual International Conference of the IEEE Engineering in Medicine and Biology Society, pp. 3095–3098. IEEE (2019). https://doi.org/10.1109/EMBC.2019.8857024. https://ieeexplore.ieee.org/document/8857024/
17. Fabri, S.G., Kadirkamanathan, V.: Functional Adaptive Control. Communications and Control Engineering. Springer, London (2001). https://doi.org/10.1007/978-1-4471-0319-6
18. Friman, O., Volosyak, I., Gräser, A.: Multiple channel detection of steady-state visual evoked potentials for brain-computer interfaces. IEEE Trans. Biomed. Eng. **54**(4), 742–750 (2007). https://doi.org/10.1109/TBME.2006.889160
19. Ge, S., Wang, R., Leng, Y., Wang, H., Lin, P., Iramina, K.: A double-partial least-squares model for the detection of steady-state visual evoked potentials. IEEE J. Biomed. Heal. Inform. **21**(4), 897–903 (2017). https://doi.org/10.1109/JBHI.2016.2546311. http://ieeexplore.ieee.org/document/7440783/
20. Ghahramani, Z., Hinton, G.E.: Variational learning for switching state-space models. Neural Comput. **12**(4), 831–864 (2000). https://doi.org/10.1162/089976600300015619. http://www.mitpressjournals.org/doi/10.1162/089976600300015619
21. Ghaleb, I., Davila, C.E., Srebro, R.: Prewhitening of background brain activity via autoregressive modeling. In: Proceedings of Sixteenth Southern Biomedical Engineering Conference, pp. 242–245 (1997). https://doi.org/10.1109/SBEC.1997.583270
22. Guger, C., et al.: How many people could use an SSVEP BCI? Front. Neurosci. **6**(169), 1–6 (2012). https://doi.org/10.3389/fnins.2012.00169

23. Han, C.H., Kim, E., Im, C.H.: Development of a brain-computer interface toggle switch with low false-positive rate using respiration-modulated photoplethysmography. Sensors **20**(2), 348 (2020). https://doi.org/10.3390/s20020348
24. Herrmann, C.S.: Human EEG responses to 1–100 Hz flicker: resonance phenomena in visual cortex and their potential correlation to cognitive phenomena. Exp. Brain Res. **137**(3–4), 346–353 (2001). https://doi.org/10.1007/s002210100682
25. Jacobs, R.A., Jordan, M.I., Nowlan, S.J., Hinton, G.E.: Adaptive mixtures of local experts. Neural Comput. **3**(1), 79–87 (1991). https://doi.org/10.1162/neco.1991.3.1.79. https://www.mitpressjournals.org/doi/abs/10.1162/neco.1991.3.1.79
26. Jeyabalan, V., Samraj, A., Kiong, L.C.: Motor imaginary signal classification using adaptive recursive bandpass filter and adaptive autoregressive models for brain machine interface designs. Int. J. Bioeng. Life Sci. **1**(5), 116–123 (2007)
27. Krusienski, D.J., McFarland, D.J., Wolpaw, J.R.: An evaluation of autoregressive spectral estimation model order for brain-computer interface applications. In: 2006 International Conference of the IEEE Engineering in Medicine and Biology Society, vol. 1, pp. 1323–1326. IEEE (2006). https://doi.org/10.1109/IEMBS.2006.259822. http://ieeexplore.ieee.org/document/4462004/
28. Lainiotis, D.: Partitioning: a unifying framework for adaptive systems, I: Estimation. Proc. IEEE **64**(8), 1126–1143 (1976). https://doi.org/10.1109/PROC.1976.10284. http://ieeexplore.ieee.org/document/1454553/
29. Lim, J.H., et al.: An emergency call system for patients in locked-in state using an SSVEP-based brain switch. Psychophysiology **54**(11), 1632–1643 (2017). https://doi.org/10.1111/psyp.12916
30. Lin, Z., Zhang, C., Wu, W., Gao, X.: Frequency recognition based on canonical correlation analysis for SSVEP-based BCIs. IEEE Trans. Biomed. Eng. **54**(6), 1172–1176 (2007). https://doi.org/10.1109/TBME.2006.889197
31. Liu, Q.: Review: Recent development of signal processing algorithms for SSVEP-based brain computer interfaces. J. Med. Biol. Eng. **34**(4), 299 (2014). https://pdfs.semanticscholar.org/fc53/b575df72edcadfc52121f84011dd8ee2c29c.pdf
32. Magill, D.: Optimal adaptive estimation of sampled stochastic processes. IEEE Trans. Automat. Control **10**(4), 434–439 (1965). https://doi.org/10.1109/TAC.1965.1098191. http://ieeexplore.ieee.org/document/1098191/
33. Meriño, L., et al.: Asynchronous control of unmanned aerial vehicles using a steady-state visual evoked potential-based brain computer interface. Brain-Comput. Interfaces **4**(1–2), 122–135 (2017). https://doi.org/10.1080/2326263X.2017.1292721
34. Minguillon, J., Lopez-Gordo, M.A., Pelayo, F.: Trends in EEG-BCI for daily-life: requirements for artifact removal. Biomed. Signal Process. Control **31**, 407–418 (2017). https://doi.org/10.1016/j.bspc.2016.09.005. https://linkinghub.elsevier.com/retrieve/pii/S1746809416301318
35. Mora, N., De Munari, I., Ciampolini, P.: Exploitation of a compact, cost-effective EEG module for plug-and-play, SSVEP-based BCI. In: 2015 7th International IEEE/EMBS Conference on Neural Engineering NER, pp. 142–145 (2015). https://doi.org/10.1109/NER.2015.7146580
36. Nakanishi, M.: 12-class joint frequency-phase modulated SSVEP dataset for estimating online BCI performance (2015). https://github.com/mnakanishi/12JFPM_SSVEP
37. Nakanishi, M., Wang, Y., Chen, X., Wang, Y.T., Gao, X., Jung, T.P.: Enhancing detection of SSVEPs for a high-speed brain speller using task-related component analysis. IEEE Trans. Biomed. Eng. **65**(1), 104–112 (2018). https://doi.org/10.1109/TBME.2017.2694818

38. Nakanishi, M., Wang, Y., Wang, Y.T., Jung, T.P.: A comparison study of canonical correlation analysis based methods for detecting steady-state visual evoked potentials. PLoS One **10**(10), e0140703 (2015). https://doi.org/10.1371/journal.pone.0140703
39. Nakanishi, M., Wang, Y., Wang, Y.T., Jung, T.P.: A dynamic stopping method for improving performance of steady-state visual evoked potential based brain-computer interfaces. In: 2015 37th Annual International Conference of the IEEE Engineering in Medicine and Biology Society, pp. 1057–1060. IEEE (2015). https://doi.org/10.1109/EMBC.2015.7318547
40. Narendra, K., Balakrishnan, J.: Adaptive control using multiple models. IEEE Trans. Autom. Control **42**(2), 171–187 (1997). https://doi.org/10.1109/9.554398. http://ieeexplore.ieee.org/document/554398/
41. Wang, N., Qian, T., Zhuo, Q., Gao, X.: Discrimination between idle and work states in BCI based on SSVEP. In: 2010 2nd International Conference on Advanced Computer Control, vol. 4, pp. 355–358. IEEE (2010). https://doi.org/10.1109/ICACC.2010.5486907. http://ieeexplore.ieee.org/document/5486907/
42. Noman, F., Salleh, S.H., Ting, C.M., Samdin, S.B., Ombao, H., Hussain, H.: A Markov-switching model approach to heart sound segmentation and classification. IEEE J. Biomed. Health Inform. **24**(3), 705–716 (2020). https://doi.org/10.1109/JBHI.2019.2925036. https://ieeexplore.ieee.org/document/8746548/
43. Ortner, R., Allison, B.Z., Korisek, G., Gaggl, H., Pfurtscheller, G.: An SSVEP BCI to control a hand orthosis for persons with tetraplegia. IEEE Trans. Neural Syst. Rehabil. Eng. **19**(1), 1–5 (2011). https://doi.org/10.1109/TNSRE.2010.2076364
44. Oster, J., Behar, J., Sayadi, O., Nemati, S., Johnson, A.E.W., Clifford, G.D.: Semisupervised ECG ventricular beat classification with novelty detection based on switching Kalman filters. IEEE Trans. Biomed. Eng. **62**(9), 2125–2134 (2015). https://doi.org/10.1109/TBME.2015.2402236
45. Pan, J., Li, Y., Zhang, R., Gu, Z., Li, F.: Discrimination between control and idle states in asynchronous SSVEP-based brain switches: a pseudo-key-based approach. IEEE Trans. Neural Syst. Rehabil. Eng. **21**(3), 435–443 (2013). https://doi.org/10.1109/TNSRE.2013.2253801. https://ieeexplore.ieee.org/document/6514128/
46. Pardey, J., Roberts, S., Tarassenko, L.: A review of parametric modelling techniques for EEG analysis. Med. Eng. Phys. **18**(1), 2–11 (1996). https://doi.org/10.1016/1350-4533(95)00024-0. https://linkinghub.elsevier.com/retrieve/pii/1350453395000240
47. Penny, W.D., Roberts, S.J.: Dynamic models for nonstationary signal segmentation. Comput. Biomed. Res. **32**(6), 483–502 (1999). https://doi.org/10.1006/cbmr.1999.1511. https://linkinghub.elsevier.com/retrieve/pii/S0010480999915112
48. Pfurtscheller, G., Neuper, C., Schlogl, A., Lugger, K.: Separability of EEG signals recorded during right and left motor imagery using adaptive autoregressive parameters. IEEE Trans. Rehabil. Eng. **6**(3), 316–325 (1998). https://doi.org/10.1109/86.712230
49. Poryzala, P., Materka, A.: Cluster analysis of CCA coefficients for robust detection of the asynchronous SSVEPs in brain-computer interfaces. Biomed. Signal Process. Control **10**, 201–208 (2014). https://doi.org/10.1016/j.bspc.2013.11.003. https://linkinghub.elsevier.com/retrieve/pii/S1746809413001602
50. Quinn, J., Williams, C., McIntosh, N.: Factorial switching linear dynamical systems applied to physiological condition monitoring. IEEE Trans. Pattern Anal. Mach. Intell. **31**(9), 1537–1551 (2009). https://doi.org/10.1109/TPAMI.2008.191. http://ieeexplore.ieee.org/document/4586385/

51. Rezaei, S., Tavakolian, K., Nasrabadi, A.M., Setarehdan, S.K.: Different classification techniques considering brain computer interface applications. J. Neural Eng. **3**(2), 139–144 (2006). https://doi.org/10.1088/1741-2560/3/2/008
52. Safi, S.M.M., Pooyan, M., Motie Nasrabadi, A.: SSVEP recognition by modeling brain activity using system identification based on Box-Jenkins model. Comput. Biol. Med. **101**(Aug), 82–89 (2018). https://doi.org/10.1016/j.compbiomed.2018.08.011
53. Suefusa, K., Tanaka, T.: Phase-based detection of intentional state for asynchronous brain-computer interface. In: 2015 IEEE International Conference on Acoustics, Speech and Signal Processing, pp. 808–812. IEEE (2015). https://doi.org/10.1109/ICASSP.2015.7178081. http://ieeexplore.ieee.org/document/7178081/
54. Vialatte, F.B., Maurice, M., Dauwels, J., Cichocki, A.: Steady-state visually evoked potentials: focus on essential paradigms and future perspectives. Prog. Neurobiol. **90**(4), 418–438 (2010). https://doi.org/10.1016/j.pneurobio.2009.11.005. https://linkinghub.elsevier.com/retrieve/pii/S0301008209001853
55. Wang, Z., Xu, P., Liu, T., Tian, Y., Lei, X., Yao, D.: Robust removal of ocular artifacts by combining independent component analysis and system identification. Biomed. Signal Process. Control **10**(1), 250–259 (2014). https://doi.org/10.1016/j.bspc.2013.10.006
56. Wolpaw, J.R., Birbaumer, N., McFarland, D.J., Pfurtscheller, G., Vaughan, T.M.: Brain-computer interfaces for communication and control. Clin. Neurophysiol. **113**(6), 767–791 (2002). https://doi.org/10.1016/S1388-2457(02)00057-3. https://linkinghub.elsevier.com/retrieve/pii/S1388245702000573
57. Xia, B., Li, X., Xie, H., Yang, W., Li, J., He, L.: Asynchronous brain–computer interface based on steady-state visual-evoked potential. Cognit. Comput. **5**(2), 243–251 (2013). https://doi.org/10.1007/s12559-013-9202-7. http://link.springer.com/10.1007/s12559-013-9202-7
58. Zerafa, R., Camilleri, T., Bartolo, K., Camilleri, K.P., Falzon, O.: Reducing the training time for the SSVEP-based music player application. Biomed. Phys. Eng. Exp. **3**(3), 034001 (2017). https://doi.org/10.1088/2057-1976/aa73e1. https://iopscience.iop.org/article/10.1088/2057-1976/aa73e1
59. Zerafa, R., Camilleri, T., Camilleri, K.P., Falzon, O.: The effect of distractors on SSVEP-based brain-computer interfaces. Biomed. Phys. Eng. Exp. 5(035031) (2019). https://doi.org/10.1088/2057-1976/ab155d
60. Zerafa, R., Camilleri, T., Falzon, O., Camilleri, K.P.: A real-time SSVEP-based brain-computer interface music player application. In: Kyriacou, E., Christofides, S., Pattichis, C.S. (eds.) XIV Mediterranean Conference on Medical and Biological Engineering and Computing 2016. IP, vol. 57, pp. 173–178. Springer, Cham (2016). https://doi.org/10.1007/978-3-319-32703-7_36
61. Zerafa, R., Camilleri, T., Falzon, O., Camilleri, K.P.: To train or not to train? A survey on training of feature extraction methods for SSVEP-based BCIs. J. Neural Eng. **15**(5) (2018). https://doi.org/10.1088/1741-2552/aaca6e
62. Zerafa, R., Camilleri, T., Falzon, O., Camilleri, K.P.: An autoregressive multiple model probabilistic framework for the detection of SSVEPs in brain-computer interfaces. In: BIOSIGNALS 2020–13th International Conference on Bio-inspired Systems and Conference on Bio-inspired Systems and Signal Processing Proceedings; Part 13th International Joint Conference on Biomedical Engineering Systems and Technologies BIOSTEC 2020 (Biostec), pp. 68–78 (2020). https://doi.org/10.5220/0008924400680078

63. Zhang, D., Huang, B., Wu, W., Li, S.: An idle-state detection algorithm for SSVEP-based brain-computer interfaces using a maximum evoked response spatial filter. Int. J. Neural Syst. **25**(07), 1550030 (2015). https://doi.org/10.1142/S0129065715500306. https://www.worldscientific.com/doi/abs/10.1142/S0129065715500306
64. Zhang, N., Tang, J., Liu, Y., Zhou, Z.: An asynchronous SSVEP-BCI based on variance statistics of Multivariate synchronization index. In: 2017 10th Biomedical Engineering International Conference, pp. 1–4. IEEE (2017). https://doi.org/10.1109/BMEiCON.2017.8229153. http://ieeexplore.ieee.org/document/8229153/
65. Zhang, W., Sun, F., Tan, C., Liu, H.: Cognitive Systems and Signal Processing. Communications in Computer and Information Science, vol. 710. Springer, Singapore (2017). https://doi.org/10.1007/978-981-10-5230-9. http://link.springer.com/10.1007/978-981-10-5230-9
66. Zhang, Y., Ji, X., Zhang, Y.: Classification of EEG signals based on AR model and approximate entropy. In: Proceedings of International Joint Conference on Neural Networks (2015). https://doi.org/10.1109/IJCNN.2015.7280840
67. Zhang, Z.M., Deng, Z.D.: A kernel canonical correlation analysis based idle-state detection method for SSVEP-based brain-computer interfaces. Adv. Mater. Res. **341–342**, 634–640 (2011). https://doi.org/10.4028/www.scientific.net/AMR.341-342.634

Exploring Inertial Sensor Fusion Methods for Direct Ergonomic Assessments

Sara Santos[1(✉)], Duarte Folgado[1], João Rodrigues[2], Nafiseh Mollaei[2], Carlos Fujão[3], and Hugo Gamboa[1,2]

[1] Associação Fraunhofer Portugal Research, Rua Alfredo Allen 455/461, 4200-135 Porto, Portugal
sara.santos@fraunhofer.pt

[2] Laboratório de Instrumentação, Engenharia Biomédica e Física da Radiação (LIBPhys-UNL), Departamento de Física, Faculdade de Ciências e Tecnologia, FCT, Universidade Nova de Lisboa, 2829-516 Caparica, Portugal

[3] Volkswagen Autoeuropa, Quinta da Marquesa, 2954-024 Quinta do Anjo, Portugal

Abstract. The industrial site, particularly assembly lines, encompass repetitive labour processes which are considered an ergonomic risk factor for the onset of musculoskeletal disorders. Direct assessments methods promote faster ergonomic feedback, supporting the development of sustainable working conditions. This work presents an upper-body motion tracker framework using inertial sensors to provide direct measurements for ergonomics research. An experimental assessment performed by 14 subjects was completed in order to evaluate the joint angle reconstruction of the proposed method while using the measures of an optical motion capture system as reference. This study investigated the results of three distinct complementary sensor fusion techniques, namely the quaternion-based complementary filter, the Mahony filter and the Madgwick filter. Furthermore, foreseeing the possibility of magnetic disturbance in industrial environments, a comparison was conducted between methods that use magnetic data, i.e. 9-axis, and other inertial-based approaches that do not require magnetic information, i.e. 6-axis. A quantitative analysis was performed using two metrics, the cumulative distribution function and the root-mean-square error, hence, providing an evaluation for the different sensor fusion approaches. The overall results suggest that the 9-axis Madgwick filter although noisier presents a more accurate angular reconstruction.

Keywords: Ergonomics · Industry · Musculoskeletal disorders · Inertial sensors · Motion capture · Sensor fusion

1 Introduction

The recent years have introduced significant changes for industries which now aim to achieve higher levels of operational efficiency and productivity while

X. Ye et al. (Eds.): BIOSTEC 2020, CCIS 1400, pp. 289–303, 2021.
https://doi.org/10.1007/978-3-030-72379-8_14

enhancing the products and production lines quality and reducing costs [10,17]. The change of paradigm, motivated by the rise of Industry 4.0, is launching smart, more flexible and collaborative factories to meet the needs of current demands of a competitive market. Although robots are becoming more common in manufacturing environments human input is still a critical resource, particularly in assembly lines, where dexterity and flexibility are required [25]. The industrial site usually comprises repetitive activities and cyclical labour [25]. Nevertheless, high repetitiveness, combined with high precision demands, may result in the frequent occurrence of non-neutral postures, as well in incremented muscular load and mental tension. The aforementioned conditions may contribute to fatigue state and prompt Work-related Musculoskeletal Disorders (WMSDs) eventually reducing the worker or system performance and product quality [25].

One of the main occupational safety and health problems in the European Union is still related to the exposure of ergonomic risk factors, despite the legislative efforts to prevent them [14]. During the past years, the attention to this issue has grown stronger becoming one of the main challenges for Strategic Framework on Health and Safety at Work 2014–2020, which recommends that work organisations should give attention to the impact of changes in terms of physical and mental health [14]. WMSDs are not only a serious widespread work-related illness but can also affect economics, as they lead to reduction of productivity levels at work and social expenses, e.g. sick leave costs [9,13].

In order to prevent occupational illnesses, tasks/workplace and/or equipment should be designed in a way that the working person does not put much physical stress in the body. Therefore, data must be adequately collected and subsequently used in a risk assessment framework to identify the ongoing risk factors. In ergonomic assessment studies, the employment of direct measurements supports the use of wearable devices, such as Inertial Measurement Units (IMUs), which are directly attached to the subject. Hence, allowing to analyse data related to pre-production and production phases presenting not only information about production line performance factors but also reporting operator's well-being in the demanding tasks [8,11]. Inertial motion tracking systems use sensor fusion techniques to derive a single and more accurate estimate of relative device orientation. The term sensor fusion implies combining the multiple IMU sensor data through complex mathematical algorithms [15].

We previously reported in [23] our work towards the development of an upper-body motion tracker framework for ergonomic risk assessment at industrial environments. Angular motion measurements are an essential parameter for ergonomic studies and the reconstruction of motion through inertial data relies on sensor fusion approaches. In this work, we report our recent research composed of a comparative study addressing the results of employing different sensor fusion techniques in the upper-body motion tracker.

This paper is structured as follows: Sect. 1 presented the context and motivation that lead to the development of this study; Sect. 2 compiles the related work found in the literature; Sect. 3 gives an overview of the proposed methodology explaining the developed upper-body motion tracker framework; In Sect. 4 we describe the experimental assessment procedures; In Sect. 5 the experimental results are presented and discussed; finally, Sect. 6 highlights relevant conclusions and points to future research directions.

2 Related Work

Over the last years, wearable inertial sensors have undergone several improvements such as miniaturisation, sensor weight and manufacturing costs reduction, connection and data processing software improvements [4,6]. These enhancements have consequently increased the number of human motion studies [2,21]. Furthermore, the enhanced battery life and data bandwidth for continuous monitoring over long periods along with the less interference with workers' natural postures, has proven inertial sensors suitable for direct measurement of postures and movements in ergonomics studies [5,27].

Before assessing the ergonomic risk of a given activity, effort must be directed into establishing a robust framework to identify situations that can compromise workers safety. Several parameters, which are fundamental for ergonomic studies, can be directly measured using inertial devices, e.g. angular trends and pose of the limbs [8,12]. A methodology to derive such useful information can be achieved by combining different signal sources through sensor fusion techniques. Popular approaches are Kalman filters and Complementary filters [12].

The Kalman filter is quite often the standard approach for orientation algorithms, such as in [3,7]. There are some variants of the filter, depending on the approached problem. Some studies employed the linear Kalman filter [7] to work on linear systems. Others, to manage nonlinearities take advantage of the Extended Kalman filter, e.g. [24]. Alternatively, the Unscented Kalman filter, e.g. [20], also provides effectiveness under non-linear systems yet, improving the estimation of the transformed probability density function [12]. Despite the referred Kalman filter effectiveness, it can be complicated to implement as suggested by the numerous solutions seen in the literature [18].

The Complementary filter has also been exploited in several studies, e.g. [28]. This filter has been subject to modifications as the Explicit Complementary filter, suggested by Mahony et al. [19], and the Gradient Descent Orientation filter proposed by Madgwick et al. [18]. Both methods use quaternion algebra for orientation estimation. Mahony's algorithm corrects the measured angular velocity using a Proportional-Integral compensator while Madgwick's is based on a Newton optimisation using an analytic formulation of the gradient that is derived from a quaternion, providing also gyroscope drift compensation. Mahony and Madgwick filters were compared in [1] where it is observed that both filters have an identical outcome and are efficient solutions providing alternative approaches to Kalman filter.

Among the recent works on the use of inertial sensors in occupational ergonomics, in [16] it is present a narrative review in which it is proposed a conceptual framework named Modeling-Sensing-Analysis-Assessment-Intervention.

The framework name suggests the essential phases in ergonomic researches, synthesising the role of the inertial sensors. In particular, the analysis stage is concerned with examining the sensor data in order to obtain measures of specific biomechanical exposures and other work-relevant information such as frequent postures and movements. The combination of sensors data through sensor fusion methods is addressed during this stage. On our previous work in [23], we presented a motion tracking framework relying on inertial information to estimate quantitative direct measurements of posture and movement for the upper-body, aiming to identify the most contributing ergonomic risk factors.

An approach to improve the performance of an ergonomic framework relying on direct measures is through the individual study of its components which may help to identify potential defect causes. This work presents a more extensive analysis regarding sensor fusion methods for the inertial upper-body motion tracking system [23]. Therefore, our work major contribution is the comparative study regarding different sensor fusion methods, based on complementary filter approaches, for the upper-body motion tracker framework. The comparative analysis takes as reference the values from the optical mocap.

3 Upper-Body Motion Tracker

The pose estimation mechanism is consistent with the detailed information from [23]. The system was designed to have the minimum invasiveness to the worker while maintaining an adequate cost/effectiveness result, thus allowing to estimate low-level metrics of ergonomic risk while not requiring a large number of sensors.

The upper-body motion tracker comprises four different segments, depicted in Fig. 1.

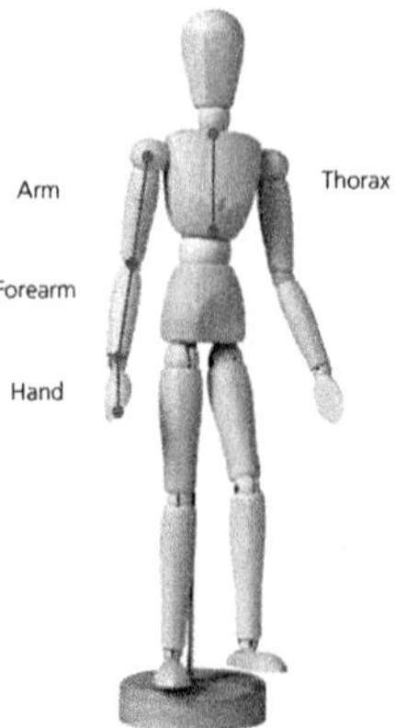

Fig. 1. The anatomical segments tracked by our upper-body motion tracking framework: thorax, arm, forearm and hand.

The segments are defined as follows: (1) the thorax, i.e. the segment between the jugular notch and the xiphoid process of the sternum, (2) the arm, i.e. the segment between shoulder and elbow joint, (3) the forearm, i.e. the segment between elbow and wrist joint, and (4) the hand, i.e. the segment between wrist and distal region of the third metacarpal. An IMU device was placed and firmly attached in each of the aforementioned segments, to collect acceleration, angular velocity and magnetic field data.

The block diagram of the motion tracker is represented in Fig. 2. After sensor acquisition, the framework comprises two major processing procedures: pre-processing and orientation estimation. The former includes temporal synchronisation and noise reduction, while the latter describes the sensor fusion approach and other necessary considerations in order to extract segments' orientation information.

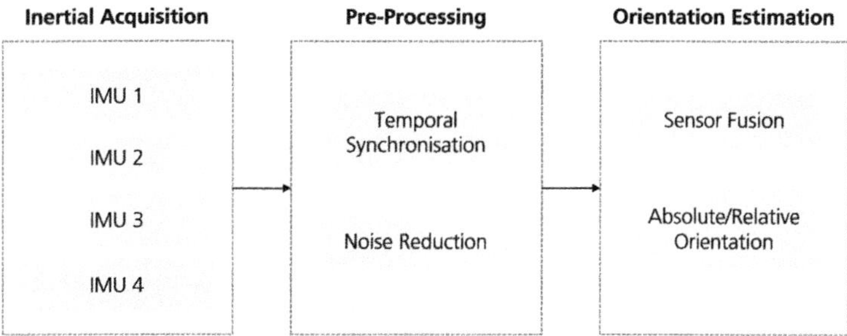

Fig. 2. Overview of the upper-body motion tracking framework.

3.1 Inertial Acquisition

The inertial collection comprises data from four IMUs, containing triaxial sensors, i.e. accelerometer, gyroscope and magnetometer. These devices collect information at a 100 Hz frequency and were positioned in thorax, arm, forearm and hand the segments. Specifically, IMU 1, IMU 2 and IMU 3 were positioned at the posterior side of the arm, forearm and hand, respectively, while IMU 4 was placed in the thorax area. All devices had commonly the Y-axis pointing up.

3.2 Pre-processing

The pre-processing pipeline includes signal synchronisation, filtering and normalisation. An unsuccessful temporal synchronisation can compromise further results of sensor fusion and even distort subsequent signal analysis since the collection of different sensors might be shifted or stretched in time. To address the synchronisation of multiple IMU devices we assured that all sensors had equal sampling frequency and were temporally aligned.

The implemented synchronisation method, represented in Fig. 3 was divided into two phases: (1) sensor level synchronisation and (2) device level synchronisation.

The built-in sensors of an IMU device may sample points with different timestamps, i.e. $t^{S1}_{Raw}, t^{S2}_{Raw}, t^{S3}_{Raw}$. At the sensor level synchronisation, the sampling frequency is adjusted, assuring that all sensors, within the same device, will share the same time domain, i.e. t^{D1} for the IMU device 1.

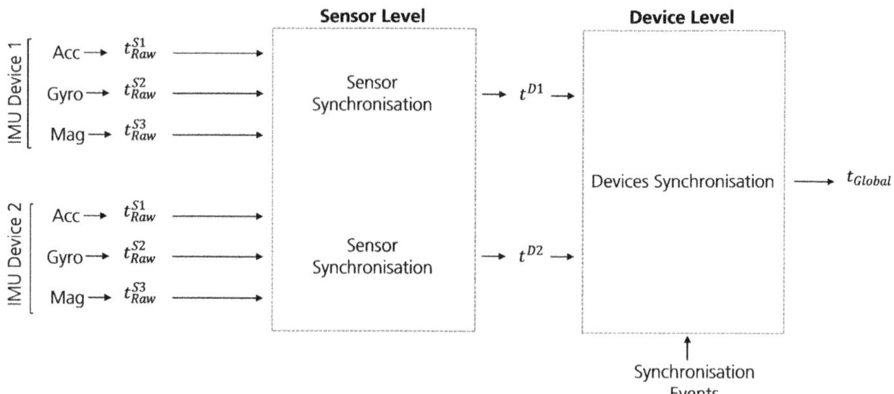

Fig. 3. Temporal synchronisation phases. Acc - accelerometer, Gyro - gyroscope, Mag - magnetometer.

Nevertheless, different devices can still present delay relative to one another. To solve the clock drift problem, at the device level we identify synchronisation events, i.e. instants in time acquired at the same instant yet shifted between different devices [22], to then calculate a common synchronised time, t_{Global}, for all devices.

Regarding noise reduction, a first-order low-pass Butterworth filter prepared for a cutoff frequency of 1 Hz [29], was applied to raw data from accelerometers and magnetometers. Afterwards, the data were normalised.

3.3 Orientation Estimation

In the orientation estimation stage, the pre-processed data is combined through sensor fusion techniques which will then allow inferring the absolute or relative limb's orientation. Several sensor fusion methods are described in the literature, differing in the sensors required or in the implemented algorithm methodology.

The combination of sensors' information can be described by quaternions, which have been widely exploited since they are a singularity-free attitude representation, and also computationally efficient.

This study will analyse and compare three different complementary filter approaches: (1) the quaternion-based complementary filter (QCF), described in [23], (2) the Mahony filter [19] and (3) the Madgwick Filter [18].

Following the sensor fusion implementation and subsequent estimation of the segment's quaternion, some angular motion assumptions can be determined. It is assumed that while IMUs are firmly secured to the limb, avoiding subtle changes in devices' locations, their axes are aligned with the anatomical axis of the body. Afterwards, using pure quaternions, which can express segments' direction vectors, and linear algebra knowledge it is possible to estimate the absolute or relative information of segments. While the absolute orientation is defined as the angle between a segment and an anatomical plane, e.g. shoulder flexion angle, the relative orientation, in its turn, represents the angle between two consecutive IMUs, e.g. wrist flexion can be expressed through the relative orientation of the hand and forearm segments. Moreover, the local axes from IMU placed on the thorax segment allowed to define the three anatomical planes, i.e. sagittal, coronal and transverse plane.

4 Experimental Overview

A compilation of upper-body movements was collected in a controlled environment. The collected dataset contains, on one side, information of inertial devices and, on the other, files of an optical motion capture (mocap) system alongside with video recordings.

The inertial estimates were compared with reference measures provided by the optical-passive mocap, Vicon system, allowing to evaluate the performance of the upper-body motion tracker.

The study comprised fourteen subjects, nine men and five women, which performed a designed experimental protocol, considering a variety of different upper-body movements. For this research we decided to track only the subjects' dominant arm. The participants had an average age of 26 ± 3 years, presented the right arm as the dominant one, and declared not to have any known musculoskeletal problem.

Two different phases comprised the experimental protocol. The first described a static evaluation, i.e. the participant is supposed to stand still while completing the protocol; the second supported a dynamic evaluation, i.e. the subject was supposed to perform a short walking exercise while performing the exercises.

Equipment and Placement. The inertial motion capture setup comprised four sensing devices, sampling at 100 Hz, positioned at the four study segments, i.e. thorax, arm, forearm and hand. The optical mocap included ten cameras. Markers were placed on participants following Vicon's Upper Limb Model Guide [26] and were tracked at 100 Hz. Vicon cameras followed calibration procedures before acquisition. In addition, two standard cameras also filmed the whole experimental protocol. Since different equipment was used temporal synchronisation was addressed during data analysis.

Dataset Composition. Data collection includes several movements which are detailed in Table 1. In particular, the thorax segment considers flexion/extension and lateral flexion/extension; the arm segment admits flexion/extension and abduction/adduction; finally, the forearm segment admits flexion/extension The inertial and Vicon data were manually annotated using video.

Table 1. Movements included in the experimental protocol.

Movement	Segment		
	Thorax	Arm	Forearm
Flexion	•	•	•
Extension	•	•	•
Lateral flexion	•		
Abduction		•	
Adduction		•	

5 Results

The selected and applied sensor fusion method is highly relevant to reconstruct the angular motion of the segments since it contributes to framework performance. Hence, different sensor fusion methods were investigated, namely the QCF, the Madgwick and Mahony filter.

An example of angular reconstruction regarding 9-axis sensor fusion techniques, i.e. methods that combine the information of accelerometer, gyroscope and magnetometer data, is represented in Fig. 4.

It can be observed that the three methods similarly reconstruct the designed motion. Additionally, it can be observed that the movement derived from Madgwick's is noisier relative to the other applied methods. During the movement execution, the three methods measures are above the values provided by the optical mocap.

The sensor fusion techniques presented in Fig. 4 relied on magnetic data, which supported the algorithms to obtain an absolute orientation reference. However, magnetometers often, influenced by buildings' ferromagnetic construction materials, lead to inaccurate results. Herewith, we also explored and implemented techniques relying solely on accelerometer and gyroscope readings, i.e. 6-axis sensor fusion. The 6-axis sensor fusion methods angular reconstruction are depicted in Fig. 5.

It can be noticed that QCF behaviour is different from the other two methods - during the abduction, QCF measures below the reference values while Mahony and Madgwick assign a higher value. Furthermore, Madgwick's signal remains noisy. Frequently, in manufacturing sites, an inhomogeneous magnetic field is observed. Thus, algorithms should be robust presenting solutions when the magnetometer information is unreliable. Although the 6-axis approaches are

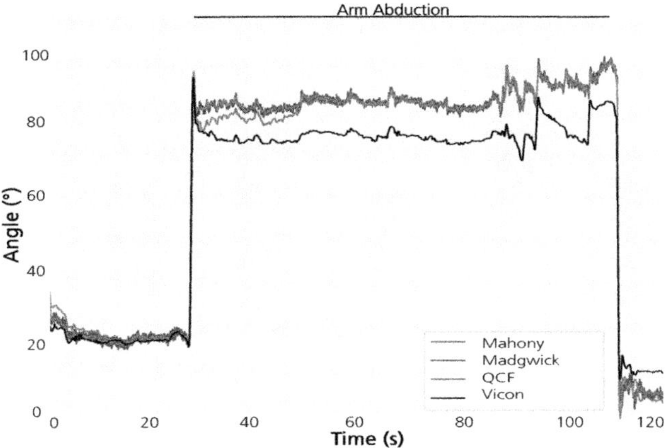

Fig. 4. Arm abduction reconstruction using 9-axis sensor fusion methods. Red - Mahony filter; Green - Madgwick filter; Blue - QCF; Black - Vicon. (Color figure online)

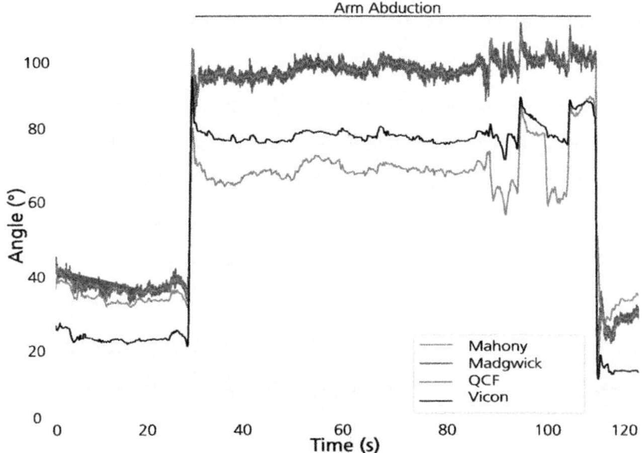

Fig. 5. Arm abduction reconstruction using 6-axis sensor fusion methods. Red - Mahony filter; Green - Madgwick filter; Blue - QCF; Black - Vicon. (Color figure online)

known to be more unstable, these could provide an alternative to situations of distorted magnetic data.

The computing time of the algorithms of both approaches, 9-axis and 6-axis, was determined. Figure 6 presents a comparison of the computing times across the different sensor fusion methods for the complete dataset.

As expected, the sensor fusion methods that combined the information of three sensors, i.e. 9-axis, require more computing time when compared to meth-

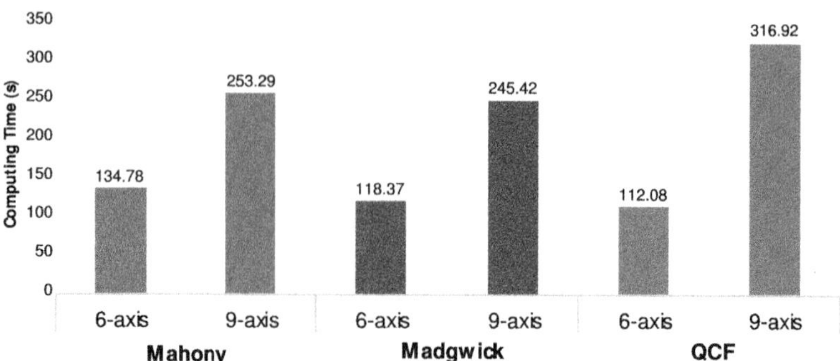

Fig. 6. Computing time across the different sensor fusion methods for the upper-body movements dataset.

ods than only fuse accelerometer and gyroscope data, i.e. 6-axis. Besides, for the considered dataset, the difference between these two approaches is close to 100 s.

Moreover, to assess which of the presented methods reconstructed the motion more accurately, the angular reconstruction was compared with the measures provided by the optical mocap. This allows performing a quantitative analysis of the reconstruction performance, which consequently characterises the employed sensor fusion method. For this analysis, we considered two evaluation metrics: the Cumulative Distribution Function (CDF), i.e. the probability that a considered variable X takes on a value less than or equal to x, and the Root-Mean-Square Error (RMSE), which provides a measure of how well an algorithm describes specific observations. Both CDF and RMSE are described, respectively, in Eqs. (1) and (2):

$$F_X(x) = \mathrm{P}(X \leq x) \tag{1}$$

where $\mathrm{P}(\mathrm{X} \leq x)$ is the probability that the considered variable X takes on a value less than or equal to x.

$$\mathrm{RMSE} = \sqrt{\frac{1}{\mathrm{T}}\sum_{t=1}^{\mathrm{T}}(y_t - \hat{y}_t)^2} \tag{2}$$

where y_t denotes the groundtruth value at time t provided by the optical mocap and $\hat{y}_t$ denotes the predicted value at time t estimated by the upper-body tracking method.

The CDF was calculated for the upper-body dataset, providing a comparison between the different sensor fusion approaches. Figure 7 represents the CDF for static exercises. The analysis of the static CDF suggests that the 6-axis QCF method presents a higher error than the other 6-axis techniques. Concerning the 9-axis sensor fusion, the Mahony filter exhibits a higher error probability. The CDF for dynamic exercises is presented in Fig. 8. Once again, the 6-axis QCF method presents less accurate results, yet, its 9-axis version is much more consistent. Moreover, all 9-axis methods behave quite similarly. It must be noted that the dynamic motion collection is smaller than the static. Therefore, an accurate comparison between these two motion consideration should not be performed due to data imbalance in the dataset. In general, the thorax movements are more accurately reconstructed, as opposed to the forearm's motion.

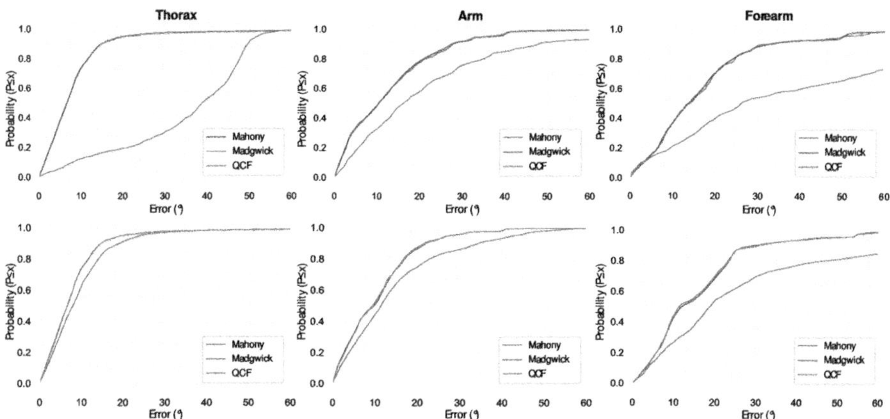

Fig. 7. Cumulative distribution function for the absolute error of Mahony, Madgwick and QCF across thorax, arm and forearm segments. Static trials. **Top:** 6-axis methods; **Bottom:** 9-axis methods.

Table 2 presents the RMSE for the different sensor fusion methods regarding both static and dynamic exercises.

Table 2. Root mean square error, in degrees, regarding the three studied sensor fusion methods: Mahony, Madgwick and QCF. Best results for static and dynamic evaluations are in bold.

Segment	RMSE (°)											
	Mahony				Madgwick				QCF			
	Static		Dynamic		Static		Dynamic		Static		Dynamic	
	6-axis	9-axis	6-axis	9-axis	6-axis	9-axis	6-axis	9-axis	6-axis	9-axis	6-axis	9-axis
Thorax	**12**	13	22	23	**12**	**12**	22	22	34	21	34	22
Arm	18	18	21	**20**	18	**15**	21	21	32	18	30	27
Forearm	26	45	18	19	**25**	26	**17**	20	44	30	43	20

In general, the 9-axis QCF method, in agreement with the CDF analysis, presents better performance than the 6-axis. Regarding the other two techniques, both 6-axis and 9-axis, the RMSE values are quite consistent.

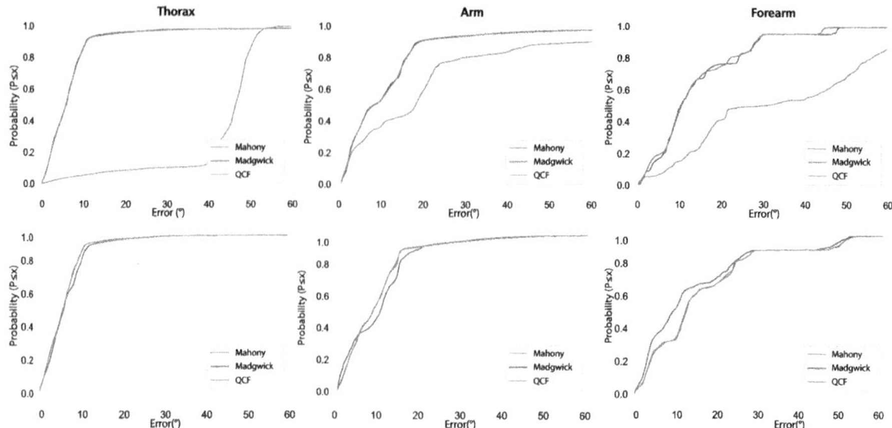

Fig. 8. Cumulative distribution function for the absolute error of Mahony, Madgwick and QCF across thorax, arm and forearm segments. Dynamic trials. **Top:** 6-axis methods; **Bottom:** 9-axis methods.

Comparing the three methods, the Madgwick filter, although noisier, is more accurate according to Vicon results than the others. Regarding the segments evaluation, the thorax movements are more accurate, while the forearm presents a higher error when compared with the optical mocap reference measures.

Furthermore, the overall inspection of the RMSE results suggests that the upper-body motion tracker has the potential to be improved. A more robust framework should be built considering biomechanical constraints. Moreover, we believe that the accuracy would certainly improve after some calibration procedures that we did not contemplate in this study. The angular reconstruction algorithm is established only considering vector knowledge, and thus the incorrect sensing device alignment with the anatomical axis of the body might have increased the segment's movements reconstruction error.

6 Conclusion

WMSDs are not only an occupational health concern but also a public issue and a demographic and social challenge, which should be addressed by developing sustainable working conditions. The arrival of the fourth industrial revolution offers the means to tackle WMSDs through the use of wearable devices in ergonomic researches. Nevertheless, to consider the use of direct measurements for ergonomic assessment, proposed wearable solutions must be reliable and accurate for not compromising the assessment and consequent intervention phases of ergonomic studies.

This research presents a more extensive analysis of complementary sensor fusion methods regarding the framework presented in [23]. Sensor fusion techniques are processes in which data from multiple physical sensors are combined, hence, diminishing single sensor associated flaws. Complementary filters have the advantage of overcoming the known problem of gyroscope drift over time which negatively impacts the accuracy of orientation estimation algorithms. This work contributed by highlighting the importance of sensor fusion techniques for estimating relevant ergonomic parameters as angular measures.

An experimental protocol was conducted with fourteen subjects wearing inertial sensors and markers from an optical mocap to collect several upper-body movements. Calculated angular measures from the optical mocap were considered as reference. We investigated the outcomes of QCF, Madgwick and Mahony sensor fusion methods for human motion reconstruction of the upper-body dataset. In particular, we studied 9-axis and 6-axis approaches for the aforementioned methods, i.e. the combination of accelerometer-gyroscope-magnetometer data and accelerometer-gyroscope fusion, respectively.

Some conclusions were drawn from the results. Concerning the computing time, the 9-axis algorithms require more time to completely calculate the segments' orientation for the assembled upper-body dataset than the 6-axis. Furthermore, the 9-axis Madgwick method presents better overall performance, meaning that this method results are more coherent concerning the measures provided by the optical mocap. Yet, all 9-axis methods are in a disadvantage in the presence of ferromagnetic materials which interfere with magnetometer readings and consequently leads to inaccurate results. In this context, an interesting finding is related to the accuracy of the 6-axis Mahony and Madgwick. Although these approaches rely solely on two sensors, they are quite effective in reconstructing the angular movement and also their RMSE values are consistent with the 9-axis approaches.

As future work, we intend to improve the presented framework, by introducing calibration procedures and performing analysis regarding biomechanical constraints. Additionally, to make the framework feasible in the manufacturing environment, we have to take into account the possibility of magnetic disturbances and thus, the algorithms should be prepared to make adjustments. A solution would be using a 6-axis sensor fusion method when magnetic data is disturbed or even introducing different classes of tracking devices, e.g. video and inertial, to periodically calibrate the system.

References

1. Alam, F., Zhaihe, Z., Jiajia, H.: A comparative analysis of orientation estimation filters using MEMS based IMU. In: 2nd International Conference on Research in Science, Engineering and Technology (ICRSET 2014) (2014). https://doi.org/10.15242/iie.e0314552
2. Alves, J., Silva, J., Grifo, E., Resende, C., Sousa, I.: Wearable embedded intelligence for detection of falls independently of on-body location. Sensor **19**(11) (2019). https://doi.org/10.3390/s19112426
3. Bancroft, J.B., Lachapelle, G.: Data fusion algorithms for multiple inertial measurement units. Sensors **11**(7), 6771–6798 (2011). https://doi.org/10.3390/s110706771

4. Barbour, N., Schmidt, G.: Inertial sensor technology trends. IEEE Sens. J. **1**(4), 332–339 (2001). https://doi.org/10.1109/7361.983473
5. Battini, D., Persona, A., Sgarbossa, F.: Innovative real-time system to integrate ergonomic evaluations into warehouse design and management. Comput. Ind. Eng. **77**, 1–10 (2014). https://doi.org/10.1016/j.cie.2014.08.018
6. Bergmann, J.H., Mayagoitia, R.E., Smith, I.C.: A portable system for collecting anatomical joint angles during stair ascent: a comparison with an optical tracking device. Dyn. Med. **8**(1), 1–7 (2009). https://doi.org/10.1186/1476-5918-8-3
7. Brückner, H.P., Spindeldreier, C., Blume, H., Schoonderwaldt, E., Altenmüller, E.: Evaluation of inertial sensor fusion algorithms in grasping tasks using real input data: comparison of computational costs and root mean square error. In: Proceedings of the 9th International Workshop on Wearable and Implantable Body Sensor Networks, BSN 2012, pp. 189–194 (2012). https://doi.org/10.1109/BSN.2012.9
8. Caputo, F., Greco, A., D'Amato, E., Notaro, I., Spada, S.: IMU-based motion capture wearable system for ergonomic assessment in industrial environment. In: Ahram, T.Z. (ed.) AHFE 2018. AISC, vol. 795, pp. 215–225. Springer, Cham (2019). https://doi.org/10.1007/978-3-319-94619-1_21
9. Cerqueira, S.M., Da Silva, A.F., Santos, C.P.: Instrument-based ergonomic assessment: a perspective on the current state of art and future trends. In: Proceedings of the 6th IEEE Portuguese Meeting on Bioengineering, ENBENG 2019, pp. 14–17 (2019). https://doi.org/10.1109/ENBENG.2019.8692514
10. Fera, M., Greco, A., Caterino, M., Gerbino, S., Caputo, F.: Line balancing assessment enhanced by IoT and simulation tools. In: Proceedings of the 2019 IEEE International Workshop on Metrology for Industry 4.0 and IoT, MetroInd 4.0 and IoT 2019, pp. 84–88 (2019). https://doi.org/10.1109/METROI4.2019.8792889
11. Fera, M., et al.: Towards digital twin implementation for assessing production line performance and balancing. Sensors **20**(1), 97 (2019)
12. Filippeschi, A., Schmitz, N., Miezal, M., Bleser, G., Ruffaldi, E., Stricker, D.: Survey of motion tracking methods based on inertial sensors: a focus on upper limb human motion. Sensors **17**(6), 1–40 (2017). https://doi.org/10.3390/s17061257
13. Isusi, I.: Work-related musculoskeletal disorders – facts and figures (syntesis of 10 national reports). European Agency for Safety and Health at Work (2020). https://doi.org/10.2802/443890. http://europa.eu
14. de Kok, J., et al.: Work-related musculoskeletal disorders : prevalence, costs and demographics in the EU. European Agency for Safety and Health at Work (2019). https://doi.org/10.2802/66947
15. Kok, M., Hol, J.D., Schön, T.B.: Using inertial sensors for position and orientation estimation. Found. Trends® Sig. Process. **11**(1–2), 1–153 (2017). https://doi.org/10.1561/2000000094
16. Lim, S., D'Souza, C.: A narrative review on contemporary and emerging uses of inertial sensing in occupational ergonomics. Int. J. Ind. Ergon. **76**, 102937 (2020).https://doi.org/10.1016/j.ergon.2020.102937. http://www.sciencedirect.com/science/article/pii/S0169814119305591
17. Lu, Y.: Industry 4.0: a survey on technologies, applications and open research issues. J. Ind. Inf. Integr. **6**, 1–10 (2017). https://doi.org/10.1016/j.jii.2017.04.005
18. Madgwick, S.O., Harrison, A.J., Vaidyanathan, R.: Estimation of IMU and MARG orientation using a gradient descent algorithm. In: IEEE International Conference on Rehabilitation Robotics, pp. 179–185 (2011). https://doi.org/10.1109/ICORR.2011.5975346

19. Mahony, R., Hamel, T., Pflimlin, J.: Nonlinear complementary filters on the special orthogonal group. IEEE Trans. Autom. Control **53**(5), 1203–1218 (2008)
20. Peppoloni, L., Filippeschi, A., Ruffaldi, E., Avizzano, C.A.: A novel 7 degrees of freedom model for upper limb kinematic reconstruction based on wearable sensors. In: Proceedings of the IEEE 11th International Symposium on Intelligent Systems and Informatics, SISY 2013, pp. 105–110 (2013). https://doi.org/10.1109/SISY.2013.6662551
21. Pereira, A., Folgado, D., Nunes, F., Almeida, J., Sousa, I.: Using inertial sensors to evaluate exercise correctness in electromyography-based home rehabilitation systems. In: 2019 IEEE International Symposium on Medical Measurements and Applications (MeMeA), pp. 1–6 (2019)
22. Santos, S.: Explaining the ergonomic assessment of human movement in industrial contexts. Master's thesis, NOVA School of Science and Technology - FCT NOVA (2019). http://hdl.handle.net/10362/88342
23. Santos, S., Folgado, D., Rodrigues, J., Mollaei, N., Fujão, C., Gamboa, H.: Explaining the ergonomic assessment of human movement in industrial contexts. In: Proceedings of the 13th International Joint Conference on Biomedical Engineering Systems and Technologies (BIOSTEC 2020), pp. 79–88 (2020). https://doi.org/10.5220/0008953800790088
24. Teufl, W., Miezal, M., Taetz, B., Frohlichi, M., Bleser, G.: Validity of inertial sensor based 3D joint kinematics of static and dynamic sport and physiotherapy specific movements. PLoS ONE **14**(2), 1–18 (2019). https://doi.org/10.1371/journal.pone.0213064
25. Tsao, L., Nussbaum, M.A., Kim, S., Ma, L.: Modelling performance during repetitive precision tasks using wearable sensors: a data-driven approach. Ergonomics **63**(7), 831–849 (2020). https://doi.org/10.1080/00140139.2020.1759700
26. Vicon Motion Systems: Upper Limb Model. Product Guide (2007). http://www.vicon.com
27. Vignais, N., Bernard, F., Touvenot, G., Sagot, J.C.: Physical risk factors identification based on body sensor network combined to videotaping. Appl. Ergon. **65**, 410–417 (2017). https://doi.org/10.1016/j.apergo.2017.05.003
28. Yi, C., et al.: Estimating three-dimensional body orientation based on an improved complementary filter for human motion tracking. Sensors **18**(11) (2018). https://doi.org/10.3390/s18113765
29. Zhou, H., Hu, H.: Upper limb motion estimation from inertial measurements. Int. J. Inf. Technol. **13**, 1–14 (2007)

PDC-MI Method for EEG Functional Conectivity Analysis

Victor H. B. Tsukahara[1](✉), Pedro V. B. Jeronymo[1], Jasiara C. de Oliveira[2], Vinícius R. Cota[2], and Carlos D. Maciel[1]

[1] Signal Processing Laboratory, Department of Electrical Engineering, University of São Paulo, São Carlos, Brazil
{vhbtsukahara,carlos.maciel}@usp.br

[2] Laboratory of Neuroengineering and Neuroscience, Department of Electrical Engineering, Federal University of São João Del-Rei, São João Del-Rei, Brazil
vrcota@ufsj.edu.br

Abstract. Epilepsy is the second most prevalent brain disorder affecting approximately 70 million people worldwide. A modern approach to developing the brain study is to model it as a system of systems, represented by a network of oscillators, in which the emergent property of synchronization occurs. Based on this perspective, epileptic seizures are processes of hyper-synchronization between brain areas. The paper develops a case study with the use of Partial Directed Coherence (PDC), Surrogate and Mutual Information (MI) to perform functional connectivity analysis observing the synchronization phenomenon. The aim is to examine the connectivity and transmission rate (R) between brain areas—cortex, hippocampus and thalamus—during basal intervals. The main contribution of this paper is the combination of both methods to study the connectivity and transmission rate between brain areas. A case study performed using 5 EEG signals from rodents showed that the applied methodology represents another appropriate alternative to existing methods for functional analysis such as Granger Causality, Transfer Entropy, providing insights on epileptic brain communication.

Keywords: Epilepsy · Signal processing · Partial directed coherence · Mutual information

1 Introduction

Epilepsy is the second most common neurological disease [28] and affects approximately 70 million people worldwide [38] representing a public health concern [26].

This work was supported by the Fundação de Amparo à Pesquisa de Minas Gerais (FAPEMIG) [grant number APQ 02485-15] and financed in part by the Coordenação de Aperfeiçoamento de Pessoal de Nível Superior - Brasil (CAPES) - Finance Code 001.

X. Ye et al. (Eds.): BIOSTEC 2020, CCIS 1400, pp. 304–328, 2021.
https://doi.org/10.1007/978-3-030-72379-8_15

It is a chronic disease of the central nervous system (CNS) that reaches people of all ages in which it is commonly associated with social difficulties [7] and can cause health loss such as premature mortality and residual disability [8]. Epilepsy-based studies usually use electroencephalography (EEG) [10,23] to check brain electrical activity, and the use of electrodes directly in brain tissue is an important option to map the electrical activity of the brain with better spatial resolution [6].

The latest approach to study epilepsy is the analysis of hyper-synchronisation of brain frequencies oscillations as a feature [47]. Olamat et al. [27] performed a nonlinear synchronisation analysis in LFP epileptic data introducing this new perspective. Weiss et al. [45] used the concept to understand seizure genesis and spreading in human limbic areas and Devinsky et al. [15] reported hyper-synchronisation to discuss epilepsy epidemiology and pathophysiology. The brain model is a complex system where each region represents a subsystem, and synchronisation is an emergent property [4]. Changes in this feature during the occurrence of epileptic seizures are an essential aspect to understand the epileptic brain network and synchronisation [24]. The abnormal hyper-synchronisation of frequencies oscillations give rise to seizures [9].

There is a hypothesis that high-frequencies oscillations have a relation with the cortical local brain information processing, whereas low-frequencies have a connection with more extensive cortical networks [3]. Consequently, brain interactions through these areas can become complicated because of interactions between oscillations at different frequency bands [3]. In this situation, functional connectivity is an option to detect dependencies among neurophysiological signals [4]. There are various methods used to infer patterns of direct influences [4]. To estimate time series dependencies [20] Mutual Information is one of them [41]. It is an Information-Theoretic and nonparametric approach that measures generalized interdependence between two variables [2]. This feature meets the accepted vision that real-world time series usually are non-linear and non-stationary [43].

Although Mutual Information detects dependence on two variables, it does not show the direction of connectivity. To assess this feature, Partial Directed Coherence may be an option due to its consolidation as a linear model to perform functional connectivity analysis [42]. It provides proper adherence to study the problem [19] being more simple then nonlinear methods such as Conditional Mutual Information which requires estimations of big order [25]. It is a frequency-domain technique based on multivariate autoregressive (MVAR) modelling [31] proposed by Baccalá & Sameshima [5] and widely used in neuroscience until nowadays [11]. The main advantage is the capability to assign active connections exhibiting the direct influences between brain areas [22] resulting in a map of its interactions [1].

Once the application of PDC, there is an issue to handle that is the development of criteria to evaluate the connectivity discovered among EEG time-series [46]. The problem usually leads to the employment of arbitrarily connectivity thresholds [33]. Surrogate technique emerges as an option to provide statistical significance to connectivity measures [12]. The method consists in building a surrogate data using the original signals keeping the same power spectrum and randomizing Fourier phases, generating uncorrelated signals. Using PDC with Surrogate can reveal what communications remain even in this situation resulting in a connectivity threshold. Then it may be compared with original signals through a hypothesis test to validate the functional analysis. It is possible to check its use for that objective in literature since Information Theoretical methods [17,34] until Granger Causality, Directed Coherence and Partial Directed Coherence [1].

The objective of this paper is, in performing a case study using Mutual Information and Partial Directed Coherence, to develop functional connectivity analysis in rodents EEG signals, investigating the connectivity, the channel capacity (C) and the transmission rate between brain areas. Also, it is applied Surrogate method to evaluate the PDC measures.

In Sect. 2, the theory related to PDC, MI and Surrogate are presented. Section 3 describes the EEG data used and the applied methodology. Section 4 presents the achieved results, and in Sect. 5, there is a discussion of the results. Finally, Sect. 6 brings forward paper conclusions.

2 Theory

This section presents the leading theory required to develop this paper. At first, the introduction of Mutual Information explaining the main concepts of channel capacity and transmission rate. Then the Partial Directed Coherence and Surrogate methods to perform functional connectivity analysis are described.

2.1 Mutual Information

To determine the measure of how deterministic is a given variable entropy (H) is used and defined by [14]:

$$H(X) = -\sum_{x \in \chi} p(x) log_a p(x) \tag{1}$$

where X is a discrete random variable, $p(x) = P\{X = x\}$ is the probability of X equal to x, $x \in \chi$, i.e. the probability mass function of X, and a is the logarithm base that provides the entropy measure in bits in the case of $a = 2$. Given a signal X and another signal Y, the Mutual Information may quantify the information shared between this signals, which means how much it is possible to reduce the uncertainty of signal X given the knowledge of signal Y [14].

The Mutual Information (MI), according to [14] is the quantification of information shared between X and Y or mathematically defined as the measure of the dependence between two random variables. Mathematically written as [41]:

$$I(X;Y) = H(X) - H(X|Y) = \sum_{xy} p(x,y) log \frac{p(x,y)}{p(x)p(y)} \tag{2}$$

According to [14] the channel capacity (C) represents the maximum measure of Mutual Information:

$$C = maxI(X, Y) \tag{3}$$

and according to [32] the channel capacity for DMI is quantified by its peak value. Also according to [32], the transmission rate estimation (R) can be written as a function of channel capacity and signal bandwidth (BW) in Hertz:

$$R = 2.BW.C \tag{4}$$

If the entropy is measured in bits, the transmission rate is going to be measured as bits/s.

2.2 Partial Directed Coherence

Partial Directed Coherence is a frequency-domain approach to denote the direct linear relationship between two different signals $x_i[n]$ and $x_j[n]$ once remarked jointly with a set of other signals [5]. Considering $X[n]$ the set of all observed time series, it can be depicted as an autoregressive model as follows:

$$X[n] = \sum_{k=1}^{p} A_k x\left[n-k\right] + E[n] \tag{5}$$

where p represents the model order, E[n] is the prediction error matrix and A_k are the coefficients matrix with a_{ij} elements in which denotes the relation between signals at lag k. E(n) has a covariance matrix ξ and their coefficients are usually a white noise with zero mean. This results in PDC factor (π_{ij}) and partial coherence function ($|\kappa_{ij}[f]|^2$) that indicates the strength and the direction of communication at frequency f. They can be stated as follows [44]:

$$\pi_{ij}[f] \triangleq \frac{\overline{A}_{ij}[f]}{\sqrt{\overline{a}_j^{-H}[f]\xi^{-1}\overline{a}_j[f]}} \tag{6}$$

$$\kappa_{ij}[f] = \pi_i^H[f]\xi^{-1}\pi_j[f] \tag{7}$$

H[f] is the Hermitian matrix which is equal to $\overline{A}^{-1}[f]$. $\overline{A}_{ij}[f]$ is the complement of $A_{ij}[f]$ and represents the transfer function from $x_j[n]$ to $x_i[n]$ being also an element of $A[f]$ matrix. Finally, $\overline{a}_j[f]$ is the jth column of $\overline{A}[f]$ and $\pi_i[f]$ is the ith row of π_{ij}. The main problem of connectivity analysis is the evaluation of the hypothesis below [5]:

$$H_0 : \pi_{ij}[f] = 0 \tag{8}$$

$$H_1 : \pi_{ij}[f] \neq 0 \tag{9}$$

The rejection of the hypothesis defined in (8) suggests that there is a direct connection from $x_j[n]$ to $x_i[n]$ in which can not be justified by the other remarked signals at the same time [44].

2.3 Surrogate for Hypothesis Test

The partial coherence function is $\kappa_{ij}[f]$ from PDC method. This is the normalized cross-spectrum that can be defined generically as follows [40]:

$$\Gamma_{xy}[f] \triangleq \frac{S_{xy}[f]}{\sqrt{S_x[f]}\sqrt{S_y[f]}} \tag{10}$$

where $S_{xy}[f]$ is the cross-power density spectrum between signals x and y, and $S_x[f]$, $S_y[f]$ are the power density spectrum of each signal respectively. The cross-spectrum can be associated with the cross-correlation function - $R_{xy}[n_1, n_0]$ which can be written as $R_{xy}[l]$ in the case of stationarity, where l is the lag (difference between indices n_1 and n_0) - through Wiener-Khinchin Theorem in which states that Fourier Transform of $R_{xy}[l]$ results in $S_{xy}[f]$. Therefore it is possible to infer that placing the correlation function in frequency-domain it represents the cross-power density spectrum [40]. Following that rationale it means that cross-correlation function measures the energy shared between signals x and y at a given frequency f [40].

Surrogate is a method to create signals keeping the same statistical properties intended to be evaluated. Subsequently it is performed the comparison of the statistical property to be evaluated with the data built. According to the deviance between them, the null hypothesis is accepted or rejected. In Neuroscience there are related literature about the use of Surrogate Data to assist the strength just as the type of interdependency among EEG signals. Adkinson et al. [1] used Surrogate to validate generalized Partial Directed Coherence measures, Faes et al. [18] used Surrogate to evaluate frequency-domain causality in multivariate time-series and Pereda et al. [30] used the method to validate nonlinear multivariate analysis in neurophysiological signals.

For method application, there are several techniques such as Random Permutation (RP) Surrogates, Fourier Transform (FT), Amplitude Adjusted Fourier Transform (AAFT) and Iterative Amplitude Adjusted Fourier Transform (IAAFT). With regard to the IAAFT technique, it was proposed by Schreiber and Schmitz [36], had the aim to overcome the AAFT technique bias [1] and it has a parallelized implementation to enhance its performance [16].

To establish the number of surrogate data to be created there is a rank-order test proposed by Theiler *et al.* [39] that can be used [37]. Let us consider Ψ the probability of false rejection then the level of significance(S) can be written as:

$$S = (1 - \Psi) \cdot 100\% \tag{11}$$

The number of surrogate data to be created(M) is defined below:

$$M = \frac{K}{\Psi} - 1 \tag{12}$$

where K is an integer number defined by the type of test - 1 if it is one-sided and 2 in the case of a two-sided test- and Ψ is the probability of false rejection. K = 1 is a common choice due to computational effort to develop surrogate data [37].

3 Methodology

The section details the methodology used to analyse the EEG signals, to assess the connectivity, channel capacity and transmission rate between brain areas. Furthermore, it describes the methods applied to acquire the EEG signals and the computational environment.

3.1 Applied Methodology

The applied methodology is in Fig. 1 and used for all five rodents, each one having three recordings from 3 different brain areas (cortex, hippocampus and thalamus) totalling 15 recordings. It is analyzed the rodent's classical EEG frequency bands[1] and the Kolmogorov-Smirnov test is used to compare the group of rodents to check if there is a statistical difference between groups. Initially, the division of the EEG signal in 10 intervals of 4096 samples. After, PDC method is applied to investigate the connectivity among cortex, hippocampus and thalamus brain areas. Using the model order of 1, the same value used in previous work [35]. To evaluate the PDC measures, Surrogate is applied. Then the graph of connectivity evolution during the time series is developed based on the model of temporal series of Holme and Saramäki [21] using a surrogate data of length 35 for each signal to provide 5% of statistical analysis significance according to Eq. 11. Finally, MI is applied to investigate the transmission rate among brain areas completing the functional connectivity analysis. To simulate it was used Python language running on a computer with Intel i7 6-core processor, 16 GB of RAM and IOS operational system.

3.2 Database for Study Case

We used EEG signals database from the Laboratory of Neuroengineering and Neuroscience from Federal University of São João Del Rei. The laboratory employs male Wistar rats weighing between 250 and 350 grams coming from the University Central Vivarium to acquire data and evaluate methods of therapeutic electrical stimulation. All described procedures are in according to ethics committee under protocol 31/2014. Signal recording is performed with the aid of electrodes (monopolar type and Teflon-coated stainless-steel wires) placed directly into the right thalamus and hippocampus of rat brain through stereotactic surgery [13]. In addition, two microsurgical screws (length 4.7 mm, diameter 1.17 mm, Fine Science Tools, Inc., North Vancouver, Canada) were implanted aiming the cortical recording of the right hemisphere and to operate as reference in frontal bone. The electrodes and screws were positioned with assistance of a neuroanatomic atlas [29].

EEG signals for each rat were recorded and animals were filmed at the same time to perform behavioral analysis (observe classic seizure features such as

[1] Δ - 0–4 Hz; θ - 4–8 Hz; α - 8–14 Hz; β - 14–30 Hz; γ^l (low gamma): 30–60 Hz; γ^h (high gamma) - 60–100 Hz; r (ripples) - 100–200 Hz; and r^f (fast ripples) - 200–300 Hz.

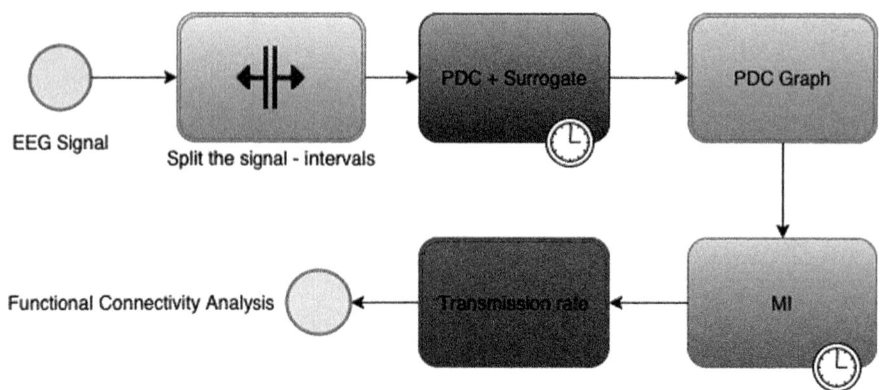

Fig. 1. The applied methodology for all rodent recordings used in this paper. Initially the signal is divided in 10 intervals (4096 samples) and then the PDC method is applied for each one, using Surrogate to evaluate the connectivity measures. Based on results the graph model evolution is developed. After MI is applied to observe the transmission rate among brain areas for all intervals using 32 bins. The choice of 32 bins was based on literature [17] in which MI with delay was applied to evaluate neural signals. The result of both methods development is the functional connectivity analysis of EEG signal.

facial automatisms, myoclonic jerk, head clonus, hind and forelimb clonus, elevation and fall, generalized tonic-clonic seizure) to allow their correlation with the electrophysiological events observed during EEG recording. EEG recording was acquired using 1 kHz sampling rate. Signals were amplified 2000 V/V and analog filtered (anti-aliasing) at 0.3 to 300 Hz using A-M Systems (model 3500) pre-amplifier and acquired on a National Instruments (PCI 6023E) A/D converter controlled by a LabView Virtual developed at LINNce. Power grid noise at 60 Hz frequency was suppressed with the aid of shielded twisted cables and Faraday cage. In order to induce seizures, animals were submitted to intravenous controlled infusion of pentylenetetrazole (PTZ), a GABAergic antagonist with, thus, proconvulsant action.

The EEG signals for each rodent was registered and filmed at the same time to perform behavioural analysis(observe classic seizure features such as facial automatisms, myoclonic concussion, head myoclonus, anterior and posterior limbs myoclonus, elevation and fall, generalized tonic-clonic seizure) to allow their correlation with the electrophysiological events observed during EEG recording. EEG recording was performed using 1 kHz sampling rate. Signals were amplified 2000 V/V through A-M Systems (model 3500) amplification system and digitalised on National Instruments (PCI 6023E) A/D converter controlled by developed LINNce Virtual Instrument from LabView platform. Sequentially they were filtered using second-order Butterworth filter (0.3 to 300 Hz band).The power grid noise at 60 Hz frequency was conditioned with use of shielded cables and Faraday cage.

4 Results

A signal sample of cortex, hippocampus and thalamus used to perform the analysis is presented in Fig. 2. The figure shows the ten intervals of 4096 samples from rodent R048 totalling 40960 samples. Cortex signal is indicated in the blue, hippocampus in red and thalamus in orange colour.

The Kolmogorov-Smirnov test performed with rodents groups indicated that there is no difference between the groups at the level of p-value equals 10%. For p-value of 5% the Kolmogorov-Smirnov test was not possible to assure this confidence level. The graphic summary of PDC results of all the five rodents is in Fig. 4. Dashed lines represent that there is no connectivity in one or more frequency bands analyzed. The connectivity measures may be checked in Tables 3, 4, 5, 6 and 7 from Appendix section. The summary table of PDC measures of all rodents is in Table 2. Figure 3 shows an example of surrogate data generated to evaluate the PDC measures developed to validate rodent R048 interval 1. The rodents EEG signal 3db bandwidth were approximately equal for all observed intervals for each rodent [41]:

- R048: Cx = 1.30 Hz, Hp = 1.49 Hz and Th = 1.23 Hz;
- R052: Cx = 1.73 Hz, Hp = 1.71 Hz and Th = 1.71 Hz;
- R064: Cx = 9.00 Hz, Hp = 10.50 Hz and Th = 8.71 Hz;
- R065: Cx = 10.00 Hz, Hp = 10.00 Hz and Th = 10.00 Hz;
- R072: Cx = 2.77 Hz, Hp = 2.75 Hz and Th = 2.74 Hz.

The MI measures (channel capacity) for each interval is presented in Tables 8, 9, 10, 11 and 12. The transmission rates are reported in Tables 13, 14, 15, 16 and 17 in Appendix. The transmission rate means with its standard deviation is presented in Table 1. The computational time spent to perform PDC with Surrogate for each rodent was approximately 90 min, and to perform MI was spent approximately 60 min. Therefore the total time was 12 h.

Table 1. Transmission rate mean (μ) among brain areas. It is reported pairwise and their respective standard deviations (σ). Due to use of base-2 log the transmission rate is given in bits/s.

Measures	Brain area					
	Hp → Cx	Th → Cx	Cx → Hp	Th → Hp	Cx → Th	Hp → Th
μ	11.06	11.36	10.77	10.68	14.26	13.11
σ	9.43	9.21	8.28	8.30	9.49	8.07

5 Discussion

Observing the graph in Fig. 4 it is possible to note that the connectivity among brain areas changes and sometimes not checked for all frequency bands. There

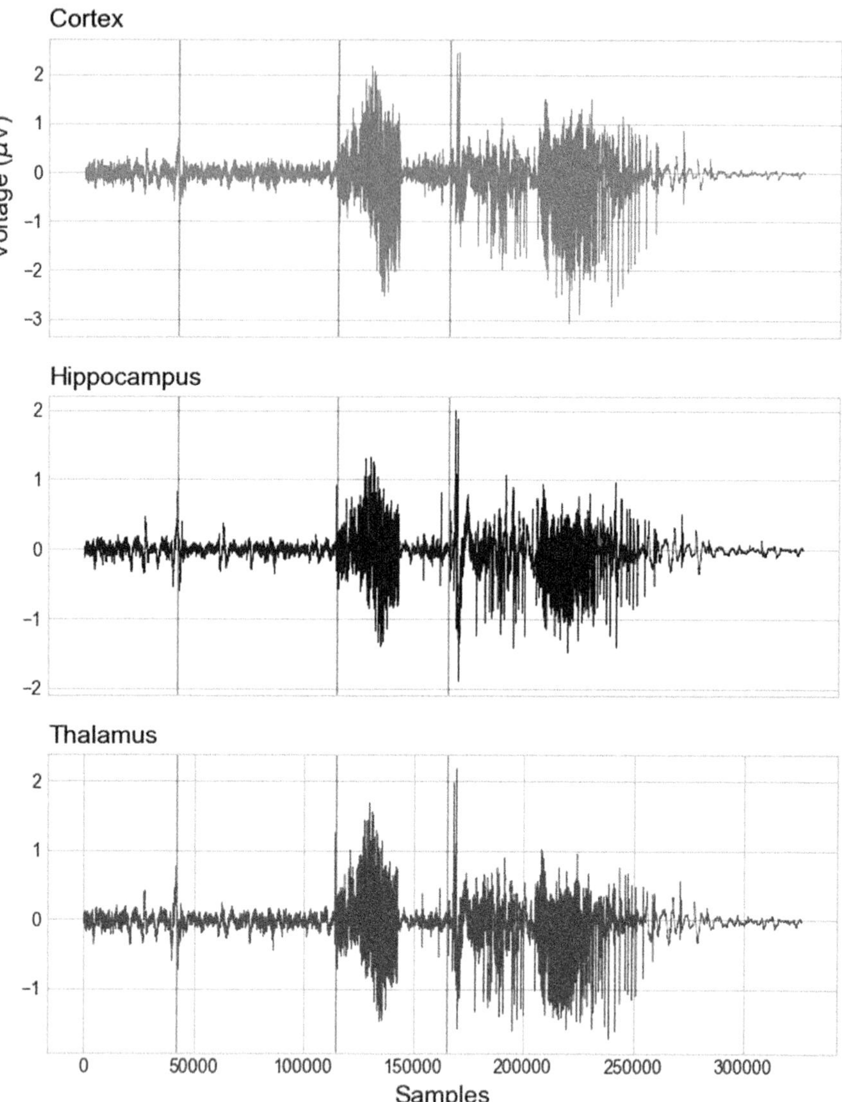

Fig. 2. Signal from rodent R048 used in this paper. It is represented the three signals acquired from cortex (blue), hippocampus (red) and thalamus brain areas (orange). The first green line represent the basal interval. From the first green line until the black line represent the infusion interval and from the second green line until the end of recording is the seizure interval. The intervals used to apply PDC and MI is the basal interval divided in 10 intervals of 4096 samples. (Color figure online)

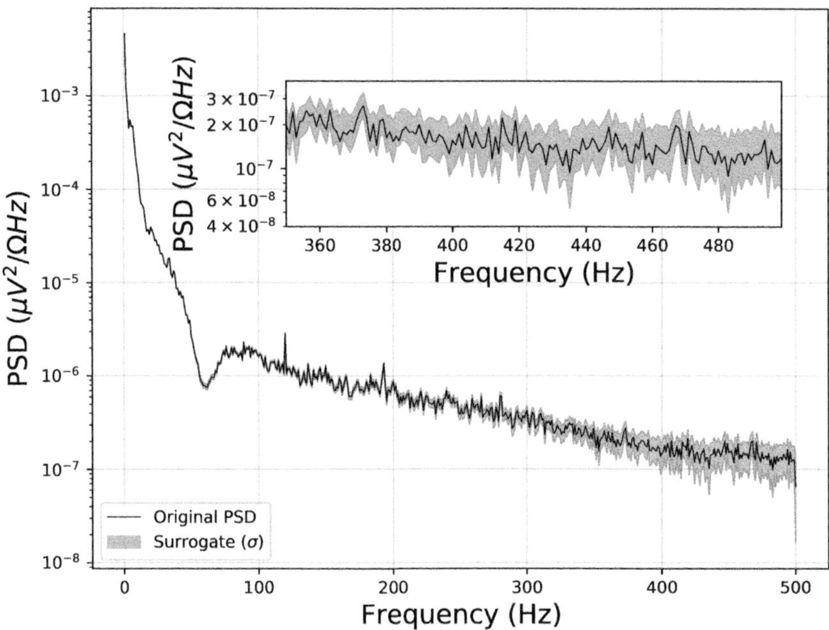

Fig. 3. Surrogate data example from interval 1 of rodent R048. Observe that power spectrum density is approximately equal indicating that the signal remain the same information despite phase change resulted from IAAFT algorithm which means that method worked as expected [41].

is different connectivity for all the five rodents, and it was expected due to the biological difference among them even being the same species of animal and present almost the same weight. However, observing Tables 3, 4, 5, 6 and 7 in Appendix there are some patterns identified through the use of PDC: the connectivity measures for lower frequencies usually is higher than observed for high-frequency bands. Another feature is when there is not full connectivity when it often happens, the high-frequency bands do not prompt communication. When there is no connectivity in lower frequencies, it is observed the lack of communication mainly in delta rhythm.

Generally, through PDC, it was possible to observe the functional connectivity during the intervals. It was possible to check ranges in which there are no connectivity brain areas for low or high frequencies, and there are only one or two rhythms of them with small values of connectivity. In this situation, it is possible to state that for low or high-frequency bands there is no connectivity even with small amounts in some frequencies. This analysis becomes more evident when observing Table 2. The standard deviation observed for rodents connectivity means is not high neither low contributing to the idea that even

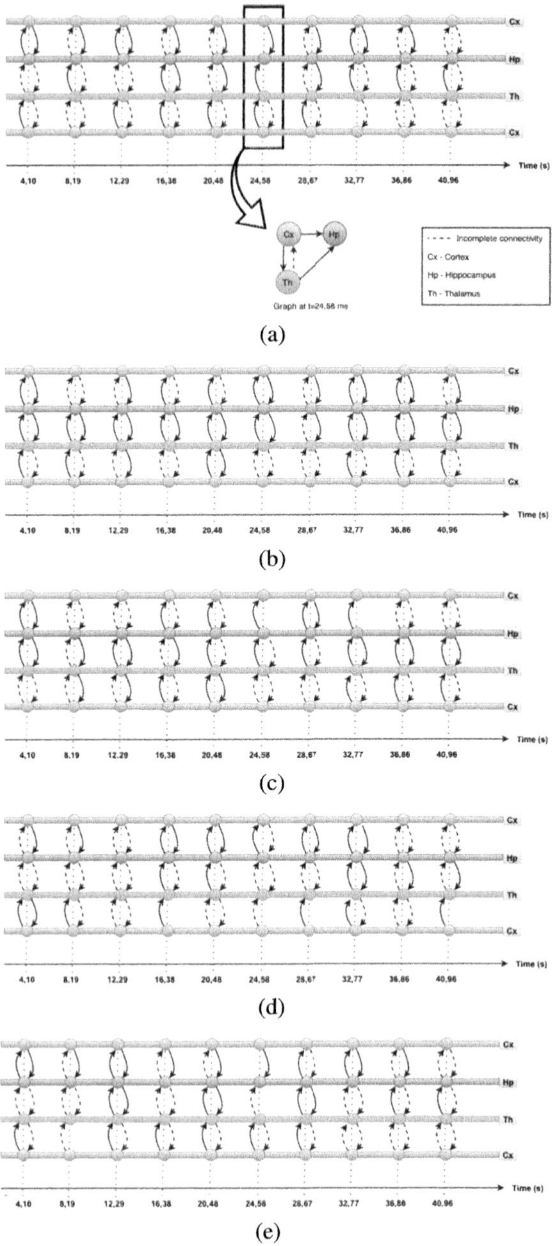

Fig. 4. Partial Directed Coherence results for rodent R048(a), R052(b), R064(c), R065(d) and R072(e). Dashed lines represent that there are no connectivity in one or more frequency bands analyzed. Please check Tables 3, 4, 5, 6 and 7 in Appendix to verify connectivity measures. Cortex signal is repeated just to turn the connectivity representation more clear.

Table 2. Connectivity measures resulted from PDC method. It is reported the connectivity mean (μ) among brain areas with their respective standard deviation (σ) considering all the classical EEG frequencies.

Brain area	Measures	Frequency							
		Delta	Theta	Alpha	Beta	Low gamma	High gamma	Ripple	Fast ripple
Hp → Cx	μ	0.79	0.82	0.70	0.58	0.50	0.46	0.44	0.50
	σ	0.29	0.25	0.18	0.14	0.16	0.18	0.17	0.19
Th → Cx	μ	0.35	0.53	0.50	0.43	0.37	0.35	0.34	0.33
	σ	0.49	0.29	0.24	0.21	0.20	0.21	0.21	0.19
Cx → Hp	μ	0.70	0.70	0.71	0.79	0.85	0.83	0.75	0.66
	σ	0.31	0.21	0.16	0.12	0.12	0.11	0.10	0.09
Th → Hp	μ	0.88	0.79	0.64	0.50	0.40	0.39	0.39	0.37
	σ	0.46	0.37	0.25	0.16	0.11	0.10	0.09	0.08
Cx → Th	μ	1.14	1.18	1.11	0.95	0.74	0.58	0.47	0.42
	σ	0.50	0.38	0.24	0.17	0.18	0.16	0.13	0.10
Hp → Th	μ	1.04	0.94	0.81	0.80	0.95	0.91	0.73	0.66
	σ	0.49	0.35	0.23	0.16	0.11	0.12	0.12	0.13

being from the same species, the rodents are slightly different physiologically presenting different connectivity measures.

Surrogate method evaluated the connectivity measures as desired, giving a threshold measure to assess the presence or absence of connectivity for frequency bands during the intervals. Observing the connectivity measures in the case of uncorrelated signals, Surrogate provided the statistical significance for PDC measures. Figure 3 showed an example of surrogate data created for rodent R048 to evaluate interval 1 PDC connectivity measures. As expected, the power spectrum density remained the same as the original signal indicating that the IAFFT method worked, changing the signal phase to create uncorrelated signals preserving the same information among them.

The transmission rate among brain areas was different for each rodent as also expected due to the physiological difference among them even being the same species. However, for each rodent, it is possible to check a transmission rate in mean approximately equal among brain areas. This result report that the brain presents a basal state of synchrony compliant with the modern theory that brain present network synchrony and epilepsy is a hypersynchrony phenomenon. The transmission means reported in Table 1 it is possible to observe that there is a slight difference in transmission rate mean among brain areas. A relative higher standard deviation indicating that there is a significant difference when comparing rodent's transmission rate even Kolmogorov-Smirnov test assuring their similarity. More transmission rate evaluation from the set of rodents used in this paper was already published in Tsukahara et al. [41].

The channel capacity observed shows that signal frequency is essential to define the transmission rate. More information results in signals with larger bandwidth increasing the transmission. It is a crucial point to understand the hyper synchronism observed during epilepsy seizure.

The PDC method provided the functional connectivity analysis showing the direction of communication during the intervals, and the MI method completed the understanding of providing the transmission rate in each situation. Together both ways depicted the brain areas communication dynamics providing some insights about the process.

6 Conclusions

The combination of PDC and MI to perform a functional connectivity analysis with rodents EEG presented insights about the communication among brain areas during the basal interval, which is before epileptic seizures. Communication dynamics among rodents were different; however, giving some patterns in common. During the basal interval, the central communication performed presents in lower frequencies, and high-frequency bands present a lower communication strength. Mainly the absence of ripples and fast ripples frequencies transmission and during the intervals evolution, it is common to observe that there is not a full communication through all frequency bands. The transmission rate investigated through MI revealed that there is a common mean of transmission, and when observing all the intervals, it is possible to check their oscillation. As expected again, it is found different transmission rates for each rodent due to the physiological difference among rodents even them being the same species. Ths result completes the idea that there is a natural brain synchronization among Cortex, Hippocampus and Thalamus contributing to the notion that epilepsy might be a hyper synchronization phenomenon. Therefore the case study results reported that combining PDC and MI seems suitable to observe communication dynamics and perform functional connectivity analysis presenting the connectivity direction among brain areas and quantifying its volume of information transited between them.

Table 5. Connectivity measures developed from PDC method, after the validation with Surrogate for rodent R064. Red measures represents that there is no connectivity between brain areas. The measures are split in intervals and reported pairwise.

Brain areas	Frequency band	Connectivity measures									
		Interval 1	Interval 2	Interval 3	Interval 4	Interval 5	Interval 6	Interval 7	Interval 8	Interval 9	Interval 10
	Delta	0.00	-0.01	-0.08	-0.02	0.08	0.16	0.00	0.06	-0.05	-0.01
	Theta	0.00	0.00	-0.07	-0.01	0.09	0.16	0.01	0.06	-0.05	-0.01
	Alpha	0.01	0.02	-0.05	-0.01	0.09	0.16	0.03	0.06	-0.04	-0.01
	Beta	0.02	0.06	0.00	0.01	0.09	0.16	0.09	0.07	-0.01	0.00
Hp→Cx	Low Gamma	0.03	0.14	0.12	0.03	0.11	0.14	0.22	0.11	0.05	0.02
	High Gamma	0.02	0.15	0.17	0.05	0.11	0.07	0.26	0.10	0.09	0.04
	Ripple	0.01	0.09	0.11	0.04	0.07	0.02	0.16	0.06	0.06	0.03
	Fast Ripple	0.00	0.06	0.07	0.02	0.05	0.00	0.10	0.04	0.04	0.02
	Delta	-0.02	0.06	0.10	0.02	0.19	0.16	-0.13	-0.05	0.19	0.18
	Theta	-0.01	0.05	0.10	0.01	0.18	0.15	-0.11	-0.05	0.17	0.17
	Alpha	0.00	0.04	0.10	-0.01	0.17	0.11	-0.07	-0.05	0.15	0.14
	Beta	-0.01	0.01	0.09	-0.04	0.11	0.04	-0.03	-0.04	0.07	0.06
Th→Cx	Low Gamma	-0.02	0.01	0.10	-0.06	0.02	-0.02	0.02	-0.02	0.00	-0.02
	High Gamma	-0.01	0.06	0.13	-0.05	0.00	-0.02	0.07	0.00	-0.01	-0.04
	Ripple	0.02	0.08	0.14	-0.02	0.01	-0.02	0.10	0.02	0.01	-0.02
	Fast Ripple	0.04	0.08	0.13	-0.01	0.02	-0.01	0.11	0.04	0.02	-0.01
	Delta	0.08	0.29	0.03	0.25	0.28	-0.02	0.12	-0.29	0.09	0.25
	Theta	0.09	0.26	0.03	0.22	0.24	-0.02	0.12	-0.28	0.07	0.2
	Alpha	0.12	0.20	0.01	0.18	0.18	-0.01	0.13	-0.26	0.03	0.12
	Beta	0.17	0.10	-0.02	0.08	0.05	-0.01	0.14	-0.21	-0.05	0.02
Cx→Hp	Low Gamma	0.22	0.02	-0.04	-0.02	-0.05	-0.01	0.15	-0.13	-0.09	-0.04
	High Gamma	0.22	-0.01	-0.03	-0.06	-0.08	-0.01	0.14	-0.07	-0.08	-0.05
	Ripple	0.18	-0.01	-0.02	-0.05	-0.06	-0.01	0.12	-0.04	-0.05	-0.04
	Fast Ripple	0.14	-0.01	-0.01	-0.04	-0.05	-0.01	0.09	-0.02	-0.03	-0.03
	Delta	0.58	0.47	0.67	0.00	0.06	0.60	0.55	0.90	0.37	0.48
	Theta	0.52	0.44	0.66	-0.01	0.05	0.56	0.51	0.75	0.36	0.46
	Alpha	0.38	0.36	0.62	-0.02	0.04	0.46	0.41	0.51	0.31	0.40
	Beta	0.20	0.18	0.49	-0.04	0.00	0.27	0.20	0.23	0.20	0.26
Th→Hp	Low Gamma	0.09	0.02	0.27	-0.03	-0.03	0.13	0.04	0.09	0.06	0.11
	High Gamma	0.07	0.02	0.15	0.02	0.02	0.11	0.04	0.07	0.04	0.09
	Ripple	0.10	0.01	0.07	0.07	0.07	0.12	0.04	0.10	0.06	0.12
	Fast Ripple	0.13	0.00	0.02	0.08	0.09	0.11	0.02	0.11	0.07	0.14
	Delta	0.30	-0.05	-0.02	0.06	0.36	-0.15	-0.22	0.09	0.20	0.22
	Theta	0.28	0.02	0.05	0.09	0.36	-0.11	-0.18	0.10	0.24	0.24
	Alpha	0.24	0.10	0.12	0.15	0.37	-0.05	-0.12	0.12	0.30	0.26
	Beta	0.16	0.16	0.19	0.25	0.37	0.01	-0.05	0.15	0.38	0.27
Cx→Th	Low Gamma	0.06	0.18	0.21	0.30	0.34	0.05	0.00	0.18	0.40	0.27
	High Gamma	0.00	0.16	0.19	0.27	0.28	0.06	0.02	0.17	0.35	0.24
	Ripple	-0.03	0.11	0.15	0.19	0.20	0.05	0.02	0.12	0.25	0.19
	Fast Ripple	-0.03	0.08	0.11	0.13	0.14	0.04	0.02	0.09	0.17	0.14
	Delta	0.02	0.10	0.13	0.40	0.46	-0.10	-0.11	0.08	0.48	0.27
	Theta	0.09	0.12	0.14	0.42	0.46	-0.04	-0.06	0.13	0.48	0.28
	Alpha	0.20	0.19	0.16	0.45	0.48	0.05	0.01	0.23	0.49	0.31
	Beta	0.43	0.37	0.25	0.57	0.54	0.26	0.17	0.45	0.54	0.44
Hp→Th	Low Gamma	0.73	0.64	0.51	0.71	0.68	0.62	0.45	0.70	0.67	0.69
	High Gamma	0.71	0.60	0.58	0.62	0.63	0.66	0.53	0.63	0.61	0.67
	Ripple	0.46	0.37	0.34	0.40	0.40	0.40	0.34	0.40	0.38	0.40
	Fast Ripple	0.29	0.23	0.21	0.26	0.25	0.25	0.21	0.26	0.24	0.25

Table 6. Connectivity measures developed from PDC method, after the validation with Surrogate for rodent R065. Red measures represents that there is no connectivity between brain areas. The measures are split in intervals and reported pairwise.

Brain areas	Frequency band	Connectivity measures									
		Interval 1	Interval 2	Interval 3	Interval 4	Interval 5	Interval 6	Interval 7	Interval 8	Interval 9	Interval 10
Hp→Cx	Delta	0.16	-0.16	0.14	0.36	0.18	0.37	0.11	0.23	0.28	0.28
	Theta	0.13	-0.16	0.09	0.29	0.16	0.32	0.08	0.20	0.24	0.26
	Alpha	0.08	-0.13	0.03	0.19	0.12	0.22	0.04	0.14	0.16	0.22
	Beta	0.01	-0.08	-0.03	0.10	0.09	0.12	0.02	0.06	0.04	0.13
	Low Gamma	-0.03	-0.04	-0.05	0.06	0.08	0.05	0.02	0.01	-0.04	0.03
	High Gamma	-0.03	-0.02	-0.05	0.06	0.09	0.04	0.03	0.01	-0.06	-0.01
	Ripple	0.00	0.00	-0.03	0.07	0.11	0.05	0.05	0.02	-0.05	-0.02
	Fast Ripple	0.03	0.02	0.00	0.09	0.15	0.07	0.07	0.04	-0.03	-0.02
Th→Cx	Delta	0.08	0.05	-0.20	0.05	0.02	-0.14	-0.12	-0.33	-0.22	-0.30
	Theta	0.08	0.03	-0.17	0.02	0.02	-0.13	-0.11	-0.30	-0.20	-0.29
	Alpha	0.07	0.01	-0.12	0.00	0.04	-0.11	-0.09	-0.23	-0.16	-0.25
	Beta	0.05	0.00	-0.05	-0.02	0.05	-0.07	-0.06	-0.11	-0.08	-0.17
	Low Gamma	0.02	-0.01	0.01	-0.02	0.04	-0.03	-0.04	-0.02	-0.01	-0.09
	High Gamma	0.01	-0.01	0.03	-0.02	0.01	-0.02	-0.03	0.01	0.02	-0.04
	Ripple	0.01	-0.01	0.02	-0.02	-0.01	-0.02	-0.02	0.02	0.03	-0.02
	Fast Ripple	0.01	-0.01	0.01	-0.02	-0.01	-0.02	-0.02	0.01	0.03	-0.01
Cx→Hp	Delta	0.24	-0.08	-0.04	-0.12	0.08	-0.04	0.00	0.16	-0.12	-0.11
	Theta	0.30	-0.04	-0.01	-0.06	0.19	0.06	0.07	0.19	-0.06	-0.08
	Alpha	0.41	0.08	0.06	0.08	0.34	0.22	0.20	0.24	0.06	-0.01
	Beta	0.54	0.30	0.21	0.29	0.55	0.40	0.42	0.32	0.23	0.11
	Low Gamma	0.60	0.48	0.33	0.42	0.66	0.49	0.57	0.36	0.34	0.21
	High Gamma	0.57	0.51	0.35	0.43	0.62	0.47	0.56	0.36	0.35	0.24
	Ripple	0.47	0.42	0.31	0.36	0.48	0.38	0.45	0.30	0.31	0.22
	Fast Ripple	0.36	0.32	0.24	0.28	0.35	0.29	0.34	0.24	0.25	0.18
Th→Hp	Delta	-0.09	-0.08	-0.26	0.09	-0.27	-0.13	-0.01	-0.17	-0.09	-0.24
	Theta	-0.07	-0.06	-0.23	0.08	-0.25	-0.11	-0.01	-0.15	-0.07	-0.23
	Alpha	-0.03	-0.02	-0.16	0.08	-0.19	-0.08	0.01	-0.10	-0.04	-0.21
	Beta	0.02	0.03	-0.05	0.07	-0.06	-0.01	0.04	-0.01	0.01	-0.14
	Low Gamma	0.06	0.08	0.06	0.06	0.07	0.04	0.04	0.05	0.06	-0.06
	High Gamma	0.07	0.08	0.10	0.05	0.10	0.05	0.04	0.06	0.07	-0.02
	Ripple	0.06	0.07	0.08	0.03	0.07	0.04	0.03	0.05	0.07	0.00
	Fast Ripple	0.04	0.05	0.06	0.02	0.05	0.03	0.02	0.04	0.06	0.00
Cx→Th	Delta	0.79	0.44	0.71	0.64	0.62	0.67	0.68	0.71	0.66	0.66
	Theta	0.73	0.45	0.71	0.64	0.60	0.64	0.67	0.71	0.64	0.65
	Alpha	0.59	0.49	0.69	0.62	0.53	0.56	0.63	0.67	0.59	0.62
	Beta	0.36	0.48	0.57	0.49	0.38	0.37	0.51	0.50	0.44	0.51
	Low Gamma	0.16	0.36	0.34	0.28	0.19	0.17	0.32	0.26	0.25	0.32
	High Gamma	0.08	0.22	0.15	0.15	0.08	0.05	0.20	0.11	0.13	0.17
	Ripple	0.05	0.13	0.04	0.07	0.02	0.00	0.12	0.03	0.06	0.07
	Fast Ripple	0.04	0.08	-0.01	0.03	0.00	-0.02	0.09	0.00	0.03	0.03
Hp→Th	Delta	0.26	0.31	0.30	0.04	0.25	-0.01	-0.15	0.47	0.28	0.41
	Theta	0.20	0.24	0.25	0.01	0.20	-0.03	-0.17	0.44	0.26	0.39
	Alpha	0.10	0.13	0.15	-0.04	0.12	-0.06	-0.18	0.35	0.20	0.33
	Beta	0.00	0.03	0.04	-0.05	0.03	-0.07	-0.14	0.20	0.12	0.21
	Low Gamma	-0.06	-0.03	-0.03	-0.03	-0.01	-0.05	-0.09	0.08	0.08	0.09
	High Gamma	-0.06	-0.05	-0.05	-0.02	-0.02	-0.03	-0.06	0.02	0.08	0.03
	Ripple	-0.03	-0.04	-0.05	0.00	0.00	-0.02	-0.04	0.01	0.09	0.02
	Fast Ripple	0.00	-0.03	-0.04	0.01	0.02	-0.01	-0.02	0.01	0.10	0.02

Table 7. Connectivity measures developed from PDC method, after the validation with Surrogate for rodent R072. Red measures represents that there is no connectivity between brain areas. The measures are split in intervals and reported pairwise.

Brain areas	Frequency band	Connectivity measures									
		Interval 1	Interval 2	Interval 3	Interval 4	Interval 5	Interval 6	Interval 7	Interval 8	Interval 9	Interval 10
Hp→Cx	Delta	0.03	0.27	0.47	0.65	0.10	0.36	0.47	0.09	0.32	0.32
	Theta	0.06	0.31	0.49	0.62	-0.03	0.35	0.46	0.12	0.36	0.33
	Alpha	0.09	0.34	0.45	0.55	-0.06	0.34	0.42	0.16	0.41	0.35
	Beta	0.11	0.30	0.31	0.40	0.00	0.33	0.31	0.21	0.42	0.35
	Low Gamma	0.10	0.22	0.18	0.22	0.06	0.33	0.20	0.21	0.33	0.30
	High Gamma	0.11	0.18	0.13	0.13	0.09	0.33	0.16	0.20	0.25	0.23
	Ripple	0.13	0.19	0.12	0.11	0.11	0.33	0.16	0.21	0.21	0.19
	Fast Ripple	0.17	0.22	0.14	0.12	0.15	0.35	0.19	0.23	0.21	0.19
Th→Cx	Delta	0.10	0.11	-0.03	0.67	-0.13	0.36	0.32	0.34	0.42	0.34
	Theta	0.10	0.10	0.02	0.60	0.05	0.28	0.28	0.32	0.46	0.32
	Alpha	0.11	0.12	0.07	0.54	0.15	0.17	0.23	0.26	0.53	0.29
	Beta	0.11	0.17	0.11	0.43	0.20	0.06	0.21	0.19	0.53	0.25
	Low Gamma	0.11	0.21	0.12	0.35	0.22	0.00	0.20	0.16	0.40	0.20
	High Gamma	0.12	0.23	0.13	0.32	0.23	-0.02	0.21	0.16	0.27	0.16
	Ripple	0.14	0.25	0.14	0.32	0.24	-0.01	0.23	0.17	0.20	0.15
	Fast Ripple	0.17	0.26	0.17	0.32	0.26	0.01	0.26	0.20	0.19	0.17
Cx→Hp	Delta	0.01	0.15	0.03	-0.21	-0.25	0.25	-0.06	0.44	0.18	0.53
	Theta	0.04	0.14	0.06	-0.18	-0.15	0.24	-0.03	0.45	0.20	0.54
	Alpha	0.07	0.14	0.12	-0.11	-0.03	0.23	0.05	0.46	0.24	0.55
	Beta	0.10	0.16	0.17	0.03	0.09	0.22	0.15	0.47	0.30	0.56
	Low Gamma	0.12	0.18	0.19	0.15	0.16	0.21	0.23	0.40	0.32	0.50
	High Gamma	0.14	0.19	0.20	0.21	0.19	0.21	0.26	0.32	0.31	0.39
	Ripple	0.17	0.21	0.22	0.25	0.22	0.22	0.28	0.27	0.29	0.28
	Fast Ripple	0.21	0.23	0.24	0.27	0.25	0.24	0.30	0.26	0.28	0.22
Th→Hp	Delta	-0.13	-0.09	0.25	-0.02	-0.27	0.27	0.14	-0.24	-0.27	0.17
	Theta	-0.10	-0.04	0.23	0.08	-0.04	0.22	0.12	-0.20	-0.23	0.18
	Alpha	-0.07	0.03	0.18	0.14	0.08	0.14	0.11	-0.13	-0.14	0.19
	Beta	-0.01	0.11	0.11	0.18	0.13	0.06	0.10	-0.02	-0.04	0.19
	Low Gamma	0.05	0.15	0.07	0.19	0.15	0.02	0.11	0.05	0.04	0.15
	High Gamma	0.08	0.17	0.06	0.20	0.16	0.01	0.11	0.08	0.07	0.12
	Ripple	0.11	0.19	0.07	0.21	0.18	0.02	0.14	0.10	0.09	0.11
	Fast Ripple	0.14	0.20	0.09	0.22	0.19	0.04	0.16	0.12	0.11	0.12
Cx→Th	Delta	0.43	0.09	-0.17	-0.13	-0.05	0.39	0.52	-0.32	-0.19	0.19
	Theta	0.39	0.10	-0.11	-0.11	-0.05	0.38	0.50	-0.29	-0.16	0.20
	Alpha	0.31	0.14	-0.01	-0.05	0.01	0.35	0.46	-0.22	-0.10	0.22
	Beta	0.20	0.18	0.11	0.06	0.10	0.31	0.37	-0.07	0.01	0.24
	Low Gamma	0.14	0.21	0.17	0.16	0.18	0.28	0.30	0.08	0.12	0.23
	High Gamma	0.14	0.23	0.20	0.21	0.21	0.28	0.28	0.17	0.20	0.21
	Ripple	0.17	0.25	0.22	0.25	0.24	0.29	0.29	0.21	0.25	0.19
	Fast Ripple	0.21	0.28	0.25	0.28	0.27	0.31	0.31	0.24	0.27	0.19
Hp→Th	Delta	0.36	0.48	0.19	0.59	0.09	0.64	0.17	-0.02	-0.31	-0.38
	Theta	0.39	0.50	0.22	0.54	-0.07	0.59	0.17	-0.01	-0.25	-0.34
	Alpha	0.39	0.48	0.22	0.48	-0.11	0.49	0.17	0.03	-0.15	-0.25
	Beta	0.29	0.36	0.16	0.34	-0.04	0.36	0.15	0.09	-0.02	-0.09
	Low Gamma	0.18	0.21	0.10	0.18	0.04	0.29	0.14	0.14	0.08	0.04
	High Gamma	0.13	0.15	0.08	0.10	0.08	0.28	0.15	0.16	0.12	0.12
	Ripple	0.14	0.14	0.08	0.08	0.11	0.28	0.18	0.19	0.15	0.16
	Fast Ripple	0.17	0.16	0.10	0.10	0.15	0.29	0.20	0.22	0.19	0.19

Table 8. Channel capacity for rodent R048 for each interval observed. They represent the MI values among brain areas and they are reported below pairwise.

	Cx → Hp	Cx → Th	Hp → Th
Interval1	1.35	1.06	1.76
Interval2	1.74	1.42	1.84
Interval3	1.51	1.18	1.70
Interval4	0.85	0.91	1.46
Interval5	1.53	1.36	2.07
Interval6	0.72	0.90	0.87
Interval7	2.38	2.34	2.76
Interval8	1.61	1.60	1.72
Interval9	0.76	0.78	1.69
Interval10	1.60	1.67	2.04

Table 9. Channel capacity for rodent R052 for each interval observed. They represent the MI values among brain areas and they are reported below pairwise.

	Cx → Hp	Cx → Th	Hp → Th
Interval1	1.27	1.49	2.06
Interval2	1.12	1.07	1.69
Interval3	1.57	1.31	1.85
Interval4	2.64	2.67	3.11
Interval5	1.78	2.06	2.16
Interval6	1.56	1.42	1.69
Interval7	0.88	0.85	1.99
Interval8	1.43	1.37	1.88
Interval9	1.21	1.17	2.00
Interval10	1.98	2.13	2.42

Table 10. Channel capacity for rodent R064 for each interval observed. They represent the MI values among brain areas and they are reported below pairwise.

	Cx → Hp	Cx → Th	Hp → Th
Interval1	0.39	0.50	1.36
Interval2	0.36	0.34	1.35
Interval3	0.32	0.40	1.54
Interval4	0.33	0.36	1.31
Interval5	0.42	0.51	1.43
Interval6	0.41	0.52	1.26
Interval7	0.40	0.48	1.17
Interval8	0.31	0.26	1.22
Interval9	0.43	0.48	1.54
Interval10	0.35	0.38	1.25

Table 11. Channel capacity for rodent R065 for each interval observed. They represent the MI values among brain areas and they are reported below pairwise.

	Cx → Hp	Cx → Th	Hp → Th
Interval1	1.40	1.33	1.19
Interval2	1.33	1.42	0.98
Interval3	1.13	1.05	0.87
Interval4	1.27	1.39	0.96
Interval5	1.5	1.22	1.10
Interval6	1.17	1.10	0.79
Interval7	1.32	1.24	1.01
Interval8	1.73	1.22	1.07
Interval9	1.35	0.95	0.89
Interval10	1.17	1.07	0.83

Table 12. Channel capacity for rodent R072 for each interval observed. They represent the MI values among brain areas and they are reported below pairwise.

	Cx → Hp	Cx → Th	Hp → Th
Interval1	2.14	2.45	2.33
Interval2	2.21	2.71	2.15
Interval3	2.23	1.91	1.73
Interval4	2.47	2.59	2.29
Interval5	1.95	2.71	1.79
Interval6	1.86	1.82	1.84
Interval7	2.61	1.91	1.84
Interval8	2.56	2.78	2.26
Interval9	2.50	2.56	2.04
Interval10	2.66	2.75	2.21

Table 13. Transmission rate for rodent R048. The measures are reported in bits/s. They are reported for each interval and pairwise according to the brain areas.

	Cx → Hp	Hp → Cx	Cx → Th	Th → Cx	Hp → Th	Th → Hp
Interval1	3.52	4.03	2.77	2.77	5.26	4.34
Interval2	4.53	5.19	3.68	3.68	5.48	4.52
Interval3	3.92	4.5	3.07	3.07	5.07	4.19
Interval4	2.2	2.52	2.37	2.37	4.34	3.59
Interval5	3.99	4.57	3.55	3.55	6.18	5.10
Interval6	1.87	2.15	2.34	2.34	2.58	2.13
Interval7	6.19	7.1	6.08	6.08	8.22	6.79
Interval8	4.18	4.79	4.16	4.16	5.12	4.23
Interval9	1.98	2.27	2.03	2.03	5.03	4.15
Interval10	4.17	4.78	4.35	4.35	6.07	5.01

Table 14. Transmission rate for rodent R052. The measures are reported in bits/s. They are reported for each interval and pairwise according to the brain areas.

	Cx → Hp	Hp → Cx	Cx → Th	Th → Cx	Hp → Th	Th → Hp
Interval1	4.39	4.33	5.17	5.11	7.05	7.05
Interval2	3.87	3.83	3.69	3.65	5.8	5.8
Interval3	5.43	5.36	4.54	4.49	6.32	6.32
Interval4	9.13	9.03	9.25	9.14	10.64	10.64
Interval5	6.15	6.08	7.11	7.03	7.37	7.37
Interval6	5.40	5.34	4.91	4.86	5.77	5.77
Interval7	3.05	3.02	2.96	2.92	6.82	6.82
Interval8	4.94	4.88	4.75	4.69	6.44	6.44
Interval9	4.20	4.15	4.06	4.01	6.85	6.85
Interval10	6.87	6.79	7.37	7.29	8.26	8.26

Table 15. Transmission rate for rodent R064. The measures are reported in bits/s. They are reported for each interval and pairwise according to the brain areas.

	Cx → Hp	Hp → Cx	Cx → Th	Th → Cx	Hp → Th	Th → Hp
Interval1	7.09	8.27	9.08	8.79	28.58	23.71
Interval2	6.56	7.65	6.09	5.89	28.3	23.48
Interval3	5.73	6.68	7.23	7.00	32.42	26.89
Interval4	6.00	7.00	6.42	6.21	27.53	22.84
Interval5	7.57	8.84	9.24	8.94	30.03	24.91
Interval6	7.42	8.66	9.40	9.09	26.44	21.93
Interval7	7.24	8.45	8.59	8.31	24.52	20.34
Interval8	5.49	6.41	4.71	4.56	25.59	21.23
Interval9	7.81	9.11	8.61	8.33	32.35	26.84
Interval10	6.34	7.40	6.84	6.62	26.26	21.79

Table 16. Transmission rate for rodent R065. The measures are reported in bits/s. They are reported for each interval and pairwise according to the brain areas.

	Cx → Hp	Hp → Cx	Cx → Th	Th → Cx	Hp → Th	Th → Hp
Interval1	27.93	27.93	26.61	26.61	23.88	23.88
Interval2	26.61	26.61	28.47	28.47	19.64	19.64
Interval3	22.61	22.61	21.04	21.04	17.49	17.49
Interval4	25.33	25.33	27.82	27.82	19.27	19.27
Interval5	30.05	30.05	24.36	24.36	21.93	21.93
Interval6	23.43	23.43	21.91	21.91	15.72	15.72
Interval7	26.46	26.46	24.77	24.77	20.11	20.11
Interval8	34.63	34.63	24.35	24.35	21.41	21.41
Interval9	27.03	27.03	19.05	19.05	17.81	17.81
Interval10	23.32	23.32	21.49	21.49	16.59	16.59

Table 17. Transmission rate for rodent R072. The measures are reported in bits/s. They are reported for each interval and pairwise according to the brain areas.

	Cx → Hp	Hp → Cx	Cx → Th	Th → Cx	Hp → Th	Th → Hp
Interval1	11.85	11.76	13.58	13.43	12.81	12.76
Interval2	12.26	12.17	15.03	14.87	11.8	11.76
Interval3	12.34	12.25	10.58	10.46	9.54	9.50
Interval4	13.69	13.59	14.34	14.19	12.57	12.52
Interval5	10.80	10.72	15.01	14.85	9.85	9.81
Interval6	10.32	10.24	10.08	9.97	10.11	10.08
Interval7	14.48	14.38	10.56	10.45	10.1	10.07
Interval8	14.16	14.06	15.39	15.22	12.44	12.39
Interval9	13.86	13.76	14.2	14.05	11.21	11.17
Interval10	14.71	14.60	15.25	15.08	12.17	12.13

References

1. Adkinson, J.A., et al.: Connectivity and centrality characteristics of the epileptogenic focus using directed network analysis. IEEE Trans. Neural Syst. Rehabil. Eng. **27**(1), 22–30 (2019). https://doi.org/10.1109/TNSRE.2018.2886211
2. Akbarian, B., Erfanian, A.: Automatic detection of PTZ-induced seizures based on functional brain connectivity network in rats. In: 2017 8th International IEEE/EMBS Conference on Neural Engineering (NER), pp. 576–579. IEEE (2017)
3. Anastasiadou, M.N., Christodoulakis, M., Papathanasiou, E.S., Papacostas, S.S., Hadjipapas, A., Mitsis, G.D.: Graph theoretical characteristics of EEG-based functional brain networks in patients with epilepsy: the effect of reference choice and volume conduction. Front. Neurosci. **13**, 221 (2019). https://doi.org/10.3389/fnins.2019.00221.https://www.frontiersin.org/article/10.3389/fnins.2019.00221
4. Avena-Koenigsberger, A., Msic, B., Sporns, O.: Communication dynamics in complex brain networks. Nat. Rev. Neurosci. **19**, 17–33 (2017). https://doi.org/10.1038/nrn.2017.149
5. Baccalá, L.A., Sameshima, K.: Partial directed coherence: a new concept in neural structure determination. Biol. Cybern. **84**(6), 463–474 (2001). https://doi.org/10.1007/PL00007990
6. Bartolomei, F., et al.: Defining epileptogenic networks: contribution of SEEG and signal analysis. Epilepsia **58**(7), 1131–1147 (2017). https://doi.org/10.1111/epi.13791. https://onlinelibrary.wiley.com/doi/abs/10.1111/epi.13791
7. Beghi, E.: Social functions and socioeconomic vulnerability in epilepsy. Epilepsy Behav. **100**, 106363–106366 (2019)
8. Beghi, E., et al.: Global, regional, and national burden of epilepsy, 1990–2016: a systematic analysis for the global burden of disease study 2016. Lancet Neurol. **18**(4), 357–375 (2019)
9. Berglind, F., Andersson, M., Kokaia, M.: Dynamic interaction of local and transhemispheric networks is necessary for progressive intensification of hippocampal seizures. Sci. Rep. **8**(1), 5669 (2018)
10. Biasiucci, A., Franceschiello, B., Murray, M.M.: Electroencephalography. Curr. Biol. **29**(3), R80–R85 (2019)

11. Cekic, S., Grandjean, D., Renaud, O.: Time, frequency, and time-varying Granger-causality measures in neuroscience. Stat. Med. **37**(11), 1910–1931 (2018)
12. Coito, A., Michel, C.M., Vulliemoz, S., Plomp, G.: Directed functional connections underlying spontaneous brain activity. Hum. Brain Mapp. **40**(3), 879–888 (2019)
13. Cota, V., Drabowski, B.M.B., de Oliveira, J.C., Moraes, M.: The epileptic amygdala: toward the development of a neural prosthesis by temporally coded electrical stimulation. J. Neurosci. Res. **94**, 463–485 (2016). https://doi.org/10.1002/jnr.23741
14. Cover, T.M., Thomas, J.A.: Elements of Information Theory. Wiley, Hoboken (2012)
15. Devinsky, O., Vezzani, A., OBrien, T.J., Scheffer, I.E., Curtis, M., Perucca, P.: Epilepsy. Nat. Rev. Dis. Primers **4** (2018). https://doi.org/10.1038/nrdp.2018.24. https://www.nature.com/articles/nrdp201824#supplementary-information
16. Dourado, J.R., Júnior, O., Maciel, C.D., et al.: Parallelism strategies for big data delayed transfer entropy evaluation. Algorithms **12**(9), 190 (2019)
17. Endo, W., Santos, F.P., Simpson, D., Maciel, C.D., Newland, P.L.: Delayed mutual information infers patterns of synaptic connectivity in a proprioceptive neural network. J. Comput. Neurosci. **38**(2), 427–438 (2015). https://doi.org/10.1007/s10827-015-0548-6
18. Faes, L., Porta, A., Nollo, G.: Testing frequency-domain causality in multivariate time series. IEEE Trans. Biomed. Eng. **57**(8), 1897–1906 (2010). https://doi.org/10.1109/TBME.2010.2042715
19. Gaxiola-Tirado, J.A., Salazar-Varas, R., Gutiérrez, D.: Using the partial directed coherence to assess functional connectivity in electroencephalography data for brain-computer interfaces. IEEE Trans. Cogn. Dev. Syst. **10**(3), 776–783 (2018). https://doi.org/10.1109/TCDS.2017.2777180
20. Gribkova, E.D., Ibrahim, B.A., Llano, D.A.: A novel mutual information estimator to measure spike train correlations in a model thalamocortical network. J. Neurophysiol. **120**(6), 2730–2744 (2018)
21. Holme, P., Saramäki, J.: Temporal networks. Phys. Rep. **519**(3), 97–125 (2012)
22. Huang, D., et al.: Combining partial directed coherence and graph theory to analyse effective brain networks of different mental tasks. Front. Hum. Neurosci. **10**, 235 (2016). https://doi.org/10.3389/fnhum.2016.00235. https://www.frontiersin.org/article/10.3389/fnhum.2016.00235
23. Ibrahim, F., et al.: A statistical framework for EEG channel selection and seizure prediction on mobile. Int. J. Speech Technol. **22**(1), 191–203 (2019). https://doi.org/10.1007/s10772-018-09565-7
24. Mei, T., et al.: Epileptic foci localization based on mapping the synchronization of dynamic brain network. BMC Med. Inform. Decis. Making **19**(1), 19 (2019)
25. Molavipour, S., Bassi, G., Skoglund, M.: Conditional mutual information neural estimator. In: ICASSP 2020–2020 IEEE International Conference on Acoustics, Speech and Signal Processing (ICASSP), pp. 5025–5029. IEEE (2020)
26. Niriayo, Y.L., Mamo, A., Gidey, K., Demoz, G.T.: Medication belief and adherence among patients with epilepsy. Behav. Neurol. **2019**, 2806341–2806347 (2019)
27. Olamat, A.E., Akan, A.: Synchronization analysis of epilepsy data using global field synchronization. In: 2017 25th Signal Processing and Communications Applications Conference (SIU), pp. 1–4 (2017). https://doi.org/10.1109/SIU.2017.7960194
28. World Health Organization, et al.: Atlas: country resources for neurological disorders 2004. World Health Organization, Geneva (2017)
29. Paxinos, G., Watson, C.: The Rat Brain in Stereotaxic Coordinates, 7th edn. Elsevier, Amsterdam (2013)

30. Pereda, E., Quiroga, R.Q., Bhattacharya, J.: Nonlinear multivariate analysis of neurophysiological signals. Prog. Neurobiol. **77**(1), 1–37 (2005). https://doi.org/10.1016/j.pneurobio.2005.10.003. http://www.sciencedirect.com/science/article/pii/S030100820500119X
31. Pester, B., Lehmann, T., Leistritz, L., Witte, H., Ligges, C.: Influence of imputation strategies on the identification of brain functional connectivity networks. J. Neurosci. Methods **309**, 199–207 (2018)
32. Proakis, J.G., Salehi, M.: Digital Communications, vol. 4. McGraw-Hill, New York (2001)
33. Sameshima, K., Baccalá, L.A.: Using partial directed coherence to describe neuronal ensemble interactions. J. Neurosci. Methods **94**(1), 93–103 (1999)
34. Santos, F.P., Maciel, C.D., Newland, P.L.: Pre-processing and transfer entropy measures in motor neurons controlling limb movements. J. Comput. Neurosci. **43**(2), 159–171 (2017). https://doi.org/10.1007/s10827-017-0656-6
35. Santos, T.M.O., Tsukahara, V.H.B., de Oliveira, J.C., Cota, V.R., Maciel, C.D.: Graph model evolution during epileptic seizures: linear model approach. In: Cota, V.R., Barone, D.A.C., Dias, D.R.C., Damázio, L.C.M. (eds.) LAWCN 2019. CCIS, vol. 1068, pp. 157–170. Springer, Cham (2019). https://doi.org/10.1007/978-3-030-36636-0_12
36. Schreiber, T., Schmitz, A.: Improved surrogate data for nonlinearity tests. Phys. Rev. Lett. **77**, 635–638 (1996). https://doi.org/10.1103/PhysRevLett.77.635
37. Schreiber, T., Schmitz, A.: Surrogate time series. Phys. D **142**(3–4), 346–382 (2000)
38. Spiciarich, M.C., von Gaudecker, J.R., Jurasek, L., Clarke, D.F., Burneo, J., Vidaurre, J.: Global health and epilepsy: Update and future directions. Curr. Neurol. Neurosci. Rep. **19**(6) (2019). Article number: 30. https://doi.org/10.1007/s11910-019-0947-6
39. Theiler, J., Eubank, S., Longtin, A., Galdrikian, B., Farmer, J.D.: Testing for nonlinearity in time series: the method of surrogate data. Phys. D Nonlinear Phenom. **58**(1), 77–94 (1992). https://doi.org/10.1016/0167-2789(92)90102-S. http://www.sciencedirect.com/science/article/pii/016727899290102S
40. Therrien, C.W.: Discrete Random Signals and Statistical Signal Processing. Prentice Hall PTR, Upper Saddle River (1992)
41. Tsukahara, V.H.B., Jeronymo, P.V.B., de Oliveira, J.C., Cota, V.R., Maciel, C.D.: Delayed mutual information to develop functional analysis on epileptic signals. In: BIOSIGNALS, pp. 89–97 (2020)
42. Varotto, G., et al.: Network characteristics in benign epilepsy with centro-temporal spikes patients indicating defective connectivity during spindle sleep: a partial directed coherence study of EEG signals. Clin. Neurophys. **129**(11), 2372–2379 (2018). https://doi.org/10.1016/j.clinph.2018.09.008. http://www.sciencedirect.com/science/article/pii/S138824571831229X
43. Wan, X., Xu, L.: A study for multiscale information transfer measures based on conditional mutual information. PLoS ONE **13**(12), e0208423 (2018)
44. Wang, G., Sun, Z., Tao, R., Li, K., Bao, G., Yan, X.: Epileptic seizure detection based on partial directed coherence analysis. IEEE J. Biomed. Health Inform. **20**(3), 873–879 (2016)
45. Weiss, S.A., et al.: Interneurons and principal cell firing in human limbic areas at focal seizure onset. Neurobiol. Dis. **124**, 183–188 (2019). https://doi.org/10.1016/j.nbd.2018.11.014. http://www.sciencedirect.com/science/article/pii/S096999611830682X

46. Yasumasa Takahashi, D., Antonio Baccal, L., Sameshima, K.: Connectivity inference between neural structures via partial directed coherence. J. Appl. Stat. **34**(10), 1259–1273 (2007)
47. Yu, H., et al.: Variation of functional brain connectivity in epileptic seizures: an EEG analysis with cross-frequency phase synchronization. Cogn. Neurodyn. **14**, 35–49 (2020). https://doi.org/10.1007/s11571-019-09551-y

Comparison of Medical Image Evaluations in Magnetic Resonance Cholangiopancreatography Through Image J

K. E. P. Pinho[1(✉)], P. M. Gewehr[1], A. C. Pinho[1], E. Milhoretto[2], A. M. Gusso[3], and C. A. Goedert[3]

[1] Federal University of Technology-Parana (UTFPR), Curitiba, Brazil
{katiaprus,gewehr,acpinho}@utfpr.edu.br
[2] Federal University of Technology (DAFIS), UTFPR, Curitiba, Brazil
edneymilhoretto@utfpr.edu.br
[3] Diagnostic Clinic (Cetac), Curitiba, Brazil

Abstract. The objective of the study was to compare the physical characteristics of the diseases of each patient participating in the MRCP exam and to carry out a detailed analysis between the score obtained by the medical evaluation, the averages obtained by the Image J® software curve. Participated in the study 64 patients (31 women, 33 men). Determination of the sequences and the procedure for the patients was defined by two radiologists from the clinic. Thus, they also analyzed the images acquired from the research, called evaluator 1 (E1) and 2 (E2). For this study, the images and scores assigned by E2, obtained with a manufactured contrast were chosen for a subset of 14 patients (21.87%) of 64. 4 being score 2 (100%) (1 woman and 3 men); 5 patients with score 3 (12.82%) (3 women and 2 men) of 39 total; and 5 (23.81%) were score 4 (2 women and 3 men) of 21 total. In the selected images, a line or rectangle was used in the region of the common bile duct. The relevance of this work is in the development of a protocol applied to available software for the identification of diseases through changes in average values of gray levels in chosen regions of organs.

Keywords: Magnetic resonance cholangiopancreatography · Comparison image · Image J · Curve averages in the region · Gray levels

1 Introduction

Magnetic Resonance Imaging (MRI) is a technique that uses high magnetic fields, allows detailing of the human body in its anatomy and physiology, does not expose the patient to ionizing radiation and is currently, alongside Multislice Computed Tomography, one of the few methods that provide images in the three orthogonal planes (axial, coronal and sagittal) without repositioning the patient [1–3]. An example of a diagnostic procedure in MRI is the Magnetic Resonance Cholangiopancreatography (MRCP or MRC) exam indicated to evaluate patients with suspected pancreatic alterations, disease or biliary complications, lithiasis (colitis and choledocholithiasis),

X. Ye et al. (Eds.): BIOSTEC 2020, CCIS 1400, pp. 329–343, 2021.
https://doi.org/10.1007/978-3-030-72379-8_16

for liver donors [4–7] and allows anatomical detailing of the accessory digestive organs (pancreas and gallbladder) (see Fig. 1).

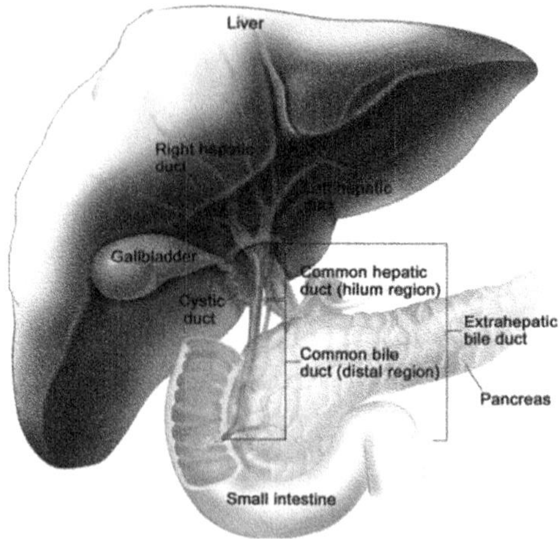

Fig. 1. Anatomical image of the gallbladder, pancreas and ducts, authorization [8].

MRCP is based on T2 weighted images, which significantly reduces the residual signal of parenchymal structures and remains only with the hyperintense (white in the image) of structures with liquid content [2]. Figure 2 indicates the arrows for essential organs in the visualization of the image in the MRCP exam with administration of the oral contrast agent, gallbladder (1), the common bile duct (2) and pancreatic duct (3). The stomach (represented by the star) and the duodenum (represented by the circle) have been completely deleted (not shown in the picture).

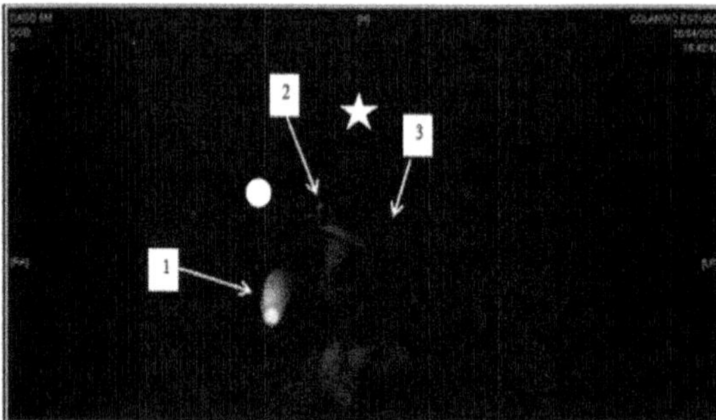

Fig. 2. CPRM image acquisition from a research volunteer using oral contrast agent, where the main organs are indicated by arrows: gallbladder (1), the common bile duct (2), pancreatic duct (3), the stomach is represented by the star and the duodenum represented by the circle.

The scan protocol may vary depending on the clinical service routine or the anatomical region to be emphasized. [9] cite that due to the high prevalence of hepatic or pancreatic parenchymal abnormalities in patients with changes in the bile and pancreatic ducts, the MRCP sequence can be part of a liver or pancreas protocol, services that include the complete abdomen examination. Variations in strongly T2 weighted sequence in two dimensions (2D), starting with multiplane acquisition locator and multiple thin slices following: Half Single Shot Turbo Echo Acquisition (HASTE); Single Shot Fast Spin Echo (SS-FSE); Single Shot Turbo Spin Echo (SS-TSE), the patient must be breath-holding during data acquisition, and the cut plane is the coronal with a cut thickness of 3 mm, with fat suppression, to improve the quality of maximum intensity. In the SS-FSE sequence, oral contrast is used to change relaxation times. Two types of oral contrast agent can be used in MRCP: natural and commercial [10, 11]. If a contrast enhances the signal from an anatomical region, it works as a positive contrast (hypersignal). But if a contrast eliminates the signals from certain anatomical regions, it works as a negative contrast (hyposignal). Oral contrasts administered at appropriate concentrations appear brilliant in T1-weighted images, as they shorten the T1 time of the tissues that absorb it. Contrasts can also shorten T2, causing hyposignal in the T2-weighted image.

The negative effect of contrast in MRCP is to eliminate the signs from the stomach and duodenum (Fig. 2) in order to better visualize anatomical structures such as the pancreas, gallbladder and the common bile duct [7, 9, 12].

The objective of the study was to compare the physical characteristics of the diseases of each patient participating in the MRCP exam and to carry out a detailed analysis between the score obtained by the medical evaluation, the averages obtained by the Image J® software curve and the existing diseases [12, 13]. For this study, only the commercial contrast agent administered to MRCP patients was considered.

2 Materials and Methods

The study was approved by UTFPR Ethics Committee and obtained authorization under the registration of CAAE 02.520.512.0.0000.5547.

2.1 MRCP Technique

Subjects. The research participants were selected at the Clinical Hospital of the Federal University of Paraná (UFPR), which provides general care in Curitiba-PR, where referrals are made via Health Units, receiving patients from the Metropolitan Region of Curitiba and from the entire State of Paraná, Brazil [12]. The research was started and concluded in about eight months, in the outpatient clinics for non-alcoholic steatopathy, alcoholic liver disease and fatty and biliary disease.

There was clearance for the follow-up of consultations and subsequent invitation to research participants (designated as patients) at the time of the consultations. Patients who agreed to participate received the Free and Informed Consent Form (ICF) and the appropriate guidance on the MR examination, as well as the contraindications [7, 12]. If the patient had any contraindication for the exam, or could not attend the two days of examination, it was excluded. Patients received confirmation and reinforcement of the guidelines two days before the scheduled date [14]. Participated in the study 64 patients (31 women, 33 men), and each participant received an identification to assist in research and preserve its anonymity. For this research, gender, followed by the order of exams, e.g., F1, M2 was used for standardization. They performed MRCP exams in 2 days, being instructed to perform a 3 hour fast, at the Diagnostic Imaging Clinic in Curitiba, Paraná, Brazil [12, 15].

Image Acquisition. The image acquisition protocol was exactly the same as the clinic already used for MRCP, starting with: locator (LOC) in three orthogonal planes (PL); following SS-FSE in apnea and; then axial lava (Liver Acquisition Volume Acceleration) T1 without fat and; finally, radial cholangio [15–17]. In addition to this protocol, multiple thin slices were acquired in the coronal plane: HASTE, TSE, followed by thick radial slices in FSE / TSE also in strong weighting in T2. The acquisitions were always made in the Coronal plans using 2D Fast Imaging Employing Steady-State (FIESTA), Axial 2D FIESTA (with fat saturation) Array Spatial Sensitivity Encoding Technique (ASSET) and the sequence of radial cholangio was the same for both days, in order to compare the effectiveness of contrasts [12, 18]. The images were obtained in 1.5T MRI system from General Electric Company (GE), model HDXT with 12 channels with the Full Fov coil, during the acquisition of the images, GE Healthcare Advantage workstation running Centricity DICOM Viewer version 3.0 software in the Clinic above [12, 16].

On the first day, the total abdomen sequence was performed, followed by MRCP, with the administration of commercial contrast (called A). On the second day, only the MRCP sequence was used, with administration of natural contrast (called B). The dose of each contrast was 200 mL divided into 2 portions of 100 mL, one dose was given after the anamnesis and another 10 min later [12, 16]. For each patient who completed the MRCP protocol, a report was issued by the clinic's doctors. The images of the two exams served for certification and identification of diseases.

2.2 Analysis of Images

The determination of the sequences and the procedure for the patients was defined by two radiologists from the clinic, responsible for carrying out these exams. Thus, they also analyzed the images acquired from the research, called evaluator 1 (E1) and 2 (E2) [12].

When the exams were completed, the images were saved in the PACS (Picture Archiving and Communication System) [12, 19] and made available on file system to each evaluator that could access and analyze the quality image with contrasts administrated (manufactured and natural), evaluating and using a scale from 1 to 4. Score 1 means that there is a hyperintensity signal of stomach and duodenum and it is not possible to evaluate these structures. Score 2: assessment occurs when there is a partial view of the structures. In score 3, hyperintensity signal does not hinder the analysis of the structures, and score 4 means that there is no signal hyperintensity for stomach and duodenum, which makes clearer the MRCP image [6, 7, 20].

The Image J® software (2019) is an image processing and analysis program with free download [21], it allows application in different areas, mainly health, as it is easy to use, it allows tools and image processing in several formats. Examples of these tools include histograms, measurements of areas, densities and others [22]. In this work, the Image J® software was employed to analyze and compare the image quality of the patients by separating a common bile duct region (according to its position, it is noteworthy that in some patients the location and size were varied), with the same dimension (selection rectangle with size approximately 58.00 mm × 5.60 mm (length)) for 12 patients and in 2 of these a line measuring 58.00 mm (length and height) was used [12, 16, 23].

In addition, the Image J® software analyzes a region demarcated in the image [24], using the plot profile tool, and thus obtaining values referring to the gray shades in axis (Y), by the distance in (mm) axis (X) plotted on a graph. In this work 91 points were used (example of Fig. 3), selecting the size mentioned above, where the central point was number 46, which should present the maximum value of the gray levels [7]. In Fig. 3, the numbers indicate: 1. Region do duodenum; 2. Region of the common bile duct and 3. Region of pancreas.

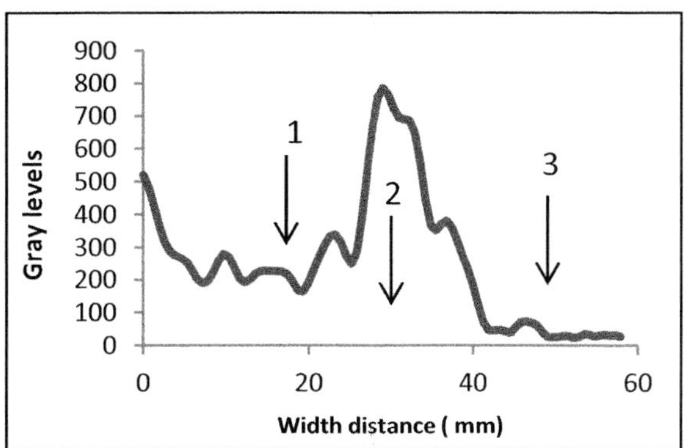

Fig. 3. Regions contiguous to the choledochal duct separated into: 1. Region of the duodenum; 2. Region of the common bile duct and 3. Region of the pancreas, from the radial cholangio examination of patient F36 with contrast A, acquired by the software Image J®.

3 Results

Analysis of Images. In the evaluation of medical images, each evaluator chose, among the sequences of images, two of them, one for each type of contrast administered (A and B), which identified with quality the region of the bile ducts and assessing whether the contrasts erased the signal of the stomach and duodenum, in order to allow a clinical analysis, making a report issue possible [7, 12].

In this study, the images and scores assigned by E2 (because he/she more reliable compared to E1) of the commercial contrast were chosen for a subset of 14 patients (21.87%) of 64. The selection of patients was carried out at random, as the purpose was to consider the image note, the diseases associated and a quantitative analysis of gray levels by the Image J® software. 4 notes being 2 (100%) (1 woman and 3 men); 5 patients with a score of 3 (12.82%) (3 women and 2 men) out of 39; and 5 (23.81%) patient with a score of 4 (2 women and 3 men) out of 21. In the selected images, a line or rectangle was used in the region of the bile duct, according to the sizes mentioned above (item 2.2), applying Image J®. Figure 4 illustrates some of these images, with score 2 (F36 and M63); 3 (F17 and M55) and 4 (F28 and M3).

For numerical analysis, as shown in Fig. 3, the average gray level for region 1 was used, this region is between 0 and 25.13 mm, with a value of 262.83; for region 2 in the range between 25.13 to 42.53 mm, the average of this range is 429.23 and for region 3 between 42.53 to 58 mm, the average is 39.12.

Figure 5 shows the curves obtained by Image J® for gray levels in relation to the distance for the 4 images obtained with E2 score 2, considering the following patients: F36, M37, M54 and M63, as well as the mean value. It can be seen in the Fig. 5 that the averages for regions 1, 2 and 3 of the F36 curve were 262.83, 429.23 and 39.12, respectively. For the M37 the values were: 151.00, 252.25 and 157.48. In the M54 the values were: 111.86, 143.51 and 91.41. For M63 the averages were: 93.68, 210.95 and 107.01. The average values obtained by means of the curves (Ave) were 154.84, 258.98 and 98.76.

When consulting the medical reports, it is emphasized that in F36 the comments were: status after cholecystectomy, and a small fluid collection around the distal choledoccus (location applied to Image J®, as shown in Fig. 4). Hepatocarcinoma (HCC) was

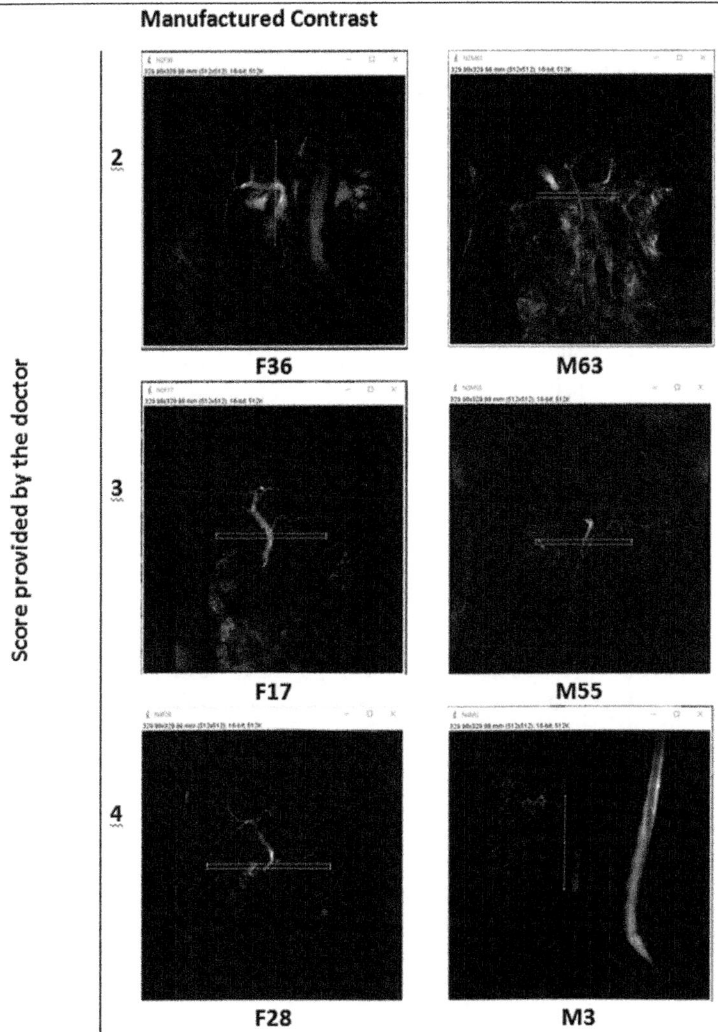

Fig. 4. Images of patients from the cholangio radial sequence of scores 2 (F36 and M63), 3 (F17 and M55) and 4 (F28 and M3) acquired with manufactured contrast obtained with evaluator 2. The rectangles in the images (M63, F17, M55 and F28) and lines (F36 and M3) indicate the area of the common bile duct, chosen for the Image J® software.

suspected in M37, in addition to portal hypertension and moderate ascites, showing that areas chosen by Image J® are altered. Patient M54 presented dilation of the common bile ducts and probable stone, accentuating the values of the curve. In M63, the medical report showed ascites, liver changes with changes to the right of the duct (region 3).

Statistical analysis was performed and the box plots are shown in Fig. 6, with the maximum and minimum values (x), intermediate values (25 and 75%) and average value (represented by the square in the figure) for the average values of regions 1, 2 and 3, following Fig. 3 and 5 for the images chosen by E2 of the 4 patients who obtained score 2. For region 1, the maximum value is for patient F36, and the others have a lower values than the average. In region 2, F36 maintains the highest average, again the other patients have a lower values than the average. And for region 3, patient M37 has the highest average and F36 the lowest average.

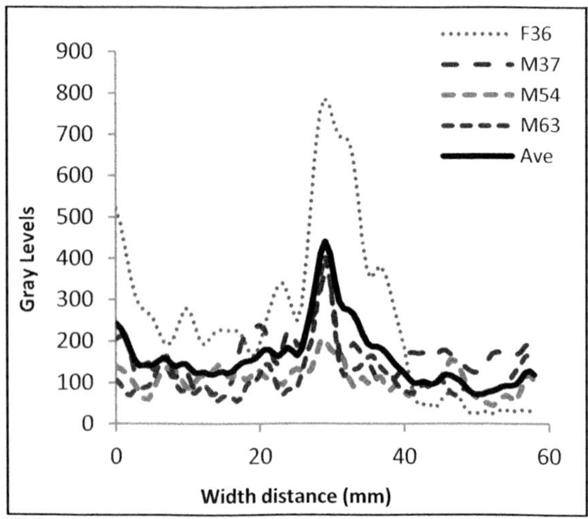

Fig. 5. The curves represent the levels of gray in relation to the distance for the A contrast, of the radial images of cholangio of the common bile duct of 4 patients with score 2, obtained with the Image J® software, as well as the average values.

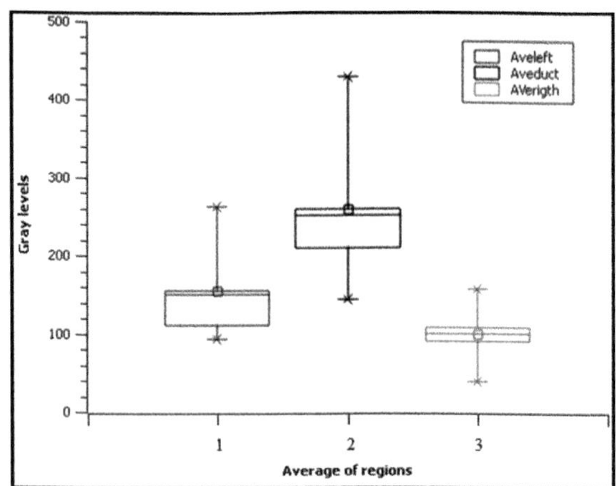

Fig. 6. Box plot of maximum, minimum, intermediate and, average value of regions 1, 2 and 3 of the 4 patients with score 2.

Figure 7 shows the curves obtained by Image J® of gray levels in relation to the distance for the 5 images obtained with score 3 of E2, for the following patients: F1, F17, F38, M25 and M55 in addition to the mean values. It can be seen in the Fig. 7 that the averages for regions 1, 2 and 3 of the F1 curve were: 39.15, 396 and 75.61, respectively. For F17 there are 39.36, 528.58 and 39.42. For patient F38, 34.15, 234.70 and 51.64 were found. For the M25, the values were: 36.25, 197.23 and 63.42. Finally, for the M55: 28.99, 90.39 and 41.14. The average values obtained by means of the curves (Ave) were 35.58, 289.38 and 54.24.

When consulting the medical reports, it was noted that F1 did not show changes in her examination. In F17, the medical report indicates slight changes in the size of the pancreas (as shown in Fig. 4). Patient F38 has post-cholecystectomy status. In M25, a small amount of free perihepatic fluid and calculous cholecystopathy were found. And M55 showed ascites, areas of ectasia and segmental stenosis involving the right and left hepatic ducts (according to Fig. 4).

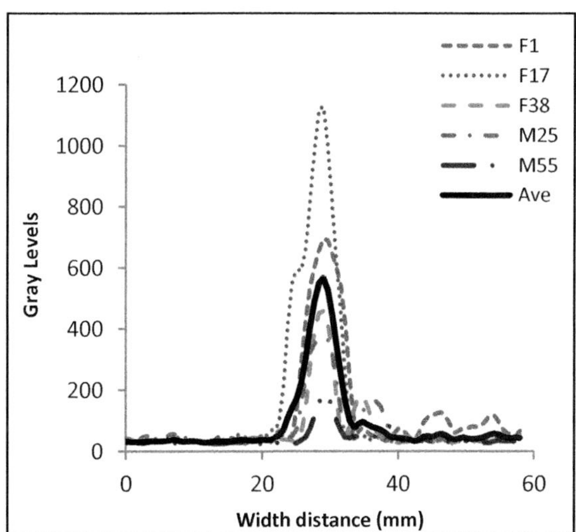

Fig. 7. The curves represent the levels of gray in relation to the distance for the A contrast, of the radial images of cholangio of the common bile duct of 5 patients with score 3, obtained with the Image J® software, as well as the average values.

The statistical analysis was performed and the box plots are shown in Fig. 8, with the maximum and minimum values (x), intermediate values (25 and 75%) and average value (represented by the square in the figure) for the average values of regions 1, 2 and 3, following Fig. 3 and 7 for the images chosen by E2 for the 5 patients who obtained score 3. For region 1, the maximum value is from patient F17 (39.15), and the minimum value is again M55 (28.99), with a difference in gray levels of 10.34. In region 2, F17 maintains the highest average and the minimum value is again M55. And for region 3 the highest value is for patient F1 (75.61) and the lowest value is for F17 (39.42).

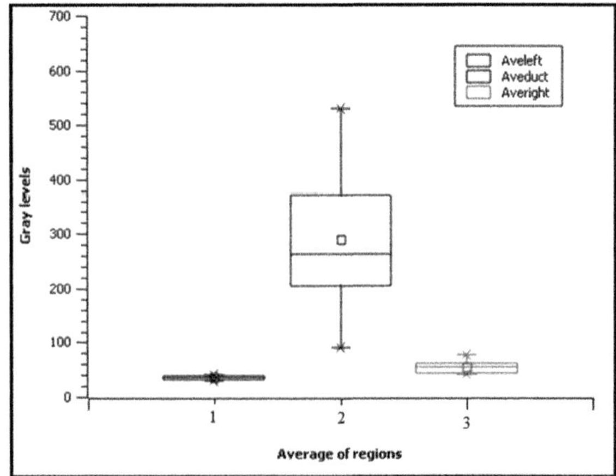

Fig. 8. Box plot of maximum, minimum, intermediate and, average value and average of regions 1, 2 and 3 of the 5 patients with score 3.

Figure 9 shows the curves obtained by Image J® of gray levels in relation to the distance for the 5 images obtained with score 4 of E2, for the following patients: F28, F58, M3, M27 and M42 and the mean values. It can be seen in the figure that the averages for regions 1, 2 and 3 of the F28 curve were: 153.58, 167.65 and 62.39, respectively. For F58, there are 54.18, 349.51 and 48.73. For patient M3, 34.09, 88.02 and 35.71 were found. For the M27, the values were: 37.63, 202.21 and 46.39. Finally, for the M42: 37.51, 99.55 and 38.95. The average values obtained by means of the curves (Ave) were 63.4, 181.39 and 46.38. When consulting the medical reports, it was noted that F28 had post-cholecystectomy status, and in region 1 (as shown in Fig. 4), the commercial contrast administered did not erase the bowel signal, which caused a value well above the average (153.8 for 63.4). In F58, the report does not indicate changes. Patient M3 presented amputation of the common hepatic duct with moderate dilation of the right and left hepatic ducts and their branches. Suspected central cholangiocarcinoma (according to Fig. 4). At M27, he presented post-cholecystectomy status. The M42 patient had no change in his examination.

Statistical analysis was performed and the box plots are shown in Fig. 10, with the maximum and minimum values (x), intermediate values (25 and 75%) and average value (represented by the square in the figure) for the average values of regions 1, 2 and 3, following Fig. 3 and 9 for the images chosen by E2 of the 5 patients who obtained score 4. For region 1, the maximum value is from patient F28 (153.58), and the minimum value is from M3 (34.09). In region 2, F58 maintains the highest average (349.51) and the minimum value is again M3 (88.02). And for region 3 the highest value is from patient F28 (62.39) and the lowest value is from M42 (38.95).

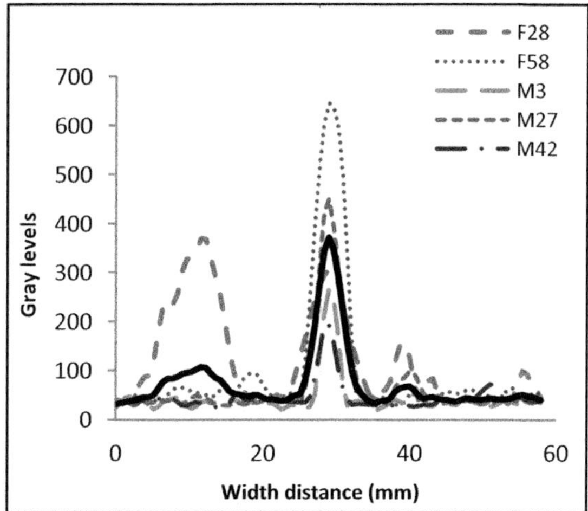

Fig. 9. The curves represent the levels of gray in relation to the distance for the A contrasts, of the radial images of cholangio of the common bile duct of 5 patients with score 4, obtained with the Image J® software, as well as the average values.

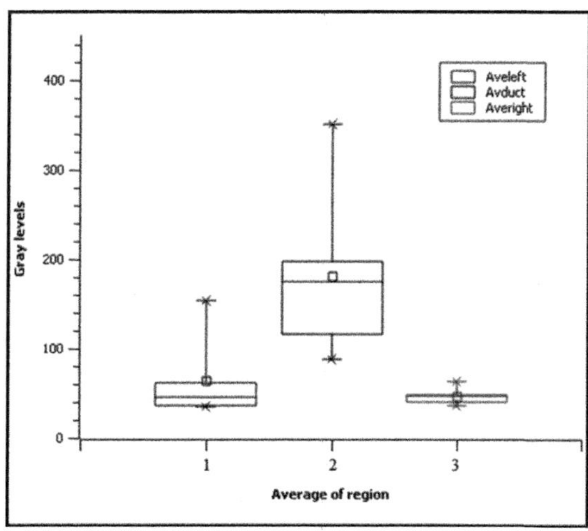

Fig. 10. Box plot of maximum, minimum, intermediate and, average value of regions 1, 2 and 3 of the 5 patients with score 4.

After presenting Fig. 5, 7 and 9, the average curves of each of are highlighted, joining them in Fig. 11. In this Fig. All the 14 patients were considered in the study, distributed them among notes 2, 3 and 4 obtained by Image J®. For score 2, the averages for regions 1, 2 and 3 were: 154.84, 258.98 and 98.76. The values for score 3 were 35.58, 289.38 and 54.24. For score 4, the mean values were 63.4, 181.39 and 46.38. As shown in Fig. 11, in regions 1 and 3 the highest averages are for score 2. In region 2 the highest average is for score 3. One can see that the lowest averages were in region 1 of score 3, and in region 2 and 3 for score 4.

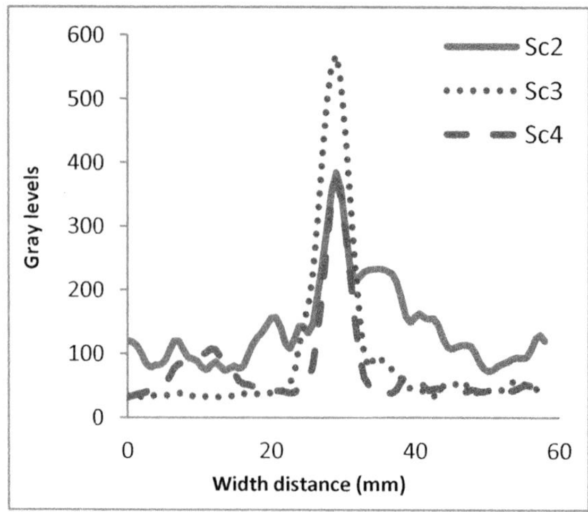

Fig. 11. Curves of the mean values for the 14 patients distributed between scores 2, 3 and 4 with overlapping.

4 Discussion

The images acquired in the MCRP sequence were evaluated by E2 giving notes from 1 to 4. There was a total of 64 patients, with score 2 there were 4 patients, with score 3 there were 39 and with score 4 there were 21 patients [16]. Of these, 14 patients were selected, subdivided as follows: 4 patients with score 2, 5 patients with score 3 and 5 patients with score 4. For a more detailed comparison of the physical characteristics of the diseases of each patient participating in the research, an analysis between the score, the averages obtained by the Image J® curve and existing diseases was performed [22, 24].

In Fig. 3, the three regions are predominantly observed, and in region 1 a lower average value is expected, because the oral contrast agent should erase the signal from the duodenum. Region 2 is the common bile duct, where the signal must be more intense (since this location is of interest to MRCP). In region 3, the mean value should be lower, as the sign of the pancreas must be erased; it only appears when there are physiological changes.

For score 2, the average values for regions 1 and 3 were 154.84 and 98.76, denoting the presence of related diseases such as: small fluid collection around the distal bile duct (F36), moderate ascites (M37) and M54 presented dilation of the pathways bile ducts and probable stones in the bile duct. Region 2 showed a variation in the average gray levels from 143.51 in patient M54 to 429.23 in patient F36, with the other patients presenting with values below the average of 258.99. The standard deviation of the gray levels averages in regions 1, 2 and 3 was 75.86, 122.02 and 48.74, respectively, with a greater variation in the gray values due to the presence of the diseases previously described.

For score 3, the mean value for region 1 was 35.58, with the highest value for patient F17, with 39.36 and the lowest value for patient M55, with 28.99 and the standard deviation was 4.27. For region 2, the mean value is 289.38, with a maximum mean for patient F17 with a value of 528.58 and a minimum mean of 90.39 for patient M55, with a standard deviation of means of 172.96. For region 3, the mean value is 54.24, with a maximum value of 75.61 for patient F1 and a minimum value of 39.42 and standard deviation of 15.32. Here in the F17 medical report there are slight changes in the size of the pancreas. With patient F38 having post-cholecystectomy status. In M25, a small amount of free perihepatic fluid and calculous cholecystopathy were found. And for M55, the report shows ascites, areas of ectasia and segmental stenosis involving the right and left hepatic ducts.

For score 4, the mean value of region 1 was 63.4, with the highest value for patient F28, with 153.58 and the lowest value for patient M3, with 34.08, with other patients having values lower than the mean, and the standard deviation was 51.01. For patient F28, the natural contrast was not able to decrease the intestinal signal, which raised the average for region 1 above all other averages for the other 4 patients. For region 2, the variation in the average gray levels varied from a minimum of 88.02 for patient M3 and a maximum of 349.50 for patient F58 and an average value of 181.39 with a standard deviation of 105.23. For region 3, the mean was 46.43, with a minimum value of 35.71 for patient M3 and a maximum value of 62.38 for patient F28, with a standard deviation of 10.37. Due to the position of the common bile duct, with a lateral view, a line was chosen in the figure by the evaluator E2 (patient M3), instead of using a rectangle. If a rectangle were chosen, it would be along the common bile duct. In this way the line crosses the bile duct up and down. When consulting the medical reports, it was noted that F28 had post-cholecystectomy status. In F58, the medical report does not indicate changes. Patient M3 presented amputation of the common hepatic duct with moderate dilation of the right and left hepatic ducts and their branches. Suspected central cholangiocarcinoma (according to Fig. 4). At M27, he presented post-cholecystectomy status. Patient M42 showed no changes in his exam.

It was proved that the mean values for the score 2 curves are higher, being 4.35 times higher than the average of score 3, in region 1. In region 3, score 2 is 2.12 times higher than score 4. That is, the signal intensity always stands out, due to the diseases existing in those patients. In region 1, the mean of score 4 is 78% higher than the mean of score 3. This is due to the image signal from patient F28 has not been properly erased (contrast or patient changes). In region 3, the mean of score 3 is 16.8% higher than the mean of score 4, due to the enhancement of the pancreatic duct.

The study limitation is due to the pandemic situation and the difficulty of exchanging information with the radiologist, because the clinic is restricting the access of people. In this study, the image database, the reports made available and the researchers experience were considered.

5 Conclusions

This study intended to present an area yet little explored, using Image J® software obtain gray level curves, in the issuance of medical reports describing the existing diseases in patients and the attribution of scores to images indicating how good they are for the emission of the medical report in MRCP exams using a commercial contrast.

From the evaluation of the averages found and the scores assigned, score 2 presented the highest averages of gray levels, compared to the averages of scores 3 and 4, because the existing diseases in these patients prevent the organ signal to be erased. This is true for both region 1 and region 3. For scores 3 and 4 the difference in averages between them is less than the average. There was a greater decrease in the signal in regions 1 and 3 for scores 3 and 4. For region 1, the mean of the signal of score 3 is less than the mean of score 4 and in region 3, the mean of score 4 was less than the mean of score 3. The medical evaluation has a certain degree of subjectivity that could not be solved in this initial quantitative assessment.

The relevance of this work is in the development of a protocol applied to available software that assists in the identification of diseases through changes in average levels of gray levels in chosen regions of organs.

Future work should improve the delimitation of regions close to the common bile duct that would facilitate the identification of existing diseases or anatomical changes.

Acknowledgements. To Araucaria Foundation from Parana State, for providing research support through project number 355/2012.

For the Hospital, Clinic and the patients who did their best to help in this study.

To Terese Winslow LLC for permission to use the anatomical image extrahepatic bile duct anatomy 06/2020.

References

1. Mazzola, A.A.: Magnetic resonance: principles of image formation and applications in functional imaging. Revista Brasileira de Física Médica **3**(1), 117–129 (2009). https://doi.org/10.29384/rbfm.2009.v3.n1.p117-129
2. Westbrook, C., Roth, C.K., Talbot, J.: MRI in Practice. 4th edn. Wiley Black Well (2011)
3. Pinheiro, Y.L.S., Costa, R.Z.V., Pinho, K.E.P., Ferreira, R.R., Schuindt, S.M.: Effects of iodinated contrast agent, xylocaine and gadolinium concentration on the signal emitted in magnetic resonance arthrography: a samples study. Radiologia Brasileira **48**(2), 69–73 (2015). https://doi.org/10.1590/0100-3984.2013.0002
4. Morita, S., et al.: Prospective comparative study of negative oral contrast agents for magnetic resonance cholangiopancreatography. Jpn. J. Radiol. **28**(2), 117–122 (2010). https://doi.org/10.1007/s11604-009-0395-3
5. Ghanaati, H., Yazdi, H.R., Jallati, A.H., Abahashemi, F., Shakiba, M., Firouznia, K.: Improvent of MR cholangiopancreatography (MRCP) images after black tea consumption. Eur. Radiol. **21**, 2551–2557 (2011). https://doi.org/10.1007/s00330-011-2217-0
6. Kim, B., et al.: Coronal 2D MR cholangiography overestimates the length of the right hepatic duct in liver transplantation donors. Eur. Radiol. **27**(5), 1822–1830 (2016). https://doi.org/10.1007/s00330-016-4572-3
7. Pinho, K.E.P., Pinho, A.C., PisanI, J.C., Goedert, C.A., Gusso, A.M., Gewehr, P.M.: Açai juice as contrast agent in MRCP exams: qualitative and quantitative image evaluation. Br. Arch. Biol. Technol. **62**, e19160697 (2019). Epub 13-Maio-2019. ISSN 1516-8913. https://doi.org/10.1590/1678-4324-2019160697
8. Terese Winslow Intrahepatic Bile Duct Anatomy for the National Cancer Institute (2015). Terese Winslow LLC https://www.teresewinslow.com/#/digestion/. Accessed 03 June 2020

9. Leyendecker, J.R., Brown, J.J., Merkle, E.M.: Abdominal & Pelvic MRI. 2nd edn. Lippincott Williams & Wilkins. Philadelphia (2011)
10. Sanchez, T.A., et al.: Clinical Feasibility of açaí (Euterpe olerácea) pulp as an oral contrast agent for magnetic resonance cholangiopancreatography. J. Comput. Assist. Tomogr. **23**(5), 666–670 (2009). https://doi.org/10.1097/RCT.0b013e31819012a0
11. Frisch, A., Walter, T.G., Griezer, C., Geisel, D., Hamm, B., Denecke, T.: Performance survey on a new standardized formula for oral signal suppression in MRCP. Eur. J. Radiol. Open **5**, 1–5 (2017). https://doi.org/10.1016/j.ejro.2017.12.002
12. Pinho, K.E.P., Pinho, A.C., Gewehr, P.M., Gusso, A.M., Goedert, C.A.: Image evaluation in Magnetic Resonance Cholangiopancreatography. In: BIOSTEC 2020 13th International Joint Conference on Biomedical Engineering Systems and Technologies. Proceedings, vol. 4, Biosignals pp. 98–105 (2020). https://www.biostec.org. Accessed 04 June 2020
13. Souza, V.B., Federizzi, M., Fernandes, D., Franco, A.R.: Avaliação quantitativa da qualidade de exame de imagem por ressonância magnética nuclear. In: XXIV Congresso Brasileiro de Engenharia Biomédica [internet] (2014). https://www.canal6.com.br/cbeb/2014/artigos/cbeb2014_submission_375.pdf
14. Rocha, N.K.S., Pinho, K.E.P.: Verificação das Imagens de Colangiopancreatografia por Ressonância Magnética com uso de Suco Natural. In: XIX Seminário de Iniciação Científica e Tecnológica, Medianeira. SICITE. UTFPR (2014)
15. Pinho, K.E.P., Pinho, A.C., Gewehr, P.M., Gusso, A.M.: Image quality in magnetic resonance cholangiopancreatography exams: study between Açai Juice and a manufactured contrast agent. In: Costa-Felix, R., Machado, J.C., Alvarenga, A.V. (eds.) XXVI Brazilian Congress on Biomedical Engineering. IP, vol. 70/2, pp. 259–264. Springer, Singapore (2019). https://doi.org/10.1007/978-981-13-2517-5_40
16. Pinho, K.E.P., Gewehr, P.M., Pinho, A.C., Pisani, J.C.: Sucos naturais como agentes de contraste para exames de colangiopancreatografia por ressonância magnética. In: XXIV Congresso de Engenharia Biomédica[internet], pp. 1685–1688 (2014). https://www.canal6.com.br/cbeb/2014/artigos/cbeb2014_submission_499.pdf
17. Sasani, H., Kayhan, A., Sasani, M.E., Sasani, M.A.: Signal analysis of pineapple according to its anatomical region in magnetic resonance cholangiopancreatography: which region is most effective in suppressing gastric fluid signal? Biomed. Res. **28**(11), 5167–5171 (2017)
18. Fukukura, Y., Fujiyoshi, F., Sasaki, M., Nakajo, M.: Pancreatic duct: morphologic evaluation with MR cholangiopancreatography after secretin stimulation. Radiology **222**, 674–680 (2002). https://doi.org/10.1148/radiol.2223010684
19. Marques, P.M.A., Caritá, E.C., Benedicto, A.A., Sanches, P.R.: Integração RIS/PACS no Hospital das Clínicas de Ribeirão Preto: Uma solução baseada em "web." Radiologia Brasileira **38**(1), 37–43 (2005). https://doi.org/10.1590/S0100-39842005000100009
20. Duarte, J.A., Furtado, A.P.A., Marroni, C.A.: Use of pineapple juice with gadopentetate dimeglumine as a negative oral contrast for magnetic resonance cholangiopancreatography: a multicentric study. Abdom. Imaging **37**, 447–456 (2012). https://doi.org/10.1007/s00261-011-9761-6
21. Image J. https://imagej.nih.gov. Accessed 12 May 2020
22. Weber, J.F., Santos, A.L.F.: Utilização do software ImageJ para avaliar área de lesão dermonecrótica. Revista de Saúde Digital e Tecnologias Educacionais **4**(1), 120–130 (2019). https://periodicos.ufc.br/resdite/index. Accessed 27 Jan 2020
23. Ferreira, T., Rasband, W.: ImageJ user Guide IJ 1.46r. 2019. https://imagej.nih.gov/ij/docs/guide/user-guide.pdf. Accessed 26 May 2019
24. Brianezi, G., Camargo, J.L.V., Miot, H.A.: Development and validation of a quantitative image analysis method to evaluate comet assay (silver staining). J. Bras. Patol. Med. Lab. **45**(4), 325–334 (2009). https://doi.org/10.1590/S1676-24442009000400010

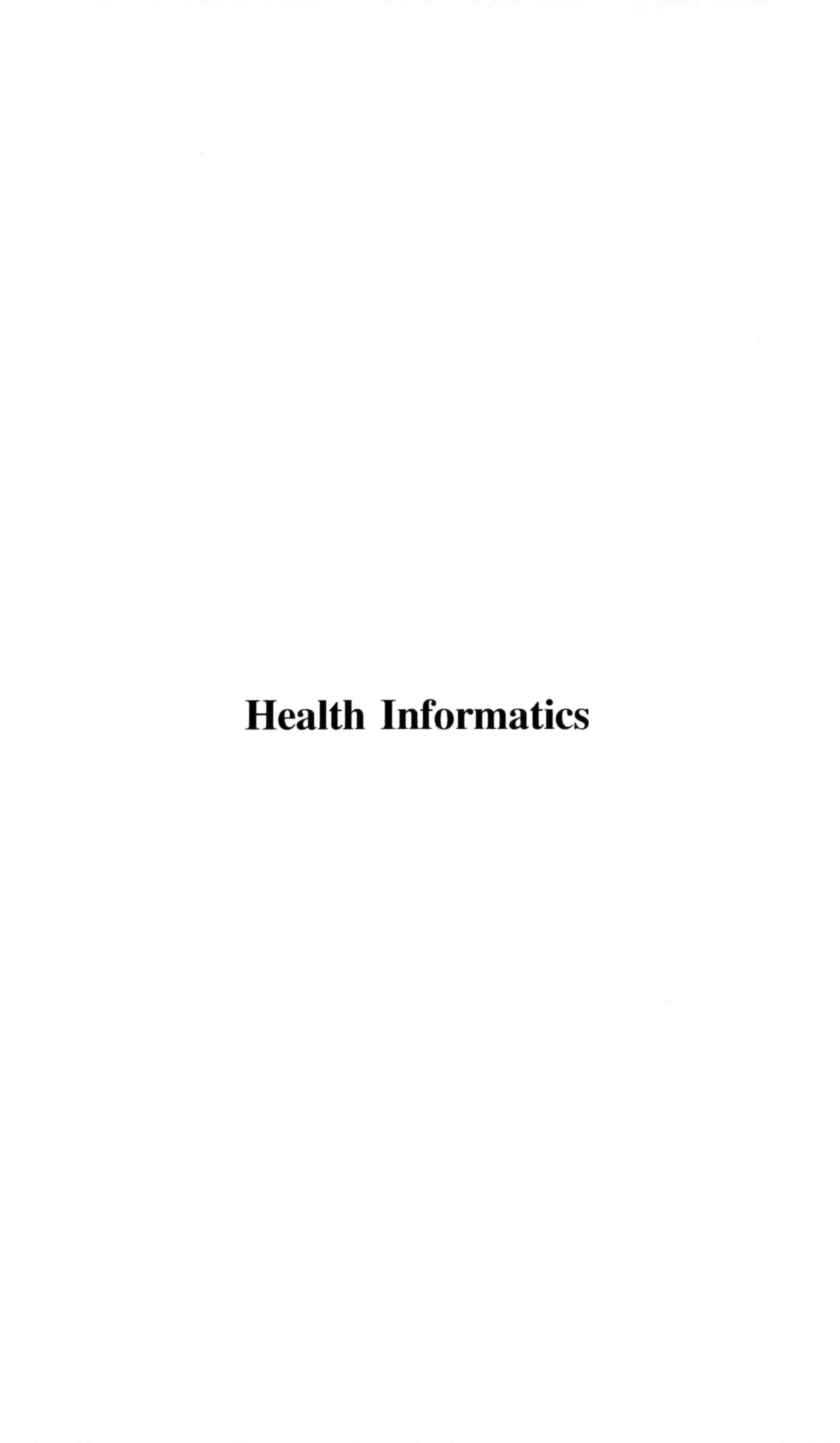

Health Informatics

Evaluating a Comparing Deep Learning Architectures for Blood Glucose Prediction

Touria El Idrissi[1] and Ali Idri[2,3(✉)]

[1] Department of Computer Sciences EMI, University Mohamed V, Rabat, Morocco

[2] Software Project Management Research Team, RITC, ENSIAS, University Mohamed V, Rabat, Morocco
ali.idri@um5.ac.ma

[3] Complex Systems Engineering, University Mohammed VI Polytechnic, Ben Guerir, Morocco

Abstract. To manage their disease, diabetic patients need to control the blood glucose level (BGL) by monitoring it and predicting its future values. This allows to avoid high or low BGL by taking recommended actions in advance. In this paper, we conduct a comparative study of two emerging deep learning techniques: Long-Short-Term Memory (LSTM) and Convolutional Neural Networks (CNN) for one-step and multi-steps-ahead forecasting of the BGL based on Continuous Glucose Monitoring (CGM) data. The objectives are twofold: 1) Determining the best strategies of multi-steps-ahead forecasting (MSF) to fit the CNN and LSTM models respectively, and 2) Comparing the performances of the CNN and LSTM models for one-step and multi-steps prediction. Toward these objectives, we firstly conducted series of experiments of a CNN model through parameters selection to determine its best configuration. The LSTM model we used in the present study was developed and evaluated in an earlier work. Thereafter, five MSF strategies were developed and evaluated for the CNN and LSTM models using the Root-Mean-Square Error (RMSE) with an horizon of 30 min. To statistically assess the differences between the performances of CNN and LSTM models, we used the Wilcoxon statistical test. The results showed that: 1) no MSF strategy outperformed the others for both CNN and LSTM models, and 2) the proposed CNN model significantly outperformed the LSTM model for both one-step and multi-steps prediction.

Keywords: Convolutional Neural Network · Long-Short-Term Memory network · Multi-step-ahead forecasting · Blood glucose · Prediction · Diabetes

1 Introduction

The diabetes mellitus disease occurs when the glucose metabolism is defected. Type 1 and Type 2 of diabetes mellitus (named T1DM and T2DM respectively) are the main types of diabetes. T1DM is due to a shortage in the insulin produced by the pancreas while T2DM is due to an inappropriate use of the produced insulin [1]. This chronic illness may cause serious health complications such as neuropathy, nephropathy, blindness and others [1]. Diabetic patients can prevent or delay the occurrence of these

X. Ye et al. (Eds.): BIOSTEC 2020, CCIS 1400, pp. 347–365, 2021.
https://doi.org/10.1007/978-3-030-72379-8_17

complications by managing their disease and maintaining their blood glucose level (BGL) within the normal range. This can be achieved by monitoring the BGL manually via sticks or automatically via continuous glucose monitoring (CGM) sensors and then predicting the future values of BGL. If the predicted values tend to be outside the normal range, the diabetic patient can act in advance toward avoiding high or low BGL [1, 2].

Several data mining techniques were investigated for the BGL prediction counting machine learning and statistical techniques [2]. Nevertheless, machine learning and especially deep learning techniques are gaining more interest as they are achieving promising results due to their aptitude to learn the data characteristics and select relevant features automatically [3, 4]. LSTM and CNN are among those emerging deep learning techniques.

BGL prediction can be considered as a time series prediction problem where the past values are provided by a CGM device. Time series forecasting can be: 1) a one-step ahead forecasting (OSF) when the prediction targets the next value, or 2) a multi-steps ahead forecasting (MSF) when the prediction targets the next H values, where H is the prediction horizon [5]. Five MSF strategies were proposed in literature [5–7]: Recursive, Direct, MIMO (for Multiple-Input Multiple-Output), DirRec that consolidates Direct and Recursive, and DirMO that consolidates Direct and MIMO. The studies [5] and [6] compared the performances of these five strategies using Neural Networks (NNs). The study [8] compared Recursive and Direct strategies using LSTM NNs and CNNs, while the study [9] compared Recursive and MIMO strategies using Recurrent NNs. The study [7] was the first to conduct an exhaustive comparison of the five MSF strategies using the LSTM. All these comparisons concluded that no strategy is better that the others in all contexts. However in [7], authors noticed that non-recursive strategies tend to be better than recursive ones.

In the present study, we evaluated and compared two deep learning models: CNN and LSTM to predict BGL based on CGM data in the context of OSF and MSF with an horizon of 30 min, which is good enough to avoid likely increase or decrease of the BGL [9]. The LSTM model we used has been developed and evaluated in our earlier work [3], while the present study develops and evaluates the CNN model using a 1D convolutional layer, followed by a Flatten layer and 2 Dense layers for OSF and MSF strategies. Thereafter, we compare the performances of both CNN and LSTM. All the evaluations and comparisons of CNN and LSTM models carried out in this study used the Root-Mean-Square Error (RMSE) and the Wilcoxon statistical test to statistically assess the differences between the performances of CNN and LSTM models. According to authors' knowledge, no study was conducted focusing on the same objectives, which motivates the current work.

This comparative study discusses five research questions (RQs):

- (RQ1): What is the best configuration of the proposed CNN model?
- (RQ2): Is there a MSF strategy that outperforms the others using the CNN model?
- (RQ3): Is the CNN model more accurate than the LSTM one in OSF?
- (RQ4): Is the CNN model more accurate than the LSTM model in MSF?
- (RQ5): Is the outperformance of a model for OSF maintained for MSF?

This paper is organized into 7 sections. Section 2 gives an overview of the MSF strategies as well as the CNN and LSTM techniques. Section 3 highlights related work.

In Sect. 4, the experimental design is detailed. Section 5 reports and discusses the results obtained. Threats to validity are presented in Sect. 6 and finally, conclusion along with future works are presented in Sect. 7.

2 Background

This section presents an overview of the MSF strategies. Thereafter, we present the two deep learning architectures LSTM and CNN we used in this study.

2.1 MSF Strategies

Let y_1 to y_N be the N past values of a time series. The time series prediction can be performed for: 1) a single period by determining the next value y_{N+1} which is called one-step ahead forecasting (OSF), or 2) multiple periods by determining y_{N+1} to y_{N+H} which correspond to the H next values, this is called multi-step ahead forecasting (MSF) [5]. The MSF problem is more difficult than the OSF one. In fact, the former is confronted to the accumulation of errors, the decreasing of accuracy and the increasing of uncertainty [5, 6].

To perform the MSF, five strategies can be used. These strategies are [5, 6]: 1) Recursive (or iterative), 2) Direct (or independent), 3) MIMO (Multi-input Multi-output), 4) DirREC combining Direct and Recursive, and 5) DirMO combining Direct and MIMO. Table 1 presents these five MSF strategies including a brief description, number of models developed and the characteristics of each MSF strategy.

Table 1. MSF strategies.

Strategy	Description	Number of models	Characteristics
Recursive (or iterative)	Prediction is iteratively performed using an OSF model. Each predicted value is used as part of input values to predict the next one	One model with single output	Intuitive and simple Risk of errors' accumulation
Direct (or independent)	Prediction for each step is independently performed from the others	H models: each one with a single output for each step	No errors' accumulation Dependencies between the estimated values may not be treated
MIMO	Prediction is performed by one model that returns the predicted values in a vector	One model with multiple output	The stochastic dependencies between the predicted values are preserved. No prediction flexibility
DirRec	For each step, the prediction is done by a corresponding model based on the past values and the predictions of previous steps	H models with single output	Using the previous estimations for each step while having more flexibility by using different models
DirMO	The prediction horizon is divided in B blocks with the same size; each block is predicted based on a MIMO model	B models with multiple output	Provide a trade-off between the high stochastic dependency of MIMO and the flexibility of Direct

Considering a time series TS, let H be the prediction horizon, d is the sampling horizon, y_i and $\widehat{y}_i$ are the observed and predicted values at the time i respectively, t is the time of the prediction, and s is an integer varying from 1 to H representing a step in the prediction horizon.

In the Recursive strategy, we start by training an OSF model M, and each value is predicted using Eq. (1).

$$\hat{y}_{t+s} = \begin{cases} M(y_{t-d+1}, \ldots, y_t) & if\ s = 1 \\ M(y_{t-d+s}, \ldots, y_t, \hat{y}_{t+1}, \ldots, \hat{y}_{t+s-1}) & if\ 2 \le s \le d \\ M(\hat{y}_{t+s-N}, \ldots, \hat{y}_{t+s-1}) & if\ s > d \end{cases} \tag{1}$$

For the Direct strategy, H models are trained. Let M_s be the model trained for the step s. The predicted value for that step is calculated using the model M_s as shown in Eq. (2).

$$\widehat{y}_{t+s} = M_s\left(y_{t-d+1}, \ldots, y_t\right)\ 1 \le s \le H \tag{2}$$

The MIMO strategy introduced in [10] considers a Multiple-Output representing a vector of the predicted values. Thus, one model M is trained to predict this vector using Eq. (3).

$$\left[\widehat{y}_{t+1}, \ldots, \widehat{y}_{t+H}\right] = M\left(y_{t-N+1}, \ldots, y_t\right) \tag{3}$$

DirRec strategy provides forecasts iteratively using H models with different input size [11]. Let M_s be the model trained for the step s, M_s provides the value of the step s using the d past values and the predicted values for the previous steps based on Eq. (4).

$$\hat{y}_{t+s} = \begin{cases} M_s(y_{t-d+1}, \ldots, y_t) & if\ s = 1 \\ M_s(y_{t-d+1}, \ldots, y_t, \hat{y}_{t+1}, \ldots, \hat{y}_{t+s-1}) & if\ 2 \le s \le N \end{cases} \tag{4}$$

DirMO strategy divides the prediction horizon in B blocks with the same size n where $B = H/n$ [12]. Each block b is directly predicted using a MIMO model M_b as shown in Eq. (5).

$$\left[\widehat{y}_{t+(b-1)*n+1}, \ldots, \widehat{y}_{t+b*n}\right] = M_b\left(y_{t-d+1}, \ldots, y_t\right) \tag{5}$$

2.2 LSTM

Hochreiter & Schmidhuber [13] introduced a novel architecture of recurrent Neural Networks (RNNs), called LSTM NNs, in order to solve the problem of vanishing or exploding gradient met in the traditional RNNs. LSTM is a recurrent neural network that contains memory cells. The memory cell has a cell state preserved over time and a gate structure containing three gates: input gate, forget gate and output gate. These gates serve for controlling and regulating the information through the memory cell. With this structure, the LSTM NNs can catch long term dependencies and treat serial data such as video, speech and time series [3, 13].

Figure 1 shows the structure of a memory cell [3] and Table 2 presents information on the memory structure. The following notations are used:

t: time or sequence number.
X_t: input vector for t.
Y_t: output vector for t.
h_t: hidden vector for t.
C_t: cell state for t.
W_i, W_f, W_o and W_c: weight matrices corresponding to each component.
b_i, b_f, b_o and b_c: bias vectors corresponding to each component..
i_t, f_t, and o_t: results of the input, forget and output gates respectively.

Note that σ and *tanh* are the sigmoid and the hyperbolic tangent functions of Eq. (6) and Eq. (7) respectively used as activation functions.

$$\sigma(x) = \frac{e^x}{1 + e^x} \tag{6}$$

$$tanh(x) = \frac{e^x - e^{-x}}{e^x + e^{-x}} \tag{7}$$

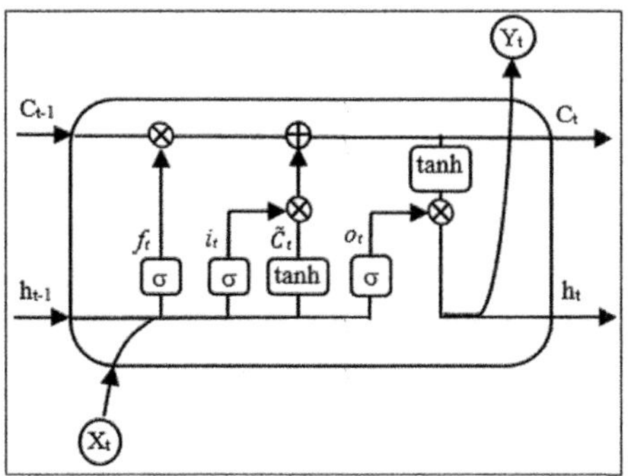

Fig. 1. Memory cell structure [3].

Table 2. LSTM memory structure.

Component	Role	Equation
Input gate	Getting the information to be retained	$i_t = \sigma(W_i * [h_{t-1}, X_t] + b_i)$
Forget gate	Getting the information to be ignored	$f_t = \sigma(W_f * [h_{t-1}, X_t] + b_f)$
Output gate	Calculating the output and updating the hidden vector	$o_t = \sigma(W_o * [h_{t-1}, X_t] + b_o)$ $h_t = o_t * tanh(C_t)$
Cell state	Maintaining the information through cells	$C_t = f_t * C_{t-1} + i_t * \tilde{C}_t$ Where $\tilde{C}_t = tanh(W_c * [h_{t-1}, X_t] + b_c)$

2.3 CNNs

The origins of the CNNs go back to the neocognitron model proposed in [14]. CNNs are based on the concept of simple and complex cells [15] that was inspired from the animal visual cortex. However, the first successful of CNNs was done by LeCun et al. in [16] who trained CNNs by the Backpropagation algorithm.

A CNN is a feed-forward NN whose main layer is a convolutional one performing a convolution operation. This latter consists of applying and sliding a filter over the input data through an elementwise multiplication [17–19]. The connection weights represent the kernel of the convolution.

The dimension of the filter depends on the type of input data. In fact, 1D is used for sequential data such as text and time series, 2D is used for images and 3D for videos [4]. Multiple filters can be used to be able to extract more useful features [18].

In the case of time series, the convolution is applied using Eq. (8).

$$C_t = f(\omega * X_{t:t+l-1} + b)\forall t \in [1, T - l + 1] \quad (8)$$

where C_t is the tth element of C, the vector resulting from the convolution, X is the time series with length T, ω is a 1D filter with length l, b is the bias parameter and f represents the activation function [18].

3 Related Work

Statistical methods and in particular autoregressive ones were widely used for prediction in diabetes including BGL prediction [2]. However, a growing trend has been observed for the use of machine learning techniques in BGL prediction and Diabetes in general [2, 9, 20]. In fact, [2] reviewed the data mining predictive techniques in diabetes self-management including BGL prediction, and reported that 57.98% of the selected studies used machine learning techniques while 50% investigated non machine learning techniques. Note that BGL was the most investigated task in diabetes self-management with 47.37% of the selected studies [21]. This interest in using machine learning techniques for BGL prediction is due to: 1) the availability of patients' data, and 2) the ability of machine learning techniques to solve complex tasks in dynamic knowledge and environment [20]. However, the use of deep learning techniques is still at its infancy in the BGL prediction: in fact, [20] reported that the deep neural networks were investigated in only 1% of the selected studies.

Table 3. BGL prediction using deep learning technique: An overview.

Reference	Technique	Architecture	Type of forecasting	HP (mn)	Findings
Mhaskar & al., 2017 [28]	Deep NN	2 layers	Not specified	30	Deep NN performed better than a shallow NN
Mirshekarian & al., 2017 [29]	LSTM	5 units LSTM Layer	MSF with Direct strategy	30, 60	LSTM performed similar to a SVR model, and was better than physician predictions
Doike & al., 2018 [30]	Deep RNN	3 hidden layers using 2000 units, one unit input layer and one unit output layer	MSF using Direct	30	BGL prediction was used for the prevention of hypoglycemia achieving 80% as accuracy
Fox & al., 2018 [9]	Deep RNN	2 layers using GRU cells	MSF with MIMO and Recursive	30	MIMO outperformed Recursive
Sun & al., 2018 [26]	LSTM	– LSTM Layer – Bidirectional LSTM layer – 3 fully connected layers	MSF with Direct strategy	15, 30, 45, 60	LSTM performed better than ARIMA and SVR baseline methods
Xie & Wang, 2018 [8]	- LSTM - CNN	– The LSTM uses 3 LSTM layers – The CNN uses 2 Temporal CNN layers	MSF using Direct and Recursive	30	For LSTM, Direct strategy has performed better than the Recursive one No conclusion for CNN
Zhu & al., 2018 [27]	CNN	3 dilated CNN blocks with 5 layers	Not specified	30	Prediction of the BGL was treated as a classification task
El Idrissi & al., 2019 [3]	LSTM	– LSTM Layer – 2 fully connected layers	One-step ahead	5	The LSTM model proposed significantly outperformed an existing LSTM model and an AutoRegressive model
El Idrissi & al., 2020 [7]	LSTM	– LSTM Layer – 2 fully connected layers	MSF with the five strategies	30	None strategy significantly outperformed others Non-recursive strategies tend to be better than recursive ones

Furthermore, deep learning techniques were successfully used in image recognition [22, 23], object detection [24], and sequential data processing such as speech [25] and in many other fields [4]. Their success is due to their ability to automatically learn the data representation from raw data and extract the relevant features [4]. In the context of BGL prediction, deep learning techniques especially LSTM and CNN were investigated and promising results were obtained [3, 26, 27].

Table 3 presents an overview of a set of selected studies dealing with deep learning for BGL prediction, including technique and architecture used, type of forecasting, horizon used and their findings.

The main findings are:

- BGL prediction using deep learning techniques provided promising results.
- The most investigated deep learning techniques were RNNs, CNN and LSTM.
- CGM data were the most frequently used.
- A horizon of 30 min was the most frequently used. However, we notice that in general the prediction horizon ranged from 5 min to 60 min.
- Direct was the most often used MSF strategy.

4 Experimental Design

This section presents the empirical design of our study, including (1) description of the dataset, the performance criterion and the statistical tests used, and (2) experimental process we followed to evaluate and compare the performances of CNN and LSTM models.

4.1 Dataset, Performance Measurement and Statistical Tests

As the current research is based on the study conducted in [7], the experiments are done on the same datasets used in [7]. These datasets are for 10 T1DM patients extracted from the dataset DirecNetInpatientAccuracyStudy available at the site [31]. Each dataset is related to a patient and contains his/her BGL measurements every 5 min using a CGM device. Note that these patients are taken randomly and a pre-processing of data was required to remove redundant records and outliers between successive records. The datasets of the Ten patients is described in Table 4.

In order to assess the performance of the investigated models, we used the performance measurement RMSE (root-mean-square error) [2] which is calculated by means of Eq. (9).

$$\mathrm{RMSE} = \sqrt{\frac{1}{\mathrm{n}}\sum\nolimits_{\mathrm{i}=1}^{\mathrm{n}} (\hat{y}_i - y_i)^2} \tag{9}$$

where y_i and $\widehat{y}_i$ represent the measured and the estimated value respectively and n represents the size of the considered sample. The RMSE value ranges in the interval $[0, +\infty[$. Note that the performance is higher when the RMSE value tends to 0.

For the statistical tests, we used the Wilcoxon statistical test which is a non-parametric test used to assess if the difference between the performances of two models is significant. This test is performed considering the null hypothesis (NH) that there is no difference between the compared models. The *p-value* of the considered NH is calculated: if the *p-value* is less than a certain significance level α, the difference is considered statistically significant [32].

In the case we need to have a ranking of the models, the sum of ranking differences (SRD) is used. It calculates the ranking of the models by summing up the difference between their ranking and an ideal ranking for the considered cases. The ideal ranking can be a reference model or the best known model. If such a model does not exist, the ideal ranking can be defined based on the minimum, the maximum or the average of the models for each case [33].

Table 4. Ten patients' data description. The BGL is in mg/dl.

Patients	P1	P2	P3	P4	P5	P6	P7	P8	P9	P10
Number of records	766	278	283	923	562	771	897	546	831	246
Min BGL	40	57	103	40	50	62	42	43	40	72
Max BGL	339	283	322	400	270	400	400	310	400	189
Mean BGL	114.78	120.96	185.89	188.44	179.71	187.45	210.26	152.88	157.50	116.51

4.2 Experimental Process

The experimental process we followed consists of four steps: 1) Data preparation, 2) Construction of the CNN and LSTM models, 3) Evaluation of the MSF strategies for the CNN and LSTM models, and 4) Comparison of the CNN and the LSTM models.

- **Step 1: Data Preparation**

When using a model, the data should be arranged in a way to fit the model's requirements. Let $X = \{s(t_i)\}$ be a time series where $s(t_i)$ is the BGL recorded at time t_i and d the sampling horizon, the time series X is decomposed into couples (X_i, y_i) where X_i and y_i are the input and the output data respectively. For OSF, y_i is the next value following the values of the vector X_i. For the MSF strategies, Table 5 presents the decomposition done for each MSF strategy to perform a 30 min ahead prediction.

- **Step 2: Construction of the CNN and LSTM Models**

The CNN model we propose for the BGL prediction is a sequential one, the first layer is a 1D convolutional layer, followed by a Flatten layer and 2 Dense layers. To determine the best configuration using this architecture, we used a Search Grid (SG) on two hyper-parameters: kernel size and the number of filters. Table 6 shows the parameters' ranges of kernel size and number of filters. Similar strategy was used in [3, 34]. This step is composed of two sub-steps which are:

- Step 2.1: For each value of the number of filters and each patient, the CNN model is trained and tested. Based on the SRD method, the best value of the number of filters is selected.
- Step 2.2: For each value of the kernel size and each patient, the CNN model with the best number of filters of Step 1.1 is trained and tested. Based on the SRD method, the best value of the kernel size is selected.

Table 5. Data preparation for MSF strategies. HP: Horizon of Prediction; mn: minutes.

MSF Strategy	Context	Decomposition
Recursive	$HP = 5$ mn	$X_i = \{s(t_{i-d+1}), \ldots, s(t_i)\}$; $y_i = s(t_{i+1})$
Direct	$HP = 30$ mn	$X_i = \{s(t_{i-d+1}), \ldots, s(t_i)\}$; $y_i = s(t_{i+6})$
MIMO	Multiple output for $HP = 30$ mn	$X_i = \{s(t_{i-d+1}), \ldots, s(t_i)\}$; $y_i = \{s(t_{i+1}), \ldots, s(t_{i+6})\}$
DirRec	6 models M_j with $HP = 5$ mn, j goes from 1 to 6	For each M_j: $X_i = \{s(t_{i-d-j+2}), \ldots, s(t_i)\}$; $y_i = s(t_{i+1})$
DirMO	Number of blocks = 2 So, 2 models are trained	For M_1: $X_i = \{s(t_{i-d+1}), \ldots, s(t_i)\}$; $y_i = \{s(t_{i+1}), \ldots, s(t_{i+3})\}$ For M_2: $X_i = \{s(t_{i-d+1}), \ldots, s(t_i)\}$; $y_i = \{s(t_{i+4}), \ldots, s(t_{i+6})\}$

Table 6. Search Grid parameters.

Parameter	Signification	Search space
Number of filters	Number of sliding windows	{2, 5, 10, 15, 20, 25}
Kernel size	Dimension of the sliding windows	{2, 3, 4, 5, 10}

For the LSTM model, we used the same architecture of [7], which is composed of one LSTM layer followed by two dense layers. It was first proposed in [3] where the best configuration was determined by tuning 3 hyper-parameters which are: 1) LSTM units, 2) dense units, and 3) sequence input length. This model significantly outperformed the LSTM proposed by [26] as well as an AutoRegressive model.

- **Step 3: Evaluation of MSF Strategies for the LSTM and CNN Models**

The objective of this step is to evaluate the performances of the MSF strategies for the two models: CNN and LSTM. Therefore, the performance of each strategy is evaluated for each patient using the RMSE criterion. The models are trained on 66% of the dataset (training dataset) and evaluated on 34% of the dataset (testing dataset). If a difference between the performances is noticed, the statistical tests are applied to statistically assess the observed differences.

- **Step 4: Comparison of the LSTM and CNN Models**

At this step, the performances of CNN and LSTM for OSF and for each of the five MSF strategies are compared. The differences between the performances are statistically assessed through the Wilcoxon test. Therefore, we consider six NHs which are:

- NH1: The CNN model does not outperform the LSTM model for OSF.
- NH2: The CNN model does not outperform the LSTM model for MSF using Direct strategy.
- NH3: The CNN model does not outperform the LSTM model for MSF using MIMO strategy.

- NH4: The CNN model does not outperform the LSTM model for MSF using Recursive strategy.
- NH5: The CNN model does not outperform the LSTM model for MSF using DirRec strategy.
- NH6: The CNN model does not outperform the LSTM model for MSF using DirMO strategy.

5 Results and Discussion

This section presents and discusses the results of the empirical evaluations carried out in the present study. The experimentations were conducted using a tool developed under Windows 10 using Python-3.6 and the framework Keras 2.2.4 with, as backend, Tensorflow 1.12.0.

5.1 Construction of the CNN and LSTM Models

The proposed CNN is a sequence of a 1D convolutional layer, a Flatten layer and 2 Dense layers. After preparing the data to fit the required input and output for OSF, we carried out a set of experiments to answer the RQ1 by varying the two hyper-parameters: 1) the number of filters, and 2) the kernel size.

Figure 2 presents the RMSE obtained for each patient and for each number of filters in Table 6. We observe that with 20 filters, the model achieves the best RMSE. Furthermore, the model with 20 filters is ranked first according to the SRD method. The results of the SRD are presented in Table 7 (the ideal ranking is obtained by considering the minimum performance). Therefore, we chose the number of filters equal to 20.

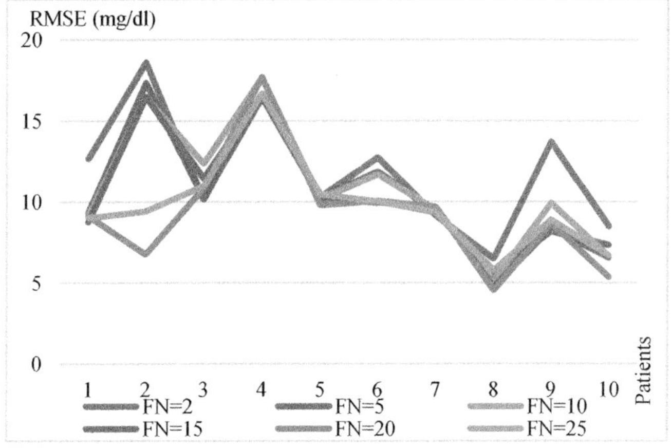

Fig. 2. RMSE values vs filters' number (FN) of CNN.

Table 7. SRD considering the variation of filters' number (FN).

Patients	FN = 2	FN = 5	FN = 10	FN = 15	FN = 20	FN = 25	Min
P1	5	4	3	0	2	1	1
P2	5	4	2	3	0	1	1
P3	0	1	5	4	2	3	1
P4	1	0	4	2	5	3	1
P5	4	3	2	1	0	5	1
P6	5	4	2	0	2	1	1
P7	0	2	3	5	4	1	1
P8	5	3	2	1	0	4	1
P9	5	0	4	1	2	3	1
P10	5	4	2	1	0	3	1
SRD	35	25	29	18	17	25	10

The same experiments were conducted by varying the kernel size according to the values in Table 6. The results of these experiments are shown in Fig. 3. As there is no clearly dominant value, the models are ranked using the SRD method. Table 8 gives the results of SRD which show that a kernel size equals to 2 provides the best ranking.

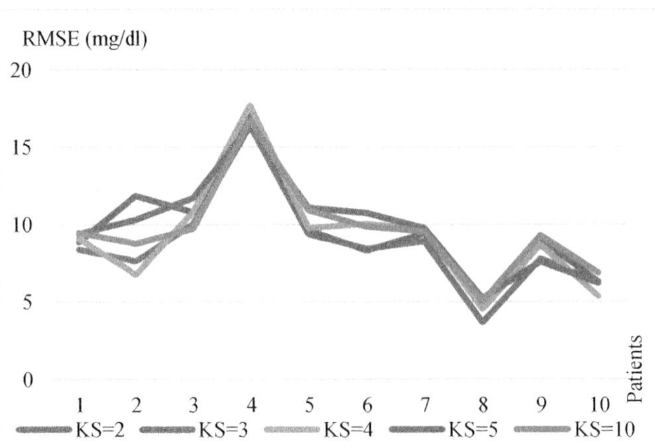

Fig. 3. RMSE values vs kernel size (KS) of CNN.

Table 8. SRD considering the variation of kernel size (KS).

Patients	KS = 2	KS = 3	KS = 4	KS = 5	KS = 10	Min
P1	0	1	2	3	4	1
P2	1	4	0	3	2	1
P3	1	2	3	4	0	1
P4	1	3	4	0	2	1
P5	0	1	2	4	3	1
P6	1	0	3	4	2	1
P7	0	1	3	4	2	1
P8	0	2	1	4	3	1
P9	1	3	2	0	4	1
P10	2	3	0	1	4	1
SRD	7	20	20	27	26	10

To sum up the results of RQ1, a number of filters equals to 20 and a kernel size equals to 2 give the best configuration of our CNN. This CNN variant will be used in the next steps of our experimental process.

For the LSTM model, we adopt the one used in [7]. It is composed of an LSTM layer and 2 dense layers with 50 LSTM units, 30 Dense units and 10 as a sequence input length based on the tuning conducted in [3].

5.2 Evaluation of MSF Strategies for the CNN and LSTM Models

a) CNN Evaluation

For each of the five MSF strategies, using the corresponding data obtained in Step 1, we train and validate the required CNN model(s) based on the configuration that we got in Step2. Figure 4 presents the performance in terms of RMSE of the five MSF strategies for the ten patients.

Figure 4 shows that there is no significant difference between the performances of the five strategies. Furthermore, considering the average of RMSE values, the means are 31.48, 30.84, 31.60, 30.22 and 31.10 for Direct, MIMO, Recursive, DirRec and DirMO respectively. Therefore, there is no need to perform a statistical test. We conclude that no MSF strategy outperforms the others using the proposed CNN. Besides, the five strategies are giving similar performances.

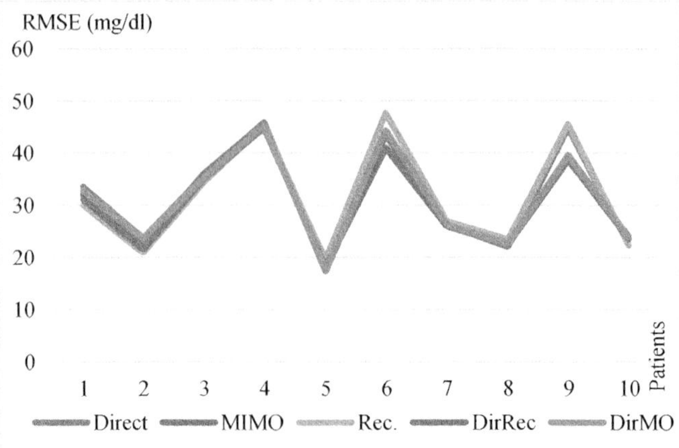

Fig. 4. RMSE values of CNN using the five strategies.

b) **LSTM Evaluation**

In [7], the authors carried out an exhaustive comparison of the five MSF strategies using the LSTM model. In fact, for each MSF strategy with the LSTM, the data were prepared for the required models as presented in Step1. Then, each model was trained and validated using RMSE for each of the 10 patients. Fig. 5 presents the results obtained in [7].

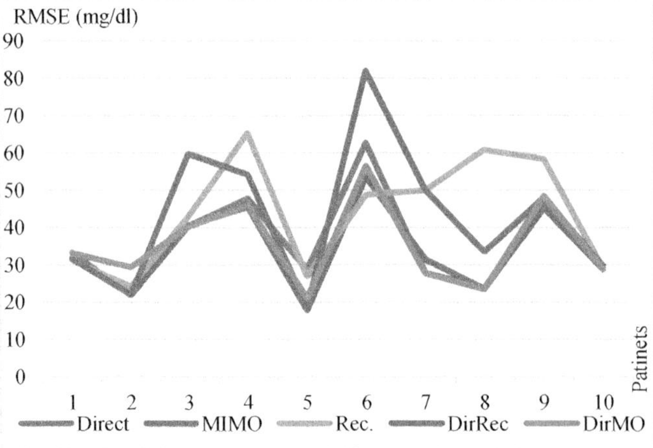

Fig. 5. RMSE values of LSTM using the five strategies [7].

As reported in [7], no MSF strategy significantly outperforms the others. However, Fig. 5 shows that strategies without recursion: Direct, MIMO and DirMO outperformed, in general, strategies with recursion which are Recursive and DirRec. In fact, the reported averages of RMSE were 36.30, 34.06 and 35.47 for Direct, MIMO and DirMO respectively; while for Recursive and DirRec, the RMSE averages were 43.76 and 42.92 respectively [7].

5.3 Comparing the CNN and LSTM Models

To compare the performances of the CNN and LSTM models, we present the results obtained in Step 2 and 3 for the OSF and for each of the MSF strategies. The results are shown in Fig. 6. Figure 6.A presents the results of OSF for both CNN and LSTM, while Fig. 6.B, to Fig. 6.F present the results of CNN and LSTM using Direct, MIMO, Recursive, DirRec and DirMO strategies respectively.

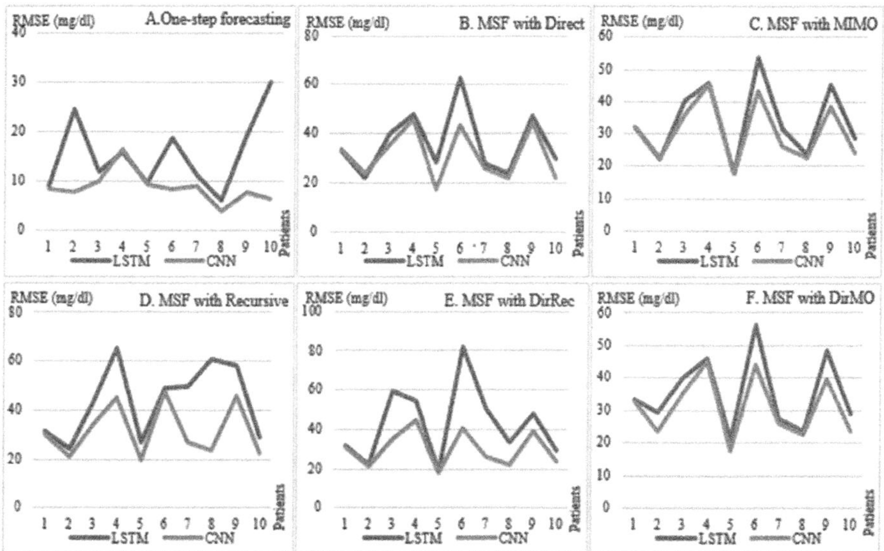

Fig. 6. CNN vs LSTM for one-step ahead forecasting (A) and multi-steps ahead forecasting (B to F).

Figure 6 shows that CNN outperformed LSTM in OSF and MSF for all the strategies. To statistically assess these findings, the p-values are calculated for the six NHs of Step 4 and presented in Table 9.

Table 9. p-value of the NHs.

NH	NH1	NH2	NH3	NH4	NH5	NH6
p-value	0.00932	0.02202	0.02852	0.00512	0.00512	0.00512

The statistical tests were Two-tailed with 0.05 as a significance level. All the p-values of Table 9 are lower than 0.05, thus the CNN significantly outperformed the LSTM for OSF and for all the MSF strategies which answers the RQ3 and RQ4.

For the RQ5, we notice from Fig. 6, that CNN is maintaining its outperformance over LSTM for OSF and all the MSF strategies.

5.4 Discussion

In [7], a comparative study was conducted between the MSF strategies using the LSTM model. As an extension of this work, we conducted a similar comparative study using a CNN model. Then, we compared the performances of the CNN and LSTM models for the OSF and the five MSF strategies. For the LSTM model, we used the same architecture used in [7] with one LSTM layer and two dense layers. Whereas, for the CNN model, we proposed a new one with one 1D convolutional layer, one Flatten layer and 2 Dense layers.

The first objective was to get the best configuration of the proposed CNN through the tuning of the two hyper-parameters: kernel size and the number of filters. Figure 2 and Fig. 3 show that each of these parameters has an influence on the model's accuracy. Therefore, a careful choice of these parameters is crucial when building a CNN model and other models [7, 19]. Our CNN model performed well in comparison to the performances found in literature and reported in [2]. Indeed, the minimum, maximum and mean of RMSE values for our CNN are 3.66, 16.4 and 8.68 respectively. Furthermore, these results are promising as regards the use of CNN in time series prediction and sequential data in general even though the CNN was traditionally conceived for image processing [4].

The second objective focuses on the evaluation of MSF strategies for the LSTM and CNN models. Toward this aim, five strategies for MSF were developed and compared using the RMSE for both LSTM and CNN. For the LSTM and as reported in [7], none of the five strategies is significantly performing better than the others, however, the non-recursive strategies tend to be better than recursive ones. This trend is not noticed for the CNN: in fact, this latter gives similar performances using these five strategies. Thus, further experiments should be carried out in order to refute or confirm this finding for CNN. In the case of confirmation, other criteria, such as simplicity and computational time, should be taken into consideration to decide on the strategy to use.

The third objective of this study was to perform a comparison between CNN and LSTM. Toward this objective, the performances of the CNN and the LSTM were compared for both OSF and MSF based on the RMSE, then the significance of performance differences are assessed using the Wilcoxon test. The results show that CNN significantly outperformed the LSTM for both OSF and MSF strategies. This can be explained by: 1) the CNN are using a small number of parameters since it uses shared weights [4], 2) there is no recurrent connections in the CNN, contrary to LSTM, which makes the process of training faster [19], and 3) the use of multiple filters in CNN helps to extract more useful features [18].

Finally, the outperformance of the CNN over the LSTM in OSF is maintained for MSF using the five strategies, which is promising as it gives some confidence in case we enlarge the prediction horizon.

6 Threats to Validity

Four threats to our study's validity are considered which are: 1) Internal validity, 2) External validity, 3) Construct validity, and 4) Statistical validity.

6.1 Internal Validity

This threat to validity takes in consideration the evaluation approach. This latter should be appropriate so as the findings of the study are valid. Toward that aim, all the models were trained and tested in different datasets. In fact, 66% of each dataset was used in the training phase while the remaining 34% was used for the evaluation phase.

6.2 External Validity

This concerns the perimeter of the study and its ability to be generalized. To ensure this, we took in a random way the datasets of ten patients from a public dataset. These datasets have different sizes. In fact, the records' number varies from 246 to 923. These datasets were previously used by [3, 7]. Note that in [2], it was reported that, in some studies, only one dataset was used.

6.3 Construct Validity

The performance is the main criterion to compare the considered models, thus it is essential to use a performance measurement that indicates how far the models are performant. In our study, we used the RMSE since it is a performance measurement used commonly in the BGL prediction [2].

6.4 Statistical Validity

In this study, we aim at determining the best model among the proposed ones through their performance's comparison. When a difference between two models is noticed, it is essential to assess statistically this difference. Therefore, we used the Wilcoxon statistical test. Besides, the SRD method is used for ranking.

7 Conclusion and Future Work

In this study, we conducted a comparison between MSF strategies using CNN and LSTM models. For the LSTM model, we used the one that has been developed and evaluated in [3] and [7]. While, for the CNN, we considered the following architecture: 1D convolutional layer, a flatten layer and two dense layers which was tuned based on the two hyper-parameters: number of filters and kernel size. Then, a performance comparison was conducted considering the CNN model and the LSTM model for one-step ahead forecasting and multi-steps ahead forecasting using the five identified MSF strategies.

The main outcomes of this work were: 1) No MSF strategy outperforms the others for CNN nor LSTM, 2) The proposed CNN significantly outperformed the LSTM model for both one-step and multi-steps prediction.

These propitious results motivate further researches in the use of the CNN model taking into consideration different challenges such as: tuning other hyper-parameters, considering other input data such as activities and medication and exploring a larger prediction horizon.

References

1. Bilous, R., Donnelly, R.: Handbook of Diabetes. Wiley, Hoboken (2010)
2. El Idrissi, T., Idri, A., Bakkoury, Z.: Systematic map and review of predictive techniques in diabetes self-management. Int. J. Inf. Manag. **46**, 263–277 (2019)
3. El Idrissi, T., Idri, A., Abnane, I., Bakkoury, Z.: Predicting blood glucose using an LSTM neural network. In: Proceedings of the 2019 Federated Conference on Computer Science and Information Systems. ACSIS, vol. 18, pp. 35–41 (2019)
4. LeCun, Y., Bengio, Y., Hinton, G.: Deep learning. Nature **521**(7553), 436–444 (2015)
5. Taieb, S.B., Bontempi, G., Atiya, A.F., Sorjamaa, A.: A review and comparison of strategies for multi-step ahead time series forecasting based on the NN5 forecasting competition. Expert Syst. Appl. **39**(8), 7067–7083 (2012)
6. An, N.H., Anh, D.T.: Comparison of strategies for multi-step-ahead prediction of time series using neural network. In: 2015 International Conference on Advanced Computing and Applications (ACOMP), pp. 142–149. IEEE, November 2015
7. El Idrissi, T., Idri, A., Kadi, I., Bakkoury, Z.: Strategies of multi-step-ahead forecasting for blood glucose level using LSTM neural networks: a comparative study. In: Proceedings of the 13th International Joint Conference on Biomedical Engineering Systems and Technologies (BIOSTEC 2020) - Volume 5: HEALTHINF, pp. 337–344 (2020)
8. Xie, J., Wang, Q.: Benchmark machine learning approaches with classical time series approaches on the blood glucose level prediction challenge. In: KHD@ IJCAI, pp. 97–102, January 2018
9. Fox, I., Ang, L., Jaiswal, M., Pop-Busui, R., Wiens, J.: Deep multi-output forecasting: learning to accurately predict blood glucose trajectories. In: Proceedings of the 24th ACM SIGKDD International Conference on Knowledge Discovery & Data Mining, pp. 1387–1395. ACM, July 2018
10. Kline, D.M.: Methods for multi-step time series forecasting neural networks. In: Neural Networks in Business Forecasting, pp. 226–250. IGI Global (2004)
11. Sorjamaa, A., Lendasse, A.: Time series prediction using DirRec strategy. In: ESANN, vol. 6, pp. 143–148, April 2006
12. Taieb, S.B., Bontempi, G., Sorjamaa, A., Lendasse, A.: Long-term prediction of time series by combining direct and mimo strategies. In: 2009 International Joint Conference on Neural Networks, pp. 3054–3061. IEEE, June 2009
13. Hochreiter, S., Schmidhuber, J.: Long short-term memory. Neural Comput. **9**(8), 1735–1780 (1997)
14. Fukushima, K., Miyake, S.: Neocognitron: a new algorithm for pattern recognition tolerant of deformations and shifts in position. Pattern Recogn. **15**(6), 455–469 (1982)
15. Hubel, D.H., Wiesel, T.N.: Receptive fields, binocular interaction and functional architecture in the cat's visual cortex. J. Physiol. **160**(1), 106–154 (1962)

16. LeCun, Y., et al.: Handwritten digit recognition with a back-propagation network. In: Proceedings of the Advances in Neural Information Processing Systems, pp. 396–404 (1990)
17. LeCun, Y., Bottou, L., Bengio, Y., Haffner, P.: Gradient-based learning applied to document recognition. Proc. IEEE **86**(11), 2278–2324 (1998)
18. Fawaz, H.I., Forestier, G., Weber, J., Idoumghar, L., Muller, P.A.: Deep learning for time series classification: a review. Data Min. Knowl. Discov. **33**(4), 917–963 (2019)
19. Li, K., Liu, C., Zhu, T., Herrero, P., Georgiou, P.: GluNet: A deep learning framework for accurate glucose forecasting. IEEE J. Biomed. Health Inform. **24**, 414–423 (2019)
20. Woldaregay, A.Z., et al.: Data-driven modeling and prediction of blood glucose dynamics: machine learning applications in type 1 diabetes. In: Artificial Intelligence in Medicine (2019)
21. El Idrissi, T., Idri, A., Bakkoury, Z.: Data mining techniques in diabetes self-management: a systematic map. In: 6th World Conference on Information Systems and Technologies, Naple, pp. 1142–1152, March 2018
22. Simonyan, K., Zisserman, A.: Very deep convolutional networks for large-scale image recognition. In: Proceedings of the International Conference on Learning Representations https://arxiv.org/abs/1409.1556 (2014)
23. Krizhevsky, A., Sutskever, I., Hinton, G.: ImageNet classification with deep convolutional neural networks. In: Proceedings of the Advances in Neural Information Processing Systems 25, pp. 1090–1098 (2012)
24. Girshick, R., Donahue, J., Darrell, T. Malik, J.: Rich feature hierarchies for accurate object detection and semantic segmentation. In: Proceedings of the Conference on Computer Vision and Pattern Recognition, pp. 580–587 (2014)
25. Hinton, G., et al.: Deep neural networks for acoustic modeling in speech recognition. IEEE Sig. Process. Mag. **29**, 82–97 (2012)
26. Sun, Q., Jankovic, M.V., Bally, L., Mougiakakou, S.G.: Predicting blood glucose with an LSTM and Bi-LSTM based deep neural network. In: 2018 14th Symposium on Neural Networks and Applications (NEUREL), pp. 1–5. IEEE, November 2018
27. Zhu, T., Li, K., Herrero, P., Chen, J., Georgiou, P.: A deep learning algorithm for personalized blood glucose prediction. In: KHD@ IJCAI, pp. 64–78 (2018)
28. Mhaskar, H.N., Pereverzyev, S.V., van der Walt, M.D.: A deep learning approach to diabetic blood glucose prediction. Front. Appl. Math. Stat. **3**, 14 (2017)
29. Mirshekarian, S., Bunescu, R., Marling, C., Schwartz, F.: Using LSTMs to learn physiological models of blood glucose behavior. In: 2017 39th Annual International Conference of the IEEE Engineering in Medicine and Biology Society (EMBC), pp. 2887–2891. IEEE, July 2017
30. Doike, T., Hayashi, K., Arata, S., Mohammad, K.N., Kobayashi, A., Niitsu, K.: A blood glucose level prediction system using machine learning based on recurrent neural network for hypoglycemia prevention. In: 2018 16th IEEE International New Circuits and Systems Conference (NEWCAS), pp. 291–295. IEEE, June 2018
31. DirecNet: Diabetes Research in Children Network (2019). https://direcnet.jaeb.org/Studies.aspx. Accessed 1 Apr 2019
32. Idri, A., Abnane, I., Abran, A.: Missing data techniques in analogy-based software development effort estimation. J. Syst. Softw. **117**, 595–611 (2016)
33. Héberger, K.: Sum of ranking differences compares methods or models fairly. TrAC Trends Anal. Chem. **29**(1), 101–109 (2010)
34. Hosni, M., Idri, A., Abran, A.: Investigating heterogeneous ensembles with filter feature selection for software effort estimation. In: Proceedings of the 27th International Workshop on Software Measurement and 12th International Conference on Software Process and Product Measurement, pp. 207–220, October 2017

Cognitive Internet of Medical Things Architecture for Decision Support Tool to Detect Early Sepsis Using Deep Learning

Mahbub Ul Alam(✉) and Rahim Rahmani

Department of Computer and Systems Sciences, Stockholm University, Stockholm, Sweden
{mahbub,rahim}@dsv.su.se

Abstract. The internet of medical things (IoMT) is a relatively new territory for the internet of things (IoT) platforms where we can obtain a significant amount of potential benefits with the combination of cognitive computing. Effective utilization of the healthcare data is the critical factor in achieving such potential, which can be a significant challenge as the medical data is extraordinarily heterogeneous and spread across different devices with different degrees of importance and authority. To address this issue, in this paper, we introduce a cognitive internet of medical things architecture with a use case of early sepsis detection using electronic health records. We discuss the various aspects of IoMT architecture. Based on the discussion, we posit that the proposed architecture could improve the overall performance and usability in the IoMT platforms in particular for different IoMT based services and applications. The use of an RNN-LSTM network for early prediction of sepsis according to Sepsis-3 criteria is evaluated with the empirical investigation using six different time window sizes. The best result is obtained from a model using a four-hour window with the assumption that data is missing-not-at-random. It is observed that when learning from heterogeneous sequences of sparse medical data for early prediction of sepsis, the size of the time window has a considerable impact on predictive performance.

Keywords: IoT · Cognitive computing · Internet of Medical Things · Edge computing · Early prediction · Machine learning · Deep learning · Health informatics · Healthcare analytics

1 Introduction

The internet of medical things (IoMT) can be summarized as a coalition of different healthcare related physical entities to perform the tasks of healthcare applications [18]. Healthcare information is connected, utilizing various network technologies [7]. The goal here is to develop an integrated healthcare system that is more dynamic, less costly, and more individual patient-centric compared to

X. Ye et al. (Eds.): BIOSTEC 2020, CCIS 1400, pp. 366–384, 2021.
https://doi.org/10.1007/978-3-030-72379-8_18

the traditional healthcare systems now [9]. Unnecessary hospital visits could be restricted, and exchanging sensitive and critical healthcare information can be exchanged among different healthcare institutions in a realtime fashion, which is extremely important in treating critical patients and immediate interventions [16]. It must be noted that, by promoting IoMT, we do not intend to replace the current healthcare systems; instead, we are proposing an external mechanism for exchanging and analyzing medical data in a robust and secured fashion [4]. We hope to ensure an improved diagnosis, which will provide better treatment and management opportunities for different stakeholders in healthcare systems.

The key challenges to make healthcare data more useful are the robust integration of different medical devices, and efficient management in the inventory sectors [13]. The architectural flexibility should be taken into account to solve these challenges in the IoMT systems design. With the ever-increasing availability of big (medical) data nowadays, the principal question we should address is how data can be converted into information on a realtime basis and with minimal human processing as possible? We must not exhaust the healthcare professionals with a plethora of information, instead, with the help of artificial intelligence, deep learning, machine learning, data analytics, and data visualization, IoMT systems should suggest only the most essential physiological anomalies, salient trends, and early prediction of the critical cases if possible [8]. If these can be done efficiently, then the current diagnosis processes can be done relatively fast, and it will ensure that the existing workflow in the healthcare institutes remains the same.

Efficient interoperability among various IoMT equipment can ensure robust and realtime data transmission [3,5]. Cognitive computing can help us in this regard as it can improve the current internet of things (internet of medical things in our case) with the utilization and application of self-learning and self-adaptation mechanisms [1,24]. These mechanisms ensure scalability and provide deep insights regarding the relevant extraction of data [23]. Therefore, with the effective utilization of the cognitive internet of medical things (CIoMT) architecture, intelligent service, and autonomous operation execution could be viable. The self-learning based on interactions with different devices and new data provides the opportunity to improve the overall system gradually and gradually accumulate and analyze information from all possible angles with minimal human interaction. This information accumulation and analysis are vital in healthcare applications, as well as symptom-related information, different hereditary, and demography-related information can also provide insights while diagnosing patients [26]. CIoMT, with the integration of machine learning analytics and data visualization components along with a clinical decision support tool, can ease this diagnosis process. One trendy example of this clinical decision support tool is early sepsis detection [11,12,25].

Sepsis is a medical condition due to the body's reaction or response to an infection. It can be attributed as one of the primary reasons for hospital morbidity and mortality [30]. Early appropriate antimicrobial treatment is the key to survival here [10], immediate decision-making is vital, which depends on the early detection of sepsis in patients. Mortality increases by 7.6% for delay of every hour in antimicrobial treatment after the sepsis onset [21], and mortality decreases with fast antimicrobial treatment response [27]. Diagnosis early detection of sepsis remains a challenge as standardization of diagnostic tests is yet to be well-acknowledged [30], and sepsis detection symptoms can also be associated with other clinical conditions [20].

Recently supervised machine learning is widely used for early detection of sepsis using large-scale annotated medical data [6,11,12,25]. In this study, we used long short-term memory based recurrent neural network (RNN-LSTM) [17] for early prediction of sepsis learning from electronic health records (EHR) data. EHR data are obtained from different medical facilities as they keep the patient records in a digital format. The data is extremely heterogeneous, including patient demographic information, diagnoses, laboratory test results, medication prescriptions, clinical notes, and medical images. Data quality, annotation of class labels, and extreme heterogeneity make it very difficult to create machine learning and deep learning-based models based on EHR data [34]. We investigated different temporal representations which divide the longitudinal EHR data into time windows of different sizes. Previous works use the time window size of length one without providing empirical justification. We posit that window size should have an insightful impact on the length of the sequence and the amount of missing data in that sequence. Therefore handling the length of the window size and missingness should be investigated. If we increase the length of the window size, we need to think of effective summarization techniques and superior missingness handling techniques. We analyzed these aspects to provide an effective decision support tool for early sepsis detection with the proposed CIoMT architecture. Our contribution can be summarized as follows,

- A cognitive internet of medical things (CIoMT) architecture is proposed to deploy the early sepsis detection clinical supporting tool on a realtime basis. We posit that, through the effective utilization of this architecture, the detection process will be robust, fast, and, thus, more effective in realtime cases.
- An RNN-LSTM model is used to model the different representations of longitudinal EHR data and predict early sepsis detection. We have observed that the time window size has a notable impact on overall predictive performance.
- Missingness is considered a random (data missing-at-random) and a non-random (data missing-not-at-random) phenomenon. We used standard averaging technique for the random case and generative adversarial imputation nets (GAIN) [35] for non-random case to model the missingness. We have observed that better performance is achieved using the later approach.

This study can be viewed as an extension of the works described in [2]. The novelty in this study compared to [2] are as follows,

- An additional cognitive internet of medical things (CIoMT) architecture is proposed to deploy the early sepsis detection clinical supporting tool.
- A completely different dataset [19] is used for all the experiments.

- Generative adversarial imputation nets (GAIN) [35] is used for non-random case to model the missingness instead of the non-random-placeholder imputation approach used in [2].

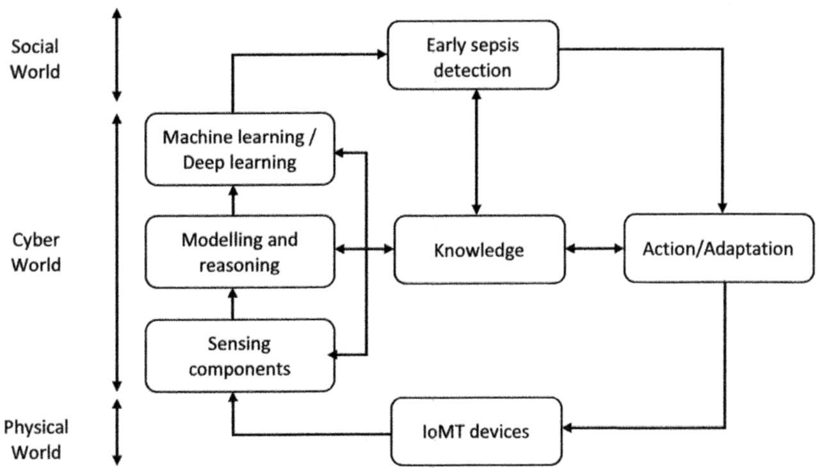

Fig. 1. Knowledge-centric cognitive IoMT architecture.

2 Cognitive IoMT Architecture for Early Sepsis Detection

Inspired by [33] we are proposing the knowledge-centric cognitive architecture described in Fig. 1. In this architecture, the cognitive computing system's central element is in the cyber world that connects the physical world with the social world. The cognitive computing system is made of three components.

- **Sensing Components.** Acquire the critical information relevant to the context of the IoMT devices, and allows the elaboration of the physical world's meta-model.
- **Modeling and Reasoning.** Use the sensed information to build models, which will serve afterward to elaborate physical and semantic reasoning.
- **Machine Learning.** Advanced learning algorithms build on the existing semantic models to provide systems with self-learning capabilities.

From the IoMT perspective, the primary focus should be given in successful acquisition, aggregation, and transmission of medical data from different sources. Medical data can come from different sources, along with EHRs. Figure 2 is illustrating the different kinds of medical data. It is vital to create a robust IoMT architecture to ensure this.

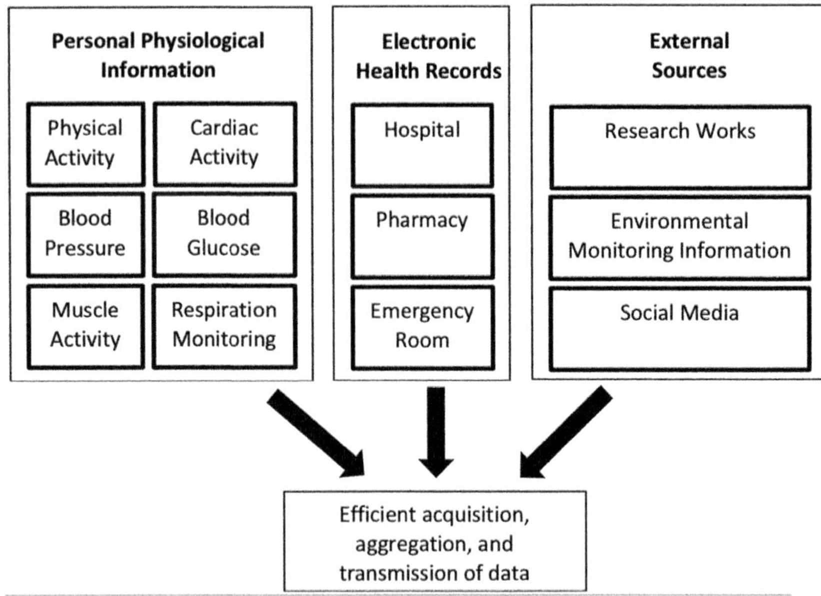

Fig. 2. Different kinds of medical data.

Figure 3 is describing such robust CIoMT architecture. By using edge and cloud frameworks, the successful integrated medical data can be analyzed using data and process cognitive engines. The knowledge-centric implementation of data and process engines is described in Fig. 1.

3 EHR Data

We used EHRs from the MIMIC-III (Multiparameter Intelligent Monitoring in Intensive Care) database, version 1.4 [19]. It comprises over 58,000 hospital admissions of over 45,000 patients between June 2001 and October 2012.

3.1 Data Selection

Acknowledging the suggestions from [30], patients older than 15 years were selected up to first sepsis onset, discharge, or death and before it of maximum 48 h. We denote one such instance in the dataset as a care episode as maximum 48 h before the first sepsis onset time.

3.2 Sepsis Definition

Sepsis is defined by the Sepsis-3 clinical criteria [28,30]. Sepsis-3 criteria is the combination of *suspected infection*, and *organ dysfunction* [28,30]. If at least two

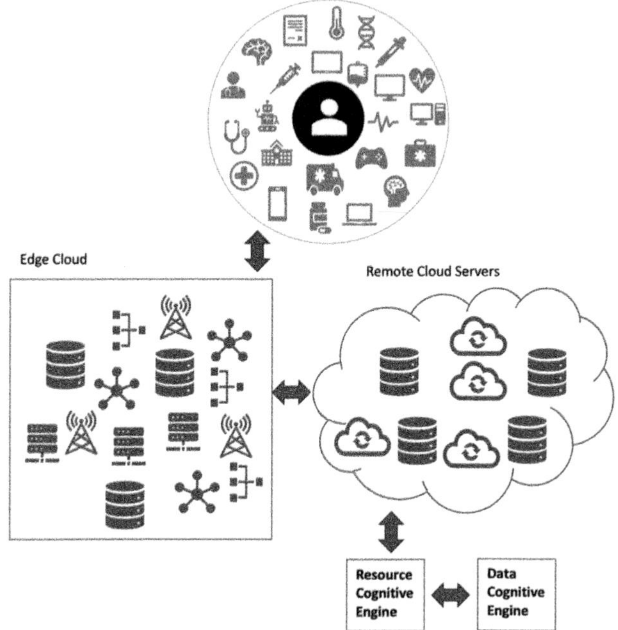

Fig. 3. Proposed CIoMT architecture.

doses of antimicrobial treatment are newly administered within a certain period and any culture is taken, then this is considered as *suspected infection*. The conditions are as follows, If antimicrobial treatment was initiated first, cultures had to be collected within 24 h. If cultures were collected first, antimicrobial treatment had to be started within 72 h after the cultures. An increase in sequential organ failure assessment (SOFA) score [32] by greater than or equal to 2 points compared to the baseline is defined as *Organ dysfunction*. It is measured 48 h before to 24 h after the onset of *suspected infection*. The latest value measured before the 72-h time window is defined as the baseline SOFA score. This is assumed to be 0 in patients not known to have a pre-existing *organ dysfunction*.

The first time-window when both *organ dysfunction* and *suspected infection* criteria are met is regarded as the sepsis onset time. We use a fixed-length time window to represent the temporality of EHR data. Therefore, we denote time zero as the particular time window in which sepsis onset occurs.

3.3 Care Episode Representation

Care episodes are transformed into sequences based on a given window (bin) size to account for the temporality of the data. Six different window sizes: 1, 2, 3, 4, 6, and 8 h are chosen to conduct experiments. Figure 5 provides an illustration regarding the implementation of a care episode based on different time windows.

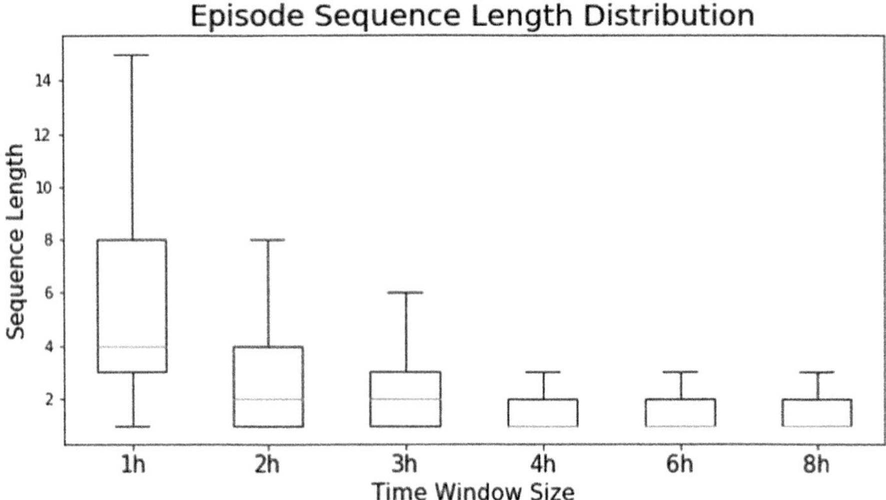

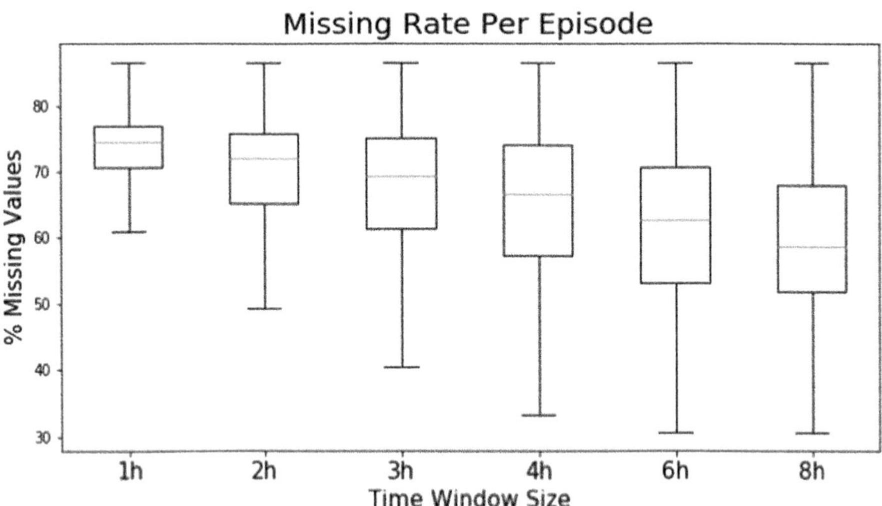

Fig. 4. Distribution of sequence length (top) and episode-wise missing rate with different time window sizes (bottom).

A time window can have multiple values for a particular variable, or it can be missing entirely. The average value is chosen from multiple such values in a time window. To handle the missing data, an essential decision is needed to be taken regarding the randomness in missing values. It could be missing-at-random or missing not-at-random [31]. We accounted for both possibilities. Missing data imputation is carried out using a generative adversarial network (based) technique [35] when data is assumed to be missing not-at-random. The

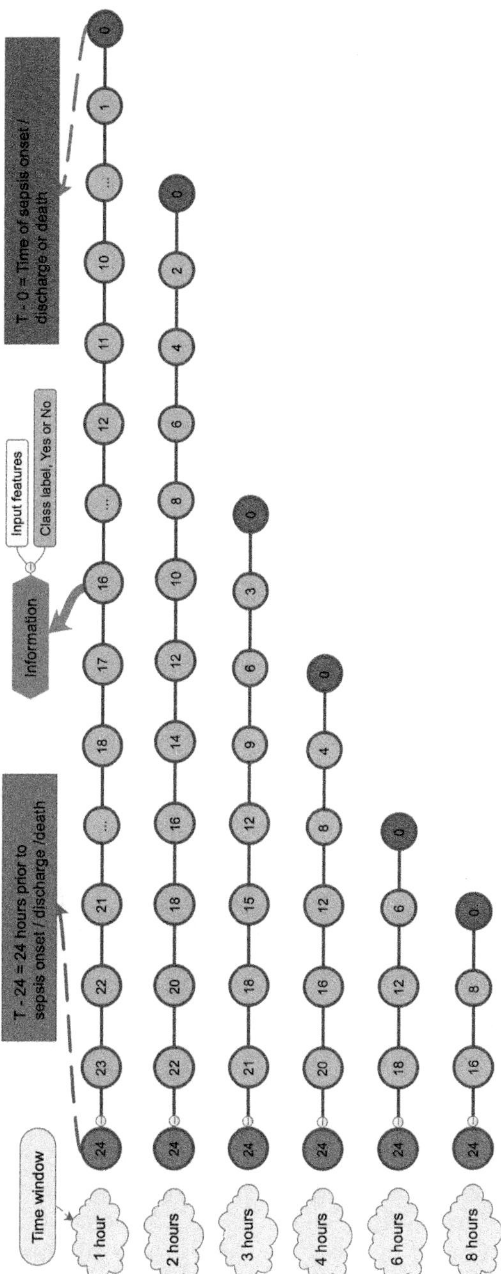

Fig. 5. Representation of a care episode of total length 24 h using different time windows.

following simple imputation strategy was carried out when data is assumed to be missing-at-random; the present value for a particular feature is carried forward to subsequent windows until another observed value is encountered, which is then carried forward on. It is imputed as a global mean of all the values in the data of a feature if there is no value for that given feature in a care episode.

Distribution of care episode lengths with different time window sizes and the episode-wise missing rate is shown in Fig. 4. We can observe a high variance in sequence length and missingness. We can also observe that the smaller time windows generate longer sequences and a higher rate of missingness compared to the larger time windows.

3.4 Feature Selection

Features are collected as demographic, vital, and lab data from the EHRs. Table 1 provides a list of all the features used in this study. We have excluded the variables which have a more than ninety percent missingness in the data in every time window based data.

4 Methods

Two deep learning methods are used in this study. Using hierarchical representations of input features, from lower-level compositions to higher-level compositions, a deep learning model learns from the input data features. This type of abstraction at multiple levels automatically allows learning features using the complex formation of functions, which map the input to the output straightforwardly without any need for human feature engineering [14].

A generative adversarial imputation network (GAIN) [35] is used to impute the missing data assuming it is missing not-at-random. We used a long short-term memory based recurrent neural network (RNN-LSTM) [17] to model the different representations of longitudinal EHR data and predict-early detection of sepsis.

4.1 Generative Adversarial Imputation Nets (GAIN)

GAIN [35] is a generalization of the generative adversarial networks (GAN) [15]. In GAIN, the generator aims to impute missing data accurately, and the discriminator aims to minimize the classification loss. In turn, the generator tries to maximize the misclassification rate of the discriminator. Thus it adapts the standard GAN architecture and provides additional information as 'hints' to ensure that the desired target is the result of this adversarial process. It has been observed that GAIN provides favorable results even when the input data contains missing values in a significant portion [35].

Table 1. List of the input features.

Vital	Laboratory
Systolic Blood Pressure	Albumin
Diastolic Blood Pressure	Bands (Immature Neutrophils)
	Bicarbonate
Mean Blood Pressure	Bilirubin
Respiratory Rate	Creatinine
Heart Rate	Chloride
SpO2 (Pulsoxymetry)	Sodium
Temperature Celsius	Potassium
Cardiac Output	Lactate
Tidal Volume Set	Hematocrit
Tidal Volume Observed	Hemoglobin
Tidal Volume Spontaneous	Platelet Count
Peak Inspiratory Pressure	Partial Thromboplastin Time
Total Peep Level	INR (Standardized Quick)
O2 flow	Blood Urea Nitrogen
FiO2 (Fraction of Inspired Oxygen)	White Blood Cells
Demographic	Creatine Kinase
Gender	Creatine Kinase MB
Admission Age	Fibrinogen
Ethnicity	Lactate Dehydrogenase
Admission Type	Magnesium
Admission Location	Calcium (free)
	pO2 Bloodgas
	pH Bloodgas
	pCO2 Bloodgas
	SO2 Bloodgas
	Glucose
	Troponin T
	Prothrombin Time (Quick)

4.2 RNN-LSTM Model

RNN-LSTM models can retain information from previous inputs in their internal memory. If needed, it also can learn from a very distant past if the information is relevant by using different gated cells (input, forget, and output) where these cells determine what information to store and what information to erase [17]. Therefore, we consider this model for performing the task to predict sepsis as early as possible based on current and past information in a given care episode.

This choice is also relevant from a clinical perspective, as typically clinical measurements and observations closer to the outcome are of higher importance.

4.3 Experimental Setup

We split the dataset into 80% for training, 10% for tuning, and 10% for testing and evaluating the tuned models. We stratify the data in each split using an equal probabilistic distribution concerning both class and sequence length; therefore, we discarded care episodes of a sequence length with five or fewer instances. We labeled positive classes or cases as care episodes in which Sepsis-3 criteria were fulfilled and comprise data from admission to sepsis onset.

Due to two approaches to handling missing values: mean imputation, and GAN imputation, we created twelve different versions of the dataset based on six different time window sizes (1h, 2h, 3h, 4h, 6h, and 8h). The model predicts a probability score regarding the presence or absence of sepsis in the patient based on current and previous information in the care episode in each time window.

We used the area under the receiver operating characteristic curve (AUROC) to evaluate the model performance. AUROC is the probability that the model will assign a larger score to the positive than to the negative episode.

Table 2 presents the hyper-parameters of the RNN-LSTM model, and the GAIN model. We chose one hundred data points to tune these parameters to search the space more effectively instead of doing a grid search in some restricted hyperparameter space. We used an oversampling method to make the distribution even (50% positive, and 50% negative) in each minibatch. We selected the tuning set with the model with the best AUROC and used the specific hyper-parameters of that model to evaluate the test set.

We evaluate earliness as the average prediction times relative to sepsis onset (in hours) for true positives with the standard decision threshold of >0.5 as a single positive prediction per care episode, retaining the first one and ignoring predictions in subsequent windows. We used three evaluation settings here:

1. <12 h before sepsis onset
2. <24 h before sepsis onset
3. <48 h before sepsis onset

Our motivation to use different settings is to restrict extremely early evaluations as they may not be that much clinically relevant.

4.4 Experiments

We carried out a series of experiments using an RNN-LSTM model for early prediction of sepsis, centered around the use of different time window sizes for representing the temporally evolving EHR data. We posit that the time window size affects (i) sequence length and (ii) missingness. We investigated the impact of these factors on the predictive performance of the RNN-LSTM model with two different approaches to handle the missing values. We conducted the following five experiments.

Table 2. Neural Network Parameters.

Name	Values/Range
Alpha	$0, 10^{-4}$
Beta one	$0, 1{-}10^{-1}$
Beta two	$0, 1{-}10^{-3}$
Hidden layers	2, 3, 4
Neurons	64, 128, 256
Drop out	0, 10, 20, 30, 40, 50, 60, 70
Epochs	1,2
Mini-batch	100
Classification function	log-softmax
Optimizer	Adam optimizer
GAIN alpha	0.1, 1, 10, 100
GAIN mini-batch	512
GAIN hint rate	0.9
GAIN total iterations	15000

Experiment 1: Different Time Window Sizes. We investigated the impact of using different window sizes on the predictive performance of the resulting model.

Experiment 2: Handling Missing Values. We investigated two imputation techniques for the missing data. For the missing not-at-random case, we used a GAN based imputation technique (GAN imputation). For the missing-at-random case, we used a simple imputation strategy based on carrying forward existing values and globally mean-imputing values that are absent at the beginning of a care episode (mean imputation). We evaluated these two approaches for each of the six time window sizes, i.e., with different degrees of missingness.

Experiment 3: Performance at Different Time Points. We evaluate the predictive performance in terms of AUROC at different time points relative to sepsis onset, starting from 24 h before onset.

Experiment 4: Evaluation of Earliness. Earliness is regarded as the time points true positive predictions are made relative to sepsis onset, for the best LSTM model. We showed this with a combination of overall AUROC scores for the particular time window size.

Experiment 5: Performance with Different Sequences Lengths. We analyzed the predictive performance in terms of area under the precision-recall curve (AUPRC) score on care episodes of different sequence lengths. We tried to learn how the best model copes with heterogeneous care episodes in terms of length of hospital stay with this experiment.

Table 3. Earliness performance in average hours before sepsis onset combined with AUROC, using test dataset, GAN and mean imputation of missing values, using different time window sizes.

Window size	GAN imputation				Mean imputation			
	Average earliness			AUROC	Average earliness			AUROC
	<12 h	<24 h	<48 h		<12 h	<24 h	<48 h	
1	2.11	3.25	4.92	87.28	4.06	7.83	6.18	84.48
2	1.19	1.19	1.62	86.65	3.6	6.47	4.25	81.39
3	0.72	1.52	1.88	86.75	1.07	1.4	2.8	79.94
4	0.64	0.88	1.98	88.54	0.97	0.97	2.13	82.28
6	0.12	0.12	0.12	83.02	0.92	2.57	4.4	53.36
8	0.3	0.3	0.3	78.07	0	3.08	3.08	58.98

5 Results

In this section, We present the results of the above experiments in terms of (i) predictive performance at different time points, (ii) earliness of true positive predictions, and (iii) predictive performance for episodes of different sequence lengths.

5.1 Temporal Analysis

We present the overall predictive performance without a specific decision threshold, in terms of AUROC, of the different models at different time points relative to sepsis onset – from as early as 24 h to sepsis onset time in Fig. 6. As can be seen, the RNN-LSTM models' performance naturally drops further from sepsis onset and does so quite rapidly. The RNN-LSTM models with GAN imputation generally perform better up to six hours before the sepsis onset time. The best results come from using a four-hour time window, with GAN imputation: at sepsis onset, the AUROC is 88.54%. The size of the window has a significant impact on the predictive performance of the resulting models. In general, assuming that data is missing not at random leads to better predictive performance compared to assuming that data are missing at random. However, the difference is generally smaller compared to the size of the time window.

5.2 Earliness

We show the average distribution of earliness (in hours) for true positive predictions of the models with different time window sizes and GAN and mean imputation in Table 3. Earliness results are reported for the three evaluation settings (<12 h, <24 h, and <48 h). The best result comes from a 1-h time window size in the mean imputation approach, 6.18 h before the sepsis onset time with a <48 h setting. We also present the overall AUROC scores of the models.

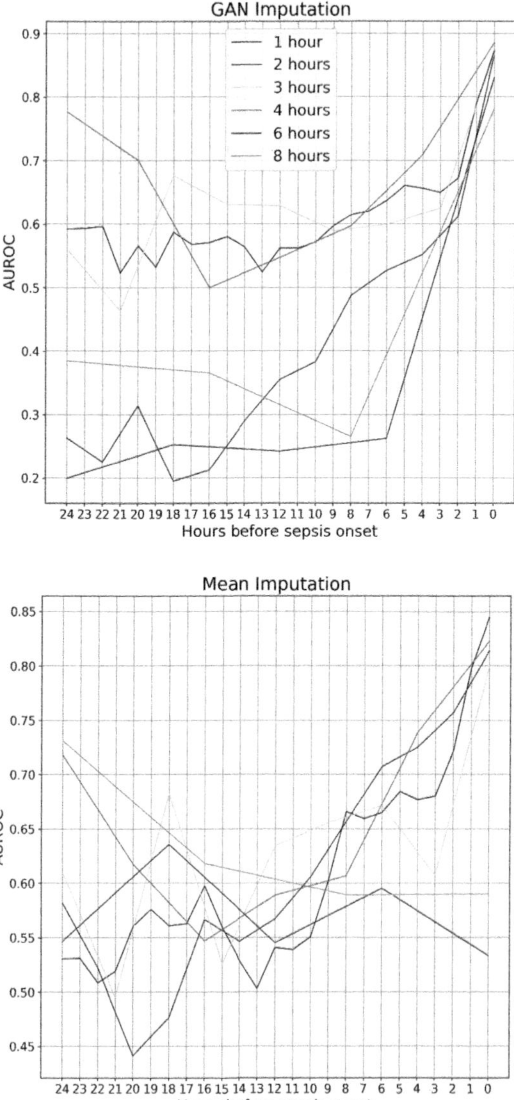

Fig. 6. AUROC for each model, using test dataset, as a function of the number of hours prior to sepsis onset/discharge. The models are colored according to the legend in the top plot.

5.3 Episode Sequence Length

We evaluate the model's predictive performance concerning sequence length as using different time window sizes has a significant impact on the length of sequences that constitute the care episodes. In Fig. 7, the AUPRC score cal-

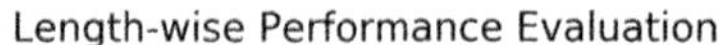

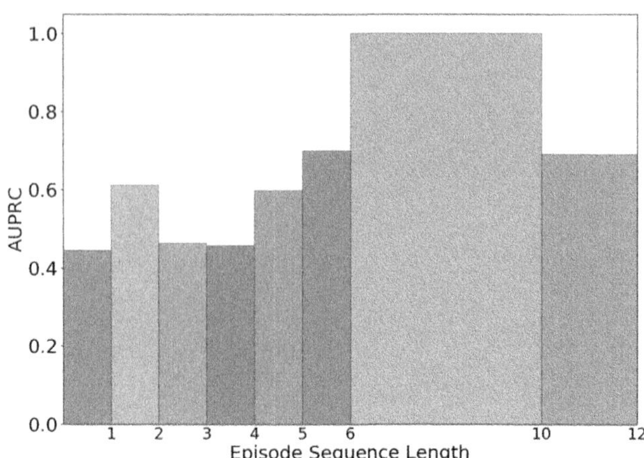

Fig. 7. Prediction performance of the best RNN-LSTM model (4 h time window, GAN imputation, evaluation setting <48 h) for episodes with different sequence lengths using the test dataset. Each bin is created such that it contains at least 10 test instances. The analysis is carried out using AUPRC score.

culated as a local scope of evaluation (described in Sect. 4.4) at the sepsis onset time (time zero) of our best model is shown. The care episodes in the test set are binned in such a way that each bin contains at least 10 test instances. In general, the model performs better on longer care episodes.

6 Discussion

We can categorize the current IoMT architectures into three primary layers, collection, transmission, and analysis. The collection layer collects and integrates information mostly through the sensors using a body area network (BAN). The gateway then sends the information to the cloud using the transmission layer. Finally, the analysis layer (usually located in the cloud) stores, visualizes, and analyzes the data and sends feedback regarding the analysis [16].

Although the IoMT devices have brought convenience to all the stakeholders in the healthcare sectors, some potential problems can be observed,

- Communication latency can increase significantly during the medical data sending time from BAN sensors to the cloud. This latency could be a problem when immediate intervention or response is required, such as early sepsis detection tasks [29].
- There is a possibility of wastage of resources if the IoMT architecture is fixed or static. It is also relatively difficult to make it more personalized according to the patient's or stakeholders customized needs [29].

Cognitive computing [1,23,24] with the successful integration of machine learning, deep learning, artificial intelligence, and natural language processing is, therefore, a promising choice for effective disease detection, pattern recognition, and deploying realtime automated decision support tools using medical data. We can also address the problems mentioned above with the successful integration of edge-based architectures as it has shown promising results [29].

To solve the above problems and thoroughly combine the various advantages of cognitive computing and edge computing, in this paper, we propose cognitive computing-based IoMT architecture for providing a decision support tool to detect sepsis early.

Rather than proposing a novel deep learning model, in this study, the key aim was to investigate time window size, and imputation of missing value to evaluate whether the empirical difference can improve the performance or not. Current state-of-the-art models [11,12,25] use one-hour time window. They treat missing data as missing-at-random without providing any theoretical or empirical justification. Therefore, extensive investigation into these matters was carried out. The effect of different sequence lengths in the prediction performance was also investigated.

We demonstrate the impact of the time window size on the predictive performance of the model. Therefore time window size selection should be justified either empirically or from a clinical point of view while designing a prediction model. It has been observed that the overall best predictive performance is achieved using a four hour time window.

It should be noted that data in the clinical setting is often should be considered as missing-not-at-random, which is not reflected in the previous studies as missingness is considered as a random phenomenon there and therefore modeled using the multitask gaussian process (MGP) adapters [11,12,25]. We can obtain important information about the condition of the patient or the treating physician's assessment in the form of missingness. How a missing value should be taken care of can also depend on different healthcare institutions' practices. If one is taken regularly in one place, and in another place, that value is only measured if it is urgent, then the missingness of that value should not be imputed globally. Our primary observation supports this notion as using generative adversarial networks (GAN) based technique provides better performance.

Previous studies [11,12,25] use the AUROC evaluation metric to predict the performance, which is a common practice in deep learning. AUROC is measured on a continuum of threshold values for the classification of patients into sepsis and no sepsis, providing a global view of predictive performance. If we want to deploy the model in a realtime setting, then we should tune the model according to the circumstances and prerequisites of the medical institution in which it will be used. We should optimize the decision threshold according to one or more performance metrics. This optimization should be based on clinical needs. False-positive tolerance is one important such example. In our study, a decision threshold of >0.5 for positive predictions was used, and it was only allowed one positive prediction per episode. We should also explore alternative ways not limiting to using a different decision threshold only. We may allow the model to make multiple predictions and silence the model for some period following a false positive, manually, by a clinical expert. We can also observe from the result that when evaluating the model from a general perspective and when employing the model in a specific manner, the optimal window sizes are different. Therefore, window size also needs to be considered in this case.

In the future, we will try to modify the neural network-based architecture based on the insights we obtained from this study, as described above. The explainability of the model is a crucial issue here as this can be utilized by different stakeholders [22]. In the future, we will also explore this explainability issue.

7 Conclusions

We proposed a cognitive internet of medical things architecture and discussed the different implementing and usability related aspects of it with a use case of early sepsis detection using electronic health records. We posited through our discussion that this architecture could provide better results in various healthcare sectors for different use cases. Missingness and different time window sizes in EHR data were investigated for the early sepsis detection task with an RNN-LSTM based deep learning model. We observed that improvement in the predictive performance could depend on the appropriate time window. It was also observed that missingness considered as a random phenomenon and subsequent modeling of it using generative adversarial networks could provide better predictive performance. In the future, we will try to implement the cognitive internet of medical things architecture to demonstrate its practicality and usability.

References

1. Afzal, A., et al.: The cognitive internet of things: a unified perspective. Mob. Netw. Appl. **20**(1), 72–85 (2015)
2. Alam, M.U., Henriksson, A., Karlsson Valik, J., Ward, L., Naucler, P., Dalianis, H.: Deep learning from heterogeneous sequences of sparse medical data for early prediction of sepsis. In: 13th International Joint Conference on Biomedical Engineering Systems and Technologies, Valletta, Malta, 24–26 February 2020, vol. 5, pp. 45–55. SciTePress (2020)
3. Bahga, A., Madisetti, V.K.: Healthcare data integration and informatics in the cloud. Computer **48**(2), 50–57 (2015)
4. Behera, R.K., Bala, P.K., Dhir, A.: The emerging role of cognitive computing in healthcare: a systematic literature review. Int. J. Med. Inform. **129**, 154–166 (2019)
5. Coccoli, M., Maresca, P.: Adopting cognitive computing solutions in healthcare. J. e-Learn. Knowl. Soc. **14**(1) (2018)
6. Delahanty, R.J., Alvarez, J., Flynn, L.M., Sherwin, R.L., Jones, S.S.: Development and evaluation of a machine learning model for the early identification of patients at risk for sepsis. Ann. Emerg. Med. **73**, 334–344 (2019)

7. Dimitrov, D.V.: Medical internet of things and big data in healthcare. Healthcare Inform. Res. **22**(3), 156–163 (2016)
8. Durga, S., Nag, R., Daniel, E.: Survey on machine learning and deep learning algorithms used in internet of things (IoT) healthcare. In: 2019 3rd International Conference on Computing Methodologies and Communication (ICCMC), pp. 1018–1022. IEEE (2019)
9. Estrela, V.V., Monteiro, A.C.B., França, R.P., Iano, Y., Khelassi, A., Razmjooy, N.: Health 4.0: applications, management, technologies and review. Med. Technol. J. **2**(4), 262–276 (2018)
10. Ferrer, R., et al.: Empiric antibiotic treatment reduces mortality in severe sepsis and septic shock from the first hour: results from a guideline-based performance improvement program. Crit. Care Med. **42**(8), 1749–1755 (2014)
11. Futoma, J., Hariharan, S., Heller, K.: Learning to detect sepsis with a multitask Gaussian process RNN classifier. In: Proceedings of the 34th International Conference on Machine Learning, vol. 70, pp. 1174–1182. JMLR.org (2017)
12. Futoma, J., et al.: An improved multi-output gaussian process RNN with real-time validation for early sepsis detection. In: Doshi-Velez, F., Fackler, J., Kale, D., Ranganath, R., Wallace, B., Wiens, J. (eds.) Proceedings of the 2nd Machine Learning for Healthcare Conference. Proceedings of Machine Learning Research, Boston, Massachusetts, vol. 68, pp. 243–254. PMLR, 18–19 August 2017. http://proceedings.mlr.press/v68/futoma17a.html
13. Gatouillat, A., Badr, Y., Massot, B., Sejdić, E.: Internet of medical things: a review of recent contributions dealing with cyber-physical systems in medicine. IEEE Internet of Things J. **5**(5), 3810–3822 (2018)
14. Goodfellow, I., Bengio, Y., Courville, A.: Deep Learning. MIT Press, Cambridge (2016)
15. Goodfellow, I., et al.: Generative adversarial nets. In: Advances in Neural Information Processing Systems, pp. 2672–2680 (2014)
16. Habibzadeh, H., Dinesh, K., Shishvan, O.R., Boggio-Dandry, A., Sharma, G., Soyata, T.: A survey of healthcare internet-of-things (HIoT): a clinical perspective. IEEE Internet of Things J. **7**, 53–71 (2019)
17. Hochreiter, S., Schmidhuber, J.: Long short-term memory. Neural Comput. **9**(8), 1735–1780 (1997)
18. Irfan, M., Ahmad, N.: Internet of medical things: architectural model, motivational factors and impediments. In: 2018 15th Learning and Technology Conference (L&T), pp. 6–13. IEEE (2018)
19. Johnson, A.E., Stone, D.J., Celi, L.A., Pollard, T.J.: The mimic code repository: enabling reproducibility in critical care research. J. Am. Med. Inform. Assoc. **25**(1), 32–39 (2018)
20. Jones, A.E., et al.: Lactate clearance vs central venous oxygen saturation as goals of early sepsis therapy: a randomized clinical trial. Jama **303**(8), 739–746 (2010)
21. Kumar, A., et al.: Duration of hypotension before initiation of effective antimicrobial therapy is the critical determinant of survival in human septic shock. Crit. Care Med. **34**(6), 1589–1596 (2006)
22. Lipton, Z.C.: The doctor just won't accept that! arXiv preprint arXiv:1711.08037 (2017)
23. Mishra, N., Lin, C.C., Chang, H.T.: A cognitive adopted framework for IoT big-data management and knowledge discovery prospective. Int. J. Distrib. Sens. Netw. **11**(10), 718390 (2015)
24. Modha, D.S., Ananthanarayanan, R., Esser, S.K., Ndirango, A., Sherbondy, A.J., Singh, R.: Cognitive computing. Commun. ACM **54**(8), 62–71 (2011)

25. Moor, M., Horn, M., Rieck, B., Roqueiro, D., Borgwardt, K.: Early recognition of sepsis with Gaussian process temporal convolutional networks and dynamic time warping. arXiv preprint arXiv:1902.01659 (2019)
26. Pagola-Lorz, I., et al.: Epidemiological study and genetic characterization of inherited muscle diseases in a northern Spanish region. Orphanet J. Rare Dis. **14**(1), 276 (2019)
27. Seymour, C.W., et al.: Time to treatment and mortality during mandated emergency care for sepsis. N. Engl. J. Med. **376**(23), 2235–2244 (2017)
28. Seymour, C.W., et al.: Assessment of clinical criteria for sepsis: for the Third International Consensus Definitions for Sepsis and Septic Shock (Sepsis-3). JAMA **315**(8), 762–774 (2016)
29. Shi, W., Dustdar, S.: The promise of edge computing. Computer **49**(5), 78–81 (2016)
30. Singer, M., et al.: The third international consensus definitions for sepsis and septic shock (Sepsis-3). JAMA **315**(8), 801–810 (2016)
31. Steele, A.J., Denaxas, S.C., Shah, A.D., Hemingway, H., Luscombe, N.M.: Machine learning models in electronic health records can outperform conventional survival models for predicting patient mortality in coronary artery disease. PloS One **13**(8), e0202344 (2018)
32. Vincent, J.L., et al.: The sofa (sepsis-related organ failure assessment) score to describe organ dysfunction/failure. Intensive Care Med. **22**(7), 707–710 (1996)
33. Wu, Q., Ding, G., Xu, Y., Feng, S., Du, Z., Wang, J., Long, K.: Cognitive internet of things: a new paradigm beyond connection. IEEE Internet of Things J. **1**(2), 129–143 (2014)
34. Xiao, C., Choi, E., Sun, J.: Opportunities and challenges in developing deep learning models using electronic health records data: a systematic review. J. Am. Med. Inform. Assoc. **25**(10), 1419–1428 (2018)
35. Yoon, J., Jordon, J., Van Der Schaar, M.: Gain: missing data imputation using generative adversarial nets. arXiv preprint arXiv:1806.02920 (2018)

Interoperability Evaluation in Building Automation and Health Smart Homes Using Tag-Based Semantic Frameworks

Bastian Wollschlaeger(✉), Elke Eichenberg, and Klaus Kabitzsch

Chair of Technical Information Systems, Technische Universität Dresden, 01062 Dresden, Germany
{bastian.wollschlaeger,elke.eichenberg,klaus.kabitzsch}@tu-dresden.de

Abstract. In recent years, Component-based Automation Systems have been increasingly used in office buildings and the residential context, which enabled innovative solutions in areas like Building Automation Systems and Health Smart Homes. However, with an abundance of heterogeneous automation components available, the engineering process is becoming increasingly complex and needs to rely on computer-based tool support. Expressive formal models of component functionality are a prerequisite for component selection and early-on interoperability assessment. This paper extends a flexible framework of semantic annotations (tags) and investigates different algorithms for interoperability evaluation. Based on their individual characteristics, suitable application areas for these algorithms are identified and discussed in the context of automated engineering. Thus, a pairwise comparison and a reasoning-based algorithm provide a cornerstone for the proliferation of computer-based design algorithms to carry out complex planning tasks in the future.

Keywords: Ambient assisted living · Health smart home · Building automation systems · Interoperability · Automated engineering

1 Introduction

Advanced technology in Component-based Automation Systems (CBAS) offer great opportunities for a variety of application areas, including Building Automation Systems (BAS) and Health Smart Homes (HSH), which are a key concept for realizing personalized health care in order to cope with future challenges for health care systems [17]. However, with an abundance of heterogeneous components available, the engineering process of CBAS is becoming increasingly complex and requires computer-based support [14,25]. In this context, special attention has to be paid to interoperability of components. Yet, achieving *interoperability* is a complex problem [24] in itself, resulting in high follow-up costs when neglected in the design phase. For the U.S. building industry alone, NIST reported annual costs of $ 15.8 billion due to incompatible components [12]. To detect potential interoperability issues as early as possible, it is necessary to

X. Ye et al. (Eds.): BIOSTEC 2020, CCIS 1400, pp. 385–406, 2021.
https://doi.org/10.1007/978-3-030-72379-8_19

include the semantics of information exchanged by components in their functional models, enabling a conceptual interoperability assessment at design time. While syntactical interoperability can be achieved by middleware approaches and standardizing the data types of programming languages or the payloads of communication protocols, semantic information describing the actual meaning of data is often neglected. Accordingly, the semantics of data is nowadays often not formally specified, despite its importance in achieving semantic interoperability in both design and operation phase. As a consequence, no automated processing of the meaning of data is possible, hampering the proliferation of automated engineering solutions.

To enable expressive modeling of semantic data types, an extensible semantic annotation framework (SAF) has been proposed in previous research [27]. But usage of a more expressive semantic modeling framework raises the issue, how interoperability for semantic specifications can be assessed, if a naïve comparison of simple semantic types is no longer possible. To this end, this work provides a further consolidation of the SAF and investigates different approaches on how interoperability can be determined for more expressive semantic frameworks. This paper is an extended version of the original conference paper [27]. It has been modified and extended by proposing several new algorithms for interoperability evaluation, investigating the trade-off between their expressiveness and performance, and inferring suitable application areas for the different approaches. Conversely, the initial work in [27] contains a detailed description of the creation process of SAF. All in all, this paper proposes the following main contributions:

1. *Extension of the semantic annotation framework* from [27] by investigating semantic types and their usage in the functional standard VDI 3813-2 [23].
2. Proposal of *different algorithms for interoperability evaluation* for expressive semantic type declarations.
3. Discussion of *suitable application areas for the individual algorithms.*

This paper is structured as follows: The next section presents information on the background of automated engineering approaches and discusses related work for semantic frameworks. Section 3 describes the extension to the semantic framework from [27]. Several algorithms suitable for interoperability evaluation for tag-based semantic models are proposed in Sect. 4. The algorithms are validated and their performance is evaluated in Sect. 5, which also includes a discussion of their potential application areas. Finally, the paper is summarized and further research areas are discussed by Sect. 6.

2 Background and State of the Art

2.1 Engineering of Building Automation Systems and Health Smart Homes

In order to achieve the high level of customization required in HSH [17] and BAS, computer-based tool support is necessary. Therefore, automated engineering approaches for CBAS have been a research topic for the domains of BAS and HSH. Dibowski et al. proposed a prototype of an automated engineering approach in the domain of room automation [9], using the abstract functionality standard VDI 3813 [23] as key vocabulary for functionality. Similarly, [29] formally defines the HSH engineering task as well as an approach and prototype for automated engineering of HSH, motivated by the prototype of Dibowski et al. [9]. Both approaches are based on functional component models and a common vocabulary of functionality. The role of automated interoperability evaluations can best be put into context, when considering these automated engineering approaches in detail. To this end, common tasks in the engineering process will be introduced below.

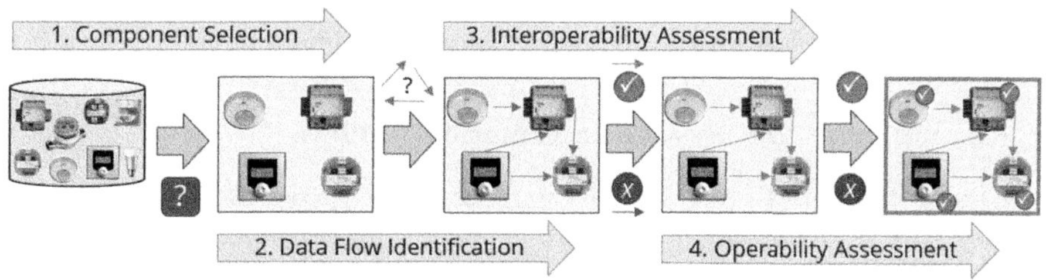

Fig. 1. Tasks for the engineering of Building Automation Systems and Health Smart Homes according to [26].

The automated engineering approaches try to match desired functionality specified by planners in a *system specification* with functionality provided by automation components, yielding several candidate system designs. Figure 1 depicts the main tasks during the process of automation engineering according to [26]. In order to come up with possible design candidates, suitable components contributing to the required functionality need to be selected from a data base of all available products (*1. Component Selection*). Subsequently, the planner's system specification is used to identify, which communication relations amongst the components should be established (*2. Data Flow Identification*). Each of these identified data flows should then be examined to determine, if the corresponding components are interoperable (*3. Interoperability Assessment*), i.e. if the exchanged data can correctly be understood and used. Finally, it needs to be determined whether each component is provided with the information required to perform its functionality (*4. Operability Assessment*). If a design candidate is still considered viable after these steps, it is a possible solution for the planner's system specification.

Such automated engineering approaches rely on a common vocabulary for a shared understanding of functionality and information types. A previous literature analysis revealed that for HSH there is currently no comprehensive standard available [28]. Since HSH is an interdisciplinary domain, prototypical approaches may resort to the BAS aspects of HSH functionality. In case of BAS, this shared understanding can be provided by the *functional standard*

VDI 3813 [23], which introduces standard functionality and information types available in room automation systems on an abstract and technology-neutral level. As representation for functionality, it defines function blocks and the information required and provided by them. However, the semantic data types of the VDI 3813 [23] are limited to a pre-defined set of 46 semantic types. A semantic type is labeled with one mnemonic name consisting of two parts hinting at the *type of information* represented and its *meaning* (e.g. A_SUN representing the angle of the sun's position). Thus, a coarse structure for attributing semantics to the information is available; yet, the two parts are often not clearly delimitated and especially the second part is used inconsistently to indicate meaning, types of information, representations, or origins of information. Further details are often only explained as unstructured text. The validity of interoperability assessment based solely on the data type names is therefore limited.

2.2 Component and System Information Models

In the aforementioned prototype of Dibowski et al. [9], the tasks 1. to 3. from Sect. 2.1 have been implemented. Different levels of interoperability are comprehensively discussed in a follow-up work [8], encompassing technical, syntactic, semantic, conceptual, and experiential interoperability. A detailed assessment of interoperability plays a vital role in automated design approaches, as interoperability can filter out a great number of false positive design candidates [8]. However, the semantic data types used in the prototypical component models were limited to a fixed set of complex composite structures. Interoperability evaluations on the semantic level were restricted to a comparison of these complex types. Therefore, the semantic models scale badly due to a high effort of vocabulary maintenance.

The work of [11] is one example of further approaches aiming at modeling components to facilitate the design process. However, none reached a level of detail or maturity comparable to the approach of Dibowski et al. [8,10].

As a different approach, *system information models* provide means to formalize specific technical system configurations. Many approaches exist for different domains, such as building automation [3] and smart homes [13]. Examples include DomoML [21], the SSN-Ontology [5], DogOnt [2], ThinkHome Ontology [16], AAL-Onto [25], or SAREF [6]. They focus on the detailed modeling of environment and context on a coarse level of granularity; however, they do not model sufficient information to attribute semantics to information for design purposes.

Similarly, abstract *reference models* such as the UniversAAL platform [22] provide a conceptual framework for systems in general, but remain too coarse on the aspect of data type semantics. The ISO/IEEE 11073 standards family [15] offers a detailed nomenclature for health information, yet largely focuses on communication in a hospital setting.

2.3 Tag-Based Semantic Frameworks

Another class of approaches for modeling systems and semantics of data are *tagging approaches*, which define semantic annotations (tags) as an easy-to-use means for modeling semantics.

The most prominent example is Project Haystack[1], which is based on a community-managed vocabulary of about 230 tags. This vocabulary is also available as an ontology [4]. This enables to create a system model organized along the hierarchies of site, equipment and (data) point. Some implicit semantics can be inferred from the modeled equipment types, such as `discharge air temp sensor`. However, fine-grained modeling of exchanged information is not in focus of this approach.

The flexibility of Haystack has inspired further work in the domain of IoT, e.g. the extended data model *BACnet XD* by the BACnet group [3], the *KNX Information Model* by the KNX Association [19], or [20] towards integration of IoT and building systems. The latter uses annotations to translate KNX system models into web service information models by means of a common meta model, which is available as an XML schema.

To improve the applicability of tagged system models, BRICK [1] introduced a *metadata schema* for buildings aimed at enabling applications such as model-predictive control or fault detection and diagnosis. BRICK offers an ontology of entities (Point, Equipment, Location, Measurement) and their relationships in order to model building automation systems and components.

These approaches aim at facilitating building analytics by adding semantic information to models of building systems. While capturing the systems' structure and metadata, they are focused on the operation phase and do not intend to use the semantic information in the design phase. In contrast to the available coarse granularity of data semantics, design tasks require a higher level of expressiveness such as shown by [26], especially for interoperability assessments.

3 Semantic Annotation Framework

3.1 Semantic Data Models in HSH Context

In order to put semantic data types into context, a conceptual framework of the assistance system aspects of HSH will be used. Based upon the conceptual core framework from [28] and the UniversAAL reference model [22], the concepts and relationships of the assistance systems are depicted in Fig. 2 in UML notation.

The classes on the left model `Automation Components` as structures for equipment, which contains a software application, modeled by `Device Application`. The software application provides a certain functionality modeled by `Function`, as part of the commonly used vocabulary of functionality. The classes on the right side – `Communication Relation` and `Semantic Data Type` – are used to model the interconnections of components in the automation system.

[1] http://project-haystack.org/.

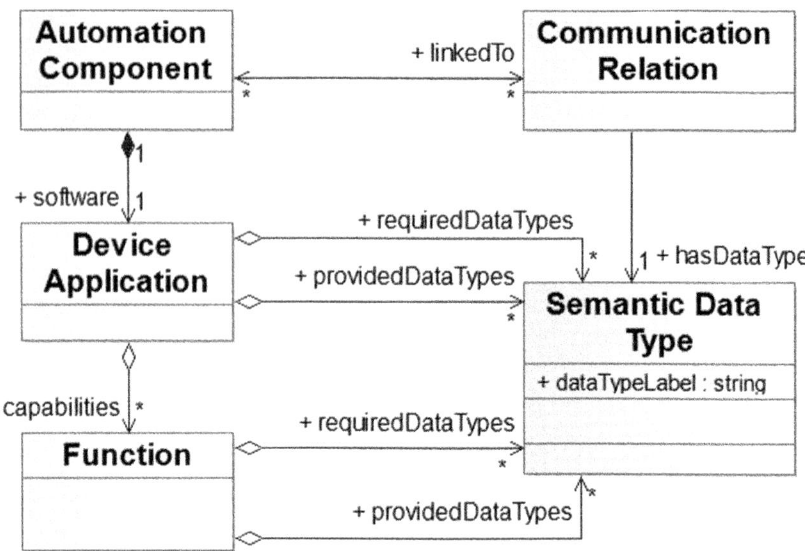

Fig. 2. Conceptual Model of Automation Systems in CBAS context.

More specifically, the components are communicating with each other in order to fulfill their functionality. A communication relation models one of the information exchanges for a set of "linked" components. Each communication relation is used to exchange a specific type of information between the components' software applications. On the other hand, these software applications need to provide information about their software interfaces. More specifically, they need to model *required data types* on the input side as well as *provided data types* on the output side.

The key concept of *interoperability* can now be investigated: the software applications exchanging information in the context of a specific communication relation need to adhere to its semantic data type. More specifically, the data types of the provided and the required side need to be *compatible* with each other. This is the case, if in a communication relation every provided semantic type is understood at the receiving end.

3.2 Summary of Initial Semantic Annotation Framework

In order to provide a more expressive and flexible framework for annotating semantic information, SAF as a multi-dimensional tag-based semantic framework was conceived in [27] by investigating and structuring the semantic data type labels of the VDI 3813 [23]. The main idea for structuring the SAF [27] was based on describing semantics along several different, non-overlapping information dimensions. This is motivated by a variety of approaches of semantic system modeling for building analytics, such as the Semantic Sensor Network Ontol-

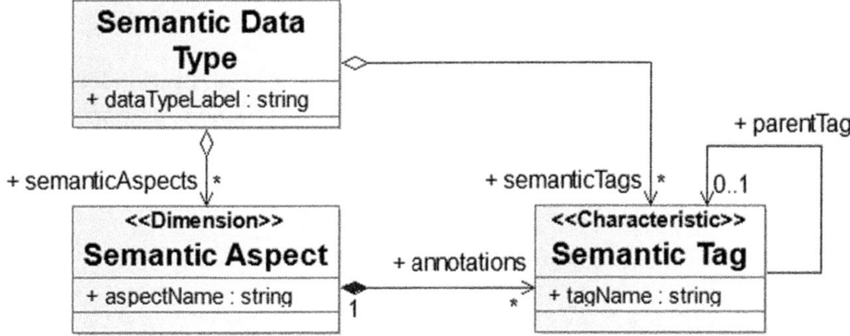

Fig. 3. Model of the Semantic Annotation Framework as created in [27].

Table 1. The following meta-characteristics were used for identifying and grouping dimensions.

Name	Explanation
Entity	What is the information referring to?
Context	In which context is the information generated and used?
Realization	How is the information encoded?

ogy, the semantic tagging approach *Project Haystack*, and the BRICK metadata schema (cf. Sect. 2.3).

Those approaches provide detailed system models by modeling entities and their relationships. We aimed to translate such expressiveness to the semantic information modeling by providing different aspects of semantics. The resulting composite semantic model allows for expressing information in much more detail than semantic models consisting of only one semantic label.

Following the structuring approach outlined above, Fig. 3 depicts a model of the initial SAF. A `Semantic Data Type` is composed of several different `Semantic Aspects`, which each are annotated with `Semantic Tags`. When regarded as a taxonomy, the aspects are taxonomy dimensions with the different annotations making up the characteristics of these dimensions.

The SAF was initially created following an established and reproducible method for taxonomy creation by Nickerson et al. [18], which is documented in more detail in [27]. In several iterations, different aspects of the semantic types used in the VDI 3813-2 [23] were analysed and clustered in order to form the independent taxonomy dimensions. These different aspects are explained in Table 1. As demanded by the taxonomy creation method [18], they were incorporated as *meta-characteristics* for guiding the identification process of the dimensions. In several iterations of increasing refinement, the initial 46 semantic types were consolidated and extended to encompass 75 semantic types at the end. All in all, the initial framework consisted of seven dimensions and a total of 63 characteristics. In order to accommodate new innovations or developments, as well as to be transferred to similar domains, each tag dimension can be extended with further characteristics.

The results from [27] propose a structure for semantic annotation frameworks that provide *more expressive* semantic data models, are able to *comprehensively* be used throughout different phases of the engineering process, and being *extensible* towards adjacent domains, such as HSH.

3.3 Refined Semantic Annotation Framework

Based on the SAF from [27], further refinements have been conducted in this paper. Extending the initial work, which was mainly focused on the semantic types' names explicitly mentioned in the standard VDI 3813-2 [23], potentially different manifestations of a semantic type could be investigated by modeling all data points of all functional blocks defined by the VDI 3813-2 [23].

Since this is the most specific context of semantics, some additional semantic types could be distinguished by these analyses. Six new semantic types related to alarm managements were added and modes for control of energy, climatisation, and ventilation systems have been streamlined.

In addition, the VARIABLE TYPE dimension was consolidated (cf. Fig. 4). It is aligned with the different roles of information in closed- as well as open-loop control systems. The central component is the controller, which is able to process measured *Values*, computed *States*, as well as *Setpoints* and *Commands*

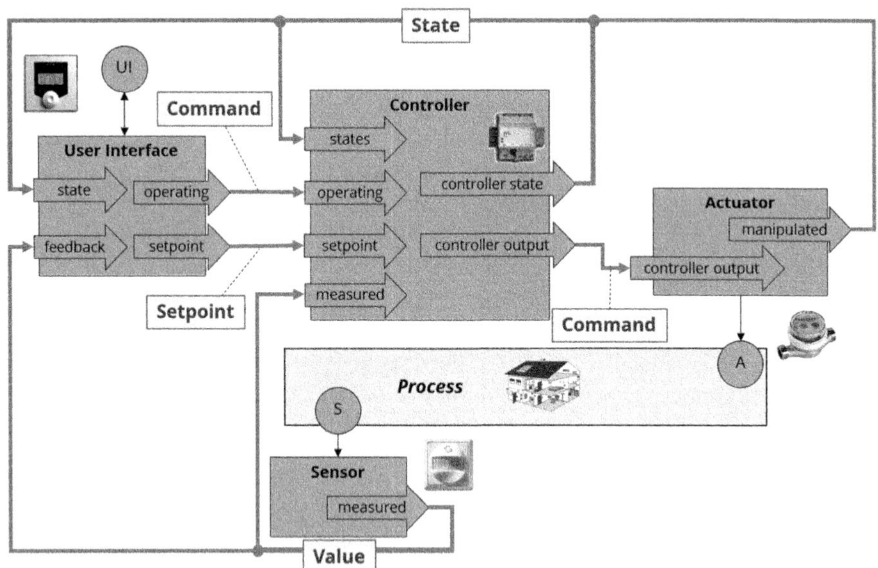

Fig. 4. The different Variable Types (bold in boxes) in a generic control system. The functionalities are displayed as function blocks according to [23].

generated by users or computation. Furthermore, *Alarm* type information is also supported.

The dimension TRIGGER TYPE has been renamed to PRIORITY to incorporate the notion of different types of sources – *automatic*, *management* (formerly associated to LOCATION) and *manual*. Finally, the dimensions REFERENCE TYPE and REPRESENTATION have been consolidated and detailed. As discussed in the initial work of [27], no further dimensions needed to be added to incorporate the more detailed analyses.

In its final version, the SAF now encompasses seven dimensions with 70 characteristics, as is depicted in Table 2. Since the described entities constitute the greatest variability of concepts, the dimensions FEATURE OF INTEREST and PHYSICAL QUALITY contain the majority of characteristics, with 20 and 27 characteristics, respectively. Dimensions regarding the context or realization aspects are more generic and require a less diverse set of characteristics (cf. Fig. 5).

3.4 Health Smart Home Tag Extension and Case Study

Unlike the domain of building automation, Health Smart Homes are much more diverse and there is no consolidated standard available that describes the common functionality as an agreed-upon vocabulary [28]. Thus, extending the SAF to HSH is currently not feasible in a comprehensive manner. Nevertheless – although the functionalities of this domain are not yet consolidated – exemplary extensions could be made to indicate the applicability of the SAF for the domain of Health Smart Homes. In order to do this, only the dimensions of the *entities*

Table 2. The updated semantic annotation framework for the room automation domain.

	Dimensions	Characteristics			
Entity	FEATURE OF INTEREST	air	calendar	climatisation	contact
		controller	drive	fan	hvac
		lamella	lamp	light	room
		shading	sun	sunblind	valve
		ventilation	water	weather	window
	PHYSICAL QUALITY	activation	angle.azimuth	angle.elevation	color
		date	dewpoint	flow	frost
		humidity	illuminance	intrusion	level
		mode.climaCtrl	mode.energyCtrl	mode.roomUsage	mode.ventCtrl
		occupancy	position	position.maint	position.prot
		precipitation	pressure	quality	rotation
		temperature	time	velocity	
Context	LOCATION	equipment	indoor	outdoor	
	VARIABLE TYPE	alarm	command	setpoint	state
		value			
Realization	PRIORITY	automatic	management	manual	
	REFERENCE TYPE	absolute	delta	offset	percentage
		step			
	REPRESENTATION	binary	continuous	interval	nominal
		ordinal	quantified	ratio	

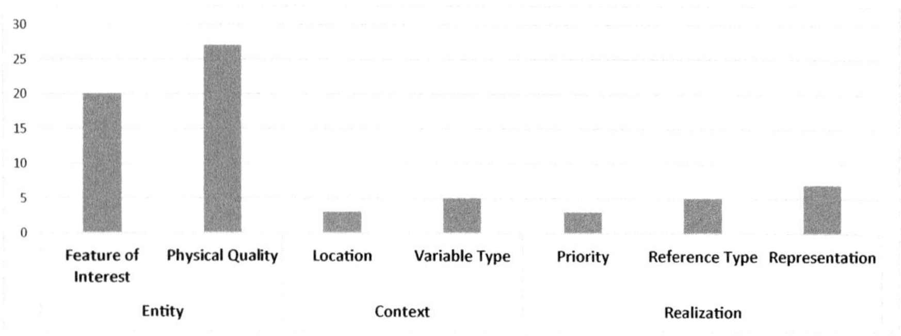

Fig. 5. Structure of the semantic annotation framework showing the number of tags (characteristics) in each aspect (dimension).

aspect (Feature of Interest, Physical Quality) needed to be extended. Table 3 depicts additional characteristics that have been proposed in [27] for some examples of HSH functionality.

Table 3. Extension to the semantic annotation framework to also address exemplary health smart home functionality.

Dimensions	Characteristics				
Feature of Interest	energy	food	medication	occupant	occupant.body
Physical Quality	activity height	amount pulse	consumptn.current rate	consumptn.total type	HbA1c weight

In this paper, a case study with functionalities from both BAS as well as HSH will be shown (cf. Fig. 6). This example is focused on night-time fall prevention and sleep monitoring, which records phases of activity and could be useful for e.g. monitoring early dementia patients. The case study consists of a motion detector installed in the hallway leading to the bedroom, the lamps in this hallway, some computation capacity for the processing of data, and an electronic "sleep diary" used to record disturbances and disruptions of the resident's sleep during the night. Based on the motion signals from the motion detector, the current occupancy state of a hallway is computed by the functionality *Occupancy Evaluation*. This occupancy state is used to automatically switch on the hallway lights (*Automatic Lighting*) to prevent falls, while a phase of interrupted sleep is recorded in the sleep diary by the function *Sleep Monitoring*.

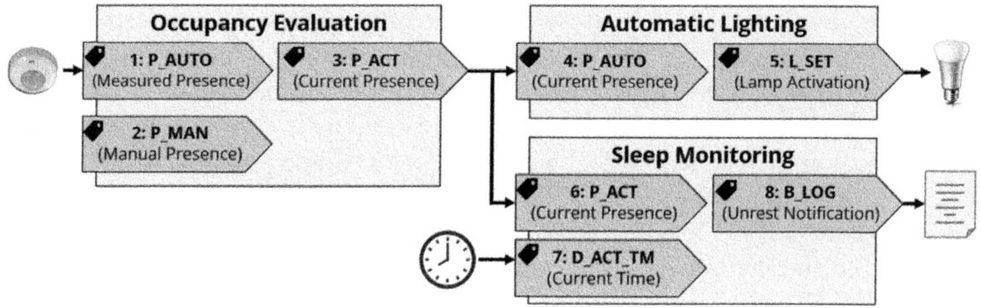

Fig. 6. Example of Room Automation and Health Smart Home Functionality. A presence detector is used to compute the current occupancy state of a hallway (*Occupancy Evaluation*). This state is used to automatically switch on the lights (*Automatic Lighting*) and to record phases of interrupted sleep (*Sleep Monitoring*).

Table 4. Tags of the data points in the case study.

Data Point	Feature of Interest	Physical Quality	Variable Type	Locality	Priority
1: P_AUTO	room	occupancy	value	indoor	automatic
2: P_MAN	room	occupancy	command	indoor	manual
3: P_ACT	room	occupancy	state	indoor	–
4: P_AUTO	room	occupancy	state	–	–
5: L_SET	lamp	activation	command	–	–
6: P_ACT	room	occupancy	state	–	–
7: D_ACT_TM	calendar	time	value	–	management
8: B_LOG	occupant	activity	state	–	–

Albeit being a small example, this case study is valuable in studying the interworking aspects of functionality from BA and HSH. As can be seen from Fig. 6, eight data points (indicated by a name and a number) are available in the example. Each data point is annotated with tags from the SAF as depicted in Table 4. Since the exemplary functions are defined on a vendor- and technology-neutral basis (similar to the VDI 3813-2 [23]), the dimensions Reference Type and Representation were left out for the sake of brevity. Besides the three different controller functionalities, the case study also contains data sources (i.e. motion detector and clock) and data sinks (i.e. lamp actuator and sleep diary), which will not be in the focus of the study.

The functionality *Occupancy Evaluation* is used for a central computation of the hallway's actual occupancy state. This computed state is then sent to the functionalities *Automatic Lighting* and *Sleep Monitoring* and acts as a trigger for their respective behavior. Thus, two of the communication relations contained in the example are considered in more detail. Specifically, the communication relation from the occupancy evaluation to automatic lighting (communication relation 1: data point 3: P_ACT to 4: P_AUTO) and sleep monitoring (communication relation 2: data point 3: P_ACT to 6: P_ACT), respectively, are used for transmission of the hallway's current occupancy state.

Communication relation 1 illustrates that only comparing the name of the data points is not sufficient for determining interoperability. Instead, when looking at the tags, it becomes clear that they are a more suitable means for assessing the compatibility of two data points. It also is apparent from Table 4 that not each dimension is specified and the number of tags associated to a data point may vary (even more so, if the additional two dimensions REFERENCE TYPE and REPRESENTATION are taken into account).

As stated in Sect. 2.1, interoperability evaluation is a vital step in course of BAS and HSH engineering. The importance of interoperability evaluations is even bigger in context of automated design approaches, as these try to come up with a selection of interacting components as design proposals, which still need to be evaluated with regard to their feasibility and validity. For this task, algorithms for interoperability evaluations for tag based semantic definitions are required. The next section will propose several algorithms, before their suitability is evaluated in Sect. 5.

4 Algorithms for Interoperability Evaluation

4.1 General Interoperability Definition

As discussed in [27], the SAF allows for an *improved interoperability assessment* by lifting the assessment from a mere comparison of names to the level of expressive semantics and subsumption hierarchies. This detailed comparison enables to spot further interoperability issues – otherwise, issues will not have been predicted and only noticed after installation, incurring high revision costs.

The downside of a more expressive semantic framework is the more difficult interoperability assessment compared to mere string comparisons. In order to assess the performance impact and the suitability of the annotation framework, potential algorithms for interoperability evaluation need to be proposed and their characteristics need to be investigated.

To formalize this understanding, let $sem()$ be a function that returns the set of semantics associated to a data point. Furthermore, let DP be the set of data points and $typename()$ be a function that returns the name of the data point type. Data points in the roles *source* and *target* will be referred to as o and i, respectively. Then, we can define a function $interop()$ indicating the general (binary) interoperability of two data points by:

$$\begin{aligned} &interop :: DP \times DP \to \mathbb{B} \\ &interop(o,i) \iff sem(o) \subseteq sem(i) \end{aligned} \tag{1}$$

Let Tag be the set of all tags and $tags :: DP \to \mathcal{P}(Tag)$ be a function that returns the set of all tags associated to a data point. With these definitions in place, we can define the following interoperability algorithms[2].

[2] Note that the presented formalizations are no algorithms per se, but rather a declarative notation that can easily be converted into an imperative algorithm.

4.2 Shallow Name Comparison

The *Shallow Name Comparison* determines (semantic) compatibility of two data points by directly comparing the associated semantic type names. As this is the state of the art evaluation of compatible semantic types, it can be regarded as a baseline for the following interoperability evaluation algorithms. The algorithm does not require the existence of semantic tags and is therefore universally applicable. Since the semantic type names are evaluated without respect to their structure, this algorithm boils down to a simple string matching (cf. the formalization in Eq. (2)). Thus, it is expected to be very efficient, but with a reduced correctness (e.g. communication relation 1 of the case study would wrongly be classified as *invalid* by the shallow name comparison).

$$interop_{shallow}(o, i) \iff typename(o) = typename(i) \tag{2}$$

4.3 Pairwise Name Comparison

The *Pairwise Name Comparison* is the first of the presented algorithms that is able to make use of the more expressive semantic definition by means of semantic tags. It requires a set of tags being annotated to data points. The tags will be interpreted on an equal level, i.e. each tag is viewed as an additional specification/restriction of the data point semantics. Complex tag expressions, such as defining alternative tags, are not supported by this algorithm.

For this structural limitation, the algorithm can efficiently check the different tag dimensions for compatibility. Since the output data point's semantics needs to be a subset of the input data point's semantics, the output semantics might be more specific than the input semantics. In other words, the output can have additional tags, while the input cannot have tags in dimensions not contained in the output semantics. Then, each dimension can be inspected independently to check, if the respective tags of output and input are equal.

As the tag dimensions are non-overlapping, this iterative approach can be abstracted to aggregating the tags of each data point in an individual tag set and checking the subset relation of these two sets. The subset relations of the sets of semantics ($sem()$) on the one hand and of the sets of tags ($tags()$) on the other hand are inverse to each other, since specifying a tag is equivalent to narrowing down the semantics. This is indicated by the formalization in Eq. (3).

$$interop_{pairwise}(o, i) \iff tags(o) \supseteq tags(i) \tag{3}$$

4.4 Classification Approach

In general, it can also be conceived that tags can be combined to form more complex tag expressions, e.g. by using conjunctive and disjunctive operators. If considering such more complex combinations of tags, computing the subset relation is much less straight-forward. In this case, semantic reasoning can be applied for declarative interoperability evaluation approaches. However, to be able to compare the algorithms introduced in this section, the reasoning approaches are presented for the structural limitations mentioned in the previous Sect. 4.3, while keeping in mind that the following two approaches are more generally applicable.

The reasoning approaches make use of formalizations of tags in description logic (DL) as both individuals and concepts. A tag individual represents the actual tag that is linked to a data point via a role $hasTag$. On the other hand, tag concepts represent a class of individual tags with the meaning of the respective tag. Using hierarchies of tag concepts, inheritance relations amongst the tags may be specified (cf. relation *parentTag* in Fig. 3). In order to represent the combined semantics of a set of tags (or a tag expression), the tag concepts can be combined to DL class expressions. Each class expression for a specific semantics represents a declarative notion of the class of all data points annotated with this specific semantics. Based on these classes of data points, different "questions" to the reasoner may be used to determine interoperability. The following two approaches will be discussed: Firstly, the *Classification Approach* is an *instance checking* decision problem, asking the reasoner if an output data point can be classified as belonging to the class of data points with semantics of the input data points. Secondly, the *Subsumption Approach* checks, if the class of data points with output semantics is a subset of the class of data points with input semantics.

For the presentation of the two approaches, the following transformation functions are introduced, making use of the role $hasTag$ associating the concept of a data point $DataPoint$ with the concept of tags. The transformation function $trans_{ClExp}()$ in Eq. (4) computes the DL class expression for the semantics of a data point. Since the tag dimensions are non-overlapping, the general role $hasTag$ can be used in constructing the DL class expression:

$$\begin{aligned} &trans_{ClExp} :: DP \rightarrow ClExpr \\ &trans_{ClExp}(dp) = (dp \doteq DataType \sqcap (\sqcap_{t \in tags(dp)}(\exists hasTag.t))) \end{aligned} \tag{4}$$

On the other hand, the transformation function $trans_{Indv}()$ in Eq. (5) computes the set of assertional axioms for representing the corresponding data point individual as additions to the ABox $\mathcal{A}$ part of the knowledge base $\mathcal{KB} = (\mathcal{T}, \mathcal{A})$. Therefore, the function $trans_{Indv}()$ makes sure that a data point is correctly represented in the knowledge base:

$$\begin{aligned} &trans_{Indv} :: DP \rightarrow \mathcal{P}(\mathcal{A}) \\ &trans_{Indv}(dp) = \{dp : DataPoint\} \cup \{(dp, t) : hasTag \mid \forall t \in tags(dp)\} \end{aligned} \tag{5}$$

With these definitions in place, the *Classification Approach* converts the semantic type of the output data point into an individual that has the relation *hasTag* linking to its respective tags. Then, it needs to be investigated, if the semantic type of the output data point is an instance of the class modeled by the DL class expression for the input semantic type. The *Classification Approach* can then be written for an initial knowledge base $\mathcal{KB} = (\mathcal{T}, \mathcal{A})$ as follows:

$$\begin{aligned} &\mathcal{KB}' = (\mathcal{T}, \mathcal{A} \cup trans_{Indv}(o)) \\ &interop_{classification}(o, i) \iff \exists \mathcal{I}\ s.th. \mathcal{I} \models (o : trans_{ClExp}(i)) \end{aligned} \tag{6}$$

Equation 6 depicts the two steps required for the *Classification Approach*: First, the knowledge base must be extended to contain the assertions for the output data point. Then, it can be checked, whether the output data point individual is an instance of the input data point class expression. In terms of DL semantics, this is related to finding at least one interpretation $\mathcal{I}$ under which the concept assertion $o : trans_{ClExp}(i)$ holds for the knowledge base $\mathcal{KB}'$.

4.5 Subsumption Approach

Similarly, the *Subsumption Approach* can be defined. In this case, the semantic types of both output and input data points are modeled as class expressions. In order to determine interoperability, it needs to be checked if the class expression of the input data point subsumes the class expression of the output data point, i.e. if the class expression of the output data point is a subclass of the class expression of the input data point. Equation 7 reflects this definition, using again an interpretation $\mathcal{I}$ for the knowledge base $\mathcal{KB}$:

$$interop_{subsumption}(o, i) \iff \exists \mathcal{I}\ s.th. \mathcal{I} \models (trans_{ClExp}(o) \sqsubseteq trans_{ClExp}(i)) \tag{7}$$

5 Validation and Performance Evaluation

5.1 Test Cases

In order to test the validity and performance of the proposed algorithms against the baseline (*Shallow*), different test scenarios have been constructed to investigate a variety of real-world situations, including differing numbers of tags and different degrees of abstraction. Table 5 summarizes the used scenarios for the test cases and indicates, which sets of tags for the test scenarios can be taken from the case study example from Sect. 3.4. For the test scenarios, we investigated the data point's semantic tags irrespective of whether it is an input or an output data point.

5.2 Test Setup

During a test session, each algorithm proposed in Sect. 4 was tested with the test cases from Sect. 5.1 and the algorithms' correctness and performance were measured. To mitigate the effects of test overhead on the performance measurements, each algorithm was executed 200 times for each test case. The algorithms *Shallow* and *Pairwise* required very little computation time, which increased the distortion due to the finite resolution of the time measurement facilities.

Table 5. Overview of Test Scenarios.

ID	Explanation	Expected Result	Example from Table 4
TC1	Same sets of tags	true	DP 3 and DP 3
TC2	Same number of tags, no matches	false	DP 5 and DP 8
TC3	Same number of tags, two mismatches	false	DP 1 and DP 2
TC4	Output more general than Input	false	DP 4 and DP 3
TC5	Input more general than Output	true	DP 3 and DP 4

Thus, for these algorithms, an additional factor of 1,000 was introduced, so that these algorithms were executed 200,000 times per test case. Each test session was repeated until 100 test iterations have been carried out.

The tests were performed on a Windows 10 computer with an Intel® Core™ i5-7200U CPU and 20 GB of RAM using Java 1.8, the OWL API library[3] and HermiT[4] as a reasoner.

5.3 Validation of Correctness

With the exception of the baseline algorithm, *Shallow*, all other algorithms yielded correct results for all test scenarios. The algorithm *Shallow* incorrectly classified TC5 as *invalid*, but classified the other test scenarios correctly. This behavior has been expected as the *Shallow* approach is only able to identify exact type matches, whereas TC5 is a scenario with the output semantics being more specific than the input semantics.

This also means that already the lightweight SAF with a DL expressivity of $\mathcal{ALC}$ is able to compute the interoperability evaluation for a variety of test scenarios. In conclusion, each of the algorithms *Pairwise*, *Classification*, and *Subsumption* provides a better correctness than the baseline algorithm.

5.4 Performance Evaluation

When selecting the best-suited interoperability algorithm, the performance impact of this algorithms has to be taken into account, besides its providing correct results. The results of the conducted performance tests are depicted as box plots in Fig. 7 and Fig. 8 (log-scaled), aggregated for the algorithms and test cases.

The baseline algorithm, *Shallow*, performs very well below a fraction of a microsecond. It can also be seen that the *Pairwise* algorithm is comparable to the baseline algorithm with a mean execution time of well below 10 μs. The algorithms relying on semantic reasoning require roughly four orders of magnitude more computation time (i.e. between 30 ms and 50 ms). Among the reasoning

[3] OWL API version 5.1.12, https://github.com/owlcs/owlapi.
[4] HermiT OWL reasoner version 1.4.5.519, http://www.hermit-reasoner.com/.

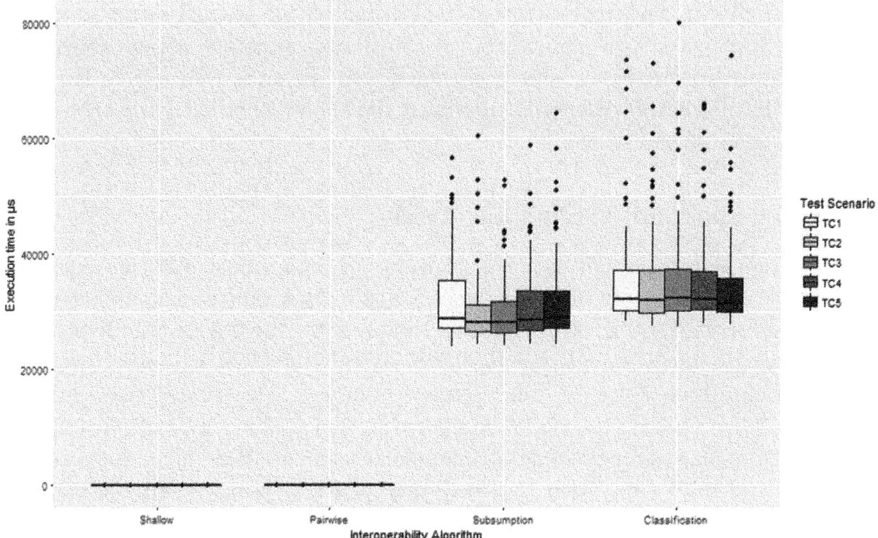

Fig. 7. Results of the performance measurements for each defined algorithm and the different test cases.

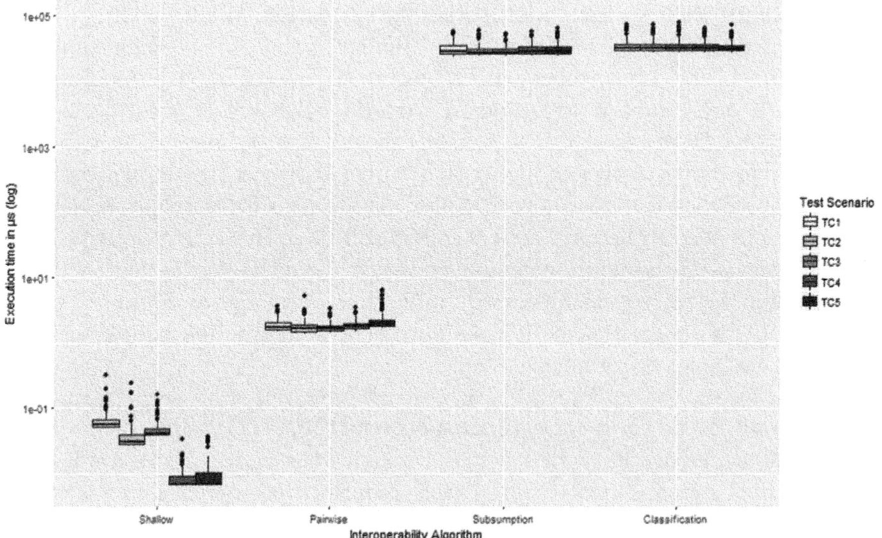

Fig. 8. Results of the performance measurements for each defined algorithm and the different test cases in logarithmic scale.

approaches, *Subsumption* seems to perform slightly better than *Classification*, which needs more computation time and also features more outliers.

Figure 8 reveals that the different test scenarios do not seem to have any significant impact on the algorithms' performance, with the exception of the baseline algorithm. However, since this algorithm takes very little time for computation, the observable differences amongst the test scenarios may be attributed to measurement inaccuracies.

5.5 Discussion and Application Areas

The baseline algorithm *Shallow* has proven to be the most efficient one; yet, it does not yield the correct results in all cases. This downside is expected to become more relevant, if the flexibilities offered by the SAF should be used. Annotating semantic models by fine-grained tags enables a more expressive semantic definition. However, once semantics cannot be reduced to a uniform and standardized name, the *Shallow* algorithm will no longer be applicable.

The *Pairwise* approach as a component-based and thus more fine-grained approach is able to cope with the flexibility of the tag-based semantic framework. Performance-wise, it is slightly less efficient than the baseline algorithm. But, with computation times of less than 10 µs it still is a viable candidate for interoperability evaluation on a restricted time budget (e.g. during automated computation of design candidates).

The *Classification* approach applies reasoning and solves an *instance checking* decision problem for each interoperability evaluation. While yielding correct results, it is the least efficient algorithm. Similarly, the *Subsumption* approach yields correct results, but comes with a huge performance impact. As discussed before, both algorithms were tested in scenarios with restrictions of the tagging structure. However, these algorithms would also be able to provide correct results for more complex tagging structures. Moreover, the implementation of both approaches is much more complex, as libraries for ontology processing and reasoning need to be used. There might still be optimization potential left, such as using pre-processing techniques in order to reduce the actual computation time for the interoperability evaluation. The *Subsumption* approach seems promising in this regard, since it does not need to change the knowledge base and might be easier to optimize.

In conclusion, the approaches *Pairwise* and *Subsumption* seem to provide the best trade-off between correctness and performance (*Pairwise*) or flexibility (*Subsumption*), respectively. In order to determine the most suitable application areas for the algorithms, the different tasks requiring interoperability evaluation need to be considered.

Firstly, interoperability needs to be assessed in the automated design approach during generating and evaluating design candidates (cf. step 3 of Fig. 1). This task needs – amongst others – to perform a massive number (up to billions) of assessments in a short time (several minutes). Thus, a single interoperability evaluation has a very strict and small time budget. In this case, the *Pairwise* approach seems to be most suitable.

Secondly, interoperability (in its more general form of *compatibility*) also needs to be assessed during the specification of the functional component models, which is done by the component manufacturer during product development. Thus, there is no strict time limit nor the need for a massive number of assessments. Instead, this task calls for a flexible manner of annotating semantics to make the component model specification process more efficient and robust, e.g. by reducing the semantic specification effort or providing suggestion mechanisms based on the detailed semantic understanding of the data types. This combination of circumstances favors the *Subsumption* approach due to its flexibility. In addition, the *Pairwise* approach might also be suitable for this task.

6 Conclusion and Future Work

In this paper, we proposed an update to a previously developed extensible semantic annotation framework that is able to add a significant level of semantic expressiveness to information types exchanged in information systems such as building automation systems and health smart homes.

With its aspect-oriented approach and the definition of different dimensions of semantic annotations, the approach is able to specify semantics in detail, surpassing the expressiveness capabilities of using mere data type names to encode semantics. Since multiple dimensions can be taken into account, the framework also allows for a seamless semantic data modeling from abstract specification to detailed component modeling, starting from a few dimensions to fully encompass all aspects of semantic data.

Furthermore, we proposed several algorithms for assessing interoperability based on the semantic annotation framework. These algorithms were tested against the state-of-the-art baseline and potential application areas have been discussed. Thus, we were able to provide the foundation for improving the quality of interoperability assessments in context of automated design approaches and for streamlining the process of specifying semantic models for automation components by enabling auxiliary suggestion functionalities.

As next steps, we intend to investigate how more complex semantic expressions can be annotated to data points to increase the flexibility during the task of functional component modeling. To account for real-world uncertainty, an investigation into more nuanced (i.e. probabilistic) notions of interoperability and individual compatibility rules for different dimensions seems to be another promising step. Non-standard DL reasoning approaches such as those presented in [7] might provide a valuable starting point for suitable interoperability evaluation mechanisms.

Furthermore, once a consolidation of functionality and data types is achieved for the whole domain of HSH, we plan to extend the framework so that it encompasses HSH as a whole. In order to integrate the SAF with existing tagging approaches, ontology matching and merging approaches might be a viable tool to consolidation of interdisciplinary semantic vocabularies (e.g. the nomenclature of health informatics provided by the IEEE 11073).

We consider the increased semantic expressiveness offered by the annotation framework as well as the possible algorithms for interoperability evaluation as vital for increasing the degree of automation of the design process of BAS and HSH and as an enabler for an increased proliferation of building automation and assistive technology applications in the future.

Acknowledgements. The work for this paper was funded by the European Social Fund and the Free State of Saxony (Grant no. 100310385).

References

1. Balaji, B., et al.: Brick: towards a unified metadata schema for buildings. In: Proceedings of the 3rd ACM International Conference on Systems for Energy-Efficient Built Environments, BuildSys 2016, pp. 41–50. ACM, New York (2016). https://doi.org/10.1145/2993422.2993577. http://doi.acm.org/10.1145/2993422.2993577
2. Bonino, D., Corno, F.: DogOnt - ontology modeling for intelligent domotic environments. In: Sheth, A., et al. (eds.) ISWC 2008. LNCS, vol. 5318, pp. 790–803. Springer, Heidelberg (2008). https://doi.org/10.1007/978-3-540-88564-1_51
3. Butzin, B., Golatowski, F., Timmermann, D.: A survey on information modeling and ontologies in building automation. In: 43rd Annual Conference of the IEEE Industrial Electronics Society, IECON 2017, pp. 8615–8621, October 2017. https://doi.org/10.1109/IECON.2017.8217514
4. Charpenay, V., Käbisch, S., Anicic, D., Kosch, H.: An ontology design pattern for IoT device tagging systems. In: 2015 5th International Conference on the Internet of Things (IOT), pp. 138–145, October 2015. https://doi.org/10.1109/IOT.2015.7356558
5. Compton, M., et al.: The SSN ontology of the W3C semantic sensor network incubator group. J. Web Semant. **17**, 25–32 (2012). https://doi.org/10.1016/j.websem.2012.05.003. http://www.sciencedirect.com/science/article/pii/S1570826812000571
6. Daniele, L., den Hartog, F., Roes, J.: Study on semantic assets for smart appliances interoperability: D-S4: Final report. European Commission, Brussels (2015)
7. Di Noia, T., Di Sciascio, E., Donini, F.M.: Semantic matchmaking as non-monotonic reasoning: a description logic approach. J. Artif. Int. Res. **29**(1), 269–307 (2007)
8. Dibowski, H.: Semantic interoperability evaluation model for devices in automation systems. In: 2017 22nd IEEE International Conference on Emerging Technologies and Factory Automation (ETFA), pp. 1–6, September 2017. https://doi.org/10.1109/ETFA.2017.8247709
9. Dibowski, H., Ploennigs, J., Kabitzsch, K.: Automated design of building automation systems. IEEE Trans. Ind. Electron. **57**(11), 3606–3613 (2010). https://doi.org/10.1109/TIE.2009.2032209. http://ieeexplore.ieee.org/stamp/stamp.jsp?arnumber=5256330
10. Dibowski, H., Kabitzsch, K.: Ontology-based device descriptions and device repository for building automation devices. EURASIP J. Embed. Syst. **2011**, 3:1–3:17 (2011)
11. Fernbach, A., Kastner, W.: Semi-automated engineering in building automation systems and management integration. In: 2017 IEEE 26th International Symposium on Industrial Electronics (ISIE), pp. 1528–1534, June 2017. https://doi.org/10.1109/ISIE.2017.8001472

12. Gallaher, M., O'Connor, A., Dettbarn, J., Gilday, L.: Cost Analysis of Inadequate Interoperability in the U.S. Capital Facilities Industry. Techreport, National Institute of Standards and Technology (2004). https://doi.org/10.6028/NIST.GCR.04-867
13. Grassi, M., Nucci, M., Piazza, F.: Ontologies for smart homes and energy management: an implementation-driven survey. In: 2013 Workshop on Modeling and Simulation of Cyber-Physical Energy Systems (MSCPES), pp. 1–3, May 2013. https://doi.org/10.1109/MSCPES.2013.6623319
14. Haux, R., Koch, S., Lovell, N.H., Marschollek, M., Nakashima, N., Wolf, K.H.: Health-enabling and ambient assistive technologies: past, present, future. Yearb Med. Inform. **Suppl. 1**(Suppl. 1), 76–91 (2016). http://www.ncbi.nlm.nih.gov/pmc/articles/PMC5171510/, 27362588[pmid]
15. ISO/IEEE 11073–10101a: Health informatics - Point-of-care medical device communication - Part 10101: Nomenclature Amendment 1: Additional Definitions (2015)
16. Kofler, M.J., Reinisch, C., Kastner, W.: A semantic representation of energy-related information in future smart homes. Energy Build. **47**, 169–179 (2012). https://doi.org/10.1016/j.enbuild.2011.11.044. http://www.sciencedirect.com/science/article/pii/S0378778811005901
17. Maeder, A.J., Williams, P.A.H.: Health smart homes: new challenges. Stud. Health Technol. Inform. **245**, 166–169 (2017)
18. Nickerson, R.C., Varshney, U., Muntermann, J.: A method for taxonomy development and its application in information systems. Eur. J. Inf. Syst. **22**(3), 336–359 (2013). https://doi.org/10.1057/ejis.2012.26
19. Pelesic, I., Fernbach, A., Granzer, W., Kastner, W.: Semantic integration in building automation a case study for KNX, oBIX and Semantic Web Applications. In: Proceedings of the KNX Scientific Conference, October 2016
20. Schachinger, D., Fernbach, A., Kastner, W.: Modeling framework for IoT integration of building automation systems. at-Automatisierungstechnik **65**(9), 630–640 (2017). https://doi.org/10.1515/auto-2017-0014. https://www.degruyter.com/view/j/auto.2017.65.issue-9/auto-2017-0014/auto-2017-0014.xml
21. Sommaruga, L., Formilli, T., Rizzo, N.: DomoML: an integrating devices framework for ambient intelligence solutions. In: Proceedings of the 6th International Workshop on Enhanced Web Service Technologies, WEWST 2011, pp. 9–15. ACM, New York (2011). https://doi.org/10.1145/2031325.2031327. http://doi.acm.org/10.1145/2031325.2031327
22. Tazari, M.R., et al.: The universAAL reference model for AAL. In: Handbook of Ambient Assisted Living (2012)
23. VDI 3813–2: Building automation and control systems (BACS). Room control functions (RA functions), May 2011
24. Vermesan, O., Friess, P., et al.: Internet of Things-from Research and Innovation to Market Deployment, vol. 29. River Publishers Aalborg (2014)
25. Welge, R., et al.: AAL-onto: a formal representation of RAALI integration profiles. In: Wichert, R., Klausing, H. (eds.) Ambient Assisted Living. ATSC, pp. 89–102. Springer, Cham (2015). https://doi.org/10.1007/978-3-319-11866-6_7
26. Wollschlaeger, B., Eichenberg, E., Kabitzsch, K.: Switching to a holistic perspective on semantic component models in building automation – tapping the full potential of automated design approaches. In: IOP Conference Series: Earth and Environmental Science, vol. 323, p. 012047, September 2019. https://doi.org/10.1088/1755-1315/323/1/012047

27. Wollschlaeger, B., Eichenberg, E., Kabitzsch, K.: Explain yourself: a semantic annotation framework to facilitate tagging of semantic information in health smart homes. In: Proceedings of the 13th International Joint Conference on Biomedical Engineering Systems and Technologies, HEALTHINF: HEALTHINF, vol. 5, pp. 133–144. INSTICC, SciTePress (2020). https://doi.org/10.5220/0008968901330144
28. Wollschlaeger, B., Kabitzsch, K.: Navigating the jungle of assistance systems: a comparison of standards for assistance functionality. In: Proceedings of the 12th International Joint Conference on Biomedical Engineering Systems and Technologies, HEALTHINF, vol. 5, pp. 359–366. INSTICC, SciTePress, February 2019. https://doi.org/10.5220/0007397903590366. https://www.scitepress.org/PublicationsDetail.aspx?ID=BWu//daTdiY=&t=1
29. Wollschlaeger, B., Kabitzsch, K.: Automated engineering for health smart homes: find a way in the jungle of assistance systems (accepted). Stud. Health Technol. Inform. **271**, 828–832 (2020)

Pathobox: The Collaborative Tele-pathology Platform with Access Management

Rui Lebre[1,2](✉), Rui Jesus[2], Pedro Nunes[2], and Carlos Costa[2,3]

[1] University of A Coruña, Campus de Elviña, La Coruña, Spain
ruilebre@ua.pt
[2] Institute of Electronics and Informatics Engineering of Aveiro, Campus Universitário de Santiago, Aveiro, Portugal
[3] University of Aveiro, Campus Universitário de Santiago, Aveiro, Portugal

Abstract. Recent technological advances in medical informatics led to the adoption of new technologies in pathology clinical area. Digital pathology is allowing the acquisition, storage, and distribution of pathological digital samples, which are gathered by scanners and displayed in network workstations. This paper discusses the opportunities and challenges of digital pathology, and how it is changing education, training, and medical practice nowadays. A new paradigm of collaborative telepathology is proposed through a cloud-based architecture, fully compliant with the DICOM standard, that integrates a cross-platform pathology viewer, collaborative tools, virtual work-spaces, and personal storage areas. Data management and privacy are ensured through the implementation of a role-based access control mechanism. The solution was designed to serve distinct use cases, including telepathology and e-academy.

Keywords: Access control · WSI · Collaborative · Digital pathology · PACS · DICOM

1 Introduction

The introduction of digital medical imaging in healthcare started when digital computers took the first steps in the seventies [25]. Later on, a new branch of medical imaging started emerging, digital pathology. Digital pathology became popular in the last years due to technological developments and to the trend regarding the adoption of digital scanners. This new branch has risen with the incorporation of digital methods to deal with pathological data. It comprises the acquisition, management, distribution, and visualization of microscopic images and their associated metadata. The processing of digital images is performed by digital pathology scanners which produce the Whole-Slide Images (WSI) [27]. WSI are acquired through the image digitization of microscope glass slides by

X. Ye et al. (Eds.): BIOSTEC 2020, CCIS 1400, pp. 407–424, 2021.
https://doi.org/10.1007/978-3-030-72379-8_20

high-resolution scanners [27,28,37]. The specially designed scanners apply multiple magnifications and focal planes, producing high-resolution digital images that can aggregate several gigabytes of data [16].

Digital pathology is quickly replacing the conventional light microscopy, potentiating new applications in education, training and diagnosis [37,40]. Opposing a traditional pathology environment, the specimen storage is cheaper as the samples do not require specialized protection carried out by trained staff.

The advantages of this emerging modern branch of medical imaging are tremendous. On one hand, there are breakthroughs regarding the production and clinical environments such as the process of storing and remote viewing, annotation, and reporting. The digital pathology allows the physician to perform diagnosis in almost any place with an internet connection. Furthermore, it leads to improvements in the diagnostic accuracy, integration with hospital information systems, and availability of distributed work processes as collaborative work and telepathology [7,28]. Besides, unlike the traditional pathology slides, the whole-slide images do not deteriorate over time and it is possible to assure homogeneity of the display quality of the images [17].

The introduction of WSI and digital pathology turns the medical diagnosis faster and simpler as the physician may navigate and dynamically view the virtual slide in their workstation, panning and zooming whenever it is necessary and appropriate [8]. Professional WSI viewers can be integrated into the hospital diagnosis network and be accessed within the network or made available for research, remote diagnosis, and consultation (second opinions, among others) [8,29]. Some authors such as Pantanowitz et al. and Chordia et al. in [9,29] report a crescent need for telepathology and digital pathology in the daily routine practice. In [9], 98% out of 247 interrogated histo-pathologists felt the need for telepathology and digital pathology. However, only 34% declared the use of telepathology in medical practice. These survey results reveal demand for solutions of telepathology and collaborative platforms not only for clinical but also for educational purposes.

WSI allows the introduction of new educational methods to teach histology and pathology in the academia that was not possible until nowadays [30,37]. The educational workflow of pathology may be highly simplified by the introduction of the digital capabilities as what was before a slide, can now be accessed simultaneously by as many teachers and students as virtually possible. Additionally, it is only required to hold a computer or a smartphone to operate the image, contrasting with the traditional physical specimen which could only be handled by an operator at a time.

The availability of a slide in the digital format allows the remote access from anywhere and from any device instantly, including previous examinations that could be hard to find in the traditional physical archives. Yet, platforms such as these demand strong access security since they can be operated in open networks and by many people. Many of the cases require confidentiality considering the sample private data related to the patient and the regulations in force [1]. The addition of security protocols and measures takes a big part in the design of such solutions.

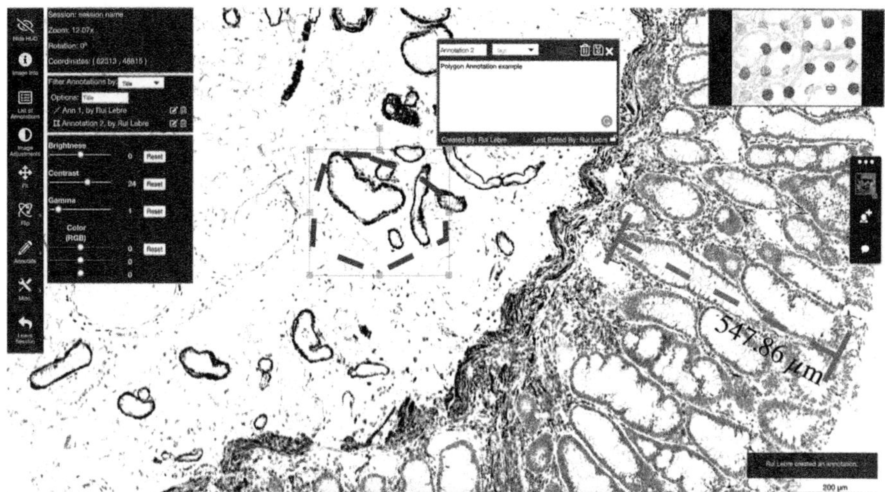

Fig. 1. Collaborative web pathology viewer screenshot. This screenshot shows the multitude of features supported, as ruler (in red), free form annotation (on purple), text annotation, chat, color and light adjustments, among others. (Color figure online)

Finally, the development of a proper user interface to aid in the adoption of these new technologies is one of the improvements that can help the teaching and collaborative diagnosis nowadays. The integration of new features impossible to include in the traditional methods became a reality, as the presence of a thumbnail to allow a fast and immediate panning, the possibility of annotate regions of interest directly in the sample and live discussion platform, for instance.

This paper proposes a collaborative pathology viewer[1] fully compatible with the Digital Imaging and Communications and Medicine (DICOM) standard. It extends [26], deploying a new refactored and improved viewer, with backend mechanisms improved in terms of performance, security, access control, and user experience. The deployed solution integrates a pure web solution supporting a pathology viewer (screenshot in Fig. 1) with an advanced security layer specially designed for DICOM compliant PACS archives [21]. The integration of both systems culminates in a secure platform where owners of the studies may give and revoke permissions to groups of users or individuals. The solution is deployed in an open-source PACS archive named Dicoogle [43].

The collaborative viewer supports new features like an image handling toolbox, shared pointers, and synchronized actions. The web pathology viewer backend archive was redesigned to support an innovative virtual multi-repository concept. Data security and privacy are ensured through the integration of an accounting mechanism specifically developed for medical imaging environments, allowing the creation of personal virtual archives. Some of the new features are, for instance, the restriction of access to only particular studies within a group

[1] Demo Video: https://www.youtube.com/watch?v=Mmsb25edcOo.

domain, among others described below. The introduction of the virtual archive feature allows the centralization of the storage. Thus, a PACS archive may serve distinct healthcare institutions simultaneously where each resource has specific permission policies giving the holder institution. In this, we discuss how crucial and pertinent the introduction of a platform as the one presented in the universities and clinical institutions is, regarding the digital and global world.

2 Background

2.1 PACS and DICOM Integration

Picture Archiving and Communication System (PACS) is a set of distinct hardware equipment and its running software connected in a network. It orchestrates the relationship between the software and hardware, the storage, and the distribution of medical data in a healthcare clinic or department. The workflow is typically divided into acquisition, distribution, and visualization of medical images [34].

The implementations of such systems have risen with the movement towards digital trend [3] and have deeply relied on the launch of the DICOM standard [24]. DICOM is one of the most popular standards in the medical imaging field [38] and provides a guide to support interoperability between multiple vendor equipment and systems [5].

DICOM was launched aiming to create a standard format for guidelines of how to handle and store radiology images [18], reflecting the real-world workflows in healthcare institutions. However, the release of new supplements keep DICOM standard constantly, keeping it updated, therefore fulfilling the users' needs over time.

Since the launch date, the adoption of DICOM among vendors was a success and supplementary modalities were added to the standard, for instance, nuclear medicine or breast tomosynthesis [3] and, in the recent past, microscopy with the release of the supplement 122 of the standard [11]. Later on, the DICOM standard committee released the supplement 145 [10]. Boosted by the development of whole-slide scanners [7], the additions and innovations of this supplement addressed the pathology in the digital form.

DICOM structures the data and associated metadata in its information model denominated DIM [33]. The organization is hierarchical and Patient-oriented [41]. The metadata associated depends on the acquisition modality. i.e., the required metadata fields in a computed tomography are distinct from the ones requested for digital pathology.

Nonetheless, supplements 122 and 145 disrupted the conventional patient-centric information model. WSI are classified by specialists as specimen centric [12,13] considering that the specimen is the relevant object. Nowadays, throughout these supplements, the DICOM standard integrates digital pathology required components and protocols as the data elements, the definition of the preparation workflow, acquisition, handling, and storage of whole-slide images [3,14].

2.2 Digital Pathology Visualization

Whole-slide scanners produce big amounts of data. In fact, the amount of data generated represents one of the biggest challenges in the displaying of whole-slide images [26]. The final scanned whole-slide image may have several gigapixels [36]. The specially designed scanners apply huge amounts of zoom so they can reproduce the physical specimen. The scanning of such a big area increases the number of pixels in the digital image. Proportional to the number of image size in pixels, also the file size increases.

The current personal computers and workstations' characteristics are still very limited and are not adequate to display locally this type of medical image [19]. Hence, DICOM standard digital pathology working group proposed a solution based on a pyramid approach. Figure 2 shows an example of this solution. The base-level image represents the full resolution scanned from the whole-slide scanners. The remaining levels are the same specimen with different levels of zoom applied, thus, more compressed stages.

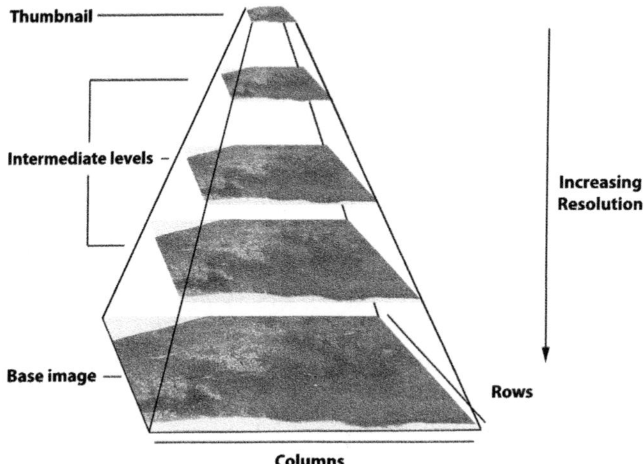

Fig. 2. DICOM supplement 145 proposes storing Whole-Slide Images in tiles from a multi resolution hierarchy in multi-frame object. The picture shows the different base level, intermediate levels and thumbnail in pyramid organization. Adapted from [26].

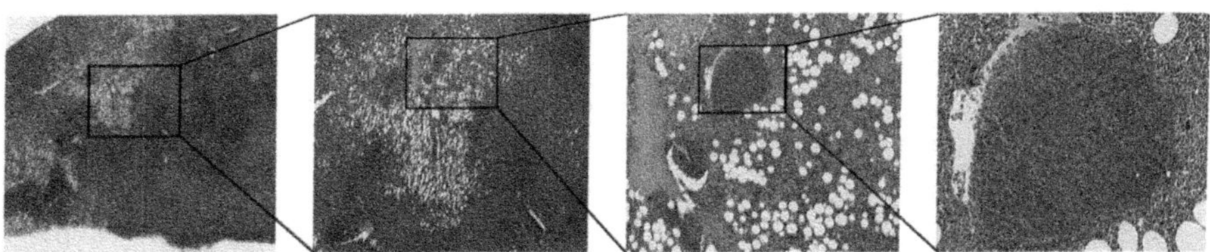

Fig. 3. Different zoom levels of an example Whole-Slide Image in the proposed viewer. From left to right: thumbnail, first intermediate level, n intermediate level, base level.

Nowadays, several solutions not only in the medical imaging field apply the same approach. Solutions as Google Maps, OpenStreetMap, or Digital Catalogs from some libraries around the world, such as the National Library of Australia, adopted the pyramid approach for handling big sized images.

The navigation in the pyramid images is achieved using the common panning and zooming tools. Selecting a part of the upper level and applying zoom, shows the next level of the pyramid in a restricted area. Figure 3 represents the workflow that may be followed by a physician while analyzing a whole-slide image, since the selection of the region of interest in the thumbnail and intermediate levels, until the reaching of the base level.

2.3 Dicoogle and Its Functionalities

Dicoogle[2] is PACS archive built with a modular architecture [43]. Dicoogle presents itself as a supporting platform for three different environments: clinical, research, and teaching. The wide applicability of Dicoogle relies on the plugin concept which allows that its base functionalities may be extended. The default provided plugins are a clear example of the extensible characteristics of Dicoogle. The default bundle provides a plugin to handle the DICOM C-Store service, for instance, and stores the received files in the local file-system. Regarding the indexing plugin, the Dicoogle team includes the Apache Lucene based plugin that indexes all the metadata contained in the received DICOM object.

The development of these plugins is supported by a software development kit (SDK). Dicoogle SDK emerged to facilitate the development of new features [43] and to assure compatibility with the intrinsic features. A Dicoogle plugin may be of many types: storage, index, query, web service, or web user interface. Storage plugins handle the storage of DICOM objects. The index plugins are typically bundled together with query plugins. This kind of modules are responsible for indexing the metadata and allow the query over the index. The default Dicoogle's web services and web interface may also be extended using plugins of type web service or web user interface, respectively.

2.4 Related Work

The ever-growing field of digital pathology, since the first steps, led to the development of distinct solutions regarding the visualization of whole-slide images. Although, most of them reproduce a representation of proprietary formats. In the scope of digital pathology viewers, an in-depth state-of-the-art analysis was done. Daniel et al. [13] state that digital pathology in the collaborative form can only be done through medical informatics accepted and widespread standard. Meanwhile, [3,13,42] authors stand that DICOM standard together with the supplements 122 and 145 provide a proper solution for a commonly accepted handling of whole-slide images and digital pathology.

[2] Available at: http://dicoogle.com/.

Carestream Health[3] [39,44] is a commercial solution for medical imaging viewing and handling. It supports radiology and cardiology modalities. However, The software is oriented for consulting and it does not support the collaborative paradigm.

In [20], the authors propose a set of tools that support the digital pathology workflow and allow the visualization of digital pathology images over the web. The authors state that the digital pathology segment is dominated by a set of vendors who have their proprietary format and viewing solutions. These vendors typically supply their viewers which are only suitable for each proprietary format.

In [6], the authors introduce iPath a Web-based digital pathology platform that allows the online presentation and discussion of cases within user groups. However, the architecture does not follow the DICOM standard.

Moreover, efforts regarding radiology have been carried out [45]. Bankhead et al. [2] propose an extensible software for medical imaging, powering users with scripting tools. However, it does not address both DICOM standard and collaborative requirements.

In [18], Godinho et al. proposed an efficient architecture for the transmission and support of digital pathology images. The authors developed an efficient web digital pathology viewer. The system allows communication with DICOM compliant PACS archives and was implemented using Dicoogle. Despite not allowing the collaborative scenario, the developed work may be extended to support it, as the deployment in Dicoogle presupposes the development in a modular architecture.

Díaz et al. propose in [15] a web-based telepathology system for pathology collaborative work. Yet, the developed platform is not DICOM compliant. Therefore, it does not support the communication with modalities that apply the same standard. Additionally, this solution does not address academic scenarios.

Liu et al. [23] proposed efficient methods for a performant transmission of medical high-resolution images in telemedicine. This method lays on a unbalance pyramid scheme based on a geometric relationship. The effort applied in multiple components allows fast transmission. However, it is not compatible with JPEG2000 and JPIP protocols.

3 Architecture

This paper proposes a set of modules that compose a collaborative platform fully DICOM compliant. The platform was integrated with the Dicoogle PACS archive, an open-source DICOM compliant PACS. The proposal features an environment for real-time collaboration between users, providing means for fully remote work, suitable for either educational or professional purposes.

3.1 Acquisition, Storage and Distribution

As the Dicoogle PACS archive is a DICOM compliant platform, it accepts communications from other data sources that implement the same standard. Dicoogle

[3] Available at https://www.carestream.com.

can act as a Service Class Provider (SCP), accepting communications from third entities like, for instance, the imaging modalities. In the digital pathology, there are already WSI scanners able to communicate through the DICOM C-Store command.

Figure 4 presents the workflows supported by Dicoogle. Once the WSI is acquired from the scanner, it can be transferred to the Dicoogle archive using distinct interfaces, including DICOM services, as STOW-RS or C-Store, or other file-sharing mechanisms made available by Dicoogle. If the received file/object is not in the DICOM format, Dicoogle is able to convert it to DICOM format. The reception of the image objects triggers the generation of the intermediate and thumbnail levels of the viewing system (see Sect. 2.2 and Fig. 2). The DICOM objects generated, corresponding to each level of the pyramid are then stored and indexed in the archive.

After being stored and indexed by Dicoogle, the examination is visible for the client sessions. The information can be queried and retrieved to be displayed in the digital pathology viewer, using the WADO-RS DICOMweb service.

3.2 Collaborative Platform

The collaborative platform architecture was constructed to be as flexible as possible foreseeing further improvements in the future. It is built using multiple modules where each one has its unit and core functionality. This kind of architecture allows us to create, update, or delete functionalities while the remaining modules keep their core functions.

Three major components compose the collaborative platform: the PACS archive described in Sects. 2.3 and 3.1; a viewer that runs on any web browser, responsible for fetching the slides of each digital pathology case study stored in the archive; and finally, an auxiliary dashboard where the management of each collaborative session can be performed either by the session manager/owner of the generality of the participants, as showed in Fig. 5.

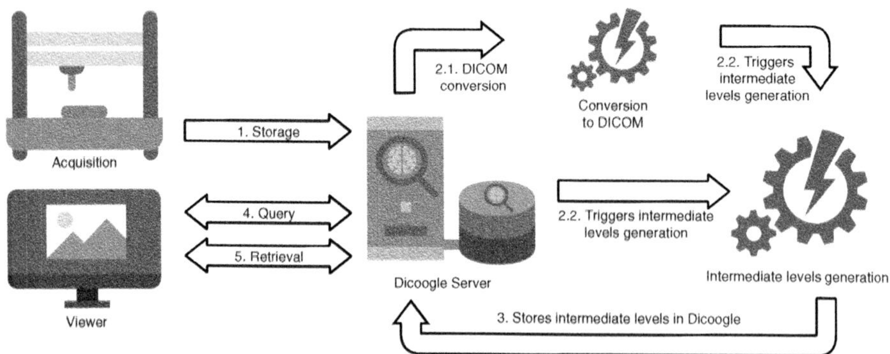

Fig. 4. Workflow of the acquisition, storage and distribution of pathology slide.

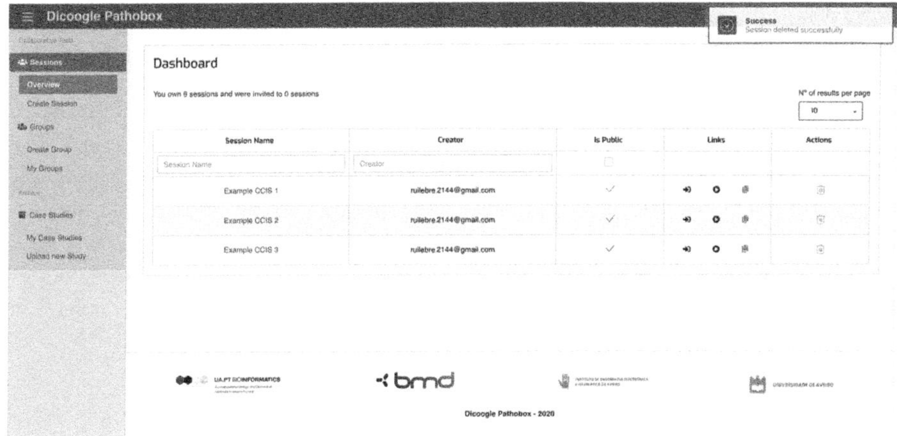

Fig. 5. Example of the main dashboard of the collaborative platform. Pathobox Demo available at: http://demo.dicoogle.com/pathobox.

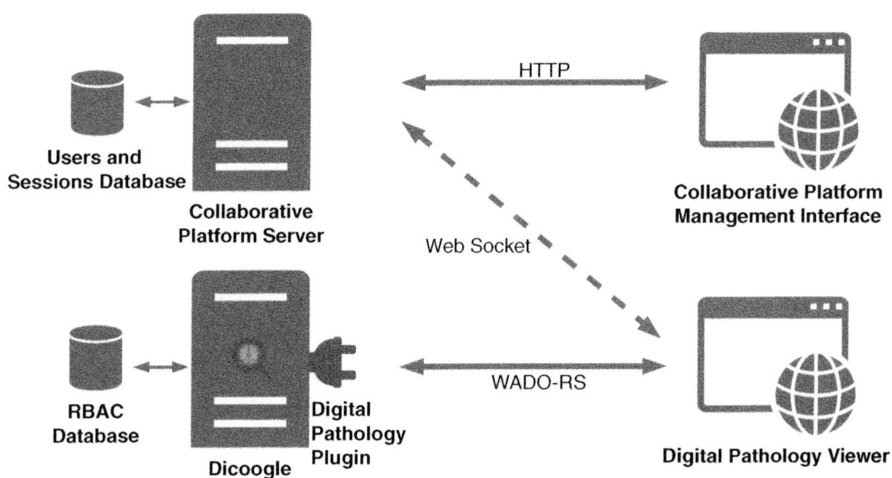

Fig. 6. System general architecture. Dicoogle and its plugins serve the Web Viewer with the WSI. Simultaneously, the viewer is connected to the collaborative platform server via WebSocket to retrieve the session details and the user's permissions. The collaborative platform management interface provides a dashboard to manage all the sessions, users, and groups. Adapted from [26].

Figure 6 represents the interactions between each component. The extension of the Dicoogle PACS archive to support the collaborative digital pathology viewer took from the base the work developed by Godinho et al. [18]. The presented work compiled both the Dicoogle PACS archive and the viewer. To support real-time collaboration between users, those elements were redesigned and new mechanisms and algorithms were developed.

The handling of the synchronization of events across all participant users is achieved with the integration of TogetherJS[4], an open-source technology that provides real-time collaboration features. This tool is responsible for managing the web viewer sessions.

The integration of the collaborative platform is independent of the web viewer. The integrated collaborative platform is a layer above the previously developed pathology viewer. Therefore, the actions taken across by multiple users throughout a session may be turned into an abstract action. I.e., the integration of the collaborative platform is independent of the source viewer where the data is originated. Thus, it is suitable for integration with other viewers.

3.3 Management of Sessions

The developed collaborative platform is responsible for the creation of the virtual working sessions and the managing of the participating users, as well as the attribution of the respective permissions. A virtual working session is a collaborative session created for one particular WSI stored in the PACS archive. The changes and adjustments to the WSI in the session are kept in the session persistence. Therefore, the WSI DICOM object is kept original.

A session consists of its creator or owner, a list of users and permissions applied to each one. Furthermore, the session is applied to an image, and stores a list of events that happened in that particular session. Additional stored information also allows the web viewer to handle the session.

One single image can have multiple sessions associated with it, with each session having its own users and events. Furthermore, one user may create multiple sessions using the same image. The unique identification of each session allows the creation of a unique URL generated so a user may join a session. Those unique URLs are created using the unique identifier of the session and the user ID of the allowed user to join. The system may, consequently, keep tracking and logging of the users who joined and participated in the session.

Figure 7 shows an example of the creation of a session. The session creation process was developed to simplify the invitation of other users. The invitation may occur by e-mail or by the sharing of a public link. In the case of the invitation by e-mail, the users are given a unique URL with personalized permissions. However, using the public link, the session join will be anonymous and the permissions to handle the image and participate in the session are limited. A maximum number of users per session may be set.

The web links allow access to a session without having to use the platform itself. Only the creator has to be logged into the platform, because of the need to proceed to initial configurations of the session. For automation of the workflow, the session emails are used as identifiers to distinguish the participants in the session. The usage of emails allows the sharing of the web links of the session automatically, turning the process of the invitation of new users transparent and agile for the session creator.

---

[4] Available at https://togetherjs.com/.

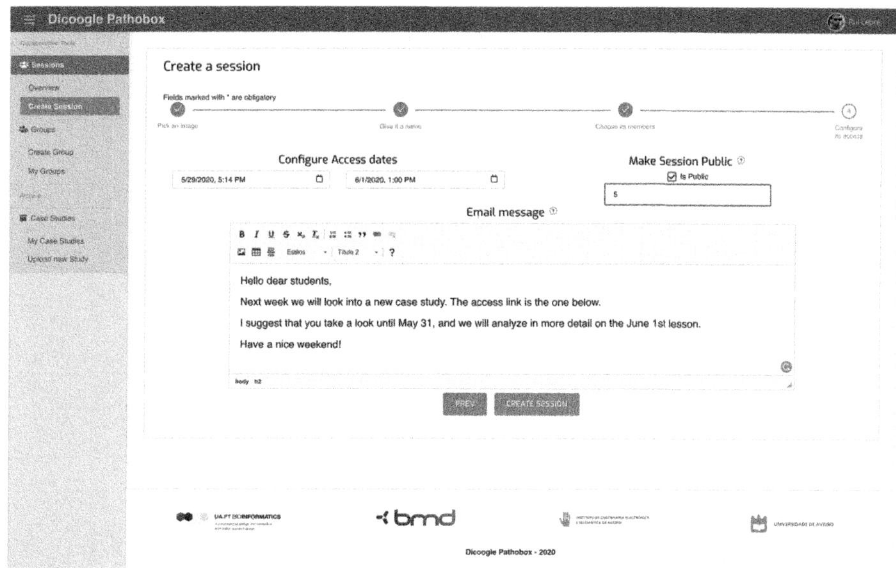

Fig. 7. Creation of a working session example with a limited window time access permission.

The sending of the session invitation links through email is naturally secured if using the proper mechanisms available, like SSL. Additionally, signing mechanisms as a digital signature may sign the email, so only the end-user, and theoretically, the e-mail owner has access to the collaborative working session.

The unique identification of each one of the web links allows the joining in the session even though the invited user does not have an account in the collaborative platform. As long as the email invited by the session creator matches the email used to sign in, the access is granted.

Regarding the viewer, the fetching is made via WADO-RS. The users access the platform through the unique web link. Thus, once the link contains information about both the user and the session, the Dicoogle permissions mechanism (more details in Sect. 3.5) checks and grants or denies access to the WSI tiles. Simultaneously, the collaborative checks constantly if the user is still logged in into the platform.

Since the session joining is based on the unique web links access, the concurrent access is restricted. There is not possible to access the same link at the same time, resulting in the restriction of one session per user at a time. Consequently, it is possible to have control of the number of users within a session. The user identity is also correct, assuming that the e-mail account was not compromised or the web link was not shared with third-parties.

Alternatively, access may be granted via a public general link that does not contain information of the user who is accessing. This modality was created looking for the broadcast of the session and sharing of the access to potential

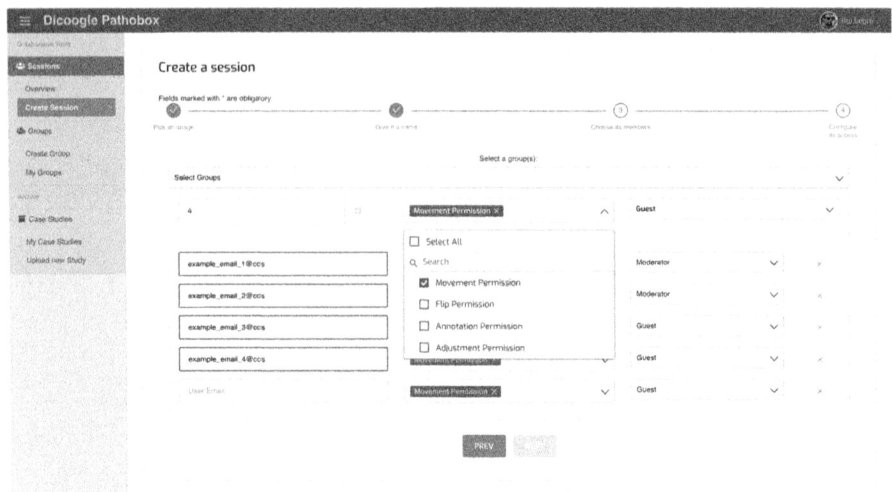

Fig. 8. Creation of a working session example in the step of inviting users.

unknown users or users whose e-mails are unknown. Yet, a limit of maximum users who may access the platform via public weblink can be set up. Similarly, the permissions may be personalized and the creation of the public link is optional. However, access to the managing platform is denied since the user must be registered to access it.

Figure 8 shows a screenshot of the step of inviting users to a session in a *Create Session* workflow.

3.4 Synchronization of User Actions

The key factor of the collaborative platform in the run-time is synchronization. The actions performed by each user, such as zooming in or changing the saturation, for instance, have to be broadcasted for the rest of the users. This synchronization is achieved via the TogetherJS framework. The developed structure allows the segregation between the entity that produces an event and the entities that replicate the same event.

The generated events are persisted in a central database. This way, the collaborative platform assures that the users that temporarily lose the connection may recover it and do not miss not saved work. The re-joining in the ongoing session retrieves all the events performed until the lost of connection and the events occurred in the downtime, keeping up the flow of the session. The storage of the occurred events allows also the replay of the session since its beginning, replicating the events chronologically.

Since many users may interact and handle the WSI simultaneously, the timestamp of the reception of the broadcasted events may differ from user to user, resulting in inconsistent states throughout the working session. An asynchronous system was developed to handle this issue. Despite the existence of multiple session states across different users, the database keeps only one final version of those events. For instance, if a user changes the brightness five times in a row, those five times are reduced and only the final brightness value is saved. This way, the broadcasted events are reduced, and eventually, all users will be in the same state.

However, only certain actions as zooming or panning the WSI create these different states. The developed algorithm makes sure that all users are set to the same state, without conflict, right after the panning or zooming event is performed. For instance, when two users perform the zooming at different levels at the same time, the users may end up on distinct zoom levels. If a third zooming operation is executed, all the remaining users will be synchronized for that zoom level.

A study for the evaluation of the usability impact of these inconsistencies was conducted. The results show that the inconsistent states stay for a very short period since the fundamental actions as color and light adjustments or annotations do not cause those inconsistencies. Thus, the addition of a delay in the propagation of an event was discarded. Therefore, the broadcasting of the user actions in the form of an event is emitted instantly after their execution.

The nature of the working sessions and the dimensions of the WSI in digital pathology may lead to huge amounts of zooming or panning type of events. Even though the panning and zooming events are minimal, it may cause visual impact. Despite the total of the broadcasted events to keep synchronization between users, when the storage in the database is performed, the events are filtered to only keep the events that lead to a noticeable visual difference from the original state. This decision prevents heavy traffic of messages between components, improves the performance of an ongoing working session, and the user experience since only the relevant information is kept.

3.5 Access Control Component

This article proposes a collaborative platform architecture that supports multiple users with associated resources, including personal data archives with sensitive information.

The General Data Protection Regulation (GDPR), in force since May 2018, defines clear guidelines to follow when developing and deploying software and hardware in healthcare, so that the risk of a security breach is attenuated (art. 32) [32]. The regulation specifies that private personal data is required to be protected from illegitimate access, destruction, damage, or accidental loss.

Following the required in the regulation, a solution of the access control mechanism was integrated into the collaborative platform. The integrated framework protects the resources from unauthorized on unwanted access by providing a resource ownership mechanism. The concept of a resource is general. I.e., an abstract resource may be DICOM objects or institution hardware.

The framework adopted is based on the work developed by Lebre et al. [22] mechanism where the authors introduce an RBAC (Role-Based Access Control)

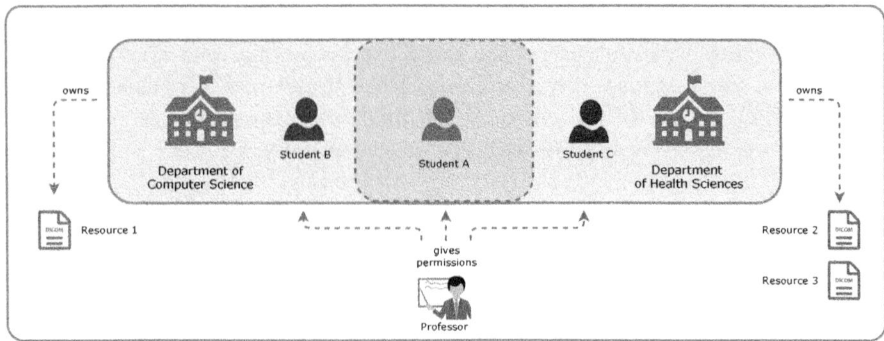

Fig. 9. Example of a academic scenario where the access control of the proposed collaborative platform is suitable.

adapted for standard DICOM archives and implemented in Dicoogle. This work is capable of managing user personal work-spaces and personalized permissions for each user. Moreover, it associates the user permissions with the PACS archive resources, allowing the set of permissions for each DICOM object and delegation of rights to third parties. The delegation of rights allows, for instance, the sharing of read or write permissions to other users.

The resulting system works as a multi-archive. The introduced framework is supported by a persistence layer and is independent of the regular DICOM workflows. Our solution introduces the resource ownership abstraction and allows the control of the access to medical imaging resources as DICOM objects. The deployment of such a framework suggests that a single PACS archive may serve different virtual archives. This way, each study stored in the PACS archive can be shared across different realms and users. The sharing feature applied to digital pathology concedes various use cases, as the sharing of a WSI to a set of users belonging to different healthcare institutions.

The integrated access control mechanism is an abstraction of real-world medical imaging environments. Figure 9 shows an example of the application of an accounting mechanism in the academic context. On it, it is represented a university, containing two departments, Department of Computer Science and Department of Health Sciences. Each department is the owner of resources, in this case, DICOM objects. Also, each department has his students, Student A belongs to both departments, Student B belongs to the Department of Computer Science, and Student C is registered in the Department of Health Sciences. The students may access the files of their associated facility. However, the administrator, in the example represented as the Professor, must give the READ permission in order for the granting to be successful.

4 Use Cases

The introduction of the collaborative digital pathology in the medical imaging domain carries multiple advantages. The deployment of a collaborative viewer, on its hand, extends its utility, improving the concept of telepathology. The WSI viewer turns itself in a workspace where several users may interact and discuss one single sample at the same time, and even in multiple sessions at a time. The collaborative pathology platform suits for three distinct domains: academic, educational, and clinical [7,28,31,37,40].

Among the multiple advantages of the collaborative platform viewer in the educational domain, the creation of collaborative classes emerge. The platform allows the creation of user groups that may represent each class. During the creation of the session, the session owner can invite a group of users and has the possibility of restricting the access to s specific schedule. These sessions may represent a case study in a class. Moreover, the session owner may also open the virtual class to public access. Finally, the students can use the replay tool to review the actions carried out throughout the session.

The clinical domain is, perhaps, the environment that benefits more from the implementation of an accounting system in the collaborative digital pathology platform. The introduction of the permission managing framework allows the regulation, control, logging, and auditing of the access requested for the PACS archive resources.

Using the collaborative digital pathology platform, it is possible to set up centralized diagnosis services where the entities can upload case and request revision services to the community. The specialist can be registered in the platform or not, to perform the service. The request can be sporadic or regular. An entity may ask for an external revision of a study, by a specialist, who can easily join into a session through an invite (e.g. email) with an access link. Or, if the center has only technicians, it can upload all examination to the central service where a predefined group of physicians will review the cases. Moreover, if the service workflow contemplates a first revision of the case and its annotation for facilitating the specialist revision, the system offers the record and replay feature. The replay session-catch service benefits the usability of the collaborative platform. This methodology consists of the fast replay of the relevant operations of a working session until the present moment.

As the security is always in mind, a session administrator may revoke access and terminate the session unilaterally. However, some security issues may occur, as the compromising of the transport layer when sending the access links. The sending of invites relies on the known secure protocols for message exchange as TLS. Moreover, the session administrator who has also access rights to the DICOM object may deny the public invitation of new users to the session. Regarding the authentication, the registered access to the platform relies on Google authentication as an additional security method.

5 Conclusions

Collaborative work is a fundamental feature in the nowadays medical imaging and diagnosis systems addressing educational and diagnosis purposes [35]. For instance, the SARS-CoV-2 pandemic at the beginning of 2020 showed to the world that humanity must be prepared for a generalized lock-down. The collaborative platforms represent a decisive role in the medical field nowadays. Digital pathology and telepathology are an emerging modality in the clinical decision-making laboratories and with the clinical staff supporting the development of new tools [4].

This paper proposes and implements an architecture for real-time collaboration in digital pathology. The system integrated an open-source PACS archive, a digital pathology viewer, and a framework to handle the access control. The concept of the developed system uses pure web technologies so the interoperability between platforms is assured. That way, a user may use the platform either on his smartphone, tablet, or computer, requiring only the internet connection to fetch the digital pathology images. The events performed in the collaborative working sessions are recorded and may be accessed later on. We analyzed the use cases of the proposed platform and presented clear potential benefits by using the digital pathology collaborative platform both on the educational point of view or the clinical practice and diagnosis perspective.

References

1. Abouelmehdi, K., Beni-Hessane, A., Khaloufi, H.: Big healthcare data: preserving security and privacy. J. Big Data **5**(1), 1 (2018). https://doi.org/10.1186/s40537-017-0110-7
2. Bankhead, P., et al.: QuPath: open source software for digital pathology image analysis. Sci. Rep. **7**, 1–7 (2017)
3. Beckwith, B.A.: Standards for digital pathology and whole slide imaging. In: Kaplan, K.J., Rao, L.K.F. (eds.) Digital Pathology, pp. 87–97. Springer, Cham (2016). https://doi.org/10.1007/978-3-319-20379-9_9
4. Bellis, M., Metias, S., Naugler, C., Pollett, A., Jothy, S., Yousef, G.M.: Digital pathology: attitudes and practices in the Canadian pathology community. J. Pathol. Inform. **4**, 3 (2013)
5. Bidgood, W.D., Horii, S.C., Prior, F.W., Van Syckle, D.E.: Understanding and using DICOM, the data interchange standard for biomedical imaging. J. Am. Med. Inform. Assoc. **4**(3), 199–212 (1997)
6. Brauchli, K., Oberholzer, M.: The iPath telemedicine platform. J. Telemed. Telecare **11**(2_suppl), 3–7 (2005)
7. Bueno, G., Fernández-Carrobles, M.M., Deniz, O., García-Rojo, M.: New trends of emerging technologies in digital pathology. Pathobiology **83**, 61–69 (2016)
8. Bueno, G., Fernández-Carrobles, M.M., Deniz, O., García-Rojo, M.: New trends of emerging technologies in digital pathology. Pathobiology **83**(2–3), 61–69 (2016). https://doi.org/10.1159/000443482
9. Chordia, T., Vikey, A., Choudhary, A., Samdariya, Y., Chordia, D.: Current status and future trends in telepathology and digital pathology. J. Oral Maxillofac. Pathol. **20**(2), 178 (2016). https://doi.org/10.4103/0973-029X.185924

10. DICOM Standards Committee: Working groups 26, pathology, "digital imaging and communications in medicine (DICOM) supplement 145: Whole slide microscopic image IOD and SOP classes" (2009)
11. DICOM Standards Committee: Working groups 26, pathology (2008)
12. Daniel, C., et al.: Standards to support information systems integration in anatomic pathology. Arch. Pathol. Lab. Med. **133**(11), 1841–1849 (2009)
13. Daniel, C., et al.: Recent advances in standards for collaborative digital anatomic pathology. In: Diagnostic Pathology, vol. 6, p. S17. BioMed Central (2011)
14. Daniel, C., et al.: Standardizing the use of whole slide images in digital pathology. Comput. Med. Imaging Graph. **35**, 496–505 (2011)
15. Díaz, D., Corredor, G., Romero, E., Cruz-Roa, A.: A web-based telepathology framework for collaborative work of pathologists to support teaching and research in Latin America. In: Lepore, N., Brieva, J., Romero, E., Racoceanu, D., Joskowicz, L. (eds.) SaMBa 2018. LNCS, vol. 11379, pp. 105–112. Springer, Cham (2019). https://doi.org/10.1007/978-3-030-13835-6_12
16. Farahani, N., Parwani, A.V., Pantanowitz, L.: Whole slide imaging in pathology: advantages, limitations, and emerging perspectives. Pathol. Lab. Med. Int. **7**, 23–33 (2015)
17. Foster, K.: Medical education in the digital age: digital whole slide imaging as an e-learning tool. J. Pathol. Inform. **1**, 14 (2010)
18. Godinho, T.M., Lebre, R., Silva, L.B., Costa, C.: An efficient architecture to support digital pathology in standard medical imaging repositories. J. Biomed. Inform. **71**, 190–197 (2017)
19. Goode, A., Gilbert, B., Harkes, J., Jukic, D., Satyanarayanan, M.: OpenSlide: a vendor-neutral software foundation for digital pathology. J. Pathol. Inform. **4**, 27 (2013)
20. Lauro, G.R., et al.: Digital pathology consultations–a new era in digital imaging, challenges and practical applications. J. Digit. Imaging **26**(4), 668–677 (2013). https://doi.org/10.1007/s10278-013-9572-0
21. Lebre, R., Godinho, T., Silva, L., Costa, C.: A performant and fully DICOM compliant web PACS for digital pathology. Int. J. Comput. Assist. Radiol. Surg. **13**, 147–148 (2018). https://doi.org/10.1007/s11548-018-1766-y
22. Lebre, R., Bastião, L., Costa, C.: Shared medical imaging repositories. In: MIE - Medical Informatics Europe, pp. 411–415 (2018)
23. Wang, L., Zhou, L., Fu, X., Liu, L., Liu, L., et al.: An efficient architecture for medical high-resolution images transmission in mobile telemedicine systems. Comput. Methods Programs Biomed. **187**, 105088 (2019)
24. Mildenberger, P.: IT innovation and big data. In: Donoso-Bach, L., Boland, G.W.L. (eds.) Quality and Safety in Imaging. MR, pp. 159–170. Springer, Cham (2017). https://doi.org/10.1007/174_2017_144
25. Mustra, M., Delac, K., Grgic, M.: Overview of the DICOM standard. In: 2008 50th International Symposium ELMAR, vol. 1, pp. 39–44. IEEE (2008)
26. Nunes., P., Jesus., R., Lebre., R., Costa., C.: Data and sessions management in a telepathology platform. In: Proceedings of the 13th International Joint Conference on Biomedical Engineering Systems and Technologies - Volume 5 HEALTHINF: HEALTHINF, pp. 455–462. INSTICC, SciTePress (2020). https://doi.org/10.5220/0008969904550462
27. Pantanowitz, L.: Digital images and the future of digital pathology. J. Pathol. Inform. **1**, 15 (2010)
28. Pantanowitz, L., et al.: Review of the current state of whole slide imaging in pathology. J. Pathol. Inform. **2**(1), 36 (2011). https://doi.org/10.4103/2153-3539.83746

29. Pantanowitz, L., Farahani, N., Parwani, A.: Whole slide imaging in pathology: advantages, limitations, and emerging perspectives. Pathol. Lab. Med. Int. 23 (2015). https://doi.org/10.2147/PLMI.S59826
30. Pantanowitz, L., Szymas, J., Yagi, Y., Wilbur, D.: Whole slide imaging for educational purposes. J. Pathol. Inform. **3**, 46 (2012)
31. Patterson, E.S., Rayo, M., Gill, C., Gurcan, M.N.: Barriers and facilitators to adoption of soft copy interpretation from the user perspective: lessons learned from filmless radiology for slideless pathology. J. Pathol. Inform. **2**, 1 (2011)
32. Pedrosa, M., Costa, C., Dorado, J.: GDPR impacts and opportunities for computer-aided diagnosis guidelines and legal perspectives. In: 2019 IEEE 32nd International Symposium on Computer-Based Medical Systems (CBMS), pp. 616–621. IEEE (2019)
33. Pedrosa, M., Silva, J.M., Silva, J.F., Matos, S., Costa, C.: SCREEN-DR: collaborative platform for diabetic retinopathy. Int. J. Med. Inform. **120**, 137–146 (2018)
34. Pianykh, O.: Digital Imaging and Communications in Medicine (DICOM), vol. 3. Springer, Heidelberg (2008). https://doi.org/10.1007/978-3-540-74571-6
35. Quintero, J.M., Aguilera, A., Abraham, M., Villegas, H., Montilla, G., Solaiman, B.: Medical decision-making and collaborative reasoning. In: Proceedings 2nd Annual IEEE International Symposium on Bioinformatics and Bioengineering (BIBE 2001), pp. 161–165. IEEE (2001)
36. Ruddle, R.A., Thomas, R.G., Randell, R., Quirke, P., Treanor, D.: The design and evaluation of interfaces for navigating gigapixel images in digital pathology. ACM Trans. Comput.-Hum. Interact. (TOCHI) **23**(1), 1–29 (2016)
37. Saco, A., Bombi, J.A., Garcia, A., Ramírez, J., Ordi, J.: Current status of whole-slide imaging in education. Pathobiology **83**(2–3), 79–88 (2016). https://doi.org/10.1159/000442391
38. Silva, J.M., Godinho, T.M., Silva, D., Costa, C.: A community-driven validation service for standard medical imaging objects. Comput. Stand. Interf. **61**, 121–128 (2019)
39. Snyder, P.D., Hasso, C.A., Masi, L.P.: Pathology dependent viewing of processed dental radiographic film having authentication data (Feb 27 2001), US Patent 6,195,474
40. Triola, M.M., Holloway, W.J.: Enhanced virtual microscopy for collaborative education. BMC Med. Educ. **11**(1), 4 (2011). https://doi.org/10.1186/1472-6920-11-4
41. Trivedi, D.N., Shah, N.D., Kothari, A.M., Thanki, R.M.: DICOM® medical image standard. Dental Image Processing for Human Identification, pp. 41–49. Springer, Cham (2019). https://doi.org/10.1007/978-3-319-99471-0_4
42. Tuominen, V.J., Isola, J.: Linking whole-slide microscope images with DICOM by using JPEG2000 interactive protocol. J. Digit. Imaging **23**(4), 454–462 (2010)
43. Valente, F., Silva, L.A.B., Godinho, T.M., Costa, C.: Anatomy of an extensible open source PACS. J. Digit. Imaging **29**(3), 284–296 (2016). https://doi.org/10.1007/s10278-015-9834-0
44. Weiss, M.: APC forum: Carestream health's IT transformation. MIS Q. Executive **11**(1), 8 (2012)
45. Zhang, J., Stahl, J.N., Huang, H.K., Zhou, X., Lou, S.L., Song, K.S.: Real-time teleconsultation with high-resolution and large-volume medical images for collaborative healthcare. IEEE Trans. Inf. Technol. Biomed. **4**(2), 178–185 (2000)

Combining Rhythmic and Morphological ECG Features for Automatic Detection of Atrial Fibrillation: Local and Global Prediction Models

Gennaro Laudato[1(✉)], Franco Boldi[2(✉)], Angela Rita Colavita[3(✉)], Giovanni Rosa[1(✉)], Simone Scalabrino[1,4(✉)], Aldo Lazich[5,6(✉)], and Rocco Oliveto[1,4(✉)]

[1] STAKE Lab, University of Molise, Pesche, IS, Italy
{gennaro.laudato,simone.scalabrino,rocco.oliveto}@unimol.it, g.rosa@studenti.unimol.it
[2] XEOS., Roncadelle, BS, Italy
franco.boldi@xeos.it
[3] ASREM, Campobasso, CB, Italy
angelarita.colavita@asrem.org
[4] Datasound srl, Pesche, IS, Italy
{rocco,simone}@datasound.it
[5] Ministero della Difesa, Rome, RM, Italy
aldo.lazich@marina.difesa.it
[6] DIAG, University of Rome "La Sapienza", Rome, Italy
lazich@diag.uniroma1.it

Abstract. Atrial fibrillation (AF) is the most common type of heart arrhythmia. AF is highly associated with other cardiovascular diseases, such as heart failure, coronary artery disease and can lead to stroke. Unfortunately, in some cases people with atrial fibrillation have no explicit symptoms and are unaware of their condition until it is discovered during a physical examination. Thus, it is considered a priority to define highly accurate automatic approaches to detect such a pathology in the context of a massive screening.

For this reason, in the recent years several approaches have been defined to automatically detect AF. These approaches are often based on machine learning techniques and—most of them—analyse the heart rhythm to make a prediction. Even if AF can be diagnosed by analysing the rhythm, the analysis of the morphology of a heart beat is also important. Indeed, during an AF events the P wave could be absent and fibrillation waves may appear in its place. This means that the presence of only arrhythmia could be not enough to detect an AF events.

Based on the above consideration we have presented MORPHYTHM, an approach that use machine learning to combine rhythm and morphological features to identify AF events. The results we achieved in an empirical evaluation seems promising. In this paper we present an extension of MORPHYTHM, called LOCAL MORPHYTHM, aiming at further improving the detection accuracy of AF events. An empirical evaluation of LOCAL

X. Ye et al. (Eds.): BIOSTEC 2020, CCIS 1400, pp. 425–441, 2021.
https://doi.org/10.1007/978-3-030-72379-8_21

Morphythm has shown significantly better results in the classification process with respect to Morphythm, particularly for what concerns the true positives and false negatives.

Keywords: Healthcare · Atrial fibrillation · Decision support system · Machine learning

1 Introduction

During the last few years has occurred a rapid technological evolution in the scientific field of the Internet of Medical Things (IoMT) and Wireless Body Area Network (WBAN). The main demands for these systems can be summarised as follows: (i) reducing the healthcare costs while keeping the quality of the services and (ii) promoting wellness programs to shift the health expenditure from treatment to prevention [3].

All the efforts in this field by the scientific research communities has made it possible to obtain electronic devices of minimal size and wearable [31]. This has created a fertile ground for telemedicine. Telemedicine can be commonly defined as the use of advanced telecommunications technologies for the purpose of supporting many medical activities. In the last years, this industry has grown and most US health institutions and hospitals are currently employing such kind of technology [12].

In this context, medical activities become responsible—beyond the knowledge and clinical skills—in handling an ample amount of data related to the patient health. Thus, appropriate elaboration of the clinical data are required to facilitate the work of experts and promote a policy of welfare. A Decision Support System (DSS) is the key component of an effective telemedicine system. Such a component is basically a layer of software that latently and continuously analyze the acquired data aimed at providing recommendations, even at patient-level, to the medical experts for the identification of a risky situation or for the diagnosis of a specific pathology [38].

In this paper we present an approach that could be integrated in a DSS of a telemedicine system aiming at supporting the identification of atrial fibrillation (AF) episodes through the analysis of ECG. AF is the most common sustained arrhythmia and is associated with significant morbidity and mortality [10]. We decided to focus on AF detection because of the incidence statistics of such a pathology. Indeed, around one third of all ischemic strokes are caused by AF [14] and the early phase of appearance is a particularly high-risk period for the development of stroke [34]. In addition, AF is often asymptomatic. Thus, it is crucial to detect onset episodes of AF with high accuracy to allow a proper intervention of cardiologist [18].

The detection of AF episodes generally involves two electrocardiogram (ECG) sources of information: (i) *beat morphology*, because during an AF episode, it is possible to observe fluctuating wave forms instead of P waves and (ii) *rhythm*, because during an AF episode it is possible to observe an irregularity of heart rate. The fact that an ECG recording of the episode is a diagnostic criterion can make the process cumbersome, especially if the arrhythmia is paroxysmal and not easily provoked during a recording session. In order to capture the episode, an extended recording time (at least 24 h) through an Holter monitoring is required [2]. These recordings from wearable ECG devices introduce an amount of data which results complicated for the physician to inspect and analyze. This recall the need of semi-automatic approaches to determine onset and duration of AF episodes.

A lot of effort in the research community has been devoted to the definition of methods to automatically detect AF. These are often based on Machine Learning techniques and—most of them—are based only on the analysis of R-R intervals (RRI), *i.e.,* they just exploit the rhythmic source of information. Even if the accuracy of such approach is generally very high in terms of accuracy (more than 95%), the proposed approach still misclassifies *fibrillant* heart beat signals as *non-fibrillant* [41]. This suggests that there is still room for improvement. Especially, our conjecture is that by combining morphological and rhythm features is possible to improve the accuracy of approaches based on just one of the two source of information.

Based on the above consideration, in a previous work we have presented MORPHYTHM [23], a new approach based on machine learning techniques where morphological and rhythmic information are fused together. MORPHYTHM showed surprising results, especially for what concerns two vital aspects of the medical classification: increment of true positives and reduction of false negatives.

In this paper we present an extension of MORPHYTHM aiming at further improving its accuracy. We first performed a rigorous feature engineering process in order to identify the features that contribute the most to the prediction of AF events. Then, we experimented most advanced machine learning techniques, including artificial neural network and deep learning techniques. Finally, we integrated in MORPHYTHM the concept of" local" prediction, successfully used in other context [28]. Especially, instead of producing a single prediction model, the new version of MORPHYTHM, called LOCAL MORPHYTHM, automatically build several prediction models based on the characteristics of the ECGs in the training set. In particular, the training set is clustered in order to put together ECGs that exhibits similar characteristics. Then, for each cluster, LOCAL MORPHYTHM builds a prediction model. When a new data point is provided, LOCAL MORPHYTHM first selects the most suitable model based on the characteristics of the new data point, and then it performs the prediction applying the selected model.

The rest of the paper is structured as follows: Sect. 2 provides details on AF and on automatic detectors of AF. Section 3 presents LOCAL MORPHYTHM, our novel approach for AF detection, while Sect. 4 reports the design and the results of the empirical study we conducted to evaluate LOCAL MORPHYTHM. Finally, Sect. 5 concludes the paper and provides suggestions for possible future research directions.

2 Background and Related Work

2.1 Atrial Fibrillation

Normally, the heart contracts and relaxes to a regular beat. In atrial fibrillation, the upper chambers of the heart (the atria) beat irregularly (quiver) instead of beating effectively to move blood into the ventricles[1]. If the ECG recording is available, AF is diagnosed by whenever an irregular heartbeat presents the following characteristics: the absence of P waves (with disorganized electrical activity in their place) and irregular R–R intervals due to irregular conduction of impulses to the ventricles [15].

The prevalence of atrial fibrillation (AF) is increasing all over the world and it is becoming one of the most important clinical issues for industrialised countries [15,42]. AF is a crucial risk factor for the occurrence of stroke. Beyond stroke, AF can lead also to congestive heart failure. Furthermore, hypertension, diabetes and heart failure are some of the most common comorbidities [24,39]. In addition, AF presents a sever influence on the global health conditions of individuals who contract it [20].

To produce a diagnosis of AF, a cardiologist checks the clinical history of the patient and the ECG signal, by at least observing a single lead during the revealing of the episode [15]. Unfortunately, AF is often paroxysmal, *i.e.,* there are recurrent episodes that stop on their own in less than seven days [15], and asymptomatic. For these reasons, the screening of such a pathology needs to become a priority.

2.2 Automatic Detection of Atrial Fibrillation

In recent years, the scientific research has provided several works aiming at automatically detect AF episodes. Most of them have shown important results by exploiting only the analysis of heart rhythm, assumed as the observation of the distances between two successive R peaks (RRI, RR intervals) [8,30,37,40]. Indeed, the detection methods based on RRI produce relatively more precise identification of AF since the R-wave peak of QRS complex is the most prominent characteristic feature of an ECG recording and the least susceptible to various kinds of noise [19,21,25,26].

In the work by Hochstadt *et al.* [18], around 18 thousand consecutive RR interval measurements were recorded in 20 patients, including about 12 thousand RR intervals during AF and 6,087 RR intervals during sinus rhythm. The automatic algorithm—based on Lorenz-plot—used by the authors distinguished AF from sinus rhythm with a sensitivity of 100% and specificity of 93.1%.

In the study by Andersen *et al.* [2], a novel approach for AF detection based on Inter Beat Intervals (IBI) extracted from long term electrocardiogram (ECG) recordings is presented. For this purpose, five time-domain features have been extracted from the IBIs and a Support Vector Machine (SVM) has been used for

[1] https://bit.ly/3dvrXJX.

classification. The proposed approach has shown a significantly reduced computation time without loss of performance, if compared to a consolidated baseline.

Afdala *et al.* [1] test the ability of simply involving the Shannon entropy in the detection of Atrial Fibrillation episodes. In their research study, they used data from a well-known public data set (Physionet MIT-BIH AFDB) and, as performance, they observed that Shannon entropy has the highest accuracy if a threshold of 0.5 is set.

In the work by Chen *et al.* [5], a new feature extraction method based on RR interval is proposed with the aim at describing an heart rhythm which will be submitted to a classification experiment. As descriptors, they used the robust coefficient of variation (RCV), the distribution shape of RR interval is described with the skewness parameter (SKP), and the complexity of RR interval is described with the Lempel-Ziv complexity (LZC). Finally, the feature vectors have been used as input into the support vector machine (SVM) classifier model to achieve automatic classification and detection of atrial fibrillation. Also in this case, the MIT-BIH atrial fibrillation database was used to verify the data. The final classification results showed a sensitivity of 95.81%, a specificity of % and an accuracy equal to 96.09%.

In the next subsection, the method chosen as baseline—and embedded in MORPHYTHM and consequently in the new approaches proposed in this paper—is described by providing the main ideas and highlighting the computational steps.

The Method Proposed by Zhou *et al.* [41]. This section provides details on the method proposed by Zhou *et al.* [41], *i.e.*, our baseline in the evaluation of LOCAL MORPHYTHM. Such an approach consists in the following steps:

- the HR sequence is converted to a symbolic sequence in a fixed interval;
- a probability distribution is constructed from the word sequence which is transformed from the symbolic sequence;
- a coarser version of Shannon entropy is employed to quantify the information size of HR sequence using the probability distribution of word sequence;
- discrimination of the heart beat type (AF or no-AF) using a threshold.

Step 1: Converting the HR Sequence. The first step of the method regards the generation of a symbolic dynamic starting from the analysis of a sequence of heart beat (hr_n). Especially, the authors encode the information included in hr_n to a sequence of fewer symbols, where each symbol aims at representing an instantaneous state of heart beating. The mapping function is the following:

$$sy_n = \begin{cases} 63, & \text{if } n \text{ hr} \geq 315 \\ \lfloor hr_n \rfloor, & \text{other cases} \end{cases}$$

where $[\lfloor \cdot \rfloor]$ represents a floor operator.

Step 2: Building the Symbolic Sequence. The authors apply a 3-symbols template in order to explore the entropic properties of the symbolic series sy_n. Thus, to examine the chaotic behavior, the word value can then be calculated as:

$$wv_n = (sy_{n-2} \times 2^1 2) + (sy_{n-1} \times 2^6) + sy_n$$

Step 3: Computing the Entropy. The authors define a coarser version of Shannon entropy $H^{''}(A)$ to quantitatively calculate the information size of wv_n. In this study, the dynamic A comprises of 127 consecutive word elements from wv_{n-126} to wv_n, as proposed in the function below:

$$H^{''}(A) = -\frac{k}{N log_2 N} \sum_{i=1}^{k} p_i log_2 p_i$$

where N and k are total number of the elements and characteristic elements in space A, respectively.

Step 4: Classification. Based on the obtained entropy value, a final beat-to-beat classification (*fibrillant* or *not-fibrillant*) is presented by applying a threshold discrimination. The optimal threshold was empirically identified at 0.639.

3 The Proposed Approach: An Overview

This section describes LOCAL MORPHYTHM, an evolution of the approach recently proposed by Laudato *et al.* [23], called MORPHYTHM. LOCAL MORPHYTHM is able—given a heart beat signal—to classify it as fibrillating or not fibrillating.

As well as MORPHYTHM, LOCAL MORPHYTHM uses supervised machine learning techniques[2] to combine rhythmic and morphological features extracted from an ECG and predict whether or not a heart beat is fibrillating or not fibrillating. However, in LOCAL MORPHYTHM, (i) a rigorous feature engineering process and (ii) a local prediction strategy have been adopted in order to identify respectively the features that best contribute to the prediction of AF episodes and to evaluate if a local approach may be preferred instead of a global one.

3.1 Pre-processing

Before extracting features, the ECG data have to be pre-processed according to [33] and [6]. The main steps involved in this phase are: (i) the detrend of the ECG signal, (ii) the application of a filtering stage (where a low and high pass filters have been applied to get rid of baseline wander and discard high frequency noise, respectively) and (iii) the normalization of the samples.

Once executed the previous steps, the Pan-Tompkins [33] QRS-detection method has been applied with the aim at segmenting the ECG in heart beat signals. In this work, as *heart beat*, it is intended the signal included between two successive R peaks. Such an interpretation is very suitable for AF detection, because it highlights the atrial activity.

[2] In the LOCAL MORPHYTHM evaluation, we experimented several supervised machine learning technique.

3.2 Feature Extraction and Selection

As the name suggests, LOCAL MORPHYTHM embeds features extracted from both the heart rhythm and the morphology of a heart beat. Rhythmic features are based on one or more heart beats and they aim at capturing aspects that mostly regard the regularity of the heart beat signal. Zhou *et al.* [41] state that the detection methods based on RRI are more useful to produce a precise and accurate identification of AF because the R-wave peak of the QRS complex is the most prominent characteristic feature of an ECG recording. Such a characteristic is less subject to noise [26].

Even if the acquisition of rhythmic features can be very reliable, such features can only help detecting arrhythmia, which is just one of the possible signs of AF. Thus, morphological features are necessary to detect anomalies in the shape of a single heart beat signal and could be particularly useful to corroborate the warnings raised by analysing the rhythm.

Thus, similarly to MORPHYTHM, also in LOCAL MORPHYTHM we consider both rhythm and morphological features. Especially, we consider the same set of features used in MORPHYTHM [23]:

- *Rhythmic Features*: we used two features based on the observation of a single heart beat signal, *i.e.,* Heart Beat Length (HBL) and Heart Beat Discrete Length (HBDL), and two additional rhythmic features that consider the information of a sequence of consecutive heart beats, *i.e.,* Heart Beat Regularity (HBR) and Entropy, as defined by [41]. HBL represents how long a single heart beat signal lasts. HBDL is a classification of the heart beat signal in three classes, based on its length: a beat is (i) *short* if it takes less than 0.5 s, (ii) *long* if it takes more than 1.2 s, and (iii) *regular* otherwise. HBR is based on HBDL. It considers a rhythmic pattern of 10 consecutive discrete heart beats lengths. Once obtained the pattern, we compute HBR simply counting the number of regular heart beats.
- *Morphological Features*: given a sequence of samples provided for a heart beat signal, we computed several features: (i) the Mean Signal Intensity (MSI), (ii) the Signal Intensity Variance (SIV), (iii) the Signal Intensity Entropy (SIE). MSI, SIV and SIE are features obtained by measuring respectively the mean, the variance and the entropy [29] of all the samples acquired in a heart beat signal. To try to enrich the knowledge of classifiers, we also used the segmented version of these last features: we divided proportionally the heart beat signal in 10 segment and for each portion we evaluated the MSI, SIV and SIE. Finally, we included the features obtained by (i) the application of the Fast Fourier Transform on 32 points and (ii) the estimation of the coefficients of the Auto-Regressive model of order 16.

For each heart beat signal we extract a total number of 76 different features (eight rhythm features and 68 morphological features). In order to select the most appropriate features for the detection of AF events we used the Weka *InfoGainAttributeEval* as Attribute Evaluator and *Ranker* as Search Method. The

Table 1. Features ranking using Information Gain.

Rank	InfoGain	Attribute	Type
1	0.86	Entropy from Zhou *et al.* [41]	Rhythmic
2	0.20	Entropy from the rhythmic pattern	Rhythmic
3	0.18	Heart beat absolute length	Rhythmic
4	0.14	Coeff. no. 10 from AR model	Morphological
5	0.13	Coeff. no. 11 from AR model	Morphological
6	0.12	Coeff. no. 7 from AR model	Morphological
7	0.11	Coeff. no. 12 from AR model	Morphological
8	0.11	Coeff. no. 1 from AR model	Morphological
9	0.11	Coeff. no. 8 from AR model	Morphological
10	0.11	Coeff. no. 9 from AR model	Morphological
11	0.11	Coeff. no. 3 from AR model	Morphological
12	0.10	Coeff. no. 6 from AR model	Morphological
13	0.10	Coeff. no. 2 from AR model	Morphological
14	0.10	Coeff. no. 4 from AR model	Morphological
15	0.10	Coeff. no. 3 from FFT model	Morphological
16	0.10	Coeff. no. 31 from FFT model	Morphological
...	...	...	...
75	0.03	Entropy of Sample Amplitudes	Morphological
76	0.01	Length discrete class	Rhythmic

former basically evaluates the worth of an attribute by measuring the information gain with respect to the class, while the latter ranks attributes by their individuals evaluations.

The feature selection process has been conducted on the MIT-BIH AF Database [16], a commonly used benchmark which contains recordings of 25 patients. Each recording in the data set lasts 10 h and contains two ECG signals sampled at 250 samples per second (12-bit resolution). Due to the embedding of morphology descriptors, the feature selection process has been performed on the $AFDB_2$, i.e., the AFDB without records 00735 and 03665 because, for such records, only information on the rhythm is available [16] and without 04936 and 05091 because—as others have shown [25]—the records 04936 and 05091 include many incorrect manual AF annotations.

The outcome of the features selection process is reported in Table 1. From the analysis of the results achieved, we observe that:

- rhythmic information in AF episodes detection represent the main contribution in terms of information gain;
- morphological features of an ECG can provide a contribution in terms of information gain for the automatic classification of heart beats. Specifically,

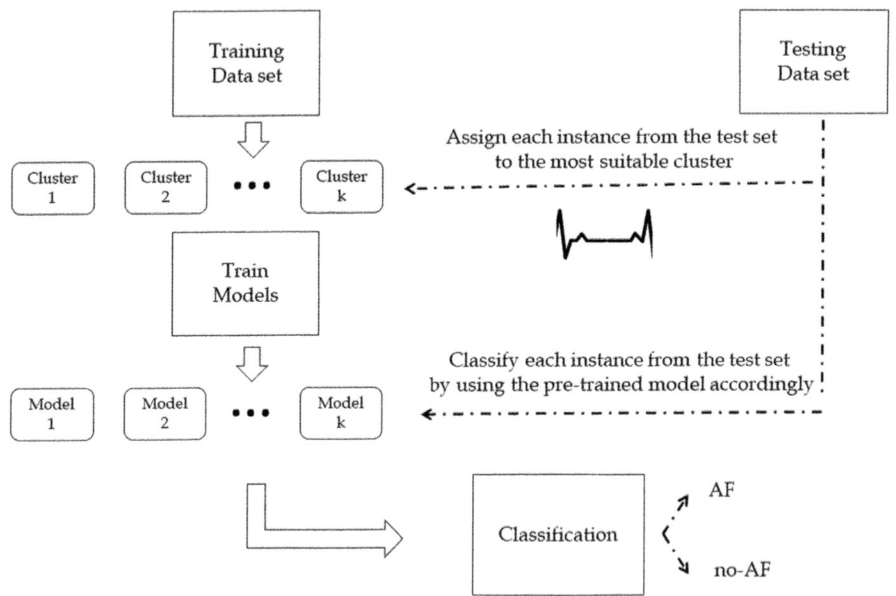

Fig. 1. Workflow of LOCAL MORPHYTHM.

these features refer to the middle and the last part of the signal, where the fibrillating rhythm appears and where the P-wave can exhibit its changes.

By selecting a fixed threshold of 0.12, we obtain a selection of a group of six features containing a balanced number of morphological and rhythmic features. Thus, we decided to incorporate in LOCAL MORPHYTHM the first six features reported in Table 1.

3.3 Making the Prediction

The main difference between LOCAL MORPHYTHM and MORPHYTHM regards the way as the prediction is performed. In MORPHYTHM, as in any canonical approach based on supervised machine learning techniques, a training set is used to build a (global) prediction model. Such a model is used on all the new data points where a prediction is required. Especially, when a new heart beat signal is provided, MORPHYTHM first computes the features on this new heart beat signal and then uses the prediction model to determine whether or not the heart beat is fibrillating or not fibrillating.

However, the heart beat signals in the training set could be quite different each other. The heterogeneity of the training set might negatively impact the accuracy of the prediction model [28]. In order to mitigate such a problem, in LOCAL MORPHYTHM we integrated a local prediction strategy [28].

LOCAL MORPHYTHM first clusters the training set into homogeneous sets of heart beat signals. Then, it builds for each cluster a specific prediction model

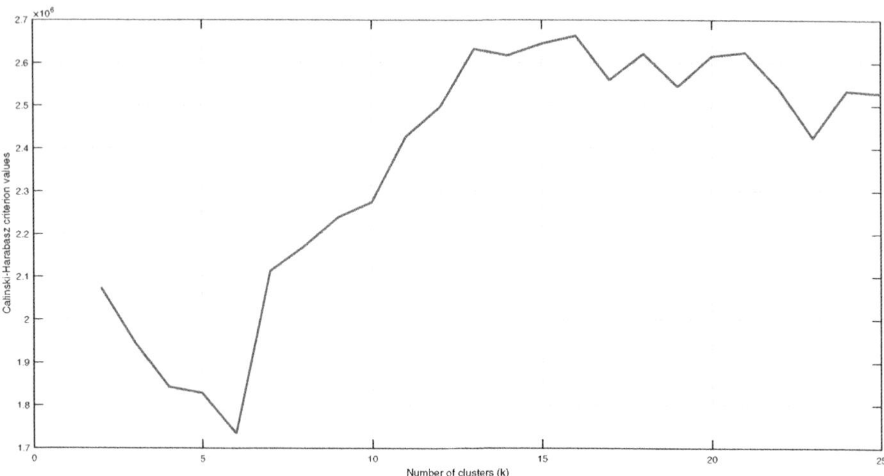

Fig. 2. Results of the Calinski-Harabasz score in order to determine the best value of k for the k-means clustering algorithm. The higher the value of the score the higher the overall quality of the clustering.

using a supervised machine learning technique. In this way, Local Morphythm does not have just one global prediction model, but it has a set of prediction models that are particularly suitable for specific heart beat signals.

When a new heart beat signal is provided, Local Morphythm first computes the features on this new heart beat signal and then it identifies the cluster of heart beat signals more similar to the new heart beat signal. Once identified such a cluster, Local Morphythm uses the model associated to the identified cluster of heart beat signals to noindent predict whether or not the new heart beat is fibrillating or not fibrillating. The workflow of Local Morphythm is depicted in Fig. 1.

In order to cluster the training set, we have exploited the k-means clustering algorithm [27]. This method follows a simple way to classify a given data set through a certain number of clusters fixed *a priori*. The main idea is to define k centroids, one for each cluster. The main steps are described below:

- Place K points into the space represented by the objects that are being clustered. These points represent initial group centroids.
- Assign each object to the group that has the closest centroid.
- When all objects have been assigned, recalculate the positions of the K centroids.
- Repeat Steps 2 and 3 until the centroids no longer move. This produces a separation of the objects into groups from which the metric to be minimized can be calculated.

We have determined the optimal value of k using the Variance Ratio Criterion (also known as Calinski-Harabasz score) [4]. Especially, we have performed the clustering of the heart beats by using different values of k from 1 to 25. For each cluster we have computed the Calinski-Harabasz score in order to determine the value of k that determines the clustering with the highest score. The plot in Figure shows that the highest Calinski-Harabasz value occurs with $k = 16$. This number has also been confirmed by involving the Silhouette method [36], an alternative method for the identification of the best k value (Fig. 2).

4 Empirical Evaluation

This section reports the empirical evaluation we conducted to evaluate the accuracy of Local Morphythm.

4.1 Design of the Study

The goal of this study is to evaluate the accuracy of Local Morphythm is classifying AF events in a patient. The perspective is both (i) of a researcher who wants to understand if a local prediction strategy to combine rhythmic and morphological features is worthwhile for detecting AF events, and (ii) of a practitioner who wants to use the most accurate and precise approach in a telemedicine application for the detection of AF events. Thus, the study is steered by the following research question:

To what extent, a local prediction model—based on the combination of rhythmic and morphological information—improves the automatic detection of AF episodes?

The context of this study is represented by the MIT-BIH AF Database [16], and specifically the $AFDB_2$, *i.e.*, the AFDB without records 00735 and 03665 because, for such records, only information on the rhythm is available [16]. Also, records 04936 and 05091 were excluded due to many incorrect manual AF annotations [25].

In the context of our study, we also experimented a large set of machine learning techniques. Indeed, for the classification performances, we have involved in our experiments—beyond the Random Forest [17], J48 [35], Logistic [9], AdaBoost M1 [13] and RepTree [11] already used by Laudato *et al.* to evaluate Morphythm [23]—Neural Networks [22], Multi Layer Perceptron [32], JRip [7] and SGD (which implements stochastic gradient descent for learning various linear models)[3].

As validation technique, we have chosen the Leave One Person Out Cross Validation (L1PO-CV). L1PO-CV means that one person at a time is left out from the training set, so that the training set contains no data specific to the individual who is being tested (the classifier was not tuned with the test data of that person). This is possible since each data segment is associated with an anonymous label corresponding to an individual.

[3] https://weka.sourceforge.io/doc.stable-3-8/weka/classifiers/functions/SGD.html.

To answer our research questions we compared:

- True Positives (TP), *i.e.,*, the number of instances classified as fibrillating by the approach and that were actually fibrillating;
- True Negatives (TN), *i.e.,*, the number of instances classified as not fibrillating by the approach and that were actually not fibrillating;
- False Positives (FP), *i.e.,*, the number of instances classified as fibrillating by the approach and that were actually not fibrillating;
- False Negatives (FN), *i.e.,*, the number of instances classified as not fibrillating by the approach and that were actually fibrillating.

In the context of telemedicine a high number of TP is desirable, because it indicates the number of AF episodes correctly detected. Also, it is desirable to have an approach that does not lose any AF episode: thus, keeping the number of FN low is very important.

4.2 Analysis of the Results

Table 2 compares the prediction accuracy, in terms of TP, TN, FP, and FN, achieved by Local Morphythm, Morphythm, and the approach proposed by Zhou *et al.* [41], the most accurate approach in the literature for the detection of AF events.

From the analysis of the results emerges that for both the approaches Morphythm and Local Morphythm the best overall accuracy is achieved when SGD is used as machine learning techniques.

Using such a technique, Local Morphythm is able to achieve the best results in terms of both TP and FN. Specifically, Local Morphythm is able to identify 8,340 TP more than the baseline (approach by Zhou *et al.*) and 1,114 TP more than Morphythm. Also, Local Morphythm is able to retrieve less FN with respect to both the baseline and Morphythm, *i.e.,* −5,533 and −569, respectively.

However, the approach proposed by Zhou *et al.* [41] is still the best in terms of TN and FP. Specifically, Local Morphythm and Morphythm generate 6,052 and 6,064 FP more than the approach by Zhou, respectively. In terms of TN, instead Local Morphythm and Morphythm retrieves less TN as compared to the baseline, *i.e.,* −8,859 and −8,326, respectively.

By looking at the results achieved at patient level, *i.e.,* by considering a single recording, we observe that Local Morphythm sensibly outperforms—in terms of every metrics—both the baseline and Morphythm for 5 out of 21 recordings (around 24%). Examples of such an improvement is reported in Table 3, where it is possible to observe the classification performances of Local Morphythm with respect to the baseline and Morphythm.

In addition, if we focus the attention on just TP and FN, Local Morphythm outperforms both the other approaches baselines in 8 out of 21 recordings (around 38% of the data set).

For the remaining recordings, the value of all the evaluation metrics are almost balanced, in the sense that no significant improvement can be observed.

Table 2. Comparison of LOCAL MORPHYTHM with MORPHYTHM (with the same features selection strategy used in LOCAL MORPHYTHM) and the approach proposed by Zhou *et al.* [41]. In boldface the best results achieved by these methods.

Approach	TP	TN	FP	FN
Zhou *et al.* on $AFDB_2$	457,001	**554,247**	**15,513**	12,966
MORPHYTHM—Random Forest	459,211	534,822	34,489	11,205
LOCAL MORPHYTHM—Random Forest	458,980	534,824	34,501	11,422
MORPHYTHM—J48	449,471	512,763	54,209	23,284
LOCAL MORPHYTHM—J48	446,947	513,453	55,259	24,068
MORPHYTHM—Logistic	463,730	545,621	22,184	8,192
LOCAL MORPHYTHM—Logistic	464,623	545,624	22,003	7,477
MORPHYTHM—AdaBoost M1	461,635	549,572	16,188	12,332
LOCAL MORPHYTHM—AdaBoost M1	461,214	547,589	18,287	12,637
MORPHYTHM—RepTree	451,962	522,829	42,931	22,005
LOCAL MORPHYTHM—RepTree	452,231	522,819	42,899	21,778
MORPHYTHM—3-layers LSTM NN	462,730	545,621	22,484	8,892
LOCAL MORPHYTHM—3-layers LSTM NN	460,076	546,799	23,081	9,771
MORPHYTHM—3-layers Conv. NN	461,319	546,032	23,260	9,116
LOCAL MORPHYTHM—3-layers Conv. NN	459,660	546,020	23,695	10,352
MORPHYTHM—MultiLayer Perceptron	457,595	544,031	26,964	11,137
LOCAL MORPHYTHM—MultiLayer Perceptron	457,606	544,017	26,992	11,112
MORPHYTHM—JRip	452,966	522,840	42,121	21,800
LOCAL MORPHYTHM—JRip	451,599	523,296	42,571	22,261
MORPHYTHM—SGD	464,227	545,921	21,577	8,002
LOCAL MORPHYTHM—SGD	**465,341**	545,388	21,565	**7,433**

Table 3. Example of records on which LOCAL MORPHYTHM outperforms both MORPHYTHM and the approach by Zhou *et al.* [41] in terms of all the considered evaluation metrics.

Record	Interval	TP	TN	FP	FN
04043	Zhou *et al.* [41]	8,690	44,299	3,063	5,862
	Best MORPHYTHM- Logistic	9,608	43,565	3,797	4,944
	LOCAL MORPHYTHM- AdaBoost M1	**10,090**	**44,991**	**2,371**	**4,462**
06426	Zhou *et al.* [41]	52,104	815	1,229	1,006
	Best MORPHYTHM- Logistic	52,633	629	1,415	477
	LOCAL MORPHYTHM- SGD	**52,576**	**901**	**1,143**	**534**

The only recording with abnormal classification performances is the recording 08378 where LOCAL MORPHYTHM presents a significant loss in terms of TP and FN with respect to the other two approaches. This suggests that on this particular recording the local prediction strategy is not worthwhile because very

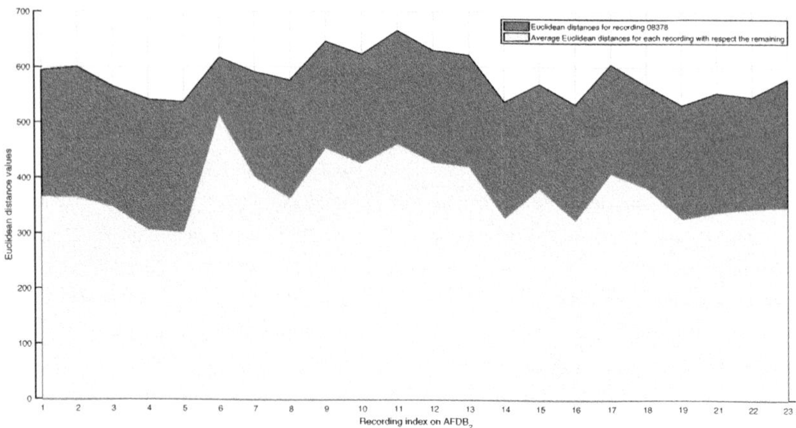

Fig. 3. Average distance between a generic recording i and all the other recordings but 08378 compared to the distance between recording i and 08378.

likely such a recording exhibits characteristics that are quite different from the other recordings in the data set.

In order to validate such a conjecture we compare the average distance between each recording and all the others but 08378 and the distance between each recording and recording 08378. In order to compute the distance between two recordings we considered them as mono dimensional vectors (by selecting the first ECG channel available for each recording) and then compute the Euclidean distance between the two vectors.

The analysis is depicted in Fig. 3. As we can see, the distance between the recording 08378 and a generic recording i is much higher that the average distance between the recording i and all the other recordings but 08378. Such a result confirms our conjecture that the recording 08378 is quite different from the others recording; thus, in this specific case, the local prediction strategy does not provide any benefits as compared to the other two approaches.

Once this recording is excluded from the data set, the classification accuracy of Local Morphythm improves even more. Indeed, Local Morphythm—especially when using the Logistic and the SGD algorithms—avoids a loss of around 1,5 thousands heart beats classified as TP and FN.

5 Conclusion and Future Work

In this paper we presented an extended version of the approach proposed by Laudato *et al.* [23], named Morphythm, where rhythmic and morphological features are combined together in order to improve the classification accuracy of AF episodes. The new approach, called Local Morphythm integrates a more rigorous feature engineering process as compared to Morphythm and more advanced machine learning techniques, including artificial neural networks.

We also extended MORPHYTHM by integrating in the approach the strategy of "local" prediction, successfully used in other contexts [28]. Especially, instead of producing a single prediction model, LOCAL MORPHYTHM automatically builds several prediction models based on the characteristics of the ECGs in the training set. In particular, the training set is clustered in order to put together ECGs that exhibits similar characteristics. Then, for each cluster, LOCAL MORPHYTHM builds a prediction model. When a new data point is provided, LOCAL MORPHYTHM first selects the most suitable model based on the characteristics of the new data point, and then it performs the prediction applying the selected model.

An experimentation conducted on the MIT-BIH AF Database [16] indicates that LOCAL MORPHYTHM is able to increase the TP and reduce the FN as compared to MORPHYTHM and the approach by Zhou *et al.* [41], one of the best approaches in the literature for the detection of AF episodes. Future work will be devoted on the one hand on the replication of the experimentation on other data sets in order to corroborate the results achieved on the MIT-BIH AF Database and on the other hand on the application of a local prediction technique in the context of automatic detection of other types of arrhythmia.

References

1. Afdala, A., Nuryani, N., Nugroho, A.S.: Automatic detection of atrial fibrillation using basic Shannon entropy of RR interval feature. J. Phys.: Conf. Ser. **795**, 012038 (2017)
2. Andersen, R.S., Peimankar, A., Puthusserypady, S.: A deep learning approach for real-time detection of atrial fibrillation. Expert Syst. Appl. **115**, 465–473 (2019)
3. Balestrieri, E., et al.: The architecture of an innovative smart T-shirt based on the internet of medical things paradigm. In: 2019 IEEE International Symposium on Medical Measurements and Applications (MeMeA), pp. 1–6. IEEE (2019)
4. Caliński, T., Harabasz, J.: A dendrite method for cluster analysis. Commun. Stat.-Theory Methods **3**(1), 1–27 (1974)
5. Chen, Z., Li, J., Li, Z., Peng, Y., Gao, X.: Automatic detection and classification of atrial fibrillation using RR intervals and multi-eigenvalue. Sheng wu yi xue gong cheng xue za zhi= J. Biomed. Eng.= Shengwu yixue gongchengxue zazhi **35**(4), 550–556 (2018)
6. Clifford, G.D., Azuaje, F., McSharry, P., et al.: Advanced Methods and Tools for ECG Data Analysis. Artech House, Boston (2006)
7. Cohen, W.W.: Fast effective rule induction. In: Machine Learning Proceedings 1995, pp. 115–123. Elsevier (1995)
8. Colloca, R., Johnson, A.E., Mainardi, L., Clifford, G.D.: A support vector machine approach for reliable detection of atrial fibrillation events. In: Computing in Cardiology 2013, pp. 1047–1050. IEEE (2013)
9. Cramer, J.S.: The origins of logistic regression (2002)
10. Dash, S., Chon, K., Lu, S., Raeder, E.: Automatic real time detection of atrial fibrillation. Ann. Biomed. Eng. **37**(9), 1701–1709 (2009). https://doi.org/10.1007/s10439-009-9740-z
11. Devasena, C.L.: Comparative analysis of random forest, REP tree and J48 classifiers for credit risk prediction. Int. J. Comput. Appl. (2014). 0975-8887

12. Elliott, T., Yopes, M.C.: Direct-to-consumer telemedicine. J. Allergy Clin. Immunol. Pract. **7**(8), 2546–2552 (2019)
13. Freund, Y., Schapire, R.E.: A desicion-theoretic generalization of on-line learning and an application to boosting. In: Vitányi, P. (ed.) EuroCOLT 1995. LNCS, vol. 904, pp. 23–37. Springer, Heidelberg (1995). https://doi.org/10.1007/3-540-59119-2_166
14. Friberg, L., Rosenqvist, M., Lindgren, A., Terént, A., Norrving, B., Asplund, K.: High prevalence of atrial fibrillation among patients with ischemic stroke. Stroke **45**(9), 2599–2605 (2014)
15. Fuster, V., et al.: ACC/AHA/ESC 2006 guidelines for the management of patients with atrial fibrillation: a report of the American college of cardiology/american heart association task force on practice guidelines and the european society of cardiology committee for practice guidelines (writing committee to revise the 2001 guidelines for the management of patients with atrial fibrillation): developed in collaboration with the European heart rhythm association and the heart rhythm society. Circulation **114**(7), e257–e354 (2006)
16. Goldberger, A.L., et al.: PhysioBank, PhysioToolkit, and PhysioNet: components of a new research resource for complex physiologic signals. Circulation **101**(23), e215–e220 (2000)
17. Ho, T.K.: The random subspace method for constructing decision forests. IEEE Trans. Pattern Anal. Mach. Intell. **20**(8), 832–844 (1998)
18. Hochstadt, A., Chorin, E., Viskin, S., Schwartz, A.L., Lubman, N., Rosso, R.: Continuous heart rate monitoring for automatic detection of atrial fibrillation with novel bio-sensing technology. J. Electrocardiol. **52**, 23–27 (2019)
19. Huang, C., Ye, S., Chen, H., Li, D., He, F., Tu, Y.: A novel method for detection of the transition between atrial fibrillation and sinus rhythm. IEEE Trans. Biomed. Eng. **58**(4), 1113–1119 (2010)
20. Kleyko, D., Osipov, E., Wiklund, U.: A comprehensive study of complexity and performance of automatic detection of atrial fibrillation: classification of long ECG recordings based on the PhysioNet computing in cardiology challenge 2017. Biomed. Phys. Eng. Express **6**(2), 025010 (2020)
21. Lake, D.E., Moorman, J.R.: Accurate estimation of entropy in very short physiological time series: the problem of atrial fibrillation detection in implanted ventricular devices. Am. J. Physiol.-Heart Circ. Physiol. **300**(1), H319–H325 (2011)
22. Lang, S., Bravo-Marquez, F., Beckham, C., Hall, M., Frank, E.: WekaDeeplearning4j : a deep learning package for Weka based on deeplearning4j. Knowl.-Based Syst. **178**, 48–50 (2019)
23. Laudato, G., et al.: Combining rhythmic and morphological ECG features for automatic detection of atrial fibrillation. In: HEALTHINF, pp. 156–165 (2020)
24. de Heuzey, J.Y., et al.: Cost of care distribution in atrial fibrillation patients: the COCAF study. Am. Heart J. **147**(1), 121–126 (2004)
25. Lee, J., Nam, Y., McManus, D.D., Chon, K.H.: Time-varying coherence function for atrial fibrillation detection. IEEE Trans. Biomed. Eng. **60**(10), 2783–2793 (2013)
26. Lian, J., Wang, L., Muessig, D.: A simple method to detect atrial fibrillation using RR intervals. Am. J. Cardiol. **107**(10), 1494–1497 (2011)
27. MacQueen, J., et al.: Some methods for classification and analysis of multivariate observations. In: Proceedings of the Fifth Berkeley Symposium on Mathematical Statistics and Probability, Oakland, CA, USA, vol. 1, pp. 281–297 (1967)
28. Menzies, T., et al.: Local versus global lessons for defect prediction and effort estimation. IEEE Trans. Softw. Eng. **39**(6), 822–834 (2012)

29. Moddemeijer, R.: On estimation of entropy and mutual information of continuous distributions. Sig. Process. **16**(3), 233–248 (1989)
30. Mohebbi, M., Ghassemian, H.: Detection of atrial fibrillation episodes using SVM. In: 2008 30th Annual International Conference of the IEEE Engineering in Medicine and Biology Society, pp. 177–180. IEEE (2008)
31. Niknejad, N., Ismail, W.B., Mardani, A., Liao, H., Ghani, I.: A comprehensive overview of smart wearables: the state of the art literature, recent advances, and future challenges. Eng. Appl. Artif. Intell. **90**, 103529 (2020)
32. Pal, S.K., Mitra, S.: Multilayer perceptron, fuzzy sets, classification (1992)
33. Pan, J., Tompkins, W.J.: A real-time QRS detection algorithm. IEEE Trans. Biomed. Eng. **3**, 230–236 (1985)
34. Procter, N.E., Stewart, S., Horowitz, J.D.: New-onset atrial fibrillation and thromboembolic risk: cardiovascular syzygy? Heart Rhythm **13**(6), 1355–1361 (2016)
35. Quinlan, J.R.: C4.5: Programs for Machine Learning. Elsevier, Amsterdam (2014)
36. Rousseeuw, P.J.: Silhouettes: a graphical aid to the interpretation and validation of cluster analysis. J. Comput. Appl. Math. **20**, 53–65 (1987)
37. Sepulveda-Suescun, J.P., Murillo-Escobar, J., Urda-Benitez, R.D., Orrego-Metaute, D.A., Orozco-Duque, A.: Atrial fibrillation detection through heart rate variability using a machine learning approach and Poincare plot features. CLAIB 2016. IP, vol. 60, pp. 565–568. Springer, Singapore (2017). https://doi.org/10.1007/978-981-10-4086-3_142
38. Sim, I., et al.: Clinical decision support systems for the practice of evidence-based medicine. J. Am. Med. Inform. Assoc. **8**(6), 527–534 (2001)
39. Stewart, S., Murphy, N., Walker, A., McGuire, A., McMurray, J.: Cost of an emerging epidemic: an economic analysis of atrial fibrillation in the UK. Heart **90**(3), 286–292 (2004)
40. Yuan, C., Yan, Y., Zhou, L., Bai, J., Wang, L.: Automated atrial fibrillation detection based on deep learning network. In: 2016 IEEE International Conference on Information and Automation (ICIA), pp. 1159–1164. IEEE (2016)
41. Zhou, X., Ding, H., Wu, W., Zhang, Y.: A real-time atrial fibrillation detection algorithm based on the instantaneous state of heart rate. PloS One **10**(9), e0136544 (2015)
42. Zoni-Berisso, M., Lercari, F., Carazza, T., Domenicucci, S.: Epidemiology of atrial fibrillation: European perspective. Clin. Epidemiol. **6**, 213 (2014)

Privacy by Design for Neuropsychological Studies Based on an mHealth App

Alexander Gabel[1(✉)], Funda Ertas[2], Michael Pleger[1], Ina Schiering[1], and Sandra Verena Müller[2]

[1] Faculty of Computer Science, Ostfalia University of Applied Sciences, Salzdahlumerstraße 46/48, Wolfenbüttel, Germany
{ale.gabel,f.ertas,mic.pleger,i.schiering,s-v.mueller}@ostfalia.de
[2] Faculty of Social Work, Ostfalia University of Applied Sciences, Salzdahlumerstraße 46/48, Wolfenbüttel, Germany

Abstract. mHealth applications provide a huge potential to integrate neuropsychological rehabilitation into the everyday life of patients with executive dysfunctions by supporting them in daily activities and achieving personal goals. In the context of intervention studies it is important to gain insight in the usage of these applications by patients as an additional measurement beside neuropsychological pre- and post-tests. On the other hand, measuring usage of mobile applications constitutes a privacy risk for users. In this article the neuropsychological intervention study is described and a concept for privacy-preserving metrics with a focus on data minimization is derived from research questions. These considerations are then incorporated in a thorough privacy by design and privacy by default design process for the mHealth app.

Keywords: mHealth · Data minimization · Privacy by design · Privacy by default · Data aggregation · Metrics · Privacy design strategies · Neuropsychology · Empirical study

1 Introduction

In the therapy of patients that have an impairment of executive function (EF) after traumatic brain injury often Goal Management Training (GMT) [4,27,43] is used effectively. These patients have deficits concerning "the selection and execution of cognitive plans, their updating and monitoring, the inhibition of irrelevant responses and problems with goal-directed behaviour usually result in disorganized behaviour, impulsivity and problems in goal management and self-regulation" [11, p. 17]. GMT is based on the central idea to divide goals into sub-goals until single tasks are identified. This central idea of GMT was realized as the mHealth application RehaGoal for mobile systems such as smartphones, smartwatches and tablets [15,36].

Since the RehaGoal app accompanies patients during daily activities, privacy is a central requirement in the design and development process of the application

X. Ye et al. (Eds.): BIOSTEC 2020, CCIS 1400, pp. 442–467, 2021.
https://doi.org/10.1007/978-3-030-72379-8_22

and also in mechanisms to support intervention studies. This is addressed by a privacy by design and privacy by default approach as demanded in the General Data Protection Regulation (GDPR) [12] based on *privacy protection goals* [20] (confidentiality, integrity and availability, transparency, unlinkability and intervenability) and *privacy design strategies* [8]. In addition privacy patterns [9] are employed to realize specific aspects in the design process.

In this paper the concept of a neuropsychological intervention study based on an mHealth app addressing executive dysfunctions is presented with corresponding research questions. Based on the RehaGoal app developed as a flexible digitized version of the goal management training, an approach for a thorough privacy by design and privacy by default strategy is presented in detail.

In Sect. 3 the study design is described. First preliminary results are stated in [13]. Detailed results of the study are currently analyzed and will be published later on. Based on the description of the goals of the study Sect. 4 describes derived research questions as a basis for the definition of metrics which are briefly summarized in Sect. 5. The metric language and metric architecture is discussed in detail in [13]. Afterwards the privacy by design process with a focus on privacy design strategies is described Sect. 6.

2 Related Work

mHealth applications are employed in various medical and psychological areas. Measurements on mental health and the mental state of patients are investigated in [18,25,38]. Beside typical medical application e.g. in the area of diabetes [7], aspects such as stress are measured [16].

Typically in a first step, raw data is gathered and then transformed by data mining approaches [35]. In this area privacy-sensitive deep learning techniques, e.g. based on differential privacy [33] or federated learning approaches using a cryptographic protocol for secure aggregation [5] are described in literature but are typically until now not broadly used in this area.

Privacy by design and data minimization were generally not prioritized based on the results of several investigations concerning security and privacy of mHealth apps [22,26,32,34,39,45]. Issues reported were among others the transmission of strong identifiers as email address and device IDs and health related data. The use of third-party advertising or analytics solutions, insecure storage, data leakage or weak server side controls were identified. Standard security measurements as end-to-end encryption are not mentioned.

3 Neuropsychological Study Based on mHealth App

3.1 Study Design and Assessment Tools

During the pilot study phase, we decided to test the RehaGoal App and the study design in a multiple case study (Fig. 1). As a first step in the study all participants underwent a neuropsychological pre-testing. These included the following tasks or questionnaires on attention, executive function and working memory:

- *Working memory (test battery to assess attention):* This task examines the control of information flow and the updating of information in working memory [2,3,48].
- *Go-NoGo (test battery to assess attention):* The Go/No-go test is used to measure under time pressure the participants capacity to respond ("go") to only one particular stimulus and withhold responses ("no-go") to all other stimuli [42,48].
- *Tower of London:* The Tower of London (TOL) is a transformation task used to assess the participants ability to plan several moves ahead in order to reach a goal (problem-solving ability) [46].
- *Semantic-categorical and formal-lexical word fluency (Regensburg Word Fluency Test (RWT)):* The RWT evaluates the formal-lexical word fluency as well as the semantic-categorical verbal fluency of the participants [1].
- *Dysexcutive Questionnaire (Behavioural Assessment of Dysexecutive Syndrome (BADS)):* The Dysexcutive Questionnaire (DEX) is a questionnaire designed to assess everyday changes to cognition, emotion, and behaviour of the participants [47].
- *Zoo Map Test (BADS):* The Zoo Map Test of the BADS battery is applied to measure planning ability as well as problem solving ability of the participants [47].
- *Modified Six Elements Test (BADS):* The Modified Six Elements Test of the BADS battery is applied to measures the abilities of planning, problem solving, prospective memory, organizing and to monitor participants own behaviour [47].
- *The Digit Span test forward span and backward span (Wechsler Adult Intelligence Scale and the Wechsler Memory Scales):* The Digit Span Test Forward span captures participants attention efficiency and capacity. The Backward span is an executive task and measures the working memory [21]
- *Trail Making Test A/B:* The Trail Making Test (TMT) A and B provides information on visual search, scanning, speed of processing, mental flexibility, and executive functions of the participants [40].
- *Goal Attainment Scaling:* Goal attainment scaling (GAS) is a technique for evaluating individual progress toward goals. GAS provides a judgement on the quality of the tasks that needs to be performed [24].

The neuropsychological pre-testing was followed by a group-based instruction to Goal Management Training and an individual instruction to the RehaGoal App. The participants were encouraged to use the RehaGoal App for five weeks in their everyday life to achieve their individual goals. Subsequently, the neuropsychological post-testing was performed (Fig. 1). Finally, the participants completed a partly standardized questionnaire (based on the System Usability Scale by John Brooke [6]), in which they were asked about their experience and opinions regarding the usage of the RehaGoal App.

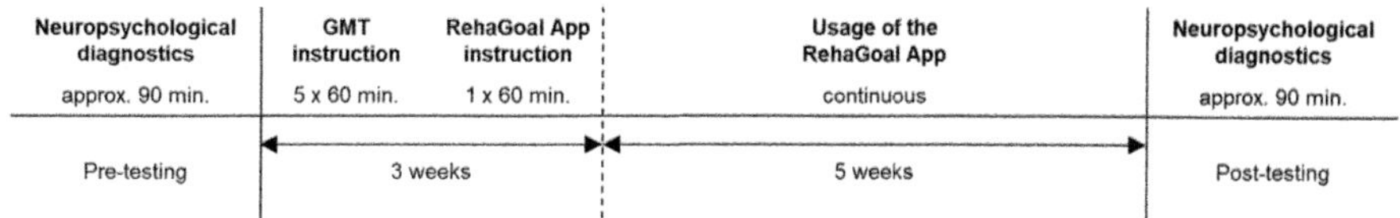

Fig. 1. Study design schema.

The obtained results should provide indications whether:

Q1 The participants improve through the interventions
$\Longrightarrow$ *Determination by neuropsychological pre- and post-testing*
Q2 The RehaGoal App is able to support the participants in their everyday life to achieve their self-defined goals.
$\Longrightarrow$ *Determination of the improvement by using GAS.*
Q3 The RehaGoal App should be improved in participants' perspective.
$\Longrightarrow$ *Determination by using a questionnaire on the App.*
Q4 The study is also appropriate to be conducted for bigger investigated groups.
$\Longrightarrow$ *Implementation of the intervention within a group.*

3.2 Participants

The inclusion criterion required the participant to have an impairment of executive function (EF) after traumatic brain injury. EF is an umbrella term that refers to a wide range of higher cognitive functions used to accomplish goals in a shifting environment. It serves as a general term and includes constructs such as planning, inhibition, cognitive flexibility, impulse control, creativity, working memory and action initiation. EF coordinate the intermediate steps of action planning and provide alternatives in case of complications [37]. Participants were excluded from the study if they had a neurodegenerative disorder or acute brain injury, were unable to understand speech and/or had substance abuse problems, severe psychiatric problems, severe cognitive comorbidity.

3.3 Intervention

Following the pre-testing, the participants received instruction into a technique for defining goals and breaking down overarching goals into sub-goals called Goal Management Training (GMT). GMT is a neurorehabilitation intervention developed by Robertson [41] and demonstrated efficacy in improving executive functions in acquired brain injury [29]. GMT focuses on improving patients organizational and goal-directed behaviours on a global level [28]. The participants received a total of five GMT sessions in a group setting with the following topics and contents:

Session 1: Errors in action
General introduction, define goals, absence of mind, errors in action, increase awareness for the consequences of action

Session 2: Automatic pilot behaviour
Define the autopilot (difference between habit and control), errors through the autopilot, stop the autopilot

Session 3: Get your goals in focus
Define the mental blackboard (working memory), use "STOP" for checking the mental blackboard, practice mindfulness

Session 4: Take decisions
Examples of concurrent goals, understanding the emotional response to concurrent goals (including indecision), To-Do lists in the "STOP"-"STATE" cycle

Session 5: Divide tasks into subtasks and monitor ("STOP")
Establish goal hierarchies, "STOP"-"STATE"-"SPLIT" cycle, identify errors in "STOP"-"STATE"-"SPLIT" cycle, Use "STOP" to monitor the ongoing action towards the formulated goal

Subsequently, the RehaGoal App was introduced in a separate session and installed onto participants mobile devices (smartphone or tablet). The RehaGoal App provides an uncomplicated option to divide tasks into sub-goals and/or sub actions, which then can be executed in smaller steps [36]. It contains a therapist and a patient view (Fig. 2 and 3), which are structured as following:

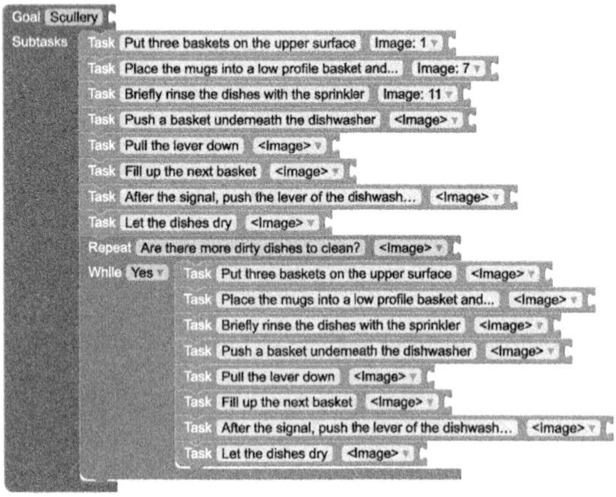

Fig. 2. Therapist view in the RehaGoal App.

Therapist View. In the therapist view, the basic structure of the workflows is displayed in an editor based on Google Blockly (Fig. 2). Using a variety of predefined blocks from a modular system the therapist is able to arrange tasks (and their sub actions with their respective sub-goals) sequentially in a modelled workflow for the patient. This allows an individual and easy creation of workflows that are able to map the daily life tasks of the patient.

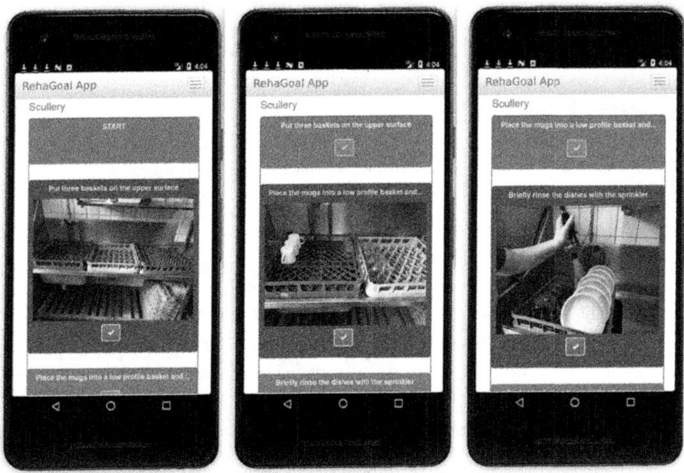

Fig. 3. Patient view to complete subgoals on a mobile device.

Patient View. The patient view of the RehaGoal App contains several informational sections and displays the previously (in the therapist view) created tasks of a workflow in an easy-to-understand and organized form. The main part of the view shows the current (active) task including possible choices where applicable. The other sections display the previous and next task to provide context to the patient.

Other features of the app include a reminder function, a task log and text-to-speech voice output for patients with limited or no reading ability. Together with the participants, a behavioural analysis was conducted to identify critical situations and/or tasks in which the app might be able to assist them. For these situations and/or tasks, individual workflows were then modeled for each participant. Those included workflows for shopping, cleaning the apartment or using public transportation to visit a friend. After the phase of using the RehaGoal App ended, the neuropsychological post-testing was performed and the participants completed a questionnaire about their experience and opinions regarding the usage of the mobile application.

4 Research Questions as a Basis for Metric Development

The RehaGoal App, as an mHealth application, is used as an intervention, since participants are encouraged to train daily life tasks with the help of it. Through the collection of usage information, so-called metrics, it strengthens the results of the study in addition to neuropsychological diagnostics.

Table 1. Research questions and associated metrics [13].

Category	Research question	Metrics
Therapeutic Results *(TR)*	*TR1:* Does the number of workflow executions correlate with changes in the goal attainment scale/neuropsychological tests/subjective well-being?	m1
	TR2: Does the repeated application of a workflow correlate with less assisted executions over time?	m2, m2a
	TR3: Does the number of completed workflow executions correlate with changes in the goal attainment scale/neuropsychological tests/subjective well-being?	m3
	TR4: Does the repeated completion of a workflow correlate with less assisted executions over time?	m4, m4a
	TR5: Does the number of canceled workflow executions correlate with changes in the goal attainment scale/neuropsychological tests/subjective well-being?	m5
	TR6: Does the repeated cancellation of workflows correlate with less assisted workflow executions over time?	m6, m6a
	TR7: Does the repeated completion of a workflow correlate with the time taken for the execution of it?	m7
	TR8: How does the amount of reminders per task change over consecutive executions?	m9, m9a, m9b, m9c_private
Usability & Therapeutic Results *(UTR)*	*UTR1:* Does the usage of TTS correlate with the number of completed/canceled workflows?	m17–m21
Usability & Workflow Design *(UW)*	*UW1:* What could be possible reasons for the active cancellation of a workflow?	m8
	UW2: How far are workflows executed when they are canceled? Are workflows canceled at specific tasks?	m22
	UW3: Does the type of presentation correlate with changes in the time taken for completing a task?	m23–m28
Usability *(U)*	*U1:* Are reminders closed once the task has been completed or as soon as the dialog appears on the device?	m10, m11, m11_private
	U2: How often was the scheduling feature used (and therefore possibly better integrated)?	m12
	U3: Is the scheduling feature canceled less over time? (and therefore possibly better integrated)?	m13
	U4: How are schedules used? How many (different) workflows are scheduled?	m14
	U5: How are schedules used? How many workflows were executed before canceling a schedule?	m15
	U6: How is the distribution of the number of workflows in completed schedules?	m16
	U7: How many (different) workflows are executed in a completed schedule?	m15, m16

As a first step towards a privacy by design process for the design of privacy-respecting metrics, research questions needed to be formulated based on the goals of the study. Then these research questions have been used as a basis to derive necessary metrics to answer research questions. Not only specific metrics regarding the target group are recorded, but also general metrics regarding the usage of the app. In consideration with the data minimization principle, only metrics were recorded which served the purpose of answering Q1–Q4 (see page 3). The research questions are summarized in Table 1.

The application of the metrics in the RehaGoal App provides the opportunity to collect additional participants data. It should be emphasized that by using the app it is also possible to determine how these are related to the neuropsychological test results, the GAS or the questionnaires. For instance, it is reasonable to check whether the workflows were started *(TR1, TR2)* finished *(TR3, TR4)* or canceled *(TR5, TR6)* several times, since the data here is useful to assess if the participants planning ability improved due to the repeated use of the workflows. More precisely, whether the participants are able to recognize workflows as an assistance for themselves and process them sequentially. Furthermore, it provides information on workflows that were actively used and whether certain workflows/tasks are repeatedly canceled *(UW1, UW2)*. The time required to complete the workflows is important because traumatic brain injury patients tend to perform their tasks very quickly and therefore are more prone to errors *(TR7)*. It is also possible to determine whether the time to completion decreases or increases during the process and further whether the way workflows are presented influences the duration of completion *(UW3)*.

The reminder function was implemented in the RehaGoal App as the participants repeatedly got lost in their tasks or forgot what stage of the task they had reached. It is therefore also reasonable to determine how often the reminder appears on the participants screen and if its frequency decreases over time *(TR8)*.

Furthermore, the handling of this function by the participants is also of interest, more precisely whether they will immediately click away the reminder after appearing on screen or wait until the completion of the task *(U1)*.

Additional metrics were recorded on the usage of the voice output and the scheduling. The voice output is important for participants who have partially or completely lost their ability to read after the trauma, as well as for participants who prefer not to read while performing a task. In this context, it is useful to examine whether the voice output has an influence on the completion or cancellation of workflows *(UTR1)*.

The scheduling allows participants to perform several tasks sequentially. It is important to determine if and how this feature is used *(U2 - U7)*.

5 Metric Language and Study Export

Table 2. Terminology (excerpt) [13].

Term	Explanation
Assignment	*Inside a metric definition*: The names of the keys under which values of a metric should be grouped. For example `['workflow', 'execution']` would mean that the metric records separate snapshots for every combination of workflow(Id) and execution(Id). Furthermore these concrete values are stored in the corresponding snapshot
Execution	A workflow is being executed, when it is being performed by a human assisted by the application. From the start of a workflow to the completion or cancellation counts as being part of the execution
Metric	Measures or computes a certain value in the context of a given assignment. Metrics may aggregate several measurements into a single value, store each measurement separately and can also trim the accuracy of a value before it is stored
Metric Type	Currently four different types are defined: number metrics (**int**eger and **float**ing point metrics) measuring primitive values, **dur**ation metrics measuring the time difference between two record points, and **meta** metrics, which compute a value based on another metric
Recording	A metric is recorded when it is triggered by a record point and measures or computes a value which is then stored in the metric database
Record Point	Named event in the program source code which may trigger the recording of several metrics. Apart from a required assignment, an optional (dynamic) value may be provided
Schedule	A schedule consists of multiple workflows which should be executed in a given order. It can be created dynamically by the user when needed
Snapshot	A snapshot consists of one or more measurements aggregated into a single value, sometimes including additional information necessary for updating the aggregate or (trimmed) timestamps. Furthermore each snapshot stores its assignment and a sequential index
Task	Simple step in a workflow, which is not being broken down into steps any more
Workflow	Representation of a task consisting of many steps performed by human, modeled using a block-based visual programming language

In order to collect measurements about the application usage in a privacy-preserving way, we decided to follow a data minimization approach. The data collection was based on research questions defined in advance (Sect. 4). Furthermore we decided to avoid the collection of raw data as much as possible and to instead aggregate the data as soon as possible, i.e. already on the participant's device. If achievable, the aggregate is also computed in an incremental fashion, i.e. intermediate values for previous aggregates cannot be reconstructed once the aggregate has been updated, or in other words we do not keep a list of all intermediate measurements but only the last aggregate and/or helper values for tracking the aggregation in a numerically stable way.

Our strategy included the translation of the research questions into multiple so-called metrics [13]. A metric in our case is a formal description of a measurement. This includes what kind of data is being measured (numeric value, duration, value derived from another metric), when it is measured and more, such as how long data should be kept, how it should be aggregated, or to what accuracy a value is stored.

To implement this concept (Fig. 4 and Table 2), we created a domain specific language for the description of such metrics. This offers a number of benefits: Firstly, we can inscribe certain questions regarding privacy into the language, in order to design a scheme for privacy-preserving metrics. Secondly, since this language is designed to be rather descriptive, it is easy to read and to understand, and it is possible to generate textual, human-readable descriptions from it. Thirdly, such a language helps to support software quality, for example the DRY (don't repeat yourself) principle is implemented, as the strategies for e.g. aggregation, management of temporary values etc. has only to be implemented once. This can also yield a better error avoidance, since mistakes can only be made in a descriptive language, while the imperative code backing the metric computation has only to be tested once by good software engineering practices.

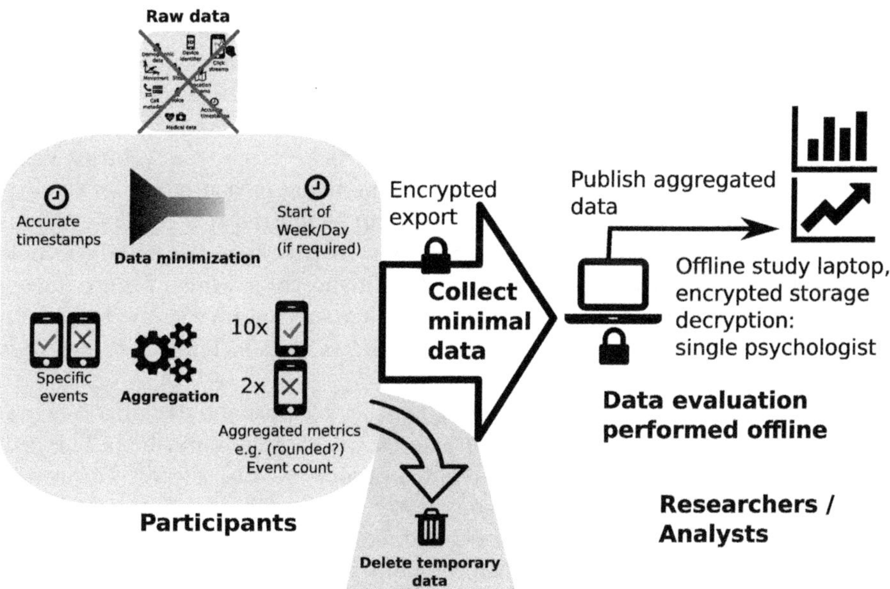

Fig. 4. Privacy-Preserving metric concept.

Our concept is centered around so-called *record points*, which can also be seen as events or certain locations in the application's source code. These are used to trigger one or more metrics, which can then record values and update existing aggregates (e.g. average). Each metric has a type, which can be either numeric (for example counting the number of occurrences, or receiving a measurement from an external source), a duration (measuring the duration between two record points), or a metric derived from one or multiple values recorded by another metric (meta metric). The accuracy of recorded values can (and should) be limited, by specifying the steps to round to (e.g. 5 s steps for a duration or an accuracy of 0.5 for a numeric metric).

Furthermore timestamps are optional and limited in precision. They are only required if the metric is aggregated over a certain time frame. For example a metric which should compute an average per week, always stores the start of the week associated to that metric value (such that the week for which the value was computed can be identified).

Other important properties regarding aggregation are the operation (e.g. mean, max, min, variance, median) and the time frame over which is being aggregated (which may also be the whole collection period).

The time frame also relates to the scope of the aggregation. For example a metric may be recorded per workflow, such that every workflow may get e.g. its own average value for that metric. Another example could be the minimal duration of an (atomic) task per execution and workflow. The latter example would produce minimum aggregates for each execution of every workflow, which would be different than asking for e.g. the minimum task duration per workflow (more coarse), or the minimum task duration per execution (same granularity, however without being grouped by workflow). We call this concept the *assignment* of a metric. It is also a required information without using the aggregation feature, since it determines what metadata is stored related to a recorded value of a metric (e.g. for which workflow is this value being measured?).

Furthermore recorded values (*snapshots*) can be limited to a certain amount, after which the oldest snapshot is overwritten. In that case the snapshot limit is also related to the assignment. This feature is mostly intended for use during therapy, e.g. such that old values from weeks ago are automatically deleted. In the study use case, the time period of recording is already limited, therefore it is not used during the study.

Some metrics (meta metrics) depend on other metrics and can only be computed at a certain point, for example once a workflow has finished. This can cause a certain amount of fine granular temporary data to gather. To prevent such excess data from being stored for longer than necessary, each metric can also specify when its values can be deleted, e.g. as they have been aggregated into a meta metric. Furthermore such temporary metrics are marked as *private*, which means they will never be exported for study evaluation, even if values were not deleted on the device for some reason.

Incomplete duration measurements (which are based on two record points: start and stop) can occur, if the stop event is never encountered. For example the duration of a completed workflow cannot be computed, if the workflow is aborted instead of being finished. In that case the metric language allows to specify events at which incomplete duration measurements can be safely deleted. In such case these measurements are also never exported.

To start the recording of metrics in the first place, the device has to enter a valid study. Studies are embedded in the application's code and consist of a name, a start and end date, as well as a PBKDF2-key which is used to verify a study password. Studies can only be entered with the knowledge of the corresponding study password and our internal policy ensures that the password is only known by study personnel. The start and end dates prevent that metrics are recorded while the study is not active, i.e. before it has started or after the study has finished. Without deliberate modification of the application/device, these protections therefore ensure that metrics are only collected on devices which are legitimately part of the study and only as long as needed.

When the study is finished, the recorded data can be exported from the device with the participant's consent. The data is always exported in an encrypted form, which is only decipherable by the study evaluation person (i.e. not even administrators or developers), due to public-key cryptography using OpenPGP. Integrity can also be verified later on by a digital signature by the participant's device. This ensures that even if the export is transmitted over an insecure channel, the personal data cannot be read by unauthorized persons and manipulations can be detected. The public key used for encryption is embedded in the application and the public key used for the signature is exported from the device when it is first set up for the study use (i.e. before data is recorded). At the end of the study the data is currently transferred to a separate study laptop, however for larger studies it would in principle be possible as well to transmit it over the internet. In comparison the usual way of only relying on transport encryption using TLS, could still allow administrators or cloud providers to decrypt the data, while in our case this is not possible without knowledge of the private study operator key, which is stored offline in a secure location.

6 Implementation of Privacy Design Strategies

Our privacy by design process is based on both the privacy protection goals (PPG) [20] and privacy design strategies (PDS) [8]. Therefore we analyzed our (continually developing) requirements to these models respectively, in order to derive principles which could be followed for an implementation. When multiple options were available, we usually decided in favour of stronger data minimization and unlinkability, except in cases where the overhead in development and usability would have been disproportionate compared to the benefit regarding privacy in the context described in Sect. 3. Utilizing privacy patterns was helpful for the implementation, which are often already categorized according to the PDS in pattern catalogues.

In retrospect, we primarily focused on the goals unlinkability and data minimization in our project. While transparency and intervenability were also kept in mind, they were assigned a lower priority, since it turned out that we could keep most data on the users device during normal usage, therefore being under control of the user. The only exception to such case were workflows shared through the online feature, which however is optional, as workflows may also be shared via file transfer instead. With regards to the study, transparency and intervenability became more important goals.

The following subsections will introduce the purpose of individual tactics for each privacy design strategy and state the corresponding privacy protection goals, following an overview of how those tactics have been implemented within the context of the application and the study use case. Each entry further provides an assessment of possible solutions which have not been, or could not been implemented given the use case. To provide a broader sense typical risks are addressed, if applicable.

6.1 MINIMISE

The *MINIMISE* strategy is about data minimization and purpose limitation. It consists of the tactics *EXCLUDE* ("refraining from processing a data subject's personal data"), *SELECT* ("decide on a case by case basis on the full or partial usage of personal data"), *STRIP* ("removing unnecessary personal data fields") and *DESTROY* ("completely removing a data subject's personal data") [8]. Concentrating on data minimization aspects, we mostly applied the *SELECT* and *DESTROY* tactics. By specifying research questions in advance and collecting only what is deemed to be necessary for answering those, we *SELECT* the kind of data that is required. Furthermore e.g. fields such as the timestamp are only recorded if necessary for the use-case and only to the required precision (see below). A different approach would be to instead collect all potentially useful data in the beginning and process it afterwards, to find out what seems necessary and what kind of questions may be answered using such data, which is more the data scientist's way of research. It may provide much more insight, however it is significantly more risky to collect, because unintended questions that might even be out of scope of the research project, may be answered as well. With more data collected, it gets also more difficult to estimate how this data could possibly be (mis)used. Using the data minimization approach instead provides a certain risk limitation.

Furthermore the possibility to opt-in into study mode, as well as making it optional to share workflows via our server during normal use fall into this tactic. Using opt-out instead, or making it non-optional to collect data or share workflows with our server, would introduce additional risks and responsibility while providing no or only a minor benefit (e.g. workflows could be made automatically available on all devices of a user, if she/he is logged in with the same credentials). Opt-in is also preferable from a user's perspective, as it provides more control about what data is being shared and sharing has to be explicitly decided. Data is only recorded during the predefined study period, afterwards recording of further data is disabled automatically. Additional data collection is simply not necessary, may be non-lawful and could increase the risk of misuse.

Even if the data is only stored on the participant's device, there is still a certain risk that it may be exfiltrated later on by an unauthorized party.

Considering the *DESTROY* tactic, we are deleting unnecessary data once it is dispensable on the users device, e.g. private metrics, which are used to derive public meta metrics, are deleted once they have been aggregated locally. Additionally, incomplete metrics such as time measurements, which have been started but not finished, are deleted automatically when they cannot be completed any more. Deletion of incomplete time measurements is especially important, as the temporary timestamps are very accurate (in order to introduce no additional error), while the final duration metrics are trimmed to the specified precision. Without this, accurate timestamps about some activities would be stored (possibly permanently) on the device (for example the accurate time when a workflow has been started, which is used later on in order to calculate the (inaccurate) average duration of a workflow). Also non-aggregated private metrics may include very fine granular event information, which is only needed temporarily in order to derive certain aggregates, therefore it is also important to delete them as soon as possible.

However, there is no automatic data deletion at the end of the study on the users device, instead the application data has to be removed manually (e.g. by application removal). An option would have been to delete data once it has been exported for the study team, however this would have come with the risk of losing study data, if for some reason the exported and encrypted data was destroyed or lost. Furthermore we intended to allow multiple exports during the study, which would not have been possible if the metric data was deleted after an export, as previous aggregates would be lost and the new values will only consist of data recorded after export, making it difficult to merge multiple exports later on. Collected pseudonymous study data is deleted according to a policy established in the application for ethics approval. Information enabling re-identification of pseudonyms is deleted once the study ends. Shared workflows, which were stored on the server are deleted when a study ends, however neither a policy nor an automatic process for how long workflows should be stored on the server apart from studies has been implemented yet. Currently, due to our data minimization approach, there is also no information stored about when a workflow has been uploaded. An alternative approach could be to store an inaccurate date about when a certain workflow was uploaded, in order to automatically delete older workflows after a certain period, without a larger impact on privacy through timestamps.

Regarding the *STRIP* tactic, an additional possibility would be to integrate the *Strip Invisible Metadata*[9] pattern in order to further reduce the amount of information which can be derived from pictures embedded into a workflow. Without this pattern it is possible that creators of a workflow can be re-identified by the metadata included in an image (such as Location information, device name and others). This has not been implemented yet, since the pictures are usually created by a therapist and therefore provide less detailed information about the study participant.

6.2 HIDE

Next up is the *HIDE* strategy, which is e.g. about unlinkability and confidentiality. It consists of the tactics *RESTRICT* ("preventing unauthorized access to personal data"), *MIX* ("processing personal data randomly within a large enough group to reduce correlation"), *OBFUSCATE* ("preventing understandability of personal data to those without the ability to decipher it") and *DISSOCIATE* ("removing the correlation between different pieces of personal data") [8].

Concerning the study, primarily the *OBFUSCATE* and *DISSOCIATE* tactics were used in our case. Depending on the size of the study, however, this may be different. For example in larger studies *MIX* may become more important, as anonymity of participants may be considered more important and possible to implement through a large enough group of participants. We apply *OBFUSCATE* by encrypting the study export for the study evaluating person with hybrid encryption (end-to-end encryption based on OpenPGP) before it is moved to external storage or transmitted. This prevents interpretation of exported data by anyone but the study evaluation person. We decided to use OpenPGP, since it has already been audited and the standard is well-established. Note that the application itself still stores the data unencrypted in its private application storage. While storage encryption would possibly offer additional confidentiality, it also requires the entry of a user-specific password (or other form of key) to be effective, e.g. every time the app starts, which reduces usability, especially for a set of people in our target group.

Instead of requiring names or other personally identifiable information, we use pseudonyms for linking the different datasets (i.e. neuropsychological test results to the automatically recorded metrics). The use of a pseudonym can be seen as applying the *DISSOCIATE* tactic, as it is a way to prevent linking other personal data to the pseudonymous data. There are many ways to generate and assign a pseudonym to a person (Pseudonymous Identity pattern [9,19]), however we decided to use a per-user on-device generated OpenPGP Key ID as the in-application pseudonym. Therefore it can be effectively treated as random and does not contain additional information like sequence number of pseudonym generation, date/time of generation or encoded personal identifiable information (e.g. initials, year of birth etc.). This can be seen as another approach to data minimization, as well as unlinkability. Alternatively using encoded personally identifiably information in the pseudonym, especially without proper encryption, may allow trivial re-identification, even for external persons who have gained access to a list of pseudonyms and suspect that a certain person is engaged in the study. Hence, even without re-identification, the data could be linked to other (possibly publicly available) datasets. For example using an email address (even if it is not based on a name) as a pseudonym could make it rather trivial for external entities to link entries in a given dataset to the study dataset.

Greater linkability also increases the risk of re-identifiability, since it produces a bigger picture of the person like puzzle pieces plugging together, and some linkable datasets of few external parties may already have established the link to the person. In case of data leakage or even misuse by an authorized person, private data of a person could become public or used for unintended purposes. In case of highly sensitive data, such as health data, this is even more critical.

We use two different pseudonyms per study participant, one when collecting the neuropsychological test data and another one for the automatic data collection using metrics. The pseudonym used for neuropsychological tests is also generated randomly. Later on these have to be linked, however this is not necessary until the actual evaluation will be conducted. It is therefore an advantage to use multiple pseudonyms per participant, as it prevents linkability between the datasets for people without knowledge of the link. In theory we could use even more pseudonyms, e.g. different pseudonyms for pre- and post-tests. This would provide even more unlinkability, however it would also make the process more complex. The use of different pseudonyms can be seen as application of the *Minimal Pseudonym Scope* pattern [14]. This brings up the question of how the pseudonyms are actually linked afterwards, when the study is evaluated. A simple solution for smaller studies, which we also use, are pseudonym tables, which map one pseudonym to another. This table should be kept separately from the data. Note, that this table is not used for re-identifying a participant, or linking the pseudonym back to an actual person, but rather to link multiple pseudonyms of a participant. This could also be realized by using encrypted identifiers as pseudonyms, where one identifier may have multiple ciphertext pseudonyms. The pseudonym table or cryptographic keys, could also be managed by a trusted third party, such that only authorized persons may link multiple pieces of data according to a policy.

Alternatively the *Pseudonym Converter* pattern [14] could be applied to let a separate entity, the Converter, link multiple pieces of data (e.g. test data and metrics), which can provide better privacy especially across organizations. However in this case there is no gain from applying this pattern, since at the end all links between the different pieces of data (pre-test, post-test, metrics) have to be resolved for the study evaluation person. However if the evaluation would only need partial data, or a subset of data, the utilization of that pattern will provide better privacy. Given that in case of a leak of the different datasets (e.g. pre-tests and post-tests), their pseudonyms will not be linkable without the help of the converter. Furthermore the evaluation person can only link data for which the converter has performed the pseudonym conversion. Especially for large systems, where data from different sources (e.g. eHealth systems consisting of multiple hospitals, general practitioners, patients and research facilities) should be only linkable when necessary, but unlinkable by default, this pattern might be useful.

It should be noted, that the entity which assigns pseudonyms to participants also usually has the ability to re-identify them, store the association or encode information for re-identification in the pseudonyms, even if this is against the policy. Therefore patterns such as *Data-owner based pseudonymisation* [14] (DISSOCIATE) or *Data hidden from pseudonymiser* [14] (OBFUSCATE) could be used to mitigate this risk. In *Data-owner based* pseudonymisation, the pseudonym is generated by the user or the user's device, therefore the pseudonym and associated data stays in control of the user upfront. It then depends on the way data is transmitted to a recipient (e.g. study team) and the included metadata to determine how much information about the pseudonym can be learned by the recipient (see MIX).

The *Data hidden from pseudonymiser* pattern prevents leaking data to the entity that assigns pseudonyms by applying cryptographic methods, such as secret sharing or encryption, which is especially useful in larger systems/studies, in order to separate pseudonym association from working with pseudonymous data.

We currently also have a "coding table" to store the association between the neuropsychological pseudonym and the identity, therefore providing re-identifiability. This is currently only used so that a participant may delete their data by request. In principle it would be possible to implement the deletion requests without the re-identifiability. For example the application could include a function to request data removal from the server, which would then send the participant's pseudonym (possibly including a digital signature to provide non-repudiation) to the study team. As this pseudonym can be linked to all data stored by the study team, this would effectively implement a data removal request.

The *Recoverable Identity* pattern [14] also describes different ways to implement re-identifiability, which provide better security/privacy guarantees in comparison to a naive implementation. For example the introduction of a trusted third party, or the use of a thresholded secret sharing scheme can provide better separation of powers and stronger enforcement of a policy for re-identification.

Unfortunately due to small number of participants and the study personnel (including evaluation person) knowing the participants (e.g. which workflows they performed) it is very likely that pseudonymous data may be re-identified by them, which cannot be prevented without losing too much data utility. A way to limit the impact of this (with higher cost for personnel) would have been to introduce a separation between the persons who interact with the patients during intervention and collect the data, and the person who is in charge of the evaluation.

Regarding the *RESTRICT* tactic, we could additionally implement a password/PIN in order to use the application, however as already mentioned this might not be usable for our target group, therefore we decided against it. On our side, the study evaluation device and decryption keys are properly secured by passwords and physical access control.

As already noted in our use case, anonymity for participants is very hard to achieve (especially without considerable data utility loss), since the study personnel interacts directly with the participants and the group of participants is also very small. Furthermore linkability between different datasets (neuropsychological pre-test, post-test and metrics) is required and therefore the data has to be at least pseudonymous. However in larger studies or datasets, anonymity or stronger pseudonymity may be achievable, by applying patterns from the *MIX* strategy. Especially metadata during transmission of pseudonymous or anonymous study data has to be reduced. For example transmitting study data over the internet includes an IP address (which could be mitigated with the *Anonymization Network* pattern [14]) and time information among other metadata, which could be used for re-identification. A simple way to hide the identities when transmitting pseudonymous data is to collect data of multiple participants at a trusted party (e.g. a therapist who is responsible for multiple patients) and then sending the data in batch (possibly in regular time intervals) to the recipient. This hides metadata such as time information of patient visits as well as IP addresses or browser metadata of patients, without requiring complex technology. A rather complex approach for hiding a patient's data, for example when asking for test results or a diagnosis, would be to send multiple fake, indistinguishable from real, data records to a server, including the real patient's data and hiding it in the noise, i.e. applying the *Use of dummies* pattern [9].

Depending on the type of data, it may be harder to generate fake records, indistinguishable from real (e.g. pictures), however with the recent advances [23] in Generative Adversarial Networks (GANs) [17], future work could support such cases. A more simplified version of this pattern would only consider leaking metadata through the network, e.g. the fact that a device is sending data to a certain server.

6.3 SEPARATE

The *SEPARATE* strategy is about "preventing correlation as much as possible by distributing or isolating". It consists of the tactics *DISTRIBUTE* ("partitioning personal data so that more access is required to process it") and *ISOLATE* ("processing parts of personal data independently, without access or correlation to related parts") [8].

Storing data such as workflows and metrics by default in a decentralized manner only on the participants' devices can be seen as application of the *ISOLATE* tactic by using the *Personal Data Store* pattern [9]. Furthermore the computation of metric results directly within the participants' devices, i.e. local aggregation, can be seen as use of the *User data confinement* pattern [9].

Instead of an on-device aggregation, we could aggregate the data on a centralized server. However this would imply that updates from the device have to be sent regularly to the server. These updates might then include the raw values over a certain time period, which at least would temporarily leave unnecessary raw data on that server.

6.4 ABSTRACT

The *ABSTRACT* strategy (previously *AGGREGATE*) targets "limiting detail as much as possible by summarizing or grouping". It consists of the tactics *SUMMARIZE* ("extracting commonalities in personal data by finding and processing correlations instead of the data itself") and *GROUP* ("inducing less detail from personal data prior to processing, by allocating into common categories") [8].

Our implementation was mainly based on the *GROUP* tactic. Values measured by our metrics are often trimmed to a low precision. Also timestamps are reduced in precision, e.g. for some measurements only the week in which a metric was recorded is stored. Lastly all values are aggregated on the participant's device (*User data confinement* pattern [9]), instead of raw data being stored and possibly transmitted for study evaluation. The aggregation is also performed incrementally (updating the previous aggregate value directly), if possible, i.e. raw values are not stored unless absolutely necessary. By using only very low precision timestamps (e.g. day or week resolution), the risk to leak detailed information about the participant's daily structure and routines can be reduced. In contrast utilizing precise timestamps and recording of more atomic events (such as most interactions with the device), this risk will be significantly higher. Furthermore it may also simplify linking to other datasets. For example if it is known that the person was performing some activity during a certain time-frame, he/she may be ruled out from other activities/places during that time. Such precise event information (e.g. every click in the app) could be used to create profiles, which could be used to match users with similar click behaviour to other applications and therefore additionally restricting the set of possible users.

To further increase privacy aspects, methods from the field of Statistical Disclosure Control (SDC) may be applied, particularly before publishing datasets. For example trimming the accuracy to discrete steps, as it is possible with our metric language, can be seen as the use of binning, which is one of the generalization methods of SDC. However, before publishing datasets, it is still necessary to verify that the risk of re-identification is low enough, i.e. that the dataset can be considered anonymous. Different models for measuring anonymity are available, such as k-anonymity [44], l-diversity [31], t-closeness [30] or differential privacy [10].

6.5 INFORM

The *INFORM* strategy provides transparency regarding data collection, processing and retention to the user. It consists of the tactics *SUPPLY*, *NOTIFY* and *EXPLAIN*. *SUPPLY* provides the user with resources about the processing of personal data, *NOTIFY* alerts the user about new information regarding the processing of personal data (e.g. data breaches or changes to data processing), while *EXPLAIN* provides concise and understandable detail on personal data processing [8].

Regarding the *SUPPLY* tactic, we inform users during their Informed Consent (additionally provided in easy German language). A privacy policy has been integrated into the application for general use (apart from the extended study use case), which includes an overview of how data is processed, along with a contact address such that users may exercise their rights.

To provide information about shared workflows, a separate dashboard could be introduced, or it could be visualized within the table of workflows that a certain workflow has been shared.

In addition information about metrics could be displayed through a privacy dashboard. This has not been implemented yet since the information is already included in the informed consent process. However, our metric language has been designed such that metrics can be specified in a descriptive manner, therefore it is possible to automatically generate human readable textual descriptions from the definitions. Additionally each metric has a descriptive name that by itself should state the scope of what is being recorded.

Considering the *EXPLAIN* tactic, a meaningful option would be to visualize the metric recording and study export process, in order to describe what kind of data does get transferred, along with what actions we take in order to preserve privacy and security properties. Metrics could e.g. be visualized as a data flow graph. However, considering that a part of our target group has congenital brain deficits, creating an understandable representation becomes much harder.

6.6 CONTROL

The *CONTROL* strategy implements intervenability for the data subjects. It includes the tactics *CONSENT* ("only processing the personal data for which explicit, freely-given, and informed consent is received"), *CHOOSE* ("allowing for the selection or exclusion of personal data, partly or wholly, from any processing"), *UPDATE* ("providing data subjects with the means to keep their personal data accurate and up to date"), as well as *RETRACT* ("honoring the data subject's right to the complete removal of any personal data in a timely fashion") [8].

As already mentioned, we utilize Informed Consent, e.g. when participants are asked whether they would like to participate in our study. Within the document it is clearly stated that consent should be freely-given, without the fear of repercussions for not participating or leaving the study prior to the intended end. Consent in easy language allows potential participants with intellectual disabilities (to a certain degree) to also understand the important facts about the study and their choice.

Participants may therefore *CHOOSE* whether they would like to participate in the study or not. There are, however, no further gradations of data collection within the study to assure comparability. Hereafter metrics could be used as part of the general therapy, to deduce information about its success by transmitting those to the therapist. Selecting what kind of data will be provided for the therapist provides further means for the participant, e.g. to choose a set of metrics or a "tracking level" of how much information should be provided. In case of workflow sharing, every user can optionally share workflows with other users through either our server or via file transfer. It is not required to store workflows on a cloud service by default.

The *RETRACT* tactic is implemented in part by allowing participants to locally delete workflows. Furthermore all study data regarding a participant (personal data/entry in coding table, entry in pseudonym mapping table, neuropsychological pre and post tests, collected metrics including encrypted data, shared workflows) can be deleted, if a participant decides to leave the study.

During the study we discussed a technical option to exit the study, i.e. stop recording of metrics and potentially even delete already recorded data by e.g. pressing a button. However, a part of our team was concerned that this button (or even a different UX pattern) is hit accidentally or without further reflection and with no possibility of undo, therefore it was decided against it. The idea was instead, that users should address the study team, or alternatively uninstall the application altogether from the device (which would delete all recorded data and users will also not be able to join the study again). The study team can also assist the participant in deleting the data from their device and uninstalling the application, if required. Currently because of our coding table we only require a participant's name in order to delete all associated data, however this could be implemented differently e.g. using only a pseudonym instead (see Subsect. 6.2). Metric results can only be deleted locally by uninstalling the application (and possibly removing already performed study export files), and not partly or wholly within the application.

6.7 ENFORCE

The *ENFORCE* strategy encompasses the creation, maintenance and upholding of policies and technical controls regarding storage, collection, retention, sharing, changes, breaches or operation on personal data. It consists of the tactics *CREATE* ("acknowledging the value of privacy and deciding policies which enable it, and processes which respect personal data"), *MAINTAIN* ("considering privacy when designing or modifying features, and updating policies and processes to better protect personal data") and *UPHOLD* ("ensuring that policies are adhered to by treating personal data as an asset, and privacy as a goal to incentivize as a critical feature") [8].

For the *CREATE* tactic, the study mode of our application has to be activated manually, i.e. the process of joining it is based on the opt-in scheme. This requires a password to be entered, which is unique per study. The password is only known to our staff, therefore it is required that both the physical device and a staff member is present in order to enter study mode. This prevents accidental study mode activation by users and therefore additional tracking. However, it has to be ensured through non-technical means, that the user actually consents to the data recording. The password is not stored in plaintext within the application due to security reasons, but rather only a PBKDF2-derived key which can be used to verify the password. This ensures that even if the application is reverse engineered, the password cannot easily be derived and circumvented without manipulation of the application.

The use of an offline, securely stored study laptop, as well as storing study-related documents in a safe can be seen as additional measures to enforce this tactic.

Necessary security updates are done on a regular basis, in order to *MAINTAIN* our privacy and security standards. During development, new features will be discussed and checked for potential privacy implications in the team. Upon introducing new features within the existing application, each merge request will be reviewed by a different developer, in order to follow a four-eye-principle. Our privacy policies and mindset are also agreed upon in our cooperation contracts, as well as in the application for ethics approval (UPHOLD).

The ENFORCE strategy gets more important, once the scope of the project and size thereof expands, or further gets incorporated within an organization.

6.8 DEMONSTRATE

The *DEMONSTRATE* strategy was established in order for the data controller to be able to show that the legal requirements are implemented as required. It can be accomplished through the tactics *LOG* ("tracking all processing of data, without revealing personal data, securing and reviewing the information gathered for any risks"), *AUDIT* ("examining all day to day activities for any risks to personal data, and responding to any discrepancies seriously.") and *REPORT* ("analyzing collected information on tests, audits, and logs periodically to review improvements to the protection of personal data").

For the *AUDIT* tactic, especially in larger projects or commercial ones, it is important to perform audits regularly, regarding security and privacy. It is important to build-up and refresh knowledge on best-practices regarding security and privacy, in order to comply with them. Privacy and security should be treated like other qualities of good products and could be marketed as an advantage in comparison to competitors.

Regarding the *LOG* tactic, due to our strict data minimization approach, our logging is rather minimal. We collect e.g. requests to our servers for downloading the software or exchanging workflows. These logs are stored only in-memory and are never written to disk, and are therefore very constrained in their storage duration.

Our software development practices also include automated integration tests as part of a continuous integration, which covers most of the functionality of the application. This includes some tests for vulnerabilities in areas such as parsing, which are known as a common source for vulnerabilities in software. Additionally, automated checks are done to *REPORT*, whether there are known security vulnerabilities in one of our dependencies, in which case the developers can act in a timely manner in order to update them.

7 Conclusion

In the context of a neuropsychological study including the use of an mHealth application it was shown how privacy by design and privacy by default principles could be included in application development and study design as a guiding principle to protect fundamental rights and freedoms of natural persons as demanded by the GDPR. This reduces also the risks for using the mHealth application afterwards in daily life activities.

Future work includes the utilization of the metrics concept in further applications. It is intended to foster communication between patient and therapist and to integrate gamification elements to enhance the motivation of patients. This will be accompanied by elements to foster transparency and intervenability via a privacy dashboard.

Acknowledgements. This work was supported by the Ministry for Science and Culture of Lower Saxony as part of SecuRIn (VWZN3224).

References

1. Aschenbrenner, S., Tucha, O., Lange, K.W.: Regensburger Wortflüssigkeits-Test. Hogrefe (2000)
2. Atkinson, R.C., Shiffrin, R.M.: The control of short-term memory. Sci. Am. **225**(2), 82–91 (1971)
3. Baddeley, A.D., Hitch, G.: Working memory. In: Bower, G.H. (ed.) Psychology of Learning and Motivation, vol. 8, pp. 47–89. Academic Press (1974). https://doi.org/10.1016/S0079-7421(08)60452-1, http://www.sciencedirect.com/science/article/pii/S0079742108604521
4. Bertens, D., Fasotti, L., Boelen, D.H., Kessels, R.P.: A randomized controlled trial on errorless learning in goal management training: study rationale and protocol. BMC Neurol. **13**(1), 64 (2013). https://doi.org/10.1186/1471-2377-13-64
5. Bonawitz, K., et al.: Practical secure aggregation for privacy preserving machine learning. Cryptology ePrint Archive, Report 2017/281 (2017). https://eprint.iacr.org/2017/281
6. Brooke, J.: SUS - a quick and dirty usability scale. Usability Eval. Ind. **189**(194), 4–7 (1996). http://www.usabilitynet.org/trump/documents/Suschapt.doc
7. Cafazzo, J.A., Casselman, M., Hamming, N., Katzman, D.K., Palmert, M.R.: Design of an mHealth App for the self-management of adolescent type 1 diabetes: a pilot study. J. Med. Internet Res. **14**(3), e70 (2012). https://doi.org/10.2196/jmir.2058
8. Colesky, M., Hoepman, J.H., Hillen, C.: A critical analysis of privacy design strategies. In: 2016 IEEE Security and Privacy Workshops (SPW), pp. 33–40 (2016). https://doi.org/10.1109/SPW.2016.23
9. Colesky, M., et al.: Privacy patterns. https://privacypatterns.org/. Accessed 10 June 2020
10. Dwork, C.: Differential privacy: a survey of results. In: Agrawal, M., Du, D., Duan, Z., Li, A. (eds.) TAMC 2008. LNCS, vol. 4978, pp. 1–19. Springer, Heidelberg (2008). https://doi.org/10.1007/978-3-540-79228-4_1
11. Emmanouel, A.: Look at the frontal side of life: anterior brain pathology and everyday executive function: assessment approaches and treatment. Ph.D. thesis, Radboud University (2017). http://repository.ubn.ru.nl/handle/2066/166754
12. Regulation (EU) 2016/679 of the European parliament and of the council of 27 April 2016 on the protection of natural persons with regard to the processing of personal data and on the free movement of such data, and repealing directive 95/46/EC (general data protection regulation). Official Journal of the European Union L119, pp. 1–88, May 2016. http://eur-lex.europa.eu/legal-content/EN/TXT/?uri=OJ:L:2016:119:TOC
13. Gabel, A., Ertas, F., Pleger, M., Schiering, I., Müller, S.: Privacy-preserving metrics for an mHealth App in the context of neuropsychological studies. In: Proceedings of the 13th International Joint Conference on Biomedical Engineering

Systems and Technologies - Volume 5: HEALTHINF, pp. 166–177. SciTePress (2020). https://doi.org/10.5220/0008982801660177, https://www.scitepress.org/DigitalLibrary/Link.aspx?doi=10.5220/0008982801660177
14. Gabel, A., Schiering, I.: Privacy patterns for pseudonymity. In: Kosta, E., Pierson, J., Slamanig, D., Fischer-Hübner, S., Krenn, S. (eds.) Privacy and Identity 2018. IAICT, vol. 547, pp. 155–172. Springer, Cham (2019). https://doi.org/10.1007/978-3-030-16744-8_11
15. Gabel, A., Schiering, I., Müller, S.V., Ertas, F.: mHealth applications for goal management training - privacy engineering in neuropsychological studies. In: Hansen, M., Kosta, E., Nai-Fovino, I., Fischer-Hübner, S. (eds.) Privacy and Identity 2017. IAICT, vol. 526, pp. 330–345. Springer, Cham (2018). https://doi.org/10.1007/978-3-319-92925-5_22
16. Garcia-Ceja, E., Osmani, V., Mayora, O.: Automatic stress detection in working environments from smartphones' accelerometer data: a first step. IEEE J. Biomed. Health Inform. **20**(4), 1053–1060 (2016). https://doi.org/10.1109/JBHI.2015.2446195
17. Goodfellow, I., et al.: Generative adversarial nets. In: Ghahramani, Z., Welling, M., Cortes, C., Lawrence, N.D., Weinberger, K.Q. (eds.) Advances in Neural Information Processing Systems 27, pp. 2672–2680. Curran Associates, Inc. (2014). https://papers.nips.cc/paper/5423-generative-adversarial-nets
18. Grünerbl, A., et al.: Smartphone-based recognition of states and state changes in bipolar disorder patients. IEEE J. Biomed. Health Inform. **19**(1), 140–148 (2015). https://doi.org/10.1109/JBHI.2014.2343154
19. Hafiz, M.: A pattern language for developing privacy enhancing technologies. Softw. Pract. Exp. **43**(7), 769–787 (2013)
20. Hansen, M., Jensen, M., Rost, M.: Protection goals for privacy engineering. In: 2015 IEEE Security and Privacy Workshops, pp. 159–166, May 2015. https://doi.org/10.1109/SPW.2015.13
21. Härting, C., Markowitsch, H.J., Neufeld, H., Calabrese, P., Deisinger, K., Kessler, J.: Wechsler Gedächtnistest - Revidierte Fassung: WMS-R (2000)
22. Huckvale, K., Prieto, J.T., Tilney, M., Benghozi, P.J., Car, J.: Unaddressed privacy risks in accredited health and wellness apps: a cross-sectional systematic assessment. BMC Med. **13**, 214 (2015). https://doi.org/10.1186/s12916-015-0444-y
23. Karras, T., Laine, S., Aittala, M., Hellsten, J., Lehtinen, J., Aila, T.: Analyzing and improving the image quality of StyleGAN. In: The IEEE/CVF Conference on Computer Vision and Pattern Recognition (CVPR), June 2020
24. Kiresuk, T.J., Sherman, R.E.: Goal attainment scaling: a general method for evaluating comprehensive community mental health programs. Community Mental Health J. **4**(6), 443–453 (1968). https://doi.org/10.1007/BF01530764
25. Kleiman, E.M., et al.: Digital phenotyping of suicidal thoughts, July 2018. https://doi.org/10.1002/da.22730, https://onlinelibrary.wiley.com/doi/abs/10.1002/da.22730
26. Knorr, K., Aspinall, D.: Security testing for Android mHealth apps. In: 2015 IEEE Eighth International Conference on Software Testing, Verification and Validation Workshops (ICSTW), pp. 1–8, April 2015. https://doi.org/10.1109/ICSTW.2015.7107459
27. Levine, B., et al.: Rehabilitation of executive functioning: an experimental-clinical validation of goal management training. J. Int. Neuropsychol. Soc. **6**(3), 299–312 (2000). https://doi.org/10.1017/S1355617700633052

28. Levine, B., et al.: Rehabilitation of executive functioning: an experimental-clinical validation of goal management training. J. Int. Neuropsychol. Soc. **6**(3), 299–312 (2000). https://doi.org/10.1017/S1355617700633052, https://www.cambridge.org/core/journals/journal-of-the-international-neuropsychological-society/article/rehabilitation-of-executive-functioning-an-experimentalclinical-validation-of-goal-management-training/79A6CAE70C3703008D083F64F34246D8
29. Levine, B., et al.: Rehabilitation of executive functioning in patients with frontal lobe brain damage with goal management training. Front. Hum. Neurosci. **5** (2011). https://doi.org/10.3389/fnhum.2011.00009, https://www.frontiersin.org/articles/10.3389/fnhum.2011.00009/full
30. Li, N., Li, T., Venkatasubramanian, S.: t-Closeness: privacy beyond k-anonymity and l-diversity. In: 2007 IEEE 23rd International Conference on Data Engineering, pp. 106–115, April 2007. https://doi.org/10.1109/ICDE.2007.367856, ISSN 2375-026X
31. Machanavajjhala, A., Kifer, D., Gehrke, J., Venkitasubramaniam, M.: L-diversity: privacy beyond k-anonymity. ACM Trans. Knowl. Discov. Data **1**(1), 3-es (2007). https://doi.org/10.1145/1217299.1217302
32. Martínez-Pérez, B., de la Torre-Díez, I., López-Coronado, M.: Privacy and security in mobile health apps: a review and recommendations. J. Med. Syst. **39**(1), 1–8 (2014). https://doi.org/10.1007/s10916-014-0181-3
33. McMahan, B., Ramage, D., Talwar, K., Zhang, L.: Learning differentially private recurrent language models. In: International Conference on Learning Representations (ICLR) (2018). https://openreview.net/pdf?id=BJ0hF1Z0b
34. Mense, A., Steger, S., Sulek, M., Jukic-Sunaric, D., Mészáros, A.: Analyzing privacy risks of mHealth applications. Stud. Health Technol. Inform. **221**, 41–45 (2016). https://doi.org/10.3233/978-1-61499-633-0-41
35. Mohr, D.L., Zhang, M., Schueller, S.M.: Personal sensing: understanding mental health using ubiquitous sensors and machine learning. Annu. Rev. Clin. Psychol. **13**, 23–47 (2017). https://doi.org/10.1146/annurev-clinpsy-032816-044949
36. Müller, S.V., Ertas, F., Aust, J., Gabel, A., Schiering, I.: Kann eine mobile Anwendung helfen abzuwaschen? Zeitschrift für Neuropsychologie **30**(2), 123–131 (2019). https://doi.org/10.1024/1016-264X/a000256
37. Müller, S.V.: Störungen der Exekutivfunktionen. Hogrefe (2013)
38. Onnela, J.P., Rauch, S.L.: Harnessing smartphone-based digital phenotyping to enhance behavioral and mental health. Neuropsychopharmacology **41**(7), 1691–1696 (2016). https://doi.org/10.1038/npp.2016.7
39. Papageorgiou, A., Strigkos, M., Politou, E., Alepis, E., Solanas, A., Patsakis, C.: Security and privacy analysis of mobile health applications: the alarming state of practice. IEEE Access **6**, 9390–9403 (2018). https://doi.org/10.1109/ACCESS.2018.2799522
40. Reitan, R.: Trail-Making Test. Reitan Neuropsychology Laboratory, Arizona (1979)
41. Robertson, I.: Goal Management Training: A Clinical Manual. PsyConsult, Cambridge (1996)
42. Schneider, W., Shiffrin, R.M.: Controlled and automatic human information processing: I. Detection, search, and attention. Psychol. Rev. **84**(1), 1–66 (1977). https://doi.org/10.1037/0033-295X.84.1.1
43. Stamenova, V., Levine, B.: Effectiveness of goal management training® in improving executive functions: a meta-analysis. Neuropsychol. Rehabil., 1–31 (2018). https://doi.org/10.1080/09602011.2018.1438294

44. Sweeney, L.: k-anonymity: a model for protecting privacy. Int. J. Uncertainty Fuzziness Knowl.-Based Syst. (2012). https://doi.org/10.1142/S0218488502001648, http://www.worldscientific.com/doi/abs/10.1142/S0218488502001648
45. Treacy, C., McCaffery, F.: Data security overview for medical mobile apps. Int. J. Adv. Secur. **9**(3 & 4), 2016 (2016)
46. Tucha, O., Lange, K.W.: TL-D: Turm von London - Deutsche Version (2004)
47. Wilson, B.A., Alderman, N., Burgess, P.W., Emslie, H., Evans, J.J.: Behavioural Assessment of the Dysexecutive Syndrome. Harcourt Assessment, San Antonio (1996)
48. Zimmermann, P., Fimm, B.: TAP Testbatterie zur Aufmerksamkeitsprüfung. Vera Fimm, Psychologische Testsysteme (2017)

Food Data Normalization Using Lexical and Semantic Similarities Heuristics

Gordana Ispirova[1,2(✉)], Gorjan Popovski[1,2], Eva Valenčič[1,2,3], Nina Hadzi-Kotarova[4], Tome Eftimov[1], and Barbara Koroušić Seljak[1]

[1] Computer Systems Department, Jožef Stefan Institute, Jamova cesta 39, 1000 Ljubljana, Slovenia
{gordana.ispirova,gorjan.popovski,eva.valencic, tome.eftimov,barbara.korousic}@ijs.si

[2] Jožef Stefan International Postgraduate School, Jamova cesta 39, 1000 Ljubljana, Slovenia

[3] School of Health Sciences, Faculty of Health and Medicine, Priority Research Centre in Physical Activity and Nutrition, The University of Newcastle, Callaghan, Australia

[4] Faculty of Computer Science and Engineering, Ss. Cyril and Methodius University, 1000 Skopje, North Macedonia

Abstract. Food is one of the main health and environmental factors in today's society. With modernization the food supply is expanding and food-related data is increasing. This type of data comes in many different forms and making it inter-operable is one of the main requirements for using in any kind of analyses. One step towards this goal is data normalization of data coming from different sources. Food-related is collected regarding various aspects – food composition, food consumption, recipe data, etc. The most commonly encountered form is food data related to food products, which in order to serve its purpose – sales and profits, is often distorted and manipulated for marketing plans of producers and retailers. This causes the data to be often misinterpreted. There exist some studies addressing the problem of heterogeneous data by data normalization based on lexical similarity of the food products' English names. We took this task a step further by considering data in non-English, low-resourced language – Slovenian. Working with such languages is challenging, as they have very limited resources and tools for Natural Language Processing (NLP). In our previously published work we considered different heuristics for matching food products: one based on lexical similarity [23], and two semantic similarity heuristics, i.e. based on word vector representations (embeddings). These data normalization approaches are evaluated once on a data set with 439 ground truth pairs of food products, obtained by matching their EAN barcodes. In this work, we extend this approach by introducing a new semantic similarity heuristic, based on sentence vector embeddings. Additionally, we extend the evaluation by taking real-world examples and tasking a subject-matter expert to rate the relevance of the top three matches for each example. The results show that using semantic similarity with the sentence embedding method yields best results, achieving 88% accuracy for the ground truth data set and 91% accuracy from the human

X. Ye et al. (Eds.): BIOSTEC 2020, CCIS 1400, pp. 468–485, 2021.
https://doi.org/10.1007/978-3-030-72379-8_23

expert evaluation, while the lexical similarity heuristic provides comparing results with 75% and 85% accuracy.

Keywords: Food data normalization · Food data linking · Food semantics · Word embeddings

1 Introduction

Working in the era of big data, there is an enormous amount of data that is available in almost every domain. This data is not only characterized by its quantity, but also by its nature, type and format, but also by the velocity and ambiguity at which it is generated and processed. In the last two decades, working with such data in most cases involves utilization of artificial intelligence (AI) methods. Such methods require information from different data sources in order to make a prediction or a decision. However, before starting to work on predictive modelling, the attributes that are shared across different data sources should be interlinked to make the data sets inter-operable. This is possible, by applying so called data normalization [28], which is the process of linking the same concepts across different data sets.

The Biomedical domain is well-researched regarding interoperability, having the Unified Medical Language System (UMLS) [3] publicly available. UMLS integrates and distributes key terminology, classification and coding standards to promote the creation of more effective and inter-operable biomedical information systems and services [29]. Additionally, it provides tools for lexical similarities to allow normalization of biomedical concepts to the standards that are part of UMLS [2]. There are also different natural language processing (NLP) workshops that are organized as a part of various international conferences, where the main focus is on developing automatic methods based on NLP and Machine Learning (ML) to support normalization of biomedical concepts such as genes, proteins, phenotype information, drugs, diseases, treatments, etc. [16,20].

In recent years, some work has been performed on the normalization of food-related data, which is heterogeneous with respect to types and formats. We should emphasize that the Food domain is still low-resourced in comparison to the Biomedical domain. There are several food ontologies that can be used for food data normalization, such as FoodOn [12], OntoFood and SNOMED CT [6]. A recently published study [27] showed that their coverage is limited, since all of them were developed to address some specific problems. Moreover, there is a semantic resource known as FoodOntoMap [26] where for each food concept, that was extracted from 1000 recipes, semantic tags from four food resources and ontologies (i.e. Hansard, SNOMED CT, FoodOn, OntoFood) are assigned. FoodOntoMap also provides links between different food ontologies that can be used for developing applications that support understanding of relations between food systems, human health, and the environment. This methodology is general and can be applied to any ontology that has a NER (Named Entity Recognition) method. Another semi-automatic system for classifying and describing English food names according to FoodEx2 [7] is StandFood [9], which was developed for the normalization of food-related data.

Food data is gathered for different aims and using different methodologies, e.g. food consumption data, food composition data, recipe data, to mention but few of them. Food product data is a type of food composition data, which is often misinterpreted due to the vast and very competitive marketing scene. Different manufacturers and retailers represent the food products in different ways to their customers to better market the product to their consumers. Additionally, this misinterpretation can be due to the variety of diet styles that people adhere to.

In our previous work, we explored methods that can be used for the normalization of food concepts specified in the Slovenian language [23]. A large subset of food concepts were extracted from data on food products from two food retailers. To link the food products, we proposed heuristics based on lexical and semantic similarities. The lexical similarity was based on the syntactic and morphological similarity, while the semantic similarity relied on word embeddings (i.e. Word2Vec [18] and GloVe [21]). In this work, we extend our previous study by including and evaluating paragraph embeddings (i.e. Doc2Vec [19]) that can be used for semantic similarity. We compared the study results with our previous results, and additionally, an evaluation by a subject-matter expert was performed to find out which of the heuristics provides the results most similar to the expert's knowledge.

The remainder of the paper is organized as follows: Sect. 2 provides an overview of the related work. Next, in Sect. 3, our proposed methodology is explained in detail, followed by an insight into the data used in Sect. 4. Then, the experimental results and discussion are presented in Sect. 4, closing with Sect. 6 where conclusions and some directions for future work are presented.

2 Related Work

Working with textual data is especially challenging due to its variability, which by the nature of language, depends on how people express themselves. Many Artificial Intelligence (AI) studies and applications involve combining different data sets that contain information about the same concepts, which are often represented in different ways. To combine this information, first the same concepts across the different data sets should be linked. To achieve this, text normalization methods should be applied. Text normalization methods are based on different types of text similarity measures, which provide a metric of similarity between two sequences of text, i.e. strings. Similarity can be measured with regard to two criteria: i) how distant two texts are both in surface form (i.e. lexical similarity) and ii) meaning (i.e. semantic similarity).

2.1 Lexical Similarity

Lexical similarity can be expressed on two levels: i) the character level and ii) the word (i.e. token) level. These measures do not take into account the meaning behind the words or the context of a phrase, but they focus on overlapping characters or words in the pair of strings being compared.

There exist several lexical similarity measures such as the*Levenshtein distance*, the *Optimal String Alignment distance*, the *Damerau-Levenshtein distance*, the *longest common substring*, the *q-gram*, the *cosine distance*, the *Jaccard distance*, the *Jaro distance*, the *Jaro-Winkler distance*, and the *skip-grams*. More details about these are presented in [13]. In the food and nutrition domain, methods based on lexical similarities that can be used for normalization based of food and nutrient names in English, have already been proposed [8–10,13]. These methods apply: (i) standard text similarity measures and (ii) a modified version of Part of Speech (POS) tagging probability-weighted method [9,10].

2.2 Semantic Similarity

Semantic similarity is a metric that determines the similarity between two strings considering their semantic meaning. It is closely related to representation learning, where each text (e.g., word, sentence, or paragraph) is represented as a vector of continuous numbers. These vectors are known as embeddings and capture the context of a word in a piece of text, as well as semantic and syntactic similarity, relation with other words, etc.

To calculate the similarity between two words, two sentences, or two paragraphs, we estimate similarity between their vectors (i.e. embeddings). To perform this, the cosine similarity between the embeddings is calculated, in order to provide the information about the angle between their vectors. The cosine distance between two vectors $\mathbf{x}$ and $\mathbf{y}$ can be calculated using the following equation:

$$cos(\mathbf{x}, \mathbf{y}) = \frac{\mathbf{xy}}{||\mathbf{x}||^2||\mathbf{y}||^2}. \quad (1)$$

This value for the cosine similarity lies in the range $[-1, 1]$, where one means the highest similarity between the texts, and -1 means the highest degree of dissimilarity. When the cosine distance is 0, it means that the vectors are orthogonal.

Word Embeddings. Word embeddings are vector representations that are learned for each word in a textual corpus. The two most commonly used word embedding methods are:

1. Word2Vec – One method for learning word embeddings is *Word2Vec* [18,19], where the authors presented a model for learning high-quality distributed vector representations that capture a large number of precise syntactic and semantic word relationships. This is the first work of this kind and it paved the way for all the work in the field of representation learning that followed. Word2Vec is a shallow neural network architecture, consisting of one hidden layer and one output layer. The Word2Vec model consists of two different architectures:

(a) Continuous Bag-of-Words architecture – This architecture aims to predict the current word based on the input context. There is a center word that should be predicted based on the words that surround it – context words. The one–hot encoded context word vectors are the input to this model. The number of dimensions of the vectors is the vocabulary size V of the corpus. The main goal is to maximize the conditional probability of the output word.
(b) Skip-gram architecture – This architecture is the opposite of the CBOW architecture. In this scenario we know the center word and we are trying to predict the preceding and succeeding words, i.e. its context. The skip-gram architecture as output will give C number of V dimensional vectors, where C is defined as the number of context words which we want the model to return and V is total vocabulary size. The skip-gram model is trained to minimize the summed prediction error and gives better word vectors when C is increased.

If we compare the two architectures, CBOW is simpler and faster to train, but skip-gram performs better with words that do not appear frequently in the data set.

2. GloVe – Another method for learning word embeddings is *GloVe* [22]. It is an unsupervised learning algorithm based on aggregated global word-word co-occurrence statistics from a given corpus, which are then used to learn word embeddings. The learned word embeddings are linear substructures of the word vector space.

Sentence Embeddings. The main difference between sentence embeddings and word embeddings is that the sentence embeddings are learned for sentences, paragraphs, and even whole documents, and not for individual words. The first such model was presented in [19].

1. Doc2Vec – In [19] the authors propose an unsupervised paragraph embedding method, called Doc2Vec, which creates vector representations of documents, regardless of their length. Doc2Vec works by concatenating the paragraph vector and word vectors in a sliding window fashion, and predicting the next word. The algorithm used for training is based on gradient decent. This algorithm also takes into account the order of words and their context.

   Doc2Vec was inspired by the Word2Vec model. The first approach is an extension of the CBOW model with an additional vector (Paragraph ID) added. This means that it uses additional document-unique features to predict the word. When training the word vectors, the document vector is trained as well. This model is called Distributed Memory version of Paragraph Vector (PV-DM). The word vectors represent the concept of a word, while the document vector represent the concept of a document.

   The second algorithm is similar to the skip-gram model and is called Distributed Bag of Words version of Paragraph Vector (PV-DBOW).

While the PV-DM method considers the concatenation of the paragraph vector with the word vectors to predict the next word in a text window, in the PV-DBOW method the context words in the input are ignored, and the model predicts words randomly sampled from the paragraph in the output. In Doc2Vec each paragraph vector is a combination of two vectors: one learned by the standard paragraph vector with distributed memory (PV-DM) and one learned by the paragraph vector with distributed bag of words (PV-DBOW). The authors also state that though the PV-DM model is superior and usually will achieve state of the art results by itself, they recommend a combination of the two models.

3 Methodology

In this section, we present both methodologies used for food data normalization, i.e. based on lexical and semantic similarity.

3.1 Lexical Similarity

For calculating lexical similarity between two food entities, we used our previously proposed approach [9,13,25] based on POS tagging combined with probability theory. If D_1 is one text segment (in our case food entity) and D_2 is another text segment, we first apply POS tagging and assign to each of the words in the text segments an appropriate Part-Of-Speech tags such as: nouns (NN, NNS, NNP, NNPS), verbs (VB, VBD, VBG, VBN, VBP, VBZ), adjectives (JJ, JJR, JJS), cardinal numbers (CD), etc. [17]. Let us define the following sets:

$$Y_{i,j} = \{tokens,\ from,\ D_i,\ that,\ belong,\ to,\ one,\ word,\ class\}, \tag{2}$$

where $j = 1, 2 \ldots, n$. The possible word classes are: nouns, adjectives, verbs, adverbs, prepositions, determiners, pronouns, conjunctions, modal verbs, particles, and numerals. Therefore, for all word classes for each text segment there is a set of tokens. For example, $Y_{i,j}$ can be a set of all tokens from D_i that are tagged as nouns. In such case, the set consists of all tokens that are tagged as NN, NNS, NNP, and NNPS. Given that we are dealing with significantly short text segments, not all of the sets for the word classes will have elements in them, and more importantly not all of them are significant for the specific problem. The set of nouns is crucial because nouns carry most of the information in the text, while all other word classes (adjectives, verbs, numbers, etc.) give an additional explanation. After extracting the set word classes that are significant, lemmatization [14] is applied to each of them. To find string similarity between both pieces of text, a probability event is defined as a product of independent events

$$X = N \prod_{j=1}^{k} Z_j, \tag{3}$$

where N is the similarity between the sets of nouns found in both pieces of text, k is the number of additional word classes that are selected and are significant for the domain, and Z_j is the similarity between the sets of word class j, found in both text. The additional word classes can be adjectives, verbs, etc.

Because these events are independent, the probability of the event X can be calculated as

$$P(X) = P(N) \prod_{j=1}^{k} P(Z_j). \tag{4}$$

To calculate it, the probabilities of the independent events need to be defined. Because the problem looks for the similarity between two sets, we use the Jaccard index J, which is used in statistics for comparing similarity and diversity of sample sets [15]. For the similarity between the nouns, the Jaccard index is used, while for the similarity between the additional word classes the Jaccard index in combination with Laplace probability estimate [4] is used. This is because in some short segments of text, the additional class sets can be empty, i.e. not contain any words. We do this to avoid probabilities equal to zero. The probabilities are calculated as

$$\begin{aligned} P(N) &= \tfrac{|N_1 \cap N_2|}{|N_1 \cup N_2|}, \\ P(Z_j) &= \tfrac{|Z_{j_1} \cap Z_{j_2}|+1}{|Z_{j_1} \cup Z_{j_2}|+2}. \end{aligned} \tag{5}$$

By substituting Eqs. 5 into Eq. 4, we obtain a weight for the matching pair.

Addressing the food domain, or specifically on the food matching problem, let D_1 and D_2 be the (in our case Slovenian, but could also be any language) names of two selected food products. As previously mentioned, the nouns carry most of the information, while the additional word classes that describe the food domain are adjectives, which explain the food item in more detail (e.g., frozen, fresh), and the verbs, which are generally related with the method of preparation (e.g., cooked, dried). Let us define

$$N_i = \{nouns\ extracted\ from\ D_i\},$$

$$A_i = \{adjectives\ extracted\ from\ D_i\}, \tag{6}$$

$$V_i = \{verbs\ extracted\ from\ D_i\} \tag{7}$$

where $i = 1, 2 \ldots, n$.

To find the similarity between the names of food products, an event is defined as a product of two other events

$$X = N \cdot (A + V), \tag{8}$$

where N is the similarity between the nouns found in N_1 and N_2, and $A + V$ is the similarity between the two sets of adjectives and verbs handled together as $A_1 + V_1$ and $A_2 + V_2$. The adjectives and verbs are handled together to avoid different forms with the same meaning. Additionally, lemmatization is applied for each extracted noun, verb and adjective, and the similarity event uses their lemmas.

Because these two events are independent, the probability of the event X can be calculated as

$$P(X) = P(N) \cdot P(A + V). \tag{9}$$

The probabilities are calculated as

$$P(N) = \frac{|N_1 \cap N_2|}{|N_1 \cup N_2|},$$
$$P(A + V) = \frac{|(A_1 \cup V_1) \cap (A_2 \cup V_2)| + 1}{|(A_1 \cup V_1) \cup (A_2 \cup V_2)| + 2} \tag{10}$$

By substituting Eqs. 10 into Eq. 9, we obtain a weight for each matching pair.

3.2 Semantic Similarity

For mapping the food products from both data sets by using semantic similarity, we explore two different embedding approaches: word embedding techniques - that generate vectors on the word level, and sentence embedding that generate vectors on the sentence/paragraph level.

In the training phase, ss in the Slovenian language one word can have different grammatical cases, we use the lemmas of the words contained in the names of the food products. This means that even if multiple words have different grammatical cases, their lemma will be the same if they are derived from the same root.

Let us have fp as the name of a food product, which is consisted of n words:

$$fp = \Big\{word_1, word_2, ..., word_n\Big\} \tag{11}$$

Then after lemmatization we have:

$$fp = \Big\{lemma_1, lemma_2, ..., lemma_n\Big\} \tag{12}$$

Heuristics for Merging Word Embeddings to Compute Paragraph/Sentence Embeddings. On word level we used two word embedding techniques – Word2Vec [18] and GloVe [22]. After applying the two algorithms, we obtained vector representations for each lemma in the food product name (Eq. 12):

$$E[lemma_a] = \Big[x_{a1}, x_{a2}, ..., x_{ad}\Big] \tag{13}$$

$a \in \{1, ..., n\}$, and d is the dimension of the generated word vectors. Because with Word2Vec and GloVe we obtain vector representations for separate words, and the text segments we want to normalize are consisted from multiple words, we need to establish a heuristic for merging the separate word vectors for all the lemmas of a name, in order to obtain the vector representation for the whole food product name. For this purpose we chose the following two heuristics:

1. Average – The vector representation for the food product is calculated by averaging the vector representations of each lemma:

$$E_{average}[fp] = \left[\frac{x_{a1} + ... + x_{n1}}{n}, ..., \frac{x_{ad} + ... + x_{nd}}{n}\right] \tag{14}$$

2. Sum – The vector representation for the food product is calculated by summing the vector representations of each lemmas:

$$E_{sum}[fp] = \left[x_{a1} + ... + x_{n1}, ..., x_{ad} + ... + x_{nd}\right] \tag{15}$$

When the heuristics for merging the separate vector representations are applied we perform the matching by calculating the cosine similarity between the vector representations of the food products by substituting Eq. 14 or Eq. 15 in Eq. 1:

$$cos(\mathbf{E}[\mathbf{fp_1}], \mathbf{E}[\mathbf{fp_2}]) = \frac{\mathbf{E}[\mathbf{fp_1}]\mathbf{E}[\mathbf{fp_2}]}{||\mathbf{E}[\mathbf{fp_1}]||^2||\mathbf{E}[\mathbf{fp_2}]||^2}, \tag{16}$$

where $E[fp_1]$ and $E[fp_2]$ are embedding vectors of two food products obtained either considering average or sum as a combining heuristic.

1. Word2Vec embeddings – When generating the Word2Vec embeddings, we considered different values for the dimension size and sliding window size. Values for the sliding window were chosen to be *[2, 3, 5]*, while the dimensions were *[100, 200]*, we also considered the two types of feature extraction available by Word2Vec – Bag of Words and skip-gram. By combining these parameter values, 12 Word2Vec models were trained, plus considering the heuristics for combining, a total of 24 models.
2. GloVe embeddings – Same as the Word2Vec parameter choice, the same values were used for the numeric parameters of GloVe, i.e. *[2, 3, 5]* for the sliding window and *[100, 200]* for the dimension size. Thus, six GloVe models were trained, when paired with the merging heuristics results in a total of 12 models.
   The sliding windows for both methods were chosen according to the average number of words per food product, which was approximately nine.

Doc2Vec Paragraph Embeddings. The second approach of generating vector embeddings for the food product names is using the Doc2Vec algorithm. If fp is the food product name with all the words lemmatized (Eq. 12) then the generated vector representation from Doc2Vec is as follows:

$$E_{Doc2Vec}[fp] = \left[x_1, x_2, ..., x_d\right] \tag{17}$$

Where d is the predefined dimension of the vectors. The similarity between two food products taking into account the Doc2Vec embeddings of the food products names is calculated by substituting Eq. 17 in Eq. 1:

$$cos(\mathbf{E_{Doc2Vec}}[\mathbf{fp_1}], \mathbf{E_{Doc2Vec}}[\mathbf{fp_2}]) = \frac{\mathbf{E_{Doc2Vec}}[\mathbf{fp_1}]\mathbf{E_{Doc2Vec}}[\mathbf{fp_2}]}{||\mathbf{E_{Doc2Vec}}[\mathbf{fp_1}]||^2||\mathbf{E_{Doc2Vec}}[\mathbf{fp_2}]||^2}. \tag{18}$$

Same as the two chosen word embedding methods, we considered different dimension sizes and sliding window sizes, specifically *[2, 3, 5]* for the sliding window and *[100, 200]* for the dimension size. We also considered the two types architectures in the Doc2Vec model – PV-DM and PV-DBOW, and we used the non-concatenative mode (separate models for the sum option, and separate for the average option) because if we used the concatenation of context vectors rather than sum/average the result would be a much-larger model. Taking into account all these parameters there are 24 Doc2Vec models trained in total.

4 Data

The data used in our experiments contains food product data from two different food retailers (for convenience and anonymity let us name them: $Retailer_1$ and $Retailer_2$). The data about each food product includes food product name in Slovenian, the EAN barcode, the food label, the lists of ingredients and allergens (if provided by the retailer), and the name of the producer. Because we are concentrating on the normalization of food data based on text similarity we are going to use the (Slovenian) names of the food products to match the data from the different retailers. The number of food products in the two data sets is different. $Retailer_1$ had 1836 available food products, while $Retailer_2$ had 6587. It is important to note that the food names were similar, but not the same (e.g. bread is named by one retailer as "bel kruh", i.e. "white bread" in English, and by another retailer as "pšenični kruh, bel", i.e. "wheat bread, white").

4.1 Data Pre-processing

Prior to applying the algorithms for obtaining semantic similarity or calculating lexical similarity, the data is pre-processed. The first step is lemmatization of the names of the food products, while the second step is assigning POS tags on the lemmatized food product names. Since we are working with words in Slovenian, the POS tagger used is a model specifically trained for the Slovenian language [11]. This tagger outputs the tagged tokens as tripples: word form, lemma, and morph-syntactic description or tag. We use the lower case lemmas for each word. The data consists of words spanning across multiple morphological types. However, only the lemmas nouns, adjectives, and verbs convey semantic information. Hence, these are the only three types that are considered while calculating lexical similarity and training the vector embedding models.

5 Evaluation

In this section we describe the two different approaches of evaluating the food data normalization methods. In the first approach we evaluate based on the ground truth data set. Because the ground truth data set comprises of only 439 instances, we included a second type of evaluation – subject-matter evaluation, where a domain expert evaluated a subset of 100 instances from the ones that are not part of the ground truth data set, i.e. for the ones that do not have EAN codes.

5.1 Experiments and Results

In order to produce a data set consisting of ground-truth values, we matched the food products by using their corresponding EAN codes, i.e. we can consider the pair with the same EAN code as a perfect match, as EAN codes are the same for the same products, regardless of where they are retailed. The format of this type of data set is shown in Table 1.

Table 1. Ground truth data set format.

Food product name from $Retailer_1$	EAN code	Food product name from $Retailer_2$
fp_{11}	bc_1	fp_{21}
$\vdots$	$\vdots$	$\vdots$
fp_{1n}	bc_n	fp_{2n}

Where fp_{1x}, $x \in 1, ...n$ are the food product names from $Retailer_1$ and analogously fp_{2x}, $x \in 1, ...n$ from $Retailer_2$, and bc is the matching EAN code. There are 439 pairs with a matching EAN code, i.e. $n = 439$.

Because of the imbalance between the data sets from the two retailers, i.e. the data set with food products from $Retailer_1$ is significantly smaller than the data set from $Retailer_2$, in order to evaluate the data normalization methods we decided to consider the following scenario:

1. For every food product from $Retailer_1$ calculate the similarity with every food product from $Retailer_2$:
   - according to Eqs. 9 and 10 for lexical similarity;
   - according to Eq. 16 for every Word2Vec and Glove model;
   - according to Eq. 18 for every Doc2Vec model.
2. Take the five most similar food products.
3. Check if one of the five corresponds to the food product matched by the EAN code in the ground truth data set (Table 1):
   - Positive - if the food product with the same EAN code is in the top five matches;
   - Negative - if the food product with the same EAN code is not in the top five matches.

After evaluating all the models, the results from the best models according to dimensionality, sliding window and architecture (for Word2Vec and Doc2Vec) are presented in Table 2 and the accuracy for the best models in Table 3. For all the embedding methods the best models were with dimensionality $d = 200$ and used a sliding window of $s = 5$. For the Word2Vec method the CBOW architecture provided better results, and for the Doc2Vec the PV-DM architecture was the best trained model. In Table 4 examples from the evaluation based on the ground

Table 2. Evaluation results for the best models.

Model	Positives	Negatives
Word2Vec average	271	168
Word2Vec sum	271	168
GloVe average	238	201
GloVe sum	238	201
Doc2Vec average	384	55
Doc2Vec sum	**385**	**54**
Lexical	329	110

Table 3. Accuracy for the best models.

Model	Accuracy
Word2Vec average	0.62
Word2Vec sum	0.62
GloVe average	0.54
GloVe sum	0.54
Doc2Vec average	0.87
Doc2Vec sum	**0.88**
Lexical	0.75

truth data set are presented. The food product name in English in the examples is *Emmental cheese snack* and the food product matches that are in bold are the matches that are positive, i.e. have the same EAN code from the ground truth data set. For this particular example, we can see that the Doc2Vec sum model gave the correct match as the first one, the lexical similarity model as the second match, the Word2Vec sum model as the third match, and the GloVe model did not provide the correct match at all. A side note here is that all the models for this example provided matches that are somewhat relevant to the product, i.e. they are all a type of cheese.

5.2 Subject-Matter Evaluation

The second approach for evaluating the methods for food data normalization is to include a subject-matter expert, i.e. nutritionist for manual evaluation. This is done because the ground-truth data set contains only 439 instances, and for the rest 1397 instances from $Retailer_1$ the EAN codes are not available, therefore we are unable to conduct the same type of evaluation. Additionally, subject-matter expert evaluation provides a real-world testing case, where a human evaluates whether the matching is relevant The human expert evaluation was done according to the following steps:

Table 4. Examples from the evaluation based on EAN code matches (bolded matches correspond to a EAN code match between that match and the food product).

(a) Word2Vec sum model	
Food product:	Sir Ementaler snack listici 150g
Match 1:	Rezani sir v listicih snack kaeserei champignon 150g
Match 2:	Topljeni sir v listicih snack kaeserei champignon 150g
Match 3:	**Topljeni sir ementaler v listicih Kaeserei Champignon 150g**
Match 4:	Topljeni sir v listicih ementalec mercator 150g
Match 5:	Topljeni sir v listicih klasik mercator 150g
(b) GloVe sum model	
Food product:	Sir Ementaler snack listici 150g
Match 1:	Poltrdi sir gauda rezine 150g
Match 2:	Svezi sir mascarpone antiche latterie 250g
Match 3:	Sir gauda starana veerger kaas 200g
Match 4:	Ovcji poltrdi sir rezine el pastor 70g
Match 5:	Poltrdi sir tilzit rezine 150g
(c) Lexical model	
Food product:	Sir Ementaler snack listici 150g
Match 1:	Topljeni sir v listicih snack kaeserei champignon 150g
Match 2:	**Topljeni sir ementaler v listicih Kaeserei Champignon 150g**
Match 3:	Rrezani sir v listicih snack kaeserei champignon 150g
Match 4:	Pasta snack z brokolijem in sirom knorr 69g
Match 5:	Topljeni sir v listicih klasik mercator 150g
(d) Doc2Vec sum model	
Food product:	Sir Ementaler snack listici 150g
Match 1:	**Topljeni sir ementaler v listicih Kaeserei Champignon 150g**
Match 2:	Sir Ementaler Meggle listici 150g
Match 3:	Topljeni sir Bel Ami Meggle 140g
Match 4:	Topljeni sir Emmental Creme Lactalis President 125g
Match 5:	Sir gauda starana Veerger Kaas 200g

1. For a random subset 100 food product from $Retailer_1$ that do not have EAN codes available, calculate the similarity with every food product from $Retailer_2$:
   - according to Eqs. 9 and 10 for lexical similarity;
   - according to Eq. 16 for every Word2Vec and Glove model;
   - according to Eq. 18 for every Doc2Vec model.
2. Take the three most similar food products.

3. Human expert evaluates each of the three most similar food products as:
   - negative - *not a match*;
   - positive - *branded product match* (total match);
   - positive - *product match* (from nutritional aspect).

In the subject-matter evaluation we included the best performing models from each method according to the first type of evaluation (Table 3), i.e.: Word2Vec CBOW, GloVe, Doc2Vec PV-DM, both heuristics – average and sum, with dimensionality $d = 200$, and a sliding window of $s = 5$.

In Table 5 the results from the subject-matter expert evaluation are presented, while in Table 6 the accuracy for each model is presented. From the tables it is evident that, asis the case with the evaluation on the ground-truth data set, that the model with the best results is the Doc2Vec PV-DM sum model. We can also see that we achieved comparative results considering the lexical similarity. This is because the subject-matter expert considered matches also based on the nutritional value of the products. Namely, two products may not be from the same brand and not have the same EAN code, but can be the same type of product, same flavour, same ingredients, etc., therefore we can notice improvement in the lexical similarity model performance compared to the previous type of evaluation. Examples from the data set for subject-matter evaluation are given in Table 7.

Table 5. Subject-matter expert evaluation results.

Model	Branded product match	Product match	Total Positives	Negatives
Word2Vec average	3	18	21	79
Word2Vec sum	5	21	26	74
GloVe average	5	13	18	82
GloVe sum	3	14	17	83
Doc2Vec average	73	18	91	9
Doc2Vec sum	**75**	**16**	**91**	**9**
Lexical	76	9	85	15

The food product names in English in the examples is *Feta cheese*, and the top three matches from the Word2Vec and GloVe models do not have any matches, i.e. all of them are of match type *no match*. Semantically, *Match 2* for Word2Vec and *Match 1* for GloVe are both types of cheeses, however they are of different nature and have different nutritional contents. Moving on to the lexical model, it produces one match of each type (*branded product match*, *product match* and *no match*). Finally, the best results were obtained by the Dov2Vec model, providing excellent results with one *branded product match* and two instances of type *product match*.

Table 6. Model accuracy from subject-matter expert evaluation.

Model	Accuracy
Word2Vec average	0.26
Word2Vec sum	0.26
GloVe average	0.18
GloVe sum	0.17
Doc2Vec average	0.91
Doc2Vec sum	**0.91**
Lexical	0.85

Table 7. Examples from the data set for human-expert evaluation.

(a) Word2Vec sum model	
Food product:	Sir Feta Kolios 200g
Match 1 (no match):	Omaka iz parmezana Dukat 200g
Match 2 (no match):	Sir Emmental Portion President 250 g pakirano
Match 3 (no match):	Sveze polnomastno mleko 3,2 m. m. Mu 1l
(b) GloVe sum model	
Food product:	Sir Feta Kolios 200g
Match 1 (no match):	Sir Edamec Zdenka rezine 200g
Match 2 (no match):	Puding s smetano bela cokolada Dany 200g
Match 3 (no match):	Nepasirana skuta 35 m. m. Mu Cuisine 1kg
(c) Lexical model	
Food product:	Sir Feta Kolios 200g
Match 1 (branded product match):	Svezi feta sir v slanici Kolios 200 g pakirano
Match 2 (product match):	Sir feta v slanici Roussas 400 g pakirano
Match 3 (no match):	Sir Edamec Mercator 300g
(d) Doc2Vec sum model	
Food product:	Sir Feta Kolios 200g
Match 1 (branded product match):	Svezi feta sir v slanici Kolios 200 g pakirano
Match 2 (product match):	Sir feta v slanici Roussas 400 g pakirano
Match 3 (product match):	Sir feta Zop Roussas 200g

6 Conclusions

Representation learning together with word and sentence embeddings have emerged as a novel way of language modeling and feature learning techniques. We explore the idea of using these techniques for data normalization of food-related data.

The term food-related data is very broad, and in this work we focus on matching food products represented by non-English (Slovenian) short text description from two different online grocery stores. The matching of the food products is done according to two different heuristics:

1. Matching food products considering lexical similarity – calculating a similarity by a modified version of our previously proposed approach [9,13];
2. Matching food products considering semantic similarity – calculating a similarity or matching score which is the cosine similarity of the learned word and sentence embedding vectors.

We previously delved into this idea [24] using only word embeddings, generated using the Word2Vec and GloVe methods, and here we extended the it by introducing sentence embeddings with the Doc2Vec method.

To evaluate our data normalization approach, we considered two different aspects:

1. Automated evaluation based on a ground-truth data set of food product matched by their EAN codes – for each pair in the ground-truth data set, we took the first product, found the five top matches based on the proposed heuristics and checked if the second product of the pair, i.e. the match based on the EAN code is in the top five matches.
2. Subject-matter evaluation – data sets from each model, with the top three matches for 100 randomly selected examples that do not have EAN codes available were evaluated by a domain expert - a nutritionist.

The EAN code evaluation follows the same method as in our previously published paper [24], while in this work we extend the evaluation by including subject-matter expert evaluation.

The results from the automated evaluation and the subject-matter evaluation show that sentence embeddings outperform word embeddings in the task of data normalization for food-related data. The Doc2Vec method provides better results in both cases, with 88% accuracy for the evaluation based of the ground truth data set, and 91% accuracy for the human-expert evaluation data set. The lexical similarity model gave good results in both cases, achieving 75% accuracy in the evaluation based on the ground truth data set, and 85% accuracy for the human-expert evaluation data set.

Taking into consideration the results from this study, for future work we plan to proceed in the direction of data normalization of food data presented in a multilingual setting. Going in this direction we intent to use Multilingual Word Embeddings (MWEs) [1,5], which represent words from multiple languages in a single distributional vector space.

Acknowledgements. This work was supported by the project from the Slovenian Research Agency (research core funding No. P2-0098), and the European Union's Horizon 2020 research and innovation programme (grant agreements No. 863059 and No. 769661).

Information and the views set out in this publication are those of the authors and do not necessarily reflect the official opinion of the European Union. Neither the European Union institutions and bodies nor any person acting on their behalf may be held responsible for the use that may be made of the information contained here.

References

1. Alaux, J., Grave, E., Cuturi, M., Joulin, A.: Unsupervised hyperalignment for multilingual word embeddings. arXiv preprint arXiv:1811.01124 (2018)
2. Aronson, A.R.: MetaMap: mapping text to the UMLS metathesaurus. Bethesda, MD: NLM, NIH, DHHS, pp. 1–26 (2006)
3. Bodenreider, O.: The unified medical language system (UMLS): integrating biomedical terminology. Nucleic Acids Res. **32**(suppl_1), D267–D270 (2004)
4. Cestnik, B., et al.: Estimating probabilities: a crucial task in machine learning. In: ECAI, vol. 90, pp. 147–149 (1990)
5. Chen, X., Cardie, C.: Unsupervised multilingual word embeddings. arXiv preprint arXiv:1808.08933 (2018)
6. Donnelly, K.: SNOMED-CT: the advanced terminology and coding system for eHealth. Stud. Health Technol. Inform. **121**, 279 (2006)
7. (EFSA), European Food Safety Authority: The food classification and description system foodex 2 (revision 2), vol. 12, no. 5, p. 804E . EFSA Supporting Publications (2015)
8. Eftimov, T., Ispirova, G., Finglas, P., Korosec, P., Korousic-Seljak, B.: Quisper ontology learning from personalized dietary web services. In: KEOD, pp. 277–284 (2018)
9. Eftimov, T., Korošec, P., Koroušić Seljak, B.: StandFood: standardization of foods using a semi-automatic system for classifying and describing foods according to FoodEx2. Nutrients **9**(6), 542 (2017)
10. Eftimov, T., Seljak, B.K.: Pos tagging-probability weighted method for matching the internet recipe ingredients with food composition data. In: 2015 7th International Joint Conference on Knowledge Discovery, Knowledge Engineering and Knowledge Management (IC3K), vol. 1, pp. 330–336. IEEE (2015)
11. Grcar, M., Krek, S., Dobrovoljc, K.: Obeliks: statisticni oblikoskladenjski oznacevalnik in lematizator za slovenski jezik. In: Zbornik Osme konference Jezikovne tehnologije, Ljubljana, Slovenia (2012)
12. Griffiths, E.J., Dooley, D.M., Buttigieg, P.L., Hoehndorf, R., Brinkman, F.S., Hsiao, W.W.: FoodON: a global farm-to-fork food ontology. In: ICBO/BioCreative (2016)
13. Ispirova, G., Eftimov, T., Korousic-Seljak, B., Korosec, P.: Mapping food composition data from various data sources to a domain-specific ontology. In: KEOD, pp. 203–210 (2017)
14. Korenius, T., Laurikkala, J., Järvelin, K., Juhola, M.: Stemming and lemmatization in the clustering of Finnish text documents. In: Proceedings of the Thirteenth ACM International Conference on Information and Knowledge Management, pp. 625–633. ACM (2004)
15. Kosub, S.: A note on the triangle inequality for the Jaccard distance. Pattern Recogn. Lett. **120**, 36–38 (2019)
16. Lu, Z., et al.: The gene normalization task in BioCreative III. BMC Bioinform. **12**(8), S2 (2011)

17. Màrquez, L., Rodríguez, H.: Part-of-speech tagging using decision trees. In: Nédellec, C., Rouveirol, C. (eds.) ECML 1998. LNCS, vol. 1398, pp. 25–36. Springer, Heidelberg (1998). https://doi.org/10.1007/BFb0026668
18. Mikolov, T., Chen, K., Corrado, G., Dean, J.: Efficient estimation of word representations in vector space. arXiv preprint arXiv:1301.3781 (2013)
19. Mikolov, T., Sutskever, I., Chen, K., Corrado, G.S., Dean, J.: Distributed representations of words and phrases and their compositionality. In: Advances in Neural Information Processing Systems, pp. 3111–3119 (2013)
20. Morgan, A.A., et al.: Overview of BioCreative II gene normalization. Genome Biol. **9**, S3 (2008). https://doi.org/10.1186/gb-2008-9-s2-s3
21. Pennington, J.A., Smith, E.C., Chatfield, M.R., Hendricks, T.C.: LANGUAL: a food-description language. Terminol. Int. J. Theoret. Appl. Issues Spec. Commun. **1**(2), 277–289 (1994)
22. Pennington, J., Socher, R., Manning, C.: Glove: global vectors for word representation. In: Proceedings of the 2014 Conference on Empirical Methods in Natural Language Processing (EMNLP), pp. 1532–1543 (2014)
23. Popovski, G., Ispirova, G., Hadzi-Kotarova, N., Valenčič, E., Eftimov, T., Seljak, B.K.: Food data integration by using heuristics based on lexical and semantic similarities. In: Proceedings of the 13th International Joint Conference on Biomedical Engineering Systems and Technologies - Volume 5 HEALTHINF: HEALTHINF, pp. 208–216. INSTICC, SciTePress (2020). https://doi.org/10.5220/0008990602080216
24. Popovski, G., Ispirova, G., Hadzi-Kotarova, N., Valenčič, E., Eftimov, T., Koroušić Seljak, B.: Food data integration by using heuristics based on lexical and semantic similarities. In: Proceedings of the 13th International Conference on Health Informatics (2020, in press)
25. Popovski, G., Kochev, S., Koroušić Seljak, B., Eftimov, T.: FoodIE: a rule-based named-entity recognition method for food information extraction. In: Proceedings of the 8th International Conference on Pattern Recognition Applications and Methods, (ICPRAM 2019), pp. 915–922 (2019)
26. Popovski, G., Koroušić Seljak, B., Eftimov, T.: FoodOntoMap: linking food concepts across different food ontologies. In: Proceedings of the 11th International Joint Conference on Knowledge Discovery, Knowledge Engineering and Knowledge Management - Volume 2: KEOD, pp. 195–202. INSTICC, SciTePress (2019). https://doi.org/10.5220/0008353201950202
27. Popovski, G., Seljak, B.K., Eftimov, T.: A survey of named-entity recognition methods for food information extraction. IEEE Access **8**, 31586–31594 (2020)
28. Pramanik, S., Hussain, A.: Text normalization using memory augmented neural networks. Speech Commun. **109**, 15–23 (2019)
29. Schuyler, P.L., Hole, W.T., Tuttle, M.S., Sherertz, D.D.: The UMLS Metathesaurus: representing different views of biomedical concepts. Bull. Med. Libr. Assoc. **81**(2), 217 (1993)

Muscle Deformation Using Position Based Dynamics

Josef Kohout[1(✉)] and Martin Červenka[2]

[1] NTIS - New Technologies for the Information Society, Faculty of Applied Sciences, University of West Bohemia, Univerzitní 8, Plzeň, Czech Republic
besoft@ntis.zcu.cz

[2] Department of Computer Science and Engineering, Faculty of Applied Sciences, University of West Bohemia, Univerzitní 8, Plzeň, Czech Republic
cervemar@kiv.zcu.cz

Abstract. This paper describes an approach to personalized musculoskeletal modelling, in which the muscle represented by its triangular mesh is subject to deformation, based on a modified position-based dynamic (PBD) method, followed by decomposition of its volume into a set of muscle fibres. The PBD was enhanced by respecting some muscle-specific features, mainly its anisotropy. The proposed method builds no internal structures and works only with the muscle surface model. It runs in real-time on commodity hardware while maintaining visual plausibility of the resulting deformation. For decomposition, the state-of-the-art Kukačka method is used. Experiments with the gluteus maximus, gluteus medius, iliacus and adductor brevis deforming during the simulation of the hip flexion and decomposed into 100 fibres of 15 line segments show that the approach is capable of achieving promising results comparable with those in the literature, at least in the term of muscle fibre lengths.

Keywords: Position based dynamics · Musculoskeletal system · Muscle deformation · Muscle fibres · Personalised model

1 Introduction

For decades, musculoskeletal modelling has been an important topic of research interest because of its ability to estimate internal loading on the human skeleton, which cannot be measured *in-vivo*. These estimations are useful, e.g., for preoperative surgical planning and postoperative assessment in orthopaedic surgery, rehabilitation procedures, prosthesis design, or prevention of injuries in professional sport.

Musculoskeletal models used in common practice (see, e.g., [1,2,6,8,11]) represent a muscle (or even a group of muscles) as one or more Hill-type one-dimensional structures, commonly referred as lines of action or fibres, connecting

This work was supported by the Ministry of Education, Youth and Sports of the Czech Republic, project SGS-2019-016 and project PUNTIS (LO1506).

X. Ye et al. (Eds.): BIOSTEC 2020, CCIS 1400, pp. 486–509, 2021.
https://doi.org/10.1007/978-3-030-72379-8_24

the origin and insertion points of the muscle, i.e., the sites at which the muscle is attached to the bone by a tendon, and passing through a couple of predefined via points, fixed to the underlying bone, or wrapping around predefined parametric objects (e.g. spheres, cylinders, or ellipsoids). Due to apparent difficulties with the specification of the locations of insertion, origin, and via points, it is common that there are no more than three fibres per muscle and they penetrate the bones in some poses. Figure 1 shows an example of models of this kind. An advantage of this approach, which makes it so popular, is its simplicity and rapid processing speed.

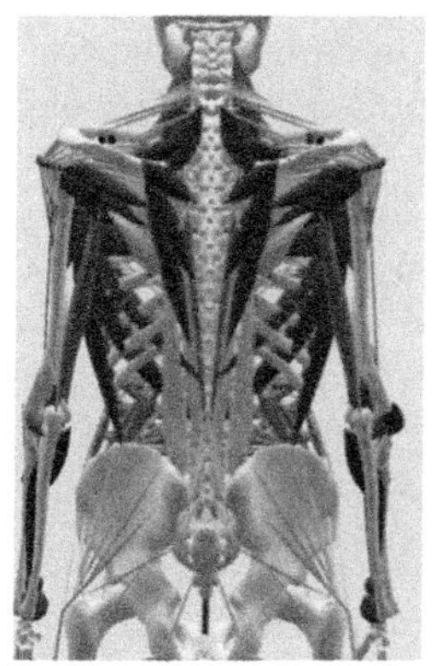
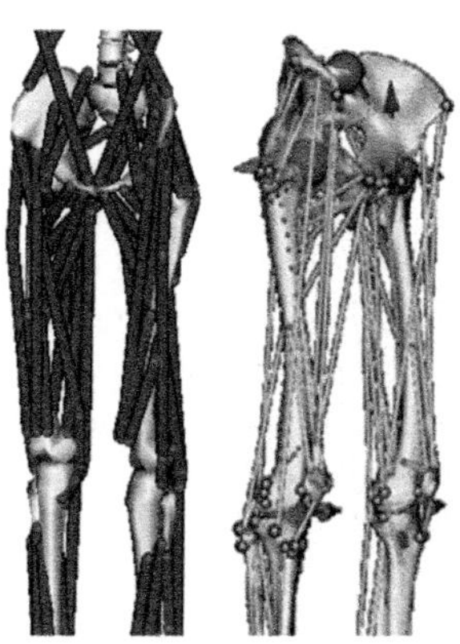

Fig. 1. Musculoskeletal models used in common practice: left – Anybody (http://www.anybodytech.com/) default model, middle – OpenSim (https://simtk.org/home/opensim) gait2392 model, right – LHDL model [22].

As acquiring complete patient-specific or subject-specific data is nearly impossible due to technological limitations of scanning devices, these musculoskeletal models have anatomical parameters derived from cadaver experiments. However, to answer specific subject-related questions, it is generally believed that a patient-specific or subject-specific model is needed. The current practice is, therefore, to take some of these generic models and adapt it to get a personalized model, which most typically consists of a non-uniform scaling (see, e.g., [38]) and a change of optimum fibre length.

Bolsterlee et al. [3] pointed out that many parameters in a model are interrelated. Adapting the model to the subject by scaling improves the anatomical resemblance between the model and the subject but may not improve force prediction. Unfortunately, it is not known how to adapt the other parameters. Several studies, e.g., [10,12,31], warn that attachment sites of muscles show high inter-subject variability, which may considerably affect muscle moment-arms because it has been shown that small differences in location of muscle attachment points often affect muscle force predictions to a great extent (see e.g., [4]).

Valente et al. [34] showed that representing a muscle, especially, a complex one, e.g., the gluteus medius, by a single line segment can produce errors up to 75% suggesting thus that the number of fibres in musculoskeletal models being in used might not be enough. Recently, Weinhandl & Bennett [37] confirmed that high number of fibres are required for the muscle surrounding the hip joint to provide an accurate estimation of joint contact forces. Modenese et al. [26] found out that representing the muscles surrounding the hip joint by fibres with none or a few via points only may limit the accuracy of hip contact force predictions.

To reduce the human effort associated with the construction of subject-specific musculoskeletal models, some researchers proposed algorithms to generate the fibres automatically providing that the surface model of a muscle is available [18,20,30]. The problem is how to update the shape of these fibres in reaction to the movement of bones. One approach to this problem is to express their vertices to be relative to the vertices of the surface mesh of the muscle, first, and then use some of the existing algorithms for surface mesh deformation proposed in the context of musculoskeletal modelling, e.g., [9,16,17,32].

In our conference paper [9], we proposed a new algorithm for muscle mesh deformation, based on position-based dynamics [28], and demonstrated its features on three hip muscles deforming during flexion of the right leg. In this paper, which is an extended version of that paper, we newly include:

- a description of the implementation details of our algorithm such as its initialization for muscle deformation, constraints calculations,
- a proposal of alternative algorithms for detecting the muscle points that should move with the bones,
- new experiments demonstrating the sensitivity of the results on its various parameters (e.g., anisotropy, number of iterations, resolution of the mesh),
- new experiments showing the lengths of fibres generated in the volume of hip muscles, and comparing them with those obtained by other approaches.

2 Position-Based Dynamics

Position-based dynamics (PBD), which is the core part of our approach, was firstly introduced in [28] as a fast, stable, and controllable alternative to mass-spring systems used in computer graphics algorithm. Since then, it has been further developed (e.g., [25] proposed recently some speed and accuracy improvements) and has found many (close to) real-time applications, not only in computer graphics, e.g., for simulations of cloth or fluids [33], but even in other domains. For example, Kotsalos et al. use PBD to model blood cells [24].

PBD represents a dynamic object, e.g., a muscle, by a set of N points, having associated mass and velocity, and a set of M constraints restricting the freedom of the movement of these points during the simulation. In their paper [28], Müller et al. presented the restraints to maintain distances among the points, the shape of the object and its volume, and to avoid collisions with other objects, however, one can use any constraint that is meaningful in their application context. Mathematically speaking, assuming that every point has the same mass, the PBD method solves Eq. 1 that describes a movement of a single point $\mathbf{p}_i$ restricted by a constraint function C with cardinality n, where $\Delta\mathbf{p}_i$ denotes the difference in position of ith point and $\nabla_{p_i} C$ is the gradient of the function C with respect to point $\mathbf{p}_i$.

$$\Delta\mathbf{p}_i = -\frac{\nabla_{p_i} C(\mathbf{p}_1, \ldots, \mathbf{p}_n)}{\sum_{j=1}^{n} \left|\nabla_{p_j} C(\mathbf{p}_1, \ldots, \mathbf{p}_n)\right|^2} \cdot C(\mathbf{p}_1, \ldots, \mathbf{p}_n) \tag{1}$$

2.1 Distance Constraint

Distance constraint is restricting each model point to change the distance from the others in its neighbourhood. It is described by Eq. 2, where d is the original distance between points $\mathbf{p}_1$ and $\mathbf{p}_2$.

$$C(\mathbf{p}_1, \mathbf{p}_2) = |\mathbf{p}_1 - \mathbf{p}_2| - d \tag{2}$$

At this point, the gradient of this function has to be determined. Calculation procedure of determining the gradient of the vector norm is shown in (3).

$$\begin{aligned}
\nabla_{\mathbf{p}_1} C(\mathbf{p}_1, \mathbf{p}_2) &= \nabla_{\mathbf{p}_1} (|\mathbf{p}_1 - \mathbf{p}_2| - d) \\
&= \frac{\left[\frac{\partial(p_{1x}-p_{2x})^2}{\partial p_{1x}} \; \frac{\partial(p_{1y}-p_{2y})^2}{\partial p_{1y}} \; \frac{\partial(p_{1z}-p_{2z})^2}{\partial p_{1z}}\right]}{2\,|\mathbf{p}_1 - \mathbf{p}_2|} \\
&= \frac{\mathbf{p}_1 - \mathbf{p}_2}{|\mathbf{p}_1 - \mathbf{p}_2|} = u \\
\nabla_{\mathbf{p}_2} C(\mathbf{p}_1, \mathbf{p}_2) &= \frac{\mathbf{p}_2 - \mathbf{p}_1}{|\mathbf{p}_1 - \mathbf{p}_2|} = -u
\end{aligned} \tag{3}$$

Coincidentally, the result is the unit directional vector u of given edge.

2.2 Volume Constraint

Volume constraint restricts the object to change its volume during the simulation process. Assuming that this object is a triangular mesh model, the constraint function is:

$$C(\mathbf{p}_1, \ldots, \mathbf{p}_n) = \sum_{i=1}^{m} \left(\mathbf{p}_{t_1^i} \cdot \left(\mathbf{p}_{t_2^i} \times \mathbf{p}_{t_3^i}\right)\right) - V_0 \tag{4}$$

where m is the number of triangles forming the mesh, V_0 is its original volume, and $p_{t_j^i}$ is jth vertex of triangle i.

To obtain complete gradient of volume constraint function, all triangles are treated independently and their results are just summed together:

$$\nabla_{\mathbf{p}_i} C(\mathbf{p}_1, \ldots, \mathbf{p}_n) = \sum_{h=1}^{t} \mathbf{p}_j \times \mathbf{p}_k; \quad i \neq j \neq k \tag{5}$$

2.3 Local Shape Constraint

Above described constraints are not enough to prevent the triangular mesh model from becoming noisy, full of unrealistic spikes. One possible solution to this problem is to use the distance constraint not only to keep the distances between adjacent points but also between the pairs of points lying on the opposite sides of the model. This would, however, need to create a 3D mesh model first, which would be quite complex to do. Another option is to ensure that the local shape is maintained. To achieve this, the dihedral angles between neighbouring triangles should stay the same during deformation.

Equation 6 presents the local shape constraint function of triangles $\mathbf{p}_1, \mathbf{p}_2, \mathbf{p}_3$ and triangle $\mathbf{p}_2, \mathbf{p}_1, \mathbf{p}_4$ sharing points $\mathbf{p}_1$ and $\mathbf{p}_2$. In this equation, $\mathbf{n}_1$ and $\mathbf{n}_2$ are normal vectors of these triangles and φ_0 is the original dihedral angle between them. Gradients are defined in (7).

$$\begin{aligned} C(\mathbf{p}_1, \mathbf{p}_2, \mathbf{p}_3, \mathbf{p}_4) &= \arccos(\mathbf{n}_1 \cdot \mathbf{n}_2) - \varphi_0 \\ &= \arccos\left(\frac{(\mathbf{p}_2 - \mathbf{p}_1) \times (\mathbf{p}_3 - \mathbf{p}_1)}{|(\mathbf{p}_2 - \mathbf{p}_1) \times (\mathbf{p}_3 - \mathbf{p}_1)|_2} \right. \\ &\quad \left. \cdot \frac{(\mathbf{p}_2 - \mathbf{p}_1) \times (\mathbf{p}_4 - \mathbf{p}_1)}{|(\mathbf{p}_2 - \mathbf{p}_1) \times (\mathbf{p}_4 - \mathbf{p}_1)|_2}\right) - \varphi_0 \end{aligned} \tag{6}$$

$$\begin{aligned} d &= \mathbf{n}_1 \cdot \mathbf{n}_2 \\ \nabla_{\mathbf{p}'_4} C &= -\frac{1}{\sqrt{1-d^2}} \left(\nabla_{\mathbf{p}'_4}(\mathbf{n}_2) \cdot \mathbf{n}_1\right) \\ \nabla_{\mathbf{p}'_3} C &= -\frac{1}{\sqrt{1-d^2}} \left(\nabla_{\mathbf{p}'_3}(\mathbf{n}_1) \cdot \mathbf{n}_2\right) \\ \nabla_{\mathbf{p}'_2} C &= -\frac{1}{\sqrt{1-d^2}} \left(\nabla_{\mathbf{p}'_2}(\mathbf{n}_1) \cdot \mathbf{n}_2 + \nabla_{\mathbf{p}'_2}(\mathbf{n}_2) \cdot \mathbf{n}_1\right) \\ \nabla_{\mathbf{p}'_1} C &= -\sum_{i=2}^{4} \nabla_{\mathbf{p}'_i} C \end{aligned} \tag{7}$$

3 Our Approach

The requested inputs of our approach are 1) a set of bones, each of which is represented by a triangular mesh and has an associated time-dependent transformation describing its movement, and 2) a muscle, also represented by a triangular mesh. We note that the first input is standard when creating any subject-specific musculoskeletal model. A muscle model is obtainable with a little effort from the medical images by segmentation (similarly as models of bones). Optionally, the user may specify a set of muscle fibres, represented by polylines, obtained, e.g., by Kohout & Kukačka [19], Kohout & Cholt [21], or Otake et al. [30] method. Furthermore, the user may also specify a set of attachment areas that describes the sites where the muscle attaches to the bones. As the muscle attachment sites

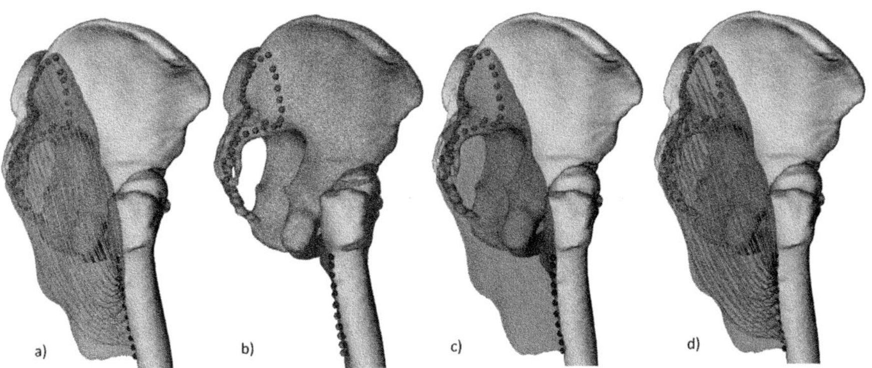

Fig. 2. Gluteus Maximus deformed by our approach: a) the input (origin and insertion attachment sites denoted by red and blue spheres), b) bones move from their initial rest-pose to the current pose (wireframe), c) the muscle surface adapted to the change of bones by PBD, d) the output. (color figure online)

are not apparent from the medical images, these are traditionally identified manually by an expert, typically as a set of landmarks fixed to the bones. Figure 2a shows an example of a typical input.

At each vertex of the muscle mesh, we create one PBD point with the mass being 1.0 and the initial velocity 0. For each pair of PBD points corresponding to the vertices connected in the muscle mesh by an edge, we establish the distance constraint (see Sect. 2.1) modified to support the anisotropic feature of muscles – see Sect. 3.1. Similarly, we create the local shape constraint (see Sect. 2.3) and the volume constraint (see Sect. 2.2). We note that we do not create any distance constraint between points of opposite sides of the muscle to avoid an unnatural change of the muscle shape during the simulation but rely solely on the latter two restraints in that.

We distinguish between two classes of PBD points: fixed and moveable, automatically detected as described in Sect. 3.3. A fixed point is bound to a single bone and moves with it at the beginning of the PBD simulation. The movement of the fixed points violates the equilibrium of the entire system, as described by the constraints, and the PBD attempts to restore it by updating, iteratively, the position of the moveable points while avoiding the penetration with the moved bones using the mechanism for collision detection and response described in Sect. 3.2 – see Fig. 2b,c.

Providing that the muscle fibres are specified, we compute the mean value coordinates of every vertex of polylines representing the fibres in the domain described by the triangular mesh of the muscle using the algorithm by Ju et al. [15]. Mathematically speaking, this operation maps the position of a muscle fibre vertex from E^3 to E^n, where n is the number of vertices of the muscle mesh. When the muscle surface deforms, the inverse mapping provides new positions of fibre vertices within the deformed domain (see Fig. 2d):

$$\mathbf{v'}_i = \sum_{j=1}^{n} w_j \cdot \mathbf{p'}_j \tag{8}$$

In the equation above, $\mathbf{v'}_i$ denotes the i-th fibre vertex, w_j are its mean value coordinates and $\mathbf{p'}_j$ is the position of the deformed muscle vertex $\mathbf{p}_j$.

The entire algorithm written in pseudocode is in Algorithm 1 and 2.

3.1 Anisotropy

The PBD algorithm has been originally proposed in the computer graphics field to model isotropic materials (e.g., cloths). However, muscles are anisotropic (may behave differently in two distinct directions), so it is appropriate to take anisotropy into account. The main idea is that muscle surface is stiffer in the direction perpendicular to the muscle fibres and more flexible in the direction parallel to these fibres. Mathematically speaking, we multiply the distance constraint (see Eq. 2) with the result of the following equation:

Algorithm 1. Pre-processing stage of our algorithm.

```
 1: procedure INIT(M, S_B, S_F, S_A)    ▷ M is a muscle triangular mesh, S_F is a
                                          set of muscle fibres, S_B is a set of bones,
                                          and S_A is a set of attachment areas
 2:   for all vertices v_i ∈ S_F do
 3:     w_i = computeMVC(v_i, M)          ▷ compute the mean value coordinates
 4:   end for

 5:   for all bones B ∈ S_B do
 6:     generateCollisionDataStructure(B)                  ▷ see Section 3.2
 7:   end for

 8:   for all vertices p_i ∈ M do
 9:     x_i = p_i, v_i = 0, m_i = 1                 ▷ initialize a PBD point
10:   end for

11:   detect fixed points                                  ▷ see Section 3.3

12:   for all edges e_i ∈ M do
13:     generateDistanceConstraint(e_i)    ▷ compute the original distance d
14:     if S_F = ∅ then
15:       k_i = 1                                   ▷ no anisotropy used
16:     else
17:       k_i = computeAnisotropyStiffness(e_i)            ▷ see Section 3.1
18:     end if
19:     generateLocalShapeConstraint(e_i)  ▷ compute the dihedral angle φ_0
20:   end for

21:   generateVolumeConstraint(M)         ▷ compute the original volume V_0
22: end procedure
```

Algorithm 2. Runtime stage of our algorithm.

```
1: procedure EXECUTE(simFrame)                 ▷ simFrame is the index of simulation frame
2:     for all bones B ∈ S_B do                                  ▷ see also Algorithm 1
3:         T = getTransform(B, simFrame)               ▷ get the transformation matrix
4:         transformMesh(B, T)
5:     end for

6:     for all PBD points i do
7:         if isFixed(i) then
8:             B = getAttachmentBoneForPoint(i)
9:             p_i = transformPoint(x_i, getTransform(B, simFrame))
10:        else
11:            v_i = v_i + Δt · f_ext(x_i) / m_i     ▷ update velocities by external forces
12:            v_i = v_i · c_damp                                ▷ apply some damping
13:            p_i = x_i + Δt · v_i
14:        end if
15:    end for

16:    loop solverIterations times
17:        for all edges e_i ∈ M do
18:            projectDistanceConstraintWithAnisotropy(e_i, k_i)          ▷ updates p_i
19:        end for
20:        projectVolumeConstraint()
21:        for all edges e_i ∈ M do
22:            projectLocalShapeConstraint(e_i)
23:        end for
24:        for all vertices i do
25:            for all bones B ∈ S_B do
26:                T = getTransform(B, simFrame)
27:                generateCollisionConstraints(B, T^{-1}, x_i, p_i)
28:            end for
29:            projectCollisionConstraints()
30:        end for
31:    end loop

32:    for all verticies i do
33:        if NotIsFixed(i) then
34:            v_i = (p_i - x_i) / Δt                         ▷ compute the velocity
35:            x_i = p_i                                       ▷ update the position
36:        end if
37:    end for

38:    for all vertices p_i ∈ M do
39:        p_i = x_i                                      ▷ update the muscle mesh
40:    end for
41:    for all vertices v_i ∈ S_F do
42:        v_i = reconstructPositionFromMVC(w_i, M)
43:    end for
44: end procedure
```

$$k_i = 1 - \mathbf{u}_i \cdot \mathbf{v}_i \tag{9}$$

The direction of ith edge is described by normalized vector $\mathbf{u}_i$, $\mathbf{v}_i$ denotes tangential direction normal vector of nearest fibre on the surface. If both vectors are collinear, the result k_i will be zero, meaning no distance is preserved. If these two vectors are perpendicular, then k_1 is equal to one and edge length will be preserved.

3.2 Collision Handling

The moving muscle and bones should not intersect each other. From several approaches to this issue we considered (see our conference paper [9]), we have opted for voxelization because of its simplicity and processing speed. In this approach, the bounding box of a bone is divided into a uniform grid of $n_x \times n_y \times n_z$ equally sized cells. For each triangle in the bone mesh, we detect the cells intersected by it and mark them as the boundary. Assuming that the mesh is closed, we mark the cells that are inside the bone using the flood-fill algorithm with 8-directions. All other cells are outside. Figure 3 shows the visualization of boundary cells when the constants n_x, n_y, and n_z are equal and when they are automatically determined from the sizes of the bounding box so that the overall number of cells is roughly equal to some given constant n_{max}.

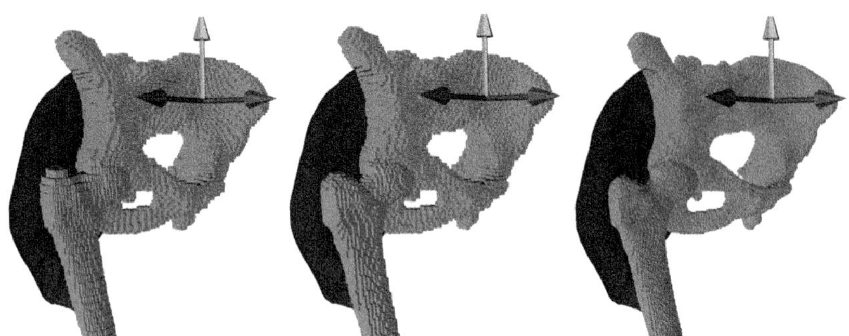

Fig. 3. Voxel representation of pelvis and femur. From left to right: $n_x = n_y = n_z = 64$ (262 144 cells, 256 KB min), n_{max} = 262 144 – pelvis = 47 × 64 × 85 (255 680 cells, 250 KB min) femur = 42 × 176 × 34 (251 328 cells, 245 KB min), $n_{max} = 8 \cdot 262\ 144 =$ 2 097 152 – pelvis = 95 × 128 × 171 (2 079 360 cells, ≈2 MB min) femur = 85 × 352 × 69 (2 064 480 cells, ≈2 MB min).

During the simulation, the algorithm identifies the cell in which a PBD point $\mathbf{p}_i$ lies. If this cell is outside the bone, the point does not collide with the bone. Otherwise, its position needs to be updated. Two scenarios have to be distinguished. In the first one, the muscle moves (e.g. because of surrounding forces) and hits a bone. As it is, the previous position of this point ($\mathbf{x}_i$) is outside the bone. The algorithm, therefore, traverses the collision data structure along the line segment from $\mathbf{p}_i$ to $\mathbf{x}_i$ until it does not find an outside cell. If this cell is the cell of $\mathbf{x}_i$, $\mathbf{p}_i$ moves back to $\mathbf{x}_i$; otherwise, it moves to the point on the line segment where the traversal stopped.

In the second scenario, a bone moves into the muscle. Therefore, even the previous position of the point ($\mathbf{x}_i$) no longer lies outside the bone. We propose a solution where $\mathbf{p}_i$ moves to $\mathbf{x}_i$ transformed by the same transformation that caused the collision.

3.3 Detecting the Fixed Points

Assuming that the muscle is, in fact, a musculotendon unit, i.e., its surface touches the bones at the attachment sites, there are three approaches to detecting the muscle points that should be fixed to some bone and move with it, each of which has its pros and cons. In our previous work [9], we used the constructed data structure for collision detection also for the identification of the fixed points. However, recent analysis shows that this algorithm may inappropriately fix also the points that are close to some bone but should slide along it – see Fig. 4. That is the real reason for the unacceptable behaviour of the iliacus muscle during the flexion of the right leg reported in the original paper.

We, therefore, have experimented with another approach. We fix all points lying in the proximity of some bone, i.e., having their distances to the surface of a bone smaller or equal to a predefined threshold. An obvious choice is to compute the average length of edges in the muscle mesh and use it as this threshold. Figure 5, however, shows that the results are not very different from the results obtained by the original algorithm. Specification of the threshold value by the user may help. Nevertheless, this is very sensitive. For example,

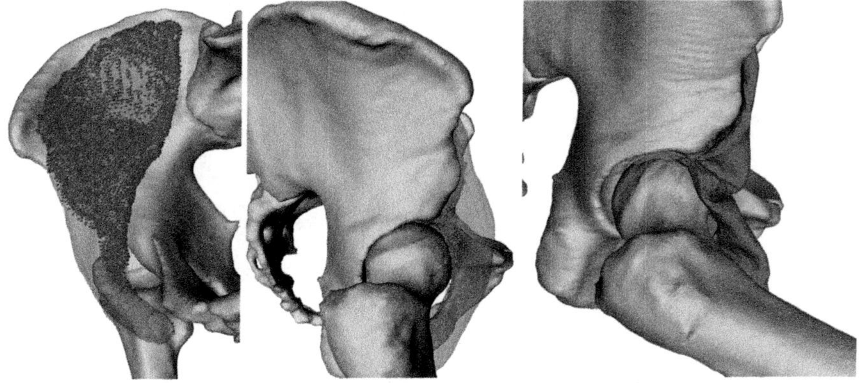

Fig. 4. Muscle vertices (red cubes) of Iliacus fixed to some bone, i.e., preserving their relative position to the bone during the simulation, as identified by the original CD-based algorithm ($n_x = n_y = n_z = 64$) causing an unsatisfactory result of the deformation (right). (Color figure online)

while 1 mm threshold seems perfect for gluteus maximus, for iliacus, a value less than 0.5 mm is needed to get something at least reasonable.

The third approach exploits the idea that muscle attachment areas are typically required for the construction of muscle fibres and, the user, therefore, have them readily available also for detection of the fixed points. We assume that an attachment area is defined by a set of landmarks that are fixed to a bone and, furthermore, they are specified in an order such that interconnecting every pair of adjacent landmarks by a line segment would produce a closed non-intersecting poly-line corresponding to the boundary of the attachment area. Following the idea described by Kohout & Kukačka in [19], we detect the patch on the muscle having the boundary corresponding to the boundary of the attachment area projected onto the muscle surface and fix all the points of this patch. As Fig. 5 demonstrates, this approach provides us with the best results.

4 Experimental Results

In this paper, a subset of a comprehensive female cadaver anatomical dataset (81 y/o, 167 cm, 63kg) is used. Specifically, pelvic and femur bones together with several muscles from the pelvic region have been selected.

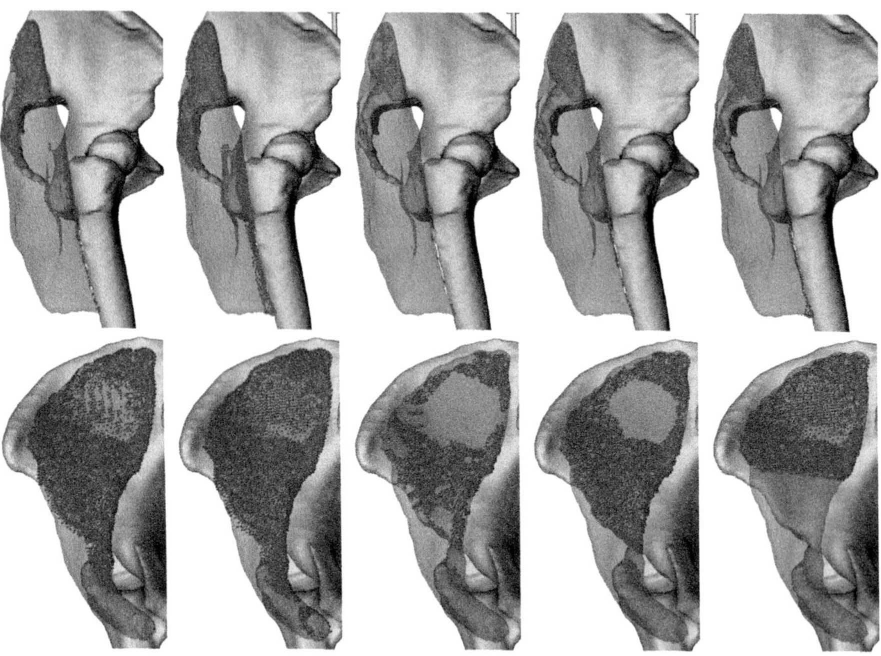

Fig. 5. Muscle vertices (red cubes) of gluteus maximus (top) and iliacus (bottom) fixed to some bone, i.e., preserving their relative position to the bone during the simulation, as identified by the original CD-based algorithm ($n_x = n_y = n_z = 64$), the muscle-bone proximity algorithm with the thresholds: average edge length, 0.5 mm, and 1 mm, and by the algorithm using muscle attachment areas input data. (Color figure online)

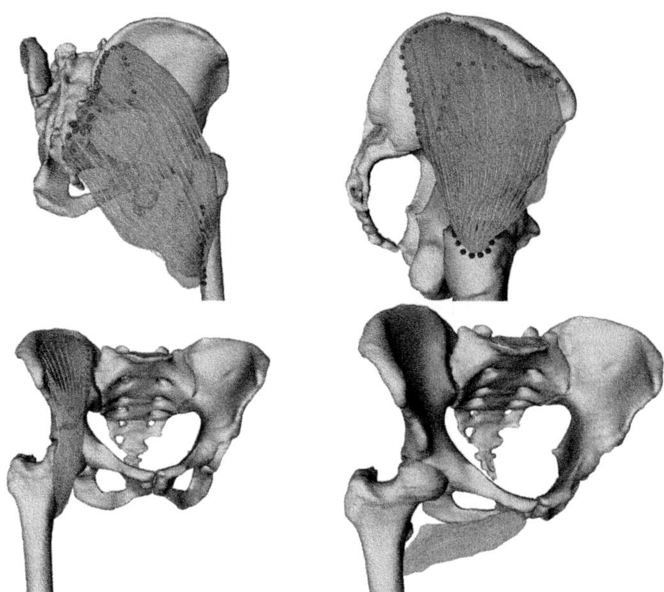

Fig. 6. Gluteus maximus (19 752 triangles (△)), gluteus medius (10 622 △), iliacus (13 858 △), and adductor brevis (17 124 △) decomposed into a set of 100 fibres composed of 15 line segments.

The complete data are publicly available in LHDL dataset [36] and has been selected because it includes high-quality surface meshes of bones and muscles. Furthermore, the dataset was improved by removing non-manifold edges, duplicated vertices and degenerate triangles followed by surface smoothing in both muscle and bone models using MeshLab [5]. The dataset also contains muscle attachment areas and geometrical paths of superficial fibres obtained from dissection [35].

To decompose the muscles into fibres, we use the Kohout & Kukačka method [19] with a slight modification: establishing the inter-contour correspondence is done by minimizing the sum of square distances between the corresponding points. This modification increases the robustness of the method even in cases when the user-specified number of straight-line segments per fibre is low.

We decomposed the surface meshes of gluteus maximus, gluteus medius, iliacus and adductor brevis into models of 100 fibres using a template with parallel fibres composed of 15 line segments – see Fig. 6. The decomposition took less than 50 ms in all cases on HP EliteDesk 800 G3 TWR (Intel Core i7-7700K @ 4.2 GHz, 64 GB RAM, Windows 10 64-bit).

Simulations of hip flexion (0° to 90°) were performed in steps of 2° via inverse kinematics. Inverse kinematics means that the location and movement of all bones are known, and muscle actual shape has to be determined according to these situations. We note this is exactly the opposite to what can be seen in real situation, where muscles control bone movement.

The default parameters in all our experiments were: $n_{max} = 8 \cdot 64 \cdot 64 \cdot 64$, the damping constant $c_{damp} = 0.99$, anisotropy on, local shape constraint stiffness = 0.9 (i.e., the solver was allowed to violate this constraint to preserve the volume and avoid the penetration between the muscle and bones).

4.1 Number of Solver Iterations

In the first experiment, we investigated the influence of the number of iterations of constraint projections (see the loop on line 16 in Algorithm 2) on the quality of the results and overall time required for the simulation. From Fig. 7, it is apparent that the average displacement of points between individual iterations quickly decreases. In a few iterations, it drops below 0.1 mm; with just 10 iterations it is below 0.01 mm.

Average time required by one simulation step (Algorithm 2) on HP EliteDesk 800 G3 TWR (Intel Core i7-7700K @ 4.2 GHz, 64 GB RAM, Windows 10 64-bit) using our, mostly unoptimized, C++ implementation is in Table 1.

Table 1. Times needed for one simulation step on average for adductor brevis using various number of PBD solver iterations (NoIters).

NoIters	1	3	5	10	25	50	100
Time [ms]	53.04	62.55	74.66	104.96	193.66	441.72	658.71

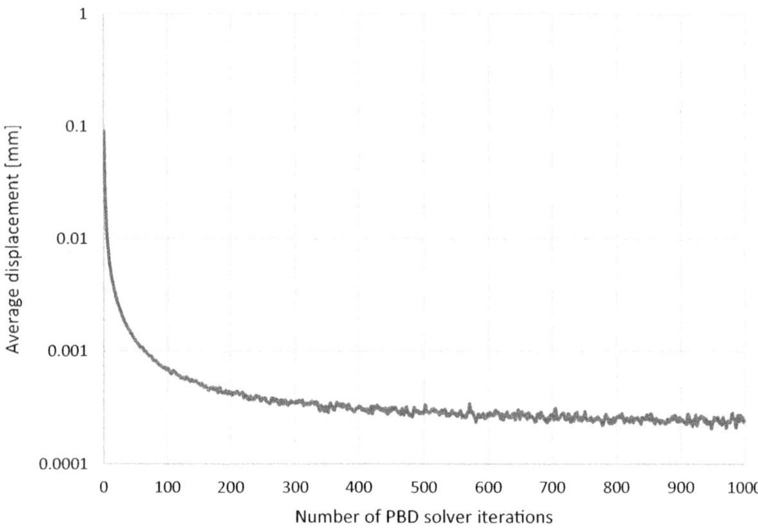

Fig. 7. The average displacement of points of adductor brevis between individual iterations of the PBD solver during the hip flexion. Note the logarithmic scale on the y-axis.

Figure 8 brings a visual comparison of the results obtained using a various number of iterations. An unrealistic bending of the muscle is apparent, especially when using a few iterations only. This behaviour has three reasons. First, the speed of the femur bone is quite high; it is 2° per simulation step, which represents the movement of the fixed points of 3.78–6.75 mm. Next, at the beginning of the simulation, the moving femur hits an unfixed part of the muscle giving it a large velocity pulling it in the direction opposite to the natural movement. Finally, the muscle mesh contains 17126 triangles, i.e., it is pretty accurate, and, therefore, a lot of iterations are required to propagate the movement from the points on the femur to those on the pelvis.

Hence, we reduced the number of triangles using the quadric edge collapse decimation implemented in MeshLab software down to 3000 (L1) and 1000 (L2). Not only visual realism improves, as Fig. 9 illustrates, but also the overall required time decreases since there are less PBD points and consequently also fewer constraints to satisfy. For L2 mesh, 1000 iterations need 349.80 ms per simulation step on average, which is even faster than 100 iterations for the original, high-resolution mesh. Naturally, this higher number of iterations improves visual appearance considerably. We note, however, that increasing the number of iterations further, e.g., to 10000, does not bring any substantial change.

4.2 Fixed Points

Figure 8 also demonstrates the effect of the algorithm used to detect the points to fix on the results of the deformation. Due to inaccuracies during the extraction of the musculotendon unit, only a very small part of the adductor brevis muscle is touching the femur. When using the original algorithm, which exploits the collision detection mechanism, a significant area on the muscle is, therefore, not fixed. As a result, the deformation algorithm produces the mesh with an unrealistic sharp spike. There is no such issue with the detection algorithm exploiting the knowledge of muscle attachment areas.

A different case happens with the iliacus muscle – see Fig. 10. Despite the relatively high resolution of the voxel data structure, many muscle points in proximity of the femur ball are fixed incorrectly to the femur. As a result, this part of the muscle moves unrealistically into the narrow space between the femur and pelvis. Using the attachment areas improves the situation but only slightly because the points in the proximity of the femur ball typically collide with the coarse voxel representation of the femur and they are, therefore, transformed using the same transformation. After turning this collision handling mechanism off, the algorithm provides us with acceptable results with a small muscle-bone penetration.

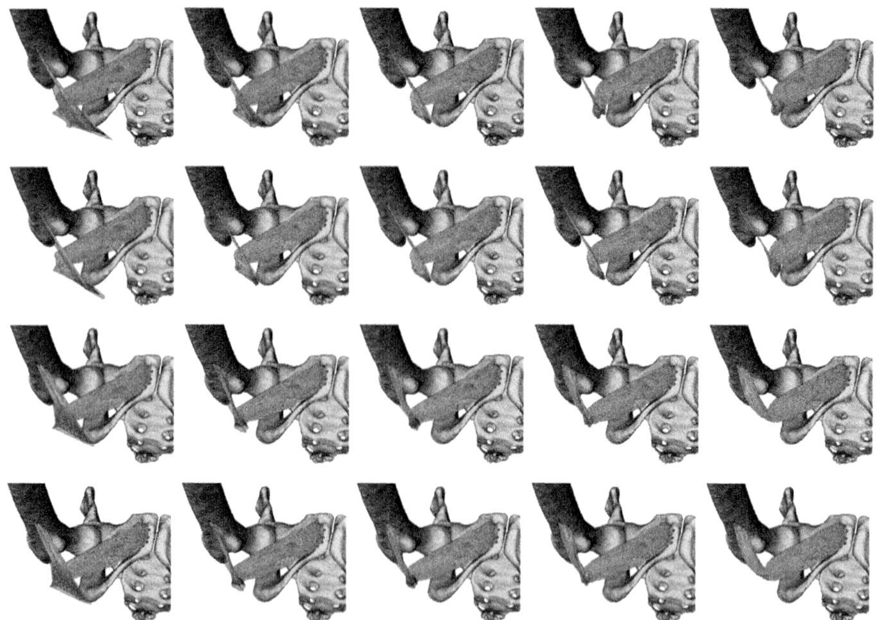

Fig. 8. Adductor brevis at flexion of 40° using 1, 3, 5, 10 or 100 PBD solver iterations (from left to right) with anisotropy off (odd rows) and on (even rows) when fixing the points by the original CD-based algorithm with $n_{max} = 8 \cdot 262\ 144$ (the first two rows) and by the algorithm using muscle attachment areas (the last two rows).

4.3 Anisotropy, Volume and Other Constraints

The impact of the anisotropy on the results is apparent in Fig. 8. Surprisingly, it is barely observable. Most probably, this is because the other constraints (especially the volume constraint) play a dominant role. Volume preservation constraint was tested by determining ratio between both original and actual volumes. Figure 11 show us the volume preservation results. As we can see, the volume is well preserved (the error is less than 1% in all cases). Other quantitative tests, e.g., preservation of the dihedral angles between two adjacent triangles and average edge extension, are presented in our original conference paper [9].

4.4 Muscle Fibre Lengths

Last but not least, we analyzed the lengths of fibres reconstructed at the end of the deformation step. To remove any noise that might be present in the data, we performed a smoothing process, repeated five times, that updates the length l_i according to the equation: $l'_i = (l_{i-1} + 4 \cdot l_i + l_{i+1})/6$. The results are present in Figs. 12, 13, and 14. Both gluteus maximus and gluteus medius behave during the hip flexion as expected. The lengths of all the gluteus maximus fibres increase. In the case of the gluteus medius, only the surface fibres extend, while the deep

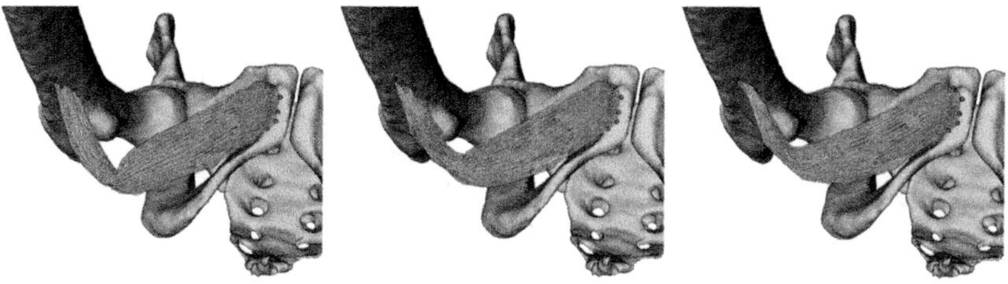

Fig. 9. Adductor brevis at flexion of 40° using 100 PBD solver iterations, anisotropy on, fixing the points at muscle attachment areas when a surface mesh with 17 124, 3 000, and 1 000 triangles is used.

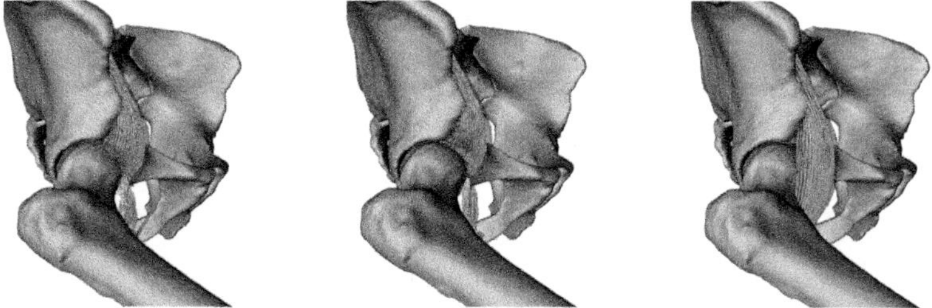

Fig. 10. Iliacus at flexion of 40° using 5 PBD solver iterations, anisotropy on, fixing the points by the original CD-based algorithm with $n_{max} = 8 \cdot 262\ 144$ (left) and by the algorithm using muscle attachment areas with (middle) and without (right) collision handling when a bone hits the muscle.

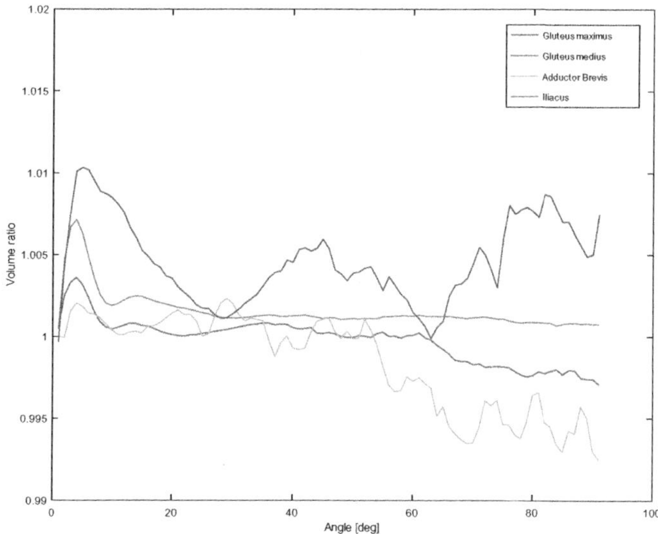

Fig. 11. Volume preservation during hip flexion using 3 PBD solver iterations.

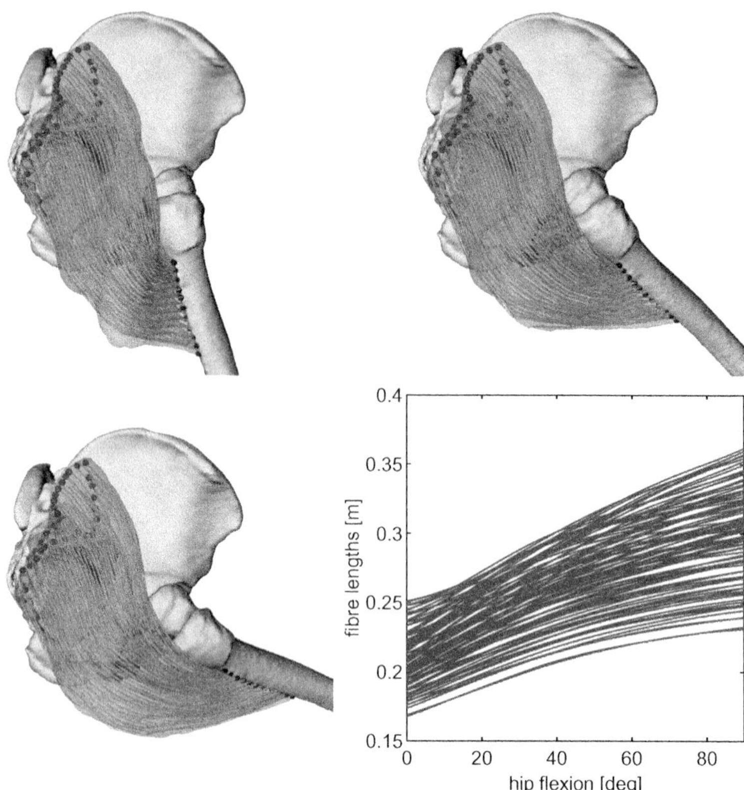

Fig. 12. Total length of each individual fibre during simulation in the gluteus maximus muscle. The visual results at 20°, 50°, and 70° are shown for illustration.

fibres contract. For the iliacus muscle, we can observe an unrealistic increase in the lengths when the flexion is greater than 70°, which is caused by the above-described issue of pushing a part of the muscle into the joint space.

4.5 Deformation Speed

The proposed method was designed to be not only precise, but mainly, fast. It was implemented in C++ using VTK toolkit. Its current version is publicly available at https://github.com/cervenkam/muscle-deformation-PBD.

Using the collision detection structure with $n_x = n_y = n_z = 64$ and three PBD solver iterations, we measured the processing speed of our implementation. All tests were performed on Intel® Core™ i7-4930K 3.40 GHz CPU, Radeon HD 8740 GPU and WDC WD40EURX-64WRWY0 4TB HDD. The results, given in FPS (Frames Per Second), i.e., the number of simulation steps per second, are listed in Table 2. As it can be seen, the FPS strictly depends on number of triangles (Spearman's $\rho = -1$). The more triangles is used, the slower the method

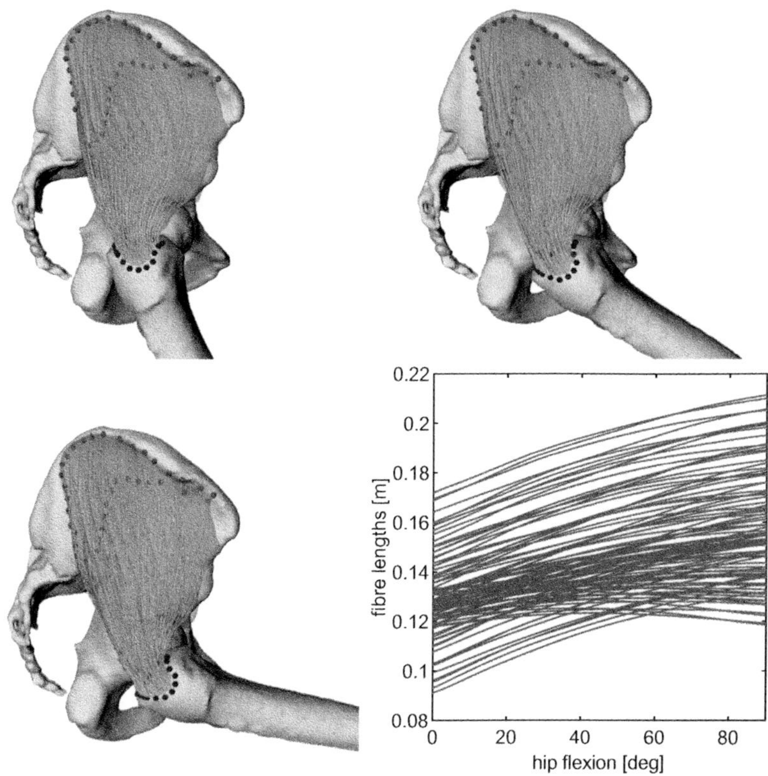

Fig. 13. Total length of each individual fibre during simulation in the gluteus medius muscle. The visual results at 20°, 50°, and 70° are shown for illustration.

Table 2. FPS of each simulation.

Deforming object	Triangle count	FPS
Gluteus maximus	19752	33.85
Abductor brevis	17124	35.89
Iliacus	13858	47.21
Gluteus medius	10622	57.12

is. Even though the program is mostly unoptimized and runs sequentially at the moment, the FPS is sufficient for considered purposes in general.

5 Discussion

In the past, several algorithms for the deformation of the surface mesh of a muscle were proposed. Most of these algorithms, however, have unreal requirements on the input, e.g., [16,17] rely on existence of a muscle skeleton (centroid)

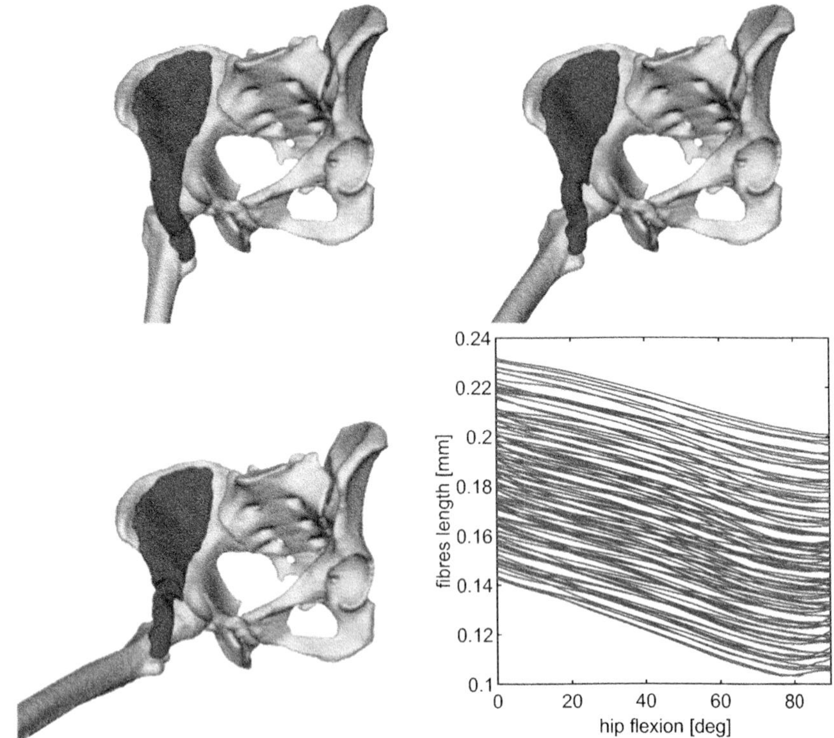

Fig. 14. Total length of each individual fibre during simulation in the iliacus muscle. The visual result at 20°, 50°, and 70° are shown for illustration. For clarity, we do not show the fibres. Readers are referred to Fig. 10 to see the produced fibres of the iliacus muscle.

having known a physiologically correct deformation, or they ignore important physiological properties such as impenetrability with bones and other muscles (e.g., [17,32]), muscle volume preservation, and anisotropy of muscles during their contraction.

Romeo et al. [32] independently to our work developed an approach similar to ours. The main differences are as follows. First, the authors build a complex internal muscle structure to better preserve the shape and volume of the muscle, while we work with the surface geometry only. Next, they do not include any mechanism to prevent penetration of muscles and bones, relying thus on manually defined various mesh-to-mesh constraints, which not only complicates the setup but also does not guarantee impenetrability. We implemented a simple and fast collision handling that avoids muscle-bone penetration in most cases. Finally, their aim is to have a visually plausible skin deformation but what is going on inside the body is not of their interest. We, on the other hand, focus on the representation of muscles for mechanical assessments.

Janak et al. [14] proposed a technique based on the mass-spring system to deform the fibres while preventing their penetration with bones and fibres of other muscles. To get reasonable results, a lot of particles are required, which causes high time and memory complexity. More importantly, the muscle volume is not preserved. This could be probably solved using the approach described in [13], however, it would increase computational time dramatically. Finally, our experiments show that although this method retains the smooth shape of iliacus muscle during flexion, it twists the part of the muscle close to the insertion. This is because, unlike our approach, the particles are in the entire volume of the muscle, which results in a model that is much more rigid, and as anisotropy is not exploited, rigid in all directions. Our method supports anisotropy, preserves the volume and runs in a fraction of time while requiring no extra parameter or input in comparison with this method.

The most complex way to solve muscle dynamics is by using the finite element method (FEM). This approach is physically the most accurate one if the muscle is well discretized (see e.g., [7]). However, computational complexity is high, meaning the FEM-based methods are unsatisfactorily slow. Therefore, it is quite impractical for real-time application or even clinical assessments. Next issue is a difficult set up of FEM methods, making them unsuitable for personalised musculoskeletal method deformation. Despite these facts, these methods can be seen in the movie industry, see e.g. Ziva VFX[1] plugin for Maya, and in muscle physiology research, see e.g. [29] or [23]. In comparison with these methods, our method is quite simple to set up and runs fast providing the promising results in most cases.

Recently, Modenese & Kohout [27] presented a simple method that calculates the kinematic position of a vertex of the fibre as a linear combination of the transformations of its rest-pose position with respect to the bones with the attachment sites of the muscle this fibre belongs to, whereas the blending weight is chosen as a function of the relative distance of this vertex from the origin point of the fibre with one user-specific parameter to minimize the penetration of the fibre with bones. Using the approach described in [18] to highly discretize the muscles of pelvic region (up to 100 fibres of 15 line segments), the fibres' moment arms of hip flexion, adduction, and internal rotation were validated against measurements and models of the same muscles from the literature with promising outcomes. Nevertheless, extending the method for muscles wrapping around multiple bones, such as *rectus femoris*, is not straightforward. Furthermore, a muscle-bone penetration cannot be avoided and in the case of the iliacus muscle, the fibres are also unrealistically pushed into the hip joint. Similarly to [14], the volume of a muscle cannot be preserved.

We compared the length of the fibres produced by Modenese & Kohout [27] with those produced by our approach using the same data. Figure 15 shows a good match between the results for the gluteus medius and the iliacus. A significant difference is apparent for the gluteus maximus. The range of lengths of our fibres is much bigger than theirs, whereas our fibres tend to be longer. One of

[1] https://zivadynamics.com/.

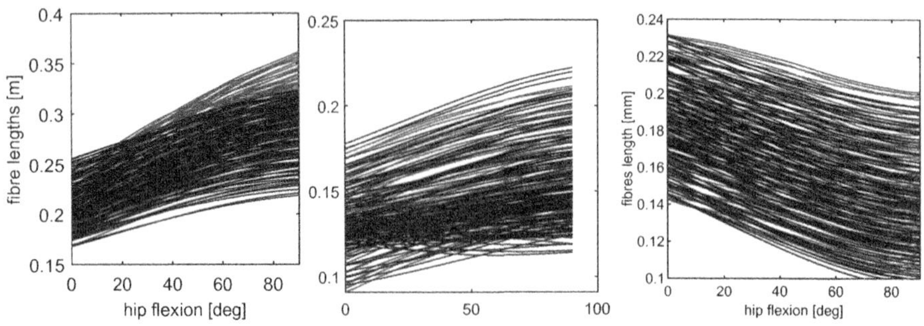

Fig. 15. Comparison of the lengths of the fibres of the gluteus maximus (left), gluteus medius (middle), and iliacus (right) muscle produced by our approach (red) and by the approach described in [27] (blue). (Color figure online)

the reasons for this difference is that our approach guarantees impenetrability between muscle and bones. As a result, all the fibres have to wrap around the joint and, naturally, they must be longer than the fibres produced by the other approach, where some fibres penetrate the femur in extreme positions. The volume preservation constraint prevents the flattening of the muscle at the greater trochanter of the femur, which means that the surface fibres are more distant from the bone than in the other approach. Consequently, they are longer.

There are some limitations of the proposed approach. First of all, the experiments have shown that detecting the muscle points that should move with bones exploiting the information about attachment areas of the muscle is superior in most cases when compared with proximity or collision-based detection. The muscle attachment sites, however, cannot be extracted automatically from the medical images and their manual specification, by an expert in anatomy, is time-consuming. Nevertheless, Fukuda et al. [10] proposed an approach to the automatic estimation of the muscle attachments that is based on applying a non-rigid transformation of the surface model of a normalized (average) bone with a normalized attachment site specified onto the surface model of the subject-specific bone. When the normalized attachment site is obtained from a probabilistic atlas built as suggested by the authors, the estimations are quite accurate, with dice coefficients reaching up to 70%.

Next, the proposed collision handling is inaccurate, which leads to an appearance of sharp spikes on the surface of the muscle, especially, when using a coarse voxel representation of bones. Naturally, as the memory complexity of this representation grows cubically, it is obvious that using a refined voxel representation is impractical. In the scenario when a bone moves into a muscle, setting the velocities of the colliding points to zero instead of using the formula on line 34 (in Algorithm 2) could help.

Finally, the results are very sensitive to the settings of the parameters. Fortunately, as the simulation runs in real-time, even using an unoptimized sequential implementation, the user may tune the values of these parameters until they are satisfied with the visual output of our approach.

6 Conclusion and Future Work

The presented approach is capable of performing a visually plausible and physically correct real-time deformation of muscles represented by triangular meshes in most cases we tested. The main issue is with the iliacus muscle, which (when deformed) looks unrealistic. Nevertheless, the qualitative and quantitative results (e.g., the length of the fibres produced in the volume of the deformed muscle) are comparable with the other state-of-the-art methods. In the future, the iliacus muscle deformation will be further analyzed and the issue with muscle tissue entering the joint is to be solved.

The implementation is written in C++ and partially included in OpenSim (a state-of-the-art simulation software) as a plugin. Its source code is available at https://github.com/cervenkam/muscle-deformation-PBD.

Acknowledgment. Authors would like to thank their colleagues and students for valuable discussion, worthful suggestions and constructive comments. Authors would like to thank also anonymous reviewers for their hints and notes provided.

References

1. Arnold, E.M., Ward, S.R., Lieber, R.L., Delp, S.L.: A model of the lower limb for analysis of human movement. Ann. Biomed. Eng. **38**(2), 269–279 (2009). https://doi.org/10.1007/s10439-009-9852-5. http://www.ncbi.nlm.nih.gov/pmc/articles/PMC2903973/
2. Audenaert, A., Audenaert, E.: Global optimization method for combined spherical-cylindrical wrapping in musculoskeletal upper limb modelling. Comput. Methods Programs Biomed. **92**(1), 8–19 (2008). https://doi.org/10.1016/j.cmpb.2008.05.005. http://www.ncbi.nlm.nih.gov/pubmed/18606476
3. Bolsterlee, B., Veeger, D.H.E.J., Chadwick, E.K.: Clinical applications of musculoskeletal modelling for the shoulder and upper limb. Med. Biol. Eng. Comput. **51**(9), 953–963 (2013). https://doi.org/10.1007/s11517-013-1099-5
4. Carbone, V., van der Krogt, M., Koopman, H., Verdonschot, N.: Sensitivity of subject-specific models to errors in musculo-skeletal geometry. J. Biomech. **45**(14), 2476–2480 (2012). https://doi.org/10.1016/j.jbiomech.2012.06.026
5. Cignoni, P., Callieri, M., Corsini, M., Dellepiane, M., Ganovelli, F., Ranzuglia, G.: MeshLab: an open-source mesh processing tool. Computing **1**, 129–136 (2008). https://doi.org/10.2312/LocalChapterEvents/ItalChap/ItalianChapConf2008/129-136
6. Delp, S.L., Loan, J.P., Hoy, M.G., Zajac, F.E., Topp, E.L., Rosen, J.M.: An interactive graphics-based model of the lower extremity to study orthopaedic surgical procedures. IEEE Trans. Biomed. Eng. **37**(8), 757–767 (1990). https://doi.org/10.1109/10.102791
7. Delp, S.: Three-dimensional representation of complex muscle architectures and geometries 1. Ann. Biomed. Eng. **33**, 1134 (2005). https://doi.org/10.1007/s10439-005-1433-7

8. Delp, S.L., Loan, J.P.: A computational framework for simulating and analyzing human and animal movement. Comput. Sci. Eng. **2**(5), 46–55 (2000)
9. Červenka, M., Kohout, J.: Fast and realistic approach to virtual muscle deformation. In: Proceedings of the 13th International Joint Conference on Biomedical Engineering Systems and Technologies. SCITEPRESS - Science and Technology Publications (2020). https://doi.org/10.5220/0009129302170227
10. Fukuda, N., et al.: Estimation of attachment regions of hip muscles in CT image using muscle attachment probabilistic atlas constructed from measurements in eight cadavers. Int. J. Comput. Assist. Radiol. Surg. **12**(5), 733–742 (2017). https://doi.org/10.1007/s11548-016-1519-8
11. Garner, B., Pandy, M.: The obstacle-set method for representing muscle paths in musculoskeletal models. Comput. Methods Biomech. Biomed. Eng. **3**(1), 1–30 (2000)
12. Herteleer, M., et al.: Variation of the clavicle's muscle insertion footprints - a cadaveric study. Sci. Rep. **9**(1), 1–8 (2019). https://doi.org/10.1038/s41598-019-52845-8
13. Hong, M., Jung, S., Choi, M.H., Welch, S.: Fast volume preservation for a mass-spring system. IEEE Comput. Graph. Appl. **26**, 83–91 (2006). https://doi.org/10.1109/MCG.2006.104
14. Janák, T., Kohout, J.: Deformable muscle models for motion simulation. In: Proceedings of the 9th International Conference on Computer Graphics Theory and Applications. pp. 301–311. SCITEPRESS - Science and and Technology Publications (2014). https://doi.org/10.5220/0004678903010311
15. Ju, T., Schaefer, S., Warren, J.: Mean value coordinates for closed triangular meshes. ACM Trans. Graph. **24**(3), 561–566 (2005). http://portal.acm.org/citation.cfm?doid=1073204.1073229
16. Kellnhofer, P., Kohout, J.: Time-convenient deformation of musculoskeletal system. In: ALGORITMY 2012, 19th Conference on Scientific Computing, Vysoke Tatry, Slovakia, 09–14 Sep 2012, pp. 239–249. Slovak Univ Technology, Bratislava (2012)
17. Kohout, J., et al.: Patient-specific fibre-based models of muscle wrapping. Interface Focus **3**(2), 20120062 (2013). https://doi.org/10.1098/rsfs.2012.0062
18. Kohout, J., Kukačka, M.: Real-time modelling of fibrous muscle. Comput. Graph. Forum **33**(8), 1–15 (2014). https://doi.org/10.1111/cgf.12354
19. Kohout, J., Kukačka, M.: Real-time modelling of fibrous muscle. In: Computer Graphics Forum [18], pp. 1–15. https://doi.org/10.1111/cgf.12354
20. Kohout, J., Cholt, D.: Automatic reconstruction of the muscle architecture from the superficial layer fibres data. Comput. Methods Programs Biomed. **150**, 85–95 (2017). https://doi.org/10.1016/j.cmpb.2017.08.002
21. Kohout, J., Cholt, D.: Automatic reconstruction of the muscle architecture from the superficial layer fibres data. In: Computer Methods and Programs in Biomedicine [20], pp. 85–95. https://doi.org/10.1016/j.cmpb.2017.08.002
22. Kohout, J., Clapworthy, G.J., Martelli, S., Viceconti, M.: Fast realistic modelling of muscle fibres. In: Csurka, G., Kraus, M., Laramee, R.S., Richard, P., Braz, J. (eds.) VISIGRAPP 2012. CCIS, vol. 359, pp. 33–47. Springer, Heidelberg (2013). https://doi.org/10.1007/978-3-642-38241-3_3
23. Kojic, M., Mijailovic, S., Zdravkovic, N.: Modelling of muscle behaviour by the finite element method using Hill's three-element model. Int. J. Numer. Meth. Eng. **43**(5), 941–953 (1998). https://doi.org/10.1002/(SICI)1097-0207(19981115)43:5⟨941::AID-NME435⟩3.0.CO;2-3

24. Kotsalos, C., Latt, J., Chopard, B.: Bridging the computational gap between mesoscopic and continuum modeling of red blood cells for fully resolved blood flow. J. Comput. Phys. **398**, 108905 (2019). https://doi.org/10.1016/j.jcp.2019.108905. cited By 0
25. Macklin, M., et al.: Small steps in physics simulation. In: Proceedings of the 18th Annual ACM SIGGRAPH/Eurographics Symposium on Computer Animation, SCA 2019, pp. 2:1–2:7. ACM, New York (2019). https://doi.org/10.1145/3309486.3340247
26. Modenese, L., Gopalakrishnan, A., Phillips, A.: Application of a falsification strategy to a musculoskeletal model of the lower limb and accuracy of the predicted hip contact force vector. J. Biomech. **46**(6), 1193–1200 (2013). https://doi.org/10.1016/j.jbiomech.2012.11.045
27. Modenese, L., Kohout, J.: Automated generation of three-dimensional complex muscle geometries for use in personalised musculoskeletal models. Ann. Biomed. Eng. **48**, 1793–1804 (2020). https://doi.org/10.1007/s10439-020-02490-4
28. Müller, M., Heidelberger, B., Hennix, M., Ratcliff, J.: Position based dynamics. J. Vis. Commun. Image Represent. **18**, 109–118 (2007). https://doi.org/10.1016/j.jvcir.2007.01.005
29. Oberhofer, K., Mithraratne, K., Stott, N.S., Anderson, I.A.: Anatomically-based musculoskeletal modeling: prediction and validation of muscle deformation during walking. Vis. Comput. **25**(9), 843–851 (2009). https://doi.org/10.1007/s00371-009-0314-8
30. Otake, Y., et al.: Patient-specific skeletal muscle fiber modeling from structure tensor field of clinical CT images. In: Descoteaux, M., Maier-Hein, L., Franz, A., Jannin, P., Collins, D.L., Duchesne, S. (eds.) MICCAI 2017. LNCS, vol. 10433, pp. 656–663. Springer, Cham (2017). https://doi.org/10.1007/978-3-319-66182-7_75
31. Pellikaan, P., et al.: Evaluation of a morphing based method to estimate muscle attachment sites of the lower extremity. J. Biomech. **47**(5), 1144–1150 (2014). https://doi.org/10.1016/j.jbiomech.2013.12.010
32. Romeo, M., Monteagudo, C., Sánchez-Quirós, D.: Muscle and fascia simulation with extended position based dynamics. Comput. Graph. Forum **39**(1), 134–146 (2019). https://doi.org/10.1111/cgf.13734
33. Shao, X., Liao, E., Zhang, F.: Improving SPH fluid simulation using position based dynamics. IEEE Access **5**, 13901–13908 (2017). https://doi.org/10.1109/ACCESS.2017.2729601
34. Valente, G., Martelli, S., Taddei, F., Farinella, G., Viceconti, M.: Muscle discretization affects the loading transferred to bones in lower-limb musculoskeletal models. Proc. Inst. Mech. Eng. Part H J. Eng. Med. **226**(2), 161–169 (2012)
35. Van Sint Jan, S.: Introducing anatomical and physiological accuracy in computerized anthropometry for increasing the clinical usefulness of modeling systems. Crit. Rev. Phys. Rehabil. Med. **17**, 149–174 (2005). https://doi.org/10.1615/CritRevPhysRehabilMed.v17.i4.10
36. Viceconti, M., Clapworthy, G., Van Sint Jan, S.: The virtual physiological human - a European initiative for in silico human modelling. J. Physiol. Sci.: JPS **58**, 441–446 (2008). https://doi.org/10.2170/physiolsci.RP009908
37. Weinhandl, J.T., Bennett, H.J.: Musculoskeletal model choice influences hip joint load estimations during gait. J. Biomech. **91**, 124–132 (2019). https://doi.org/10.1016/j.jbiomech.2019.05.015
38. Zhao, Y., et al.: Laplacian musculoskeletal deformation for patient-specific simulation and visualisation. In: 2013 17th International Conference on Information Visualisation. IEEE (2013). https://doi.org/10.1109/iv.2013.67

An Assessment of National Health Information Systems in Ireland Using Nationally Agreed Standards

Sarah Craig(✉)

Health Research Board, Dublin, Ireland
scraig@hrb.ie

Abstract. This paper presents findings of a research project undertaken to assess four national health information systems in Ireland and their compliance with nationally agreed health information standards. The review was undertaken in the Health Research Board (HRB) which is a State-funded agency with responsibility for the collection, analysis and reporting of national health data. The aim of the review was to identify the extent to which the HRB was compliant with the national standards for health information agreed by Ireland's health information regulatory body, the Health Information and Quality Authority (HIQA). The methods used focused on the application of a self-assessment tool (SAT) to the HRB's health information systems. This involved documentary analysis of written materials about the systems from both primary and secondary data sources. The findings show high levels of compliance with the standards identified but that some areas need to be addressed to ensure that all aspects of the standards are met. The research shows the value of having nationally agreed standards for health information that can be applied to a diverse range of health data sources and systems.

Keywords: National health information systems · Data quality · National standards · Ireland

1 Introduction

The recognised importance of information and data within the health care area in the last number of years has led to the emergence of a separate, related discipline, that of health informatics which has been described as 'a multi-disciplinary, multi-dimensional field that seeks to facilitate the effective collection, management and use of information in the health care environment' [1]. In the last three decades this has developed as expectations have grown about the role that health information and technology can play in improving health care outcomes.

With the increasing interest in health information has been a focus on the need to improve the quality and effectiveness of the data. HIQA [2] has identified that there are four key overarching objectives relating to health information which emphasize the need for improvement: 1) health information should be used to deliver and monitor safe and high quality care for everyone; 2) health information should be of the highest quality and where appropriate collected as close as possible to the point of care; 3)

X. Ye et al. (Eds.): BIOSTEC 2020, CCIS 1400, pp. 510–520, 2021.
https://doi.org/10.1007/978-3-030-72379-8_25

health information should be collected once and used many times and 4) data collection should be fit for purpose and cost-effective.

Building on best practice internationally, this paper presents the findings of a review of four national health information systems using a self-assessment tool (SAT) [3] which was developed by Ireland's health information regulatory body, the Health Information and Quality Authority and which have since become an agreed set of information management standards for evaluating national health and social care data collections [4]. HIQA, in developing the tool notes: 'safe, reliable health and social care depends on access to, and use of, data and information that is accurate, valid, reliable, timely, relevant, legible and complete' [3]. Initial results from the assessment were presented at the BIOSTEC Healthinf conference in February 2020 [5] but this paper draws from the broader context for health information in Ireland and attempts to locate the findings of the review into a broader discussion about the need for data quality guidelines at a national level.

The value of having key standards for monitoring data quality is well-recognised in the literature [6–8]. In other jurisdictions, a number of evaluations of public health surveillance systems have been undertaken [9–11] which Ngugi et al. [10] suggest is 'to ensure that problems of health importance are being monitored efficiently, effectively, and regularly' (p. 304).

In recent years, several guidelines and tools have been developed to assist the managers of health information systems to ensure good information governance and data quality are at the heart of their processes [12–14]. In Ireland in recent years, HIQA developed its self-assessment tool (SAT) built largely on a review of international evidence for use on national health information systems. This assessment tool is in process of being rolled out within the major Irish health and social care data collections [15–18].

The research questions for the study were:

a) Do the Health Research Board's (HRB) systems comply with the HIQA standards? If so,
b) What areas is there most/least compliance?
c) What does a SAT tell us about improving and shaping health information data quality into the future?

The paper explores the role that national standards, that are informed by international best practice, can play in assisting national bodies in their achievement of better-quality data. The perceived benefits have been identified in research [19] as better data which in turn results in improved service planning at the national and local level, safer, better care for patients and service users and improved population health.

2 Background

2.1 Health Information in Ireland

The management and delivery of health information in Ireland is the responsibility of several agencies including the Health Research Board (HRB). The information systems managed by the HRB and others have developed over a long period in an ad hoc manner usually in response to particular policy developments or service needs. As a result, there is no single or standardised approach to the management and delivery of health information and there is no scope for data sharing and data linkage. Previous research [19, 20] has highlighted that Ireland lags behind its international counterparts in relation to health information policy and practice.

2.2 Health Information and the HRB

The HRB is a public service body under the remit of the Department of Health in Ireland. It collects data in the areas of drugs and alcohol (the National Drug Treatment Reporting System (NDTRS) and the National Drug-related Deaths Index (NDRDI)); in relation to disability (the National Ability Supports System (NASS)) and mental health (the National Psychiatric In-patient Reporting System (NPIRS)).

Data collection in the HRB began in the 1960s in the mental health area, and systems to collect drug treatment and disability data were developed in the 1990s and a drug-related deaths index was set up in 2005. Appendix 1 presents a summary overview of the four systems. A staff complement of twenty-five is employed to work on the health information systems and is made up of researchers, data analysts and data administrators. The annual budget for the health information area is around €2 million. All the systems generate data at a national level to assist with service planning and monitoring of key policies in the mental health, disability and drugs areas and annual reporting is a feature at national, EU and international levels.

2.3 Data Quality: Audit and Evaluation

To ensure data quality, it has been recommended that a process of audit and evaluation needs to be included as an integral part of any information system [4]. Over the last number of years, the HRB has given some attention to this area of its work and one of the organisation's strategies proposed that all systems would be evaluated during the strategy period [21]. The level of investment in evaluation and audit has, however, been poor. In the last five-year period, only one of the HRB's information systems was formally externally evaluated and in the last ten-year period, only one other was audited [22, 23], hence the need to undertake to review the systems.

2.4 Data Quality: The Role of HIQA

The Health Information and Quality Authority (HIQA) is the independent statutory authority in Ireland that was established to promote safety and quality in the provision of health and social care services for the benefit of the health and welfare of the public in Ireland. One of its key strategic roles relates to health information governance: 'advising on the efficient and secure collection and sharing of information … about the delivery and performance of Ireland's health and social care services' [24].

Its role in health information centres on provision of advice about the efficient and secure collection and sharing of health information, setting standards, evaluating information resources and publishing information on the delivery and performance of

Ireland's health and social care services. Much of HIQA's recent endeavours in its health information function has been on developing resources for the managers of health information systems that are designed to support the implementation of common standards in relation to information governance and data quality [11, 12].

The SAT devised by HIQA is based on six broad themes which are then broken down into ten standards (see Table 1) [3].

Table 1. Themes and national standards.

Theme	Standard
Person-centred	Arrangements to protect privacy of people
Governance, leadership and management	Effective governance Publicly available statement of purpose Compliance with relevant legislation
Use of data	Compliance with health information standards Monitors quality of data Effective and appropriate dissemination strategies
Information governance	Effective information governance
Workforce	Workforce to deliver objectives
Use of resources	Effective allocation of resources

Source: Craig, 2020

The themes and standards were developed in consultation with key stakeholders in the health information area in Ireland and by using international evidence of good practice [5, 10]. The details of the standards and how to apply them are set out in the self-assessment tool.

3 Methods

The method adopted was documentary analysis where key documents for each of the systems were reviewed and the SAT was completed based on this written evidence as well as staff knowledge about practices within each system. A project team was formed to oversee the research and to ensure a standardised approach to the completion of the SAT. The project team was chaired by a staff member from HIQA and consisted of HRB staff working in each of the four systems as well as the HRB's Head of National Health Information Systems who oversaw the research. Staff worked in teams of two to complete the SAT; each team had a staff member that was very familiar with the system under review.

Written materials were consulted for each of the HRB's four national health information systems and the self-assessment pro forma was completed for each system. Sources of data reviewed included primary sources such as protocols for data collection and collation, data validation and reporting and secondary sources such as external reviews of the systems and research undertaken with system users. The project took 3 months to complete.

4 Findings of the Self-assessment

The findings of the assessment are presented below using the thematic headings as set out in the SAT.

4.1 Person-Centredness

The first standard relates to person-centredness and centres on how organisations like the HRB take steps to protect the privacy of the individuals about whom data are collected [3]. One of the best ways of exhibiting this is that data subjects are made aware of what is being collected and how it is likely to be used. This is generally achieved in the organisation's statement of information practice and by the organisation undertaking privacy impact assessments on a regular basis.

The research findings in relation to this standard found that there were privacy policies in place in the HRB and that there was a clear statement of information practice that had been worked on by the staff working in the health information area. Information leaflets are available to data subjects that tell them how their information will be used. The research found, however, that although these statements, policies and leaflets have been developed, they are not widely promoted by the organisation and that, for example, placing them on the organisation's website would ensure their wider circulation.

4.2 Governance, Leadership and Management

The research examined the governance, leadership and management arrangements that were in place at the level of the organization. Good practice in this area points to the need for a designated member of staff at a sufficiently senior level in the organization that has overall responsibility for the data collection and that a statement of purpose exists for each information system. Each system should also have its own management structure and stakeholder engagement.

The study rated the HRB's national health information systems highly in this area, but that practice was not consistent across all of the systems. Only two of the four systems had a formalised approach to stakeholder engagement.

The findings highlighted that the HRB does not currently publish reports on the effectiveness of the national data collections although all publications from these systems make reference to the quality of the data, their coverage and completeness. The research recommended that the organisation needs to develop its own metrics for assessing data quality.

While statements of purpose have been developed for each of the HRB's four information systems, there was no evidence of them being reviewed or updated on a regular basis. In addition, the study pointed to the need for staff engagement on key pieces of legislation such as data protection.

4.3 Use of Data

Within its information management standards, HIQA [4] recommends that the use of the information is optimized to achieve the best value for money and to maximize social gain. This includes ensuring accuracy, completeness, legibility, relevance, reliability and timeliness of the data. HIQA also recommends that data dictionaries be published and that a framework for data quality should be agreed with stakeholders. It also refers to the value of incorporating international classifications to enable cross-country comparisons.

All but one of the HRB's information systems include the International Classification of Disease (ICD) to record diagnosis. A data dictionary is also available for each system, but the assessment found that it should be made more widely available.

Similarly, within the HRB, there is a recognition of the need for quality data in all the information systems and considerable time and effort go in to ensuring the quality of the data. However, there is no formalized data quality framework in place. There is evidence that some internal audit of systems has been undertaken and two of the HRB's systems commissioned external evaluations, but this was some time ago and many of the recommendations have not been implemented. The SAT findings highlight the need to invest in more evaluation at the level of the information system.

The assessment found that, although the HRB's compliance in this area is high, more is needed, for example, to support users of the data. In addition, the HRB needs to develop data quality statements and should develop a calendar for the year setting out when reports from the systems will be available. The assessment also found that users of the data would benefit from training on the use of the data. In addition, a log of all requests for data received is in existence but is not recording the timeliness of the response to requests.

4.4 Information Governance

The assessment also reviewed the HRB's information governance within its information systems or how it incorporates processes to promote security and privacy in the collection and reporting of data. This may include, for example, obtaining consent from the data subject where it is necessary, having statements of information practices, arrangements around the appropriate sharing of information and ongoing audit on information governance practice.

The assessment found that there are ongoing efforts within the HRB to ensure good information governance but that more work is required on information governance audits and training for staff on information governance issues.

As noted earlier, the four systems managed by the HRB have a publicly available statement of purpose, setting out how the objectives of each system are achieved. The statement is maintained by the staff responsible for managing each system and is reviewed regularly to ensure that it is fit-for-purpose. All statements are published in HIQA's catalogue of health and social care data collections [21].

4.5 Workforce

A key consideration in the management of health information is having staff with appropriate skills and expertise, HIQA defines the workforce standard to include all of those who work in or for the national health information system and recommends that staff with specialist skills and qualifications are needed and that there is good workforce planning to deal with expected and unexpected events. It is about having the 'right people with the right knowledge' [2].

Within the HRB, workforce planning is undertaken annually in consultation with the organisation's parent body, the Department of Health. In addition, an annual training programme is devised and agreed to reflect necessary organisational and individual training and upskilling needs.

4.6 Use of Resources

HIQA defines resources as including human, physical, financial and ICT resources [2] and recommends that organisations involved in the collection and reporting of health data should strive to ensure that its resources are adequate to ensure the sustainability, continual relevance and maximum impact of the data for which they are responsible.

The assessment of the HRB's health information systems found that there are adequate levels of input into the planning and management of the necessary resources. This is particularly the case in relation to skills audit, succession planning and staff training and development.

5 Discussion

Through an examination of each of the themes set out in the SAT, the evaluation process highlighted several issues. First, regarding effective arrangements in place to protect the privacy of people about whom it holds information, compliance is high. However, there is a need to ensure greater transparency with stakeholders and with users of the data. On effective governance, leadership and management arrangements, the HRB also rated highly in the assessment. However, two of the systems do not have oversight committees and all four do not currently have formalised arrangements in place with data providers. In addition, the NHIS does not currently publish reports on the effectiveness of the national data collections it holds although all NHIS publications refer to the quality of the data contained within.

Privacy and confidentiality were seen to be important to the HRB in the assessment, but the findings showed that, again, more transparency is needed on how statements of purpose are reviewed. In general, there was high levels of compliance with legislation such as data protection legislation, but the assessment highlighted that more proactive identification of risks and issues in upcoming legislation was needed.

The SAT examines the extent to which health information systems have international classifications so as to allow for some comparison across countries. The assessment found that all but one HRB system have incorporated international classifications. In addition, whilst a data dictionary is in place for each system it is not currently made publicly available, but the SAT recommends that is should be.

Data quality is recognized as a core feature of health information systems in HIQA's SAT. The assessment found that there is a recognition of the need for quality data in all the HRB systems and considerable time and effort go in to ensuring the quality of the data collected. However, there is no formalized data quality framework in place. In addition, some work on audit and evaluation has been undertaken internally but there has been less activity on commissioning external audit and evaluation.

With regard to dissemination of data there is a high level of compliance in the HRB but the research found that a more formalized approach could be applied to record timeliness of responses to requests for data, training for users of the data, data quality statements and notifying, in advance, on an annual basis what publications will be available.

Similarly, there are high levels of compliance with the standard on information governance, but more work is required on information governance audits and training for staff.

Finally, high levels of compliance were found regarding the workforce in the HRB and its suitability to the work in hand as well as in relation to the allocation and use of resources including ICT.

The completion of the SAT was recognised by those involved as a valuable exercise in ensuring that the national standards as set by HIQA need to an integral part of the work of the HRB in its management of health data. Those involved agreed the need for an improvement plan to address the areas of weakness that the process has revealed. The improvement plan contained several recommended actions including:

- Publishing statements of information practice for each of the four systems on the HRB's website.
- Setting up oversight committees for the two systems that don't currently have this oversight in place.
- Putting in place formalised agreements with data providers.
- Reporting system performance/effectiveness in all publications.
- Developing an annual process to review statements of purpose.
- Identifying a process for reviewing upcoming legislation relevant to the HRB data collections.
- Publishing data dictionaries for each system.
- Formalizing a data quality framework for the information systems that incorporates the elements of good practice already applied to the data and including more detailed data quality statements in each HRB publication.

- Planning for further internal and external audit of the data and consider the use of the data quality framework dimensions as an audit framework.
- Using the organization's website monitoring to record access to health information publications.
- Developing metrics to monitor the use of the data such as tracking the number of times data are accessed on the HRB's website.
- Providing training to data users around the value of the HRB's data.
- Monitoring the timeliness of response to all requests for data received by the HRB.
- Developing an annual calendar on publication of reports from the HRB's systems.
- Devising a schedule for internal and external audit of the HRB systems.
- Devising a training programme for staff on information governance.

6 Conclusions

This study set out to undertake an assessment of the HRB's health information systems using a self-assessment tool developed by HIQA, the body charged with the regulation and improvement of health data in Ireland. The research questions were:

a) Do the HRB systems comply with the HIQA standards? If so,
b) What areas is there most/least compliance?
c) What does a SAT tell us about improving and shaping health information data quality into the future?

Overall, the findings indicate that there is compliance with the standards across all four systems but that practices can vary from system to system. Overall, the study highlights the value of having agreed national standards for health information systems that are based on international best practice. Of key importance to any health information system is the focus on data quality and the need for a data quality framework.

The review of the HRB's health information systems was undertaken internally over a short period of time. Since then, HIQA has begun its inspection of other national information systems including those for cancer screening and health in-patient reporting. The results of these inspections are published on HIQA's website and much can be learned from the practice of other bodies involved in the collection and management of health data. Ultimately, the aim is to improve the health information landscape in Ireland from a piecemeal one where variable practice is applied, to a much more integrated one where national standards are applied and are assessed regularly for their relevance. The findings of this assessment show the value of this standardised approach to the data quality improvement process.

Appendix

Appendix 1. Overview of HRB systems.

	Objectives	Activity
National Drug Treatment Reporting System (NDTRS)	To gather data on treated drug and alcohol misuse in Ireland that can be used by policy makers and service providers	30,000 records annually Data items: 64
National Drug-related Deaths Index (NDRDI)	To collect information on drug and alcohol-related deaths and deaths among drug and alcohol users in Ireland	600 deaths annually Data items: 70 15,000 coroners' files consulted each year
National Ability Supports System (NASS)	To capture details of current service provision and the future service requirements of individuals with a disability	30,000 records Data items: 200
National Psychiatric In-patient Reporting System (NPIRS)	To collect and report on all admissions and discharges to inpatient psychiatric units both public and private. A regular psychiatric census is carried out	38,000 records annually - 19,000 admissions and 19,000 discharges 67 sites Number of data items: 28

References

1. Whetton, S.: Health Informatics: A Socio-technical Perspective. Oxford University Press, Melbourne (2005)
2. HIQA: Guiding Principles for National Health and Social Care Data Collections. HIQA, Dublin (2013)
3. HIQA: Self-Assessment Tool for National Health and Social Care Data Collections. HIQA, Dublin (2017)
4. HIQA: Information management standards for national health and social care data collections. HIQA, Dublin (2017)
5. Craig, S.: Using a self-assessment tool (SAT) to review national health information systems in Ireland. Paper presented at Biostec 2020, 13th International Joint Conference on Biomedical Engineering Systems and Technologies, Valletta, Malta, 24–26 February 2020 (2020)
6. Australian Institute of Health Welfare: Data Governance Framework. AIHW, Canberra (2014)
7. Canadian Institute for Health Information: The CIHI Data Quality Frame work. CIHI, Ottawa (2009)
8. Anderka, M., Mai, C.T., Romitti, P.A., et al.: Development and implementation of the first national data quality standards for population-based birth defects surveillance programs in the United States. BMC Public Health **15**, 925 (2015). https://doi.org/10.1186/s12889-015-2223-2

9. Doktorchik, C., Mingshan, L., Quan, H.: A qualitative evaluation of clinically coded data quality from health information manager perspectives. Health Inf. Manag. J. **49**(1), 19–27 (2020)
10. Ngugi, B., Harrington, B., Porcher, E., Wamai, R.: Data quality shortcomings with the US HIV/AIDS surveillance system. Health Inform. J. **25**(2), 304–314 (2017)
11. Buehler, J.W., Hopkins, R.S., Overhage, J.M.: Framework for evaluating public health surveillance systems for early detection of outbreaks: recommendations from the CDC working group. Report no. 53(RR05), 7 May 2004. Centers for Disease Control and Prevention, Atlanta (2004)
12. Health and Social Care Information Centre: Information Governance Toolkit. HSCIC, London (2015)
13. American Health Information Management Association: Health Data Analysis Toolkit. AHIMA, Chicago (2011)
14. German, R.R., Westmoreland, D., Armstrong, G.: Updated guidelines for evaluating public health surveillance systems: recommendations from the guidelines working group-CDC. Report no. 50(RR13), 27 July 2001. Center for Disease Control and Prevention, Atlanta (2001)
15. HIQA: Review of information management practices in the HSE CIDR system. HIQA, Dublin (2019)
16. HIQA: Review of information management practices in the HSE PCRS. HIQA, Dublin (2019)
17. HIQA: Review of information management practices in the HIPE scheme. HIQA, Dublin (2019)
18. HIQA: Guidance on a data quality framework for health and social care. HIQA, Dublin (2018)
19. Craig, S.: The state of health information in Ireland: a socio-technical analysis, unpublished doctoral thesis, University College Dublin (2015)
20. Craig, S., Kodate, N.: Understanding the state of health information in Ireland: a qualitative study using a socio-technical approach. Int. J. Med. Inform. **114**, 1–5 (2018)
21. Health Research Board: Research, Evidence, Action. HRB Strategy 2016–2020. HRB, Dublin (2016)
22. Work Research Centre: An Evaluation of the HRB's National Psychiatric In-Patient Reporting System: Final report. HRB, Dublin (2012)
23. Dodd, P., Craig, S., Kelly, F., Guerin, S.: An audit of the Irish national intellectual disability database. Res. Dev. Disabil. **31**(2), 446–451 (2010)
24. HIQA: HIQA Catalogue for national health and social care data collections. HIQA, Dublin (2017)

Leveraging Clinical Notes for Enhancing Decision-Making Systems with Relevant Patient Information

João Rafael Almeida[1,2](✉), João Figueira Silva[1], Alejandro Pazos Sierra[2], Sergio Matos[1], and José Luís Oliveira[1]

[1] DETI/IEETA, University of Aveiro, Aveiro, Portugal
{joao.rafael.almeida,joaofsilva,aleixomatos,jlo}@ua.pt
[2] Department of Information and Communications Technologies, University of A Coruña, A Coruña, Spain
alejandro.pazos@udc.es

Abstract. Personalised treatment is usually needed for hospitalised patients afflicted by secondary illnesses that demand daily medication. Even though clinical guidelines were designed to consider those circumstances exist, current decision-support features fail to assimilate detailed relevant patient information. This creates opportunities for the development of systems capable of performing a real-time evaluation of such data against existing knowledge and providing recommendations during clinical treatments. Herein, we describe a proposal for a new feature to be integrated with electronic health record (EHR) systems which can enrich the health treatment process through the automatic extraction of information from patient medical notes and the aggregation of this novel information in clinical protocols. The purpose of this work is to exploit the historical component of the patient trajectory to improve the performance of clinical decision support systems.

Keywords: EHR · CDSS · NLP · Clinical notes · Clinical decision-making · Treatment guidance

1 Introduction

Throughout the years technology and its breakthroughs have proved fruitful for the field of medicine and health care, fostering an enhanced quality of life for the general population. Tools and data sources originated from the fusion of technology with medicine have led to improvements in disease prevention, diagnosis and treatment, and can play a vital role in clinical pipelines by assisting physicians in tasks such as clinical decision making and patient follow-up. Moreover, the increased access to medical data enables the shift towards the more patient-centric view of personalised medicine.

J. F. Silva—Contributed equally with the first author to this work.

X. Ye et al. (Eds.): BIOSTEC 2020, CCIS 1400, pp. 521–540, 2021.
https://doi.org/10.1007/978-3-030-72379-8_26

Technology brought scale along with diversity to medical data, comprising numerous data types such as laboratory analysis, medical imaging or genomic data, which must be stored and organised. Electronic health records (EHRs) provide an electronic infrastructure to aggregate administrative and medical data from various sources and to centralise information at the patient level [9,16], enabling the documentation of a patient's health status throughout time and representing the patient trajectory. Furthermore, EHRs can be important in supporting the medical act since by having a longitudinal view of the patient medical history accessible in a single structure, they can provide physicians with important contextual information.

EHR information can vary in type and structure, and considering the latter EHRs can contain structured and unstructured data. Structured data can be found in forms, and it is typical in patient demographics data where patient information is organised in form fields, but can also be found in certain medical reporting forms where codes from coding standards such as ICD (International Classification of Diseases) [37], SNOMED-CT (Systematized Nomenclature of Medicine - Clinical Terms) [31] or RxNorm [23] can be used. These standards accomplish the process of structuring text data by performing a mapping from medical concepts on symptoms, diagnosis, treatments and procedures, to unique identifying codes which can be easily processed. Despite their utility, coding standards do also have limitations hindering their use, namely the amount of time needed by clinical staff to sift through the standards to select the most suitable code, or the ambiguity or lack of specificity in certain terms.

On the other hand, unstructured data such as free text is commonly found in clinical notes such as patient discharge reports, progress notes or clinical appointment reports. Free text is written in natural language thus overcoming the limitations of structured text as it provides a flexible convoy for physicians to record comprehensive descriptions of the patient health status. Such descriptions contain the context and rationale behind the selected diagnosis or treatment, thus containing valuable information for the processes of clinical decision making and patient follow-up.

As a result of the above, free text in clinical notes accounts for a large amount of the data contained in EHRs, being particularly evident in chronic diseases where clinical notes dominate over structured data [27]. In fact, the importance of free text extends beyond that, being acknowledged that clinical free text can often encompass information otherwise not obtainable from other data sources [15], but much of this potential remains underexplored owing to the nature of clinical text that renders it particularly challenging to process and explore [24]. Historically, relevant data has been extracted from free text through manual review from clinical experts, a process that inherently faces scalability and cost issues when considering the increasing rate of generation of novel medical data [27]. Nonetheless, during the past years there has been a continuous growth in interest in this domain, with some research efforts having already been made on fields such as clinical natural language processing (NLP) to develop solutions for annotating and summarising relevant data in clinical notes [26].

In spite of the many opportunities that stemmed from the increased involvement of technology in healthcare, many challenges did also surface. For instance, the increased availability of medical data, which can aid physicians in their decisions, also led to a heavier burden for physicians who must search through larger amounts of less relevant data to find information of their actual interest. An illustrative example of this can be found in clinical notes, where the increased easiness of replicating information through actions such as copy-paste has resulted in more redundant information (which can sometimes even be erroneous), hence resulting on lower data quality which can ultimately compromise the quality of the medical act [8,30].

It comes naturally that solutions such as clinical decision support systems (CDSSs) can play an important role if they manage to assimilate the large amounts of existing EHR data and provide physicians with only key information for patient diagnosis and prognosis. However, to do so these systems must deal with the natural challenges associated with medical data, namely its high heterogeneity and poor quality (data is frequently incomplete, noisy and sparse) which are worsened by non-standardised physician practices [13].

Concerning data sources, these systems can explore single and multi modality - the latter combining various sources and being reckoned as a particularly challenging task [20] - and also structured and/or unstructured data. While structured data is more frequently used since it is generally more straightforward to exploit, the inclusion of EHR unstructured data such as clinical notes can provide key content to improve the performance of previously existing systems. However, applications with free text are still relatively scarce.

Shifting from a data to a medical process perspective, clinical practice guidelines (CPGs) consist of systematically developed statements which were created to assist physicians by providing recommendations for diagnosis and treatment guidance [21]. In spite of the relevance of their goal, CPGs failed to achieve the expected impact on health care which can be explained by certain factors, namely the lack of time by physicians to learn them or the fact that CPGs lack manageable workflows which could effectively help putting recommended tasks to practice. EHR-based CDSSs can assist in treatment guidance, but to succeed they should integrate detailed relevant patient data, perform an on the fly evaluation against prior knowledge and provide recommendations which physicians can act upon [32].

Furthermore, to have an increased impact in health care, CDSSs should be deployed with slight adjustments in clinic workflow and staff duty, and should be further explored for appointment planning instead of only providing information towards the end of clinical appointments. Several EHR-based CDSSs have already been tested in the past for patients suffering from illnesses such as diabetes, hypertension and others, with the goal of improving key intermediate clinical outcomes of chronic disease care. However, most systems failed because they did not address many of the above-mentioned key aspects [25].

In our previous work we explored clinical notes for extracting new information, which was integrated in clinical protocols in an existing open-source clinical decision support tool. The objective of this work was to leverage rich unexplored data for reducing existing gaps in treatment prescriptions and providing better treatment guidance [4]. This work extends that methodology and streamlines its implementation. While we focused and validated this methodology in the endocrinology field, with these adjustments, the work became more solid and extensible for other medical specialties.

2 Methods and Materials

The proposed methodology uses different components which have already been used and validated in other scenarios. This section is divided into: 1) the analysis and description of the NLP component used to extract relevant information from clinical notes; 2) the conversion of clinical guidelines into a computational-friendly format; and 3) the use of clinical decision support systems for treatment guidance combined with the information extracted from notes.

2.1 Extracting Patient Information from Clinical Notes

Clinical notes are very important for physicians as they keep record of patient trajectories in a readily accessible format, which makes them relevant for aiding in processes of clinical decision making and patient follow-up. The concept of patient trajectory in clinical notes can be particularly evident as these notes can be produced in different stages of health care (e.g. patient admission, discharge, clinical appointment). In spite of storing a large amount of relevant patient information (e.g. family history, diagnosis, medication, recommended or followed procedure), many clinical notes are stored and left unexplored due to the challenges associated with processing free text.

To extract information from clinical free text, a similar pipeline can be followed to that used for common text, which can usually be divided in two steps: NER (Named Entity Recognition) where entities such as drugs, dosages or diseases are identified in the text, and NEN (Named Entity Normalization) where identified entities can be disambiguated and normalised to unique identities. In clinical text, NEN can explore coding standards such as ICD, RxNorm or the UMLS (Unified Medical Language System) Metathesaurus - a thesaurus that aggregates multiple lexical sources - to convert detected entities into normalised text which can be stored as structured data. Furthermore, these steps can explore different approaches to process text, namely heuristic and NLP approaches.

Structured text is easier to integrate in CDSSs and prediction modelling, hence it is crucial to extract relevant patient information from medical narratives and store it as structured data. Considering the abovementioned points, different types of information were extracted from clinical notes. Firstly, heuristics and NLP techniques were combined to extract entities related with several classification criteria, namely cardiovascular diseases, medication taken to prevent a given disease, HbA1c values, among others [5].

Secondly, considering the family history component of clinical notes, a methodology based on heuristics and NLP was used to extract information regarding family members, their association to diseases and living status. Here, clinical text was preprocessed using Stanford CoreNLP [18] dependency parsing and co-reference resolution steps. A lexicon with possible family members was compiled and the co-reference graph was used in combination with a rule set to identify mentions of family members. A disease dictionary compiled from the UMLS was used with Neji, a biomedical text annotation server [19], to identify disease mentions. The shortest path in the dependency graph was used to associate disease mentions to family members and to determine the living status [3].

Finally, considering the NEN component, a system was used for clinical concept normalisation which used dictionary matching approaches, with exact and partial matching mechanisms, combined with word embedding similarity to normalise relevant entities in clinical notes. With this approach, identified entities were mapped to their respective concept unique identifier (CUI) from the UMLS Metathesaurus [29].

The above mentioned extraction methodologies were developed under the scope of several research challenges focused on leveraging clinical text, and were validated with datasets from the 2018 n2c2 track on cohort selection for clinical trials, 2019 n2c2/OHNLP track on family history extraction and 2019 n2c2/OHNLP track on clinical concept normalisation [10–12].

All relevant patient information resulting from the combined use of these strategies was organised in a data structure ready to be supplied to the CDSS during clinical treatments.

2.2 Combining Protocols with Text Data

Clinical guidelines were developed to assist health professionals during the treatment of specific pathologies. These guidelines consist of recommendations and procedures that should be addressed during patient evaluation and treatment. Previously, these guidelines only existed in paper format and were transmitted through textbooks or teaching. However, with the increase of new and more personalised clinical guidelines, traditional methods became obsolete due to protocol variance and complexity. While medical specialists can follow complex guidelines to treat illnesses specific to their field without the need for a CDSS, general practitioners following the same guidelines can greatly benefit from the assistance of a CDSS [7]. Moreover, these systems keep the patient history in the EHR, optimising treatments by reducing execution time and increasing precision. Besides, it is easy for a computer to identify anomalies, for instance, medications that cannot be prescribed together. Therefore, the digitisation of clinical guidelines and the use of CDSSs is a valuable resource to simplify and optimise health care professionals' tasks.

The digitisation of clinical guidelines in CDSSs requires a convention in how these guidelines should be digitally represented. Currently, this process can be

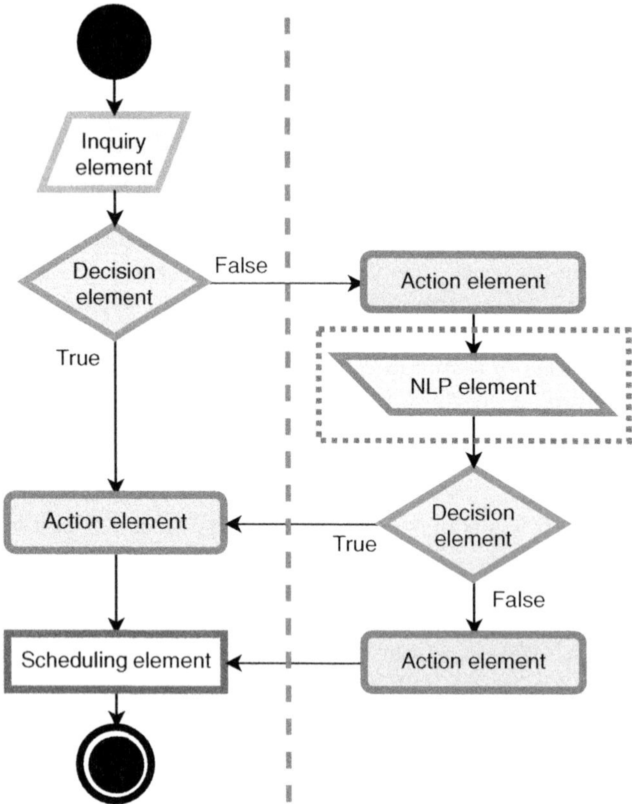

Fig. 1. Protocol components in the digital format representation. Surrounded by the red box is the main element for the proposed methodology. (Color figure online)

performed with existing methodologies such as the Guideline Interchange Format version 3 (GLIF3), which is a model designed to represent shareable computer-interpretable guidelines in the medical field. This model intends to represent different types of guidelines by specifying them following some low-level primitives, which could be applied in screening, diagnosis, and treatment in primary or speciality unit care [6]. The process of converting treatment guidelines into a digital format can be accomplished using only four different types of elements [1], which are represented in the left side of Fig. 1.

The workflow begins with the Inquiry element, where the physician collects patient information (*e.g.*, constantly updating medical variables that influence the treatments guidelines). Nevertheless, some of the patient information can be collected during the treatment, since depending on patient state it may be required to perform other measurements. Then, the Decision element, represented in the IF-THEN format, uses the collected information in a conditional operation that returns true or false. For instance, the physician collects the patient's blood glucose and based on that value the guideline will follow a different path. Any other element can be subsequent to the Decision element, which will create a workflow capable of fulfilling all the possibilities defined in the guidelines.

Treatment recommendations are described using Action elements, which are usually instructions for the procedures to perform in the treatment or the medication dosages based on patient state. Using again blood glucose as an example, the insulin dosages for a diabetic inpatient are calculated based on that current value, the patient's diet, among other factors that are collected during or prior to the treatment. The final element is the Scheduling element which determines when the patient must be checked again by the physician or nurse. This element ensures that the medical staff is reminded about the treatment schedules.

The proposed approach uses these elements and includes a fifth, the NLP element (marked with a red box on the right side of Fig. 1). This element is used to optimise time spent during treatment when the patients' information is collected, and was designed to access information from clinical notes. It is capable of identifying information in the patient history that can be relevant to mention when the system gives a treatment recommendation. Besides, this type of element also reduces the number of inquiry elements in the protocol by providing suggestions that were previously recorded in the clinical notes as free text. This simplifies interactions with the system in complex protocols that may require significant patient information that is not yet inserted in the system.

The use of the NLP element can automatically provide information to the system that is relevant to the treatment. A possible scenario can be that of patients who are taking medication at home and inform the clinical staff during the admission stage about their situation. Commonly, medications being taken and their respective dosages can have an impact on the treatments that are prescribed. For instance, type 2 diabetic inpatients may need to be medicated daily with insulin dosages, but depending on the insulin product used at home, the treatment in the hospital must be adjusted.

Another scenario is the history of relatives with certain hereditary diseases. With this information the system can alert the physician to inform the patient about several risks based on their current condition. For instance, patients with irregular blood pressure and diabetic family members are more prone to suffer from diabetes or cardiac diseases in the future. This information can be provided when measurements are done combined with the patient family history.

A final possible scenario concerns protocols for surgery preparation that, depending on the patient state, can lead to a surgery postponement. The system can detect that the patient took a specific medication in past visits and forgot to mention that in a more recent appointment. However, the medication described in their history combined with their current clinical state could indicate that the patient is unable to withstand surgery.

2.3 Treatment Guidance with the Assistance of a CDSS

The use of CDSSs to assist in treatment guidance has become an essential piece in continuing care units, since it helps improving the quality of patient care and disease prevention, and supports scientific discoveries. These systems are usually part of the EHR features, but some standalone solutions do also exist. However, an EHR with decision-making capabilities is not necessarily capable of providing treatment guidance features, thus, some standalone systems were developed. Typically, a CDSS designed for treatment assistance must be able to manage and provide guidance to the medical staff. However, this is only possible if the treatment guidelines are represented in a digital format.

The proposed methodology uses a standalone and open-source CDSS designated as GenericCDSS. This system is a web-based solution specifically designed to create, manage and execute clinical protocols for guiding treatments [2]. The tool has an easy-to-use protocol editor that allows the specialist to define the best treatments for the diseases in their medical field. In this editor, it is simple to prescribe recommendations based on patient status. Besides, the tool also alerts the health professional about treatment schedules and when patients need to be checked again, based on their current situation. During protocol execution, the tool requests information about the patient clinical state and then provides several recommendations about the treatment in question. To evaluate the suitability of the system, four key requirements were defined:

- Protocol conversion to digital format;
- Treatment guidance;
- Automatic therapeutic recommendation;
- Patient and treatment history for future references.

The typical behaviour of this tool begins by processing the protocol according to the workflow structure principles described in Sect. 2.2. There is an admission stage, in which the patient is registered in the system and assigned the first observation. In this first observation, a protocol is executed which collects information about the patient current status and defines when the physician should observe/treat the patient. During each protocol execution, collected information is used to provide a set of treatment suggestions that have been defined previously. The original system input (Inquiry elements) required structured information that could be provided in run-time. However, some of that information can be found in the patient diary (in free text) and could be aggregated to the protocol workflow during treatments.

Therefore, the previously defined NLP element was added to this tool, which can access the information extracted from the clinical reports from admitted patients. This new feature has different roles during system execution:

1. Provide suggestions for some of the required patient data that must be collected during treatments;
2. Cross information with collected data to find possible undetected alerts (for instance, incompatible medication);

3. Present the annotated notes so that physicians can validate extracted information in case of doubts.

The features implemented in the system allowed us to assess the impact of enhancing treatment protocols with relevant information from clinical notes on treatment recommendations. We observed that patient clinical state can be complemented with patient history information to obtain better treatments. Therefore, by using patient history in GenericCDSS, we were able to enrich the protocols and provide more accurate suggestions.

3 Results

In the previous sections we described in detail the different pieces of the proposed methodology and explained the selection of each component. Figure 2 presents the different stages of this workflow, from guideline conversion and system configuration to treatment guidance, using those components. However, this workflow is divided in three temporal stages. The first stage (grey box in Fig. 2) of this pipeline is focused on the digitisation of the clinical guidelines into the CDSS.

The second stage (orange box in Fig. 2) begins with the admission of the patient into the health institution. This is done by a physician after the initial triage when it is defined that the patient will be hospitalised. During patient admission the physician collects patient information such as medication taken at home, family history information and other clinical information relevant to the admission. This data is inserted into the EHR and can be stored in structured format and in free text (clinical notes).

After the patient is admitted and all additional exams are performed, the patient is hospitalised if necessary. In parallel, the system processes the clinical notes to supply the CDSS with additional relevant information. In this stage of the workflow, notes relevant to the protocol are made available to the CDSS to optimise the process, for when a treatment is required later on.

The last stage (green box in Fig. 2) of the proposed methodology is the treatment guidance supported by the CDSS. Here, the nurse or physician can provide the system with the necessary measurements taken from the patient, which are mostly vital signals and variables that change over time. Clinical information extracted from the admission notes is also provided to the CDSS, reducing considerably the information requested by the system and warning for possible associated risks.

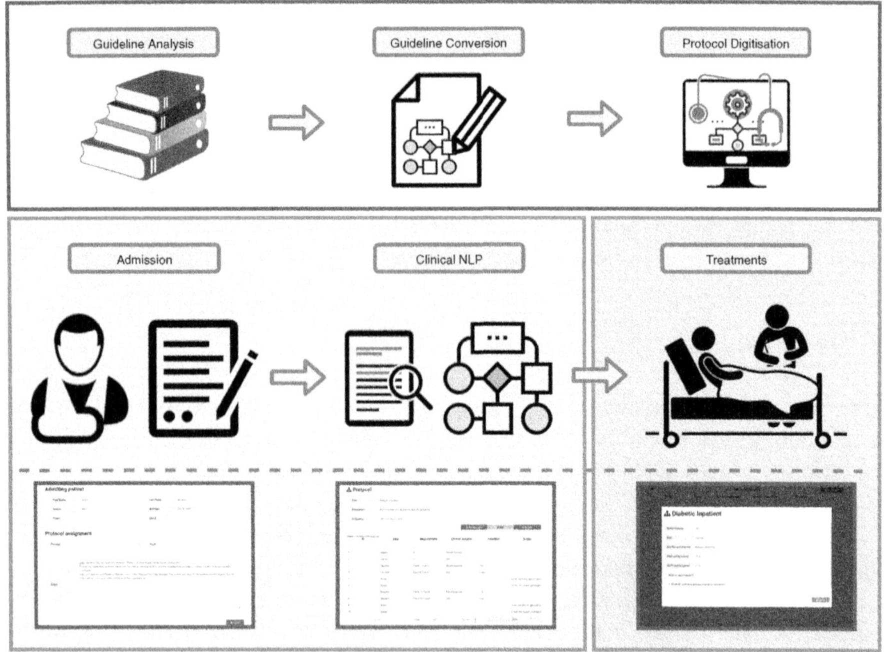

Fig. 2. Methodology overview, from guideline conversion and system configuration to treatment guidance using the GenericCDSS tool with the clinical NLP element integrated for the analysis of clinical notes.

3.1 Guidelines Digitisation

Guidelines digitisation is crucial for the success of this methodology. Although the system provided a user-friendly interface for this task, converting text into a diagram may not be a trivial task for the medical specialist. Therefore, we defined a methodology for this initial stage.

The first step consists in identifying the necessary patient variables for each protocol. During the definition of these variables it is important to see the variable type (numeric, text or choice value) and the range of possible values. Then, for each variable, it is necessary to identify the conditions for the different inputs received during the treatments. Based on the outputs of these conditions, actions must be taken (for instance, a treatment recommendation). This allows the organisation of the text into a decision-diagram, which if represented in paper format is very difficult for a human to read during the treatments, whereas for the computational system the responses are instantaneous.

The following example consists of the most common and simple protocol applied in diabetic inpatients suffering from hypoglycemia. This is a fast-acting protocol where the measurement interval is quite short, *i.e.* measurements ought to be made every 15 min if patient blood glucose is below 80 mg/dl. This protocol requires the following patient information:

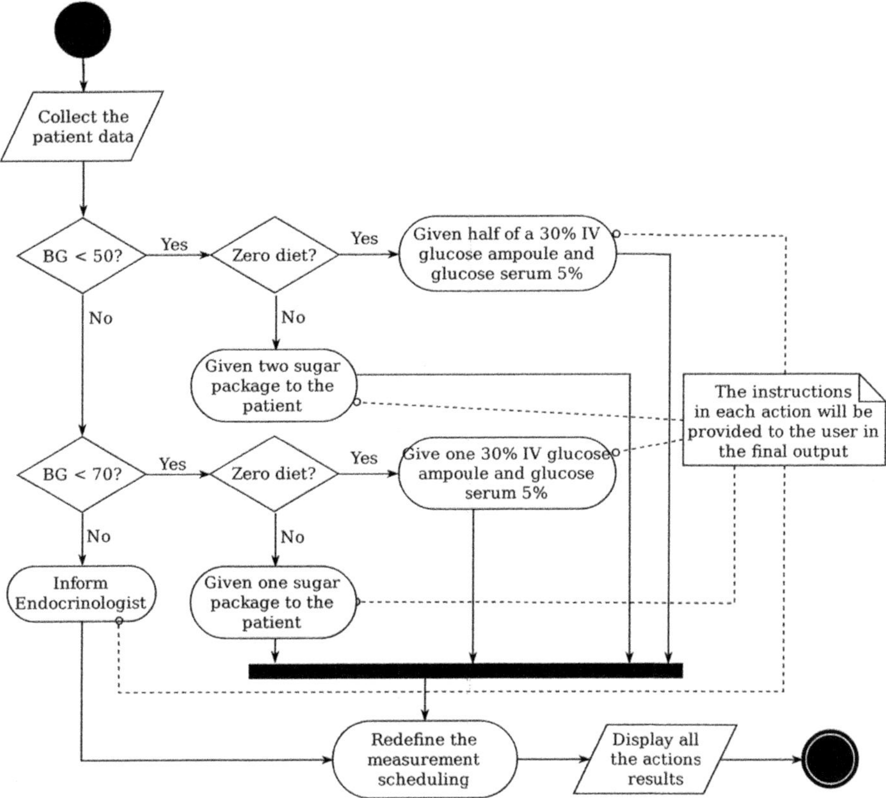

Fig. 3. Flowchart representing the hypoglycemic protocol before being inserted in the system.

- **Blood Glucose:** this variable indicates if the protocol should proceed or not. When this value is less than 80 mg/dl, the application of this protocol is required based on the current value.
- **Diet:** The diet type is a condition that decides what the physician should do in the treatment. This is a choice variable that indicates if the patient is eating or not.

When the patient can eat and the blood glucose value is between 50 and 70 mg/dl, the patient receives one sugar packet (which contains approximately 6 grams of sugar). However, if the blood glucose value is less than 50 mg/dl, the patient receives two sugar packets. A patient on a zero diet receives half of a 30% Intravenous (IV) glucose ampoule and glucose serum 5% when the blood glucose value is between 50 and 70 mg/dl, and a 30% IV glucose ampoule and glucose serum 5% when it is less than 50 mg/dl. In addition, the need for this protocol suggests that there is something wrong with this patient, and the endocrinologist

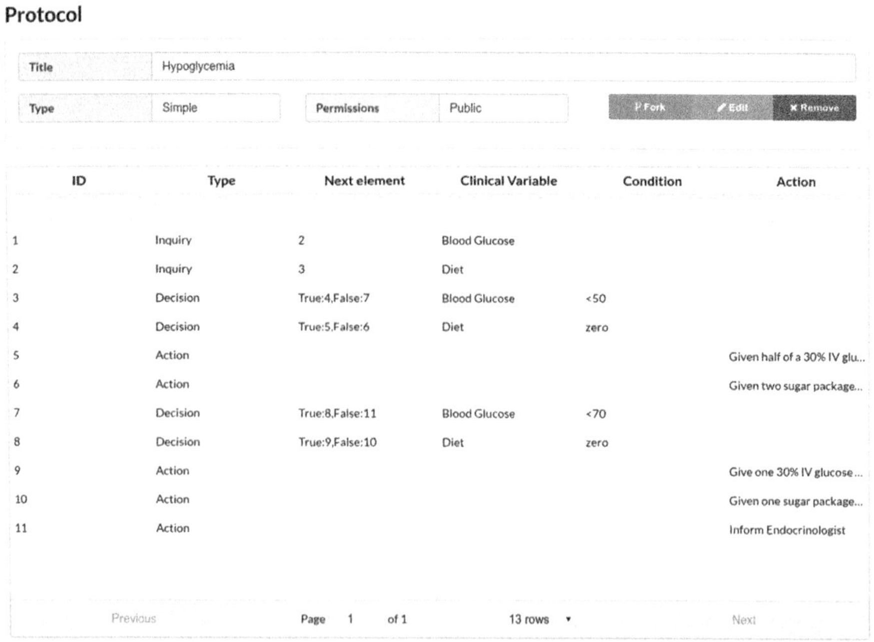

Protocol

Title	Hypoglycemia		
Type	Simple	Permissions	Public

Fork / Edit / Remove

ID	Type	Next element	Clinical Variable	Condition	Action
1	Inquiry	2	Blood Glucose		
2	Inquiry	3	Diet		
3	Decision	True:4,False:7	Blood Glucose	<50	
4	Decision	True:5,False:6	Diet	zero	
5	Action				Given half of a 30% IV glu...
6	Action				Given two sugar package...
7	Decision	True:8,False:11	Blood Glucose	<70	
8	Decision	True:9,False:10	Diet	zero	
9	Action				Give one 30% IV glucose...
10	Action				Given one sugar package...
11	Action				Inform Endocrinologist

Previous Page 1 of 1 13 rows Next

Fig. 4. Protocol editor showing the hypoglycemic protocol implemented.

must be informed about the patient state to perform some adjustments in the current therapeutic scheme.

Figure 3 presents this protocol in the flowchart format, which contains all the possible variants for this guideline. After this initial conversion from text to diagram, the protocol is inserted in the system following a tabular view. This is presented in Fig. 4, where it is possible to observe the system protocol editor with this protocol implemented.

While the presented protocol contains only two variables and a small set of conditions, the remaining implemented protocols are much more extensive. For instance, the protocol applied for diabetic inpatients uses 12 patient conditions to decide upon which is the best treatment. Some of these conditions can be extracted from information already present in the clinical notes.

3.2 Clinical Notes Format

The initial goal for the concept extraction component of this methodology was to process clinical notes in free text without considering clinical note structure. However, some EHRs provide these notes with an internal structure, which simplifies and optimises text analysis. Therefore, we used simple rules to detect structural segments, such as the occurrence of keywords isolated in lines that ended with a colon. In the example presented in Fig. 5 it is possible to see highlighted in blue the section "History of Present Illness:". Then, the system

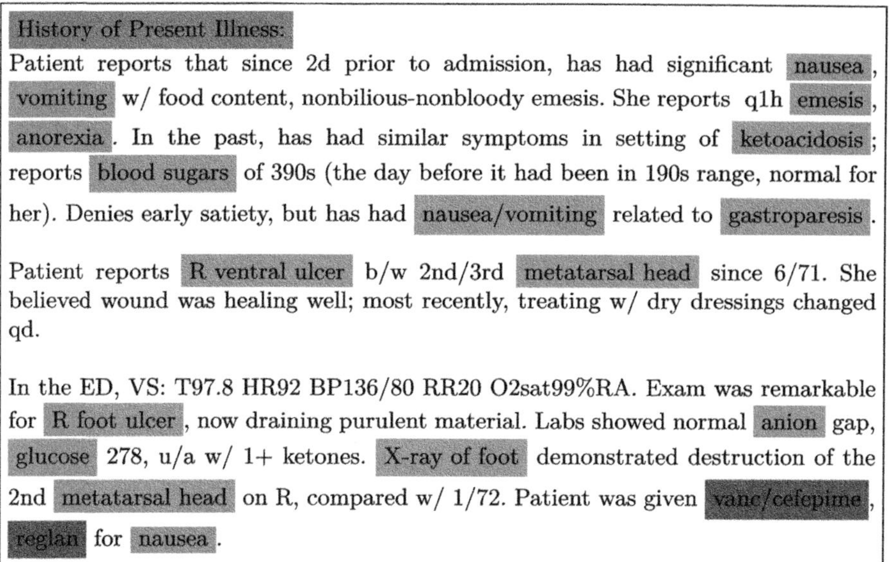

History of Present Illness:
Patient reports that since 2d prior to admission, has had significant nausea, vomiting w/ food content, nonbilious-nonbloody emesis. She reports q1h emesis, anorexia. In the past, has had similar symptoms in setting of ketoacidosis; reports blood sugars of 390s (the day before it had been in 190s range, normal for her). Denies early satiety, but has had nausea/vomiting related to gastroparesis.

Patient reports R ventral ulcer b/w 2nd/3rd metatarsal head since 6/71. She believed wound was healing well; most recently, treating w/ dry dressings changed qd.

In the ED, VS: T97.8 HR92 BP136/80 RR20 O2sat99%RA. Exam was remarkable for R foot ulcer, now draining purulent material. Labs showed normal anion gap, glucose 278, u/a w/ 1+ ketones. X-ray of foot demonstrated destruction of the 2nd metatarsal head on R, compared w/ 1/72. Patient was given vanc/cefepime, reglan for nausea.

Fig. 5. Small excerpt of history section from clinical note provided in the 2014 n2c2 track 2 on identifying risk factors for heart disease over time, annotated with the NLP component described in the methodology. (Color figure online)

extracted medical concepts in the following text which, if necessary, can be presented to the physician during the treatment. This considerably reduces the amount of text to interpret since specific sections need to be analysed instead of a full 4-page clinical note.

In this analysis, the system detected different types of mentions, *i.e.* it identified sections, medications, medical observations and negations of those. These were marked with different colours as shown in the two examples (Fig. 5 and Fig. 6) of excerpts from one clinical note provided in the 2014 n2c2 track 2 on identifying risk factors for heart disease over time. Green is used to highlight medical observations that were extracted but not used in the guidelines, and yellow represents the negations of those observations. On the other hand, in red it is exhibited the medications which are important to analyse and may be useful during the treatments. In the excerpt presented in Fig. 6, the "Medications" section was detected and the system extracted each line under this section. Then, it tried to detect which parts of the text refer to the drugs and dosages. The inference of the right dosage still needs improvements due to the existing diversity in its medical text representation. However, the most important information was extracted, which is the medication in use.

Finally, it is important to consider that some clinical notes may not follow any structure. In those cases the system does not detect sections in the text, and the NLP component performs an analysis considering all text present in the clinical note.

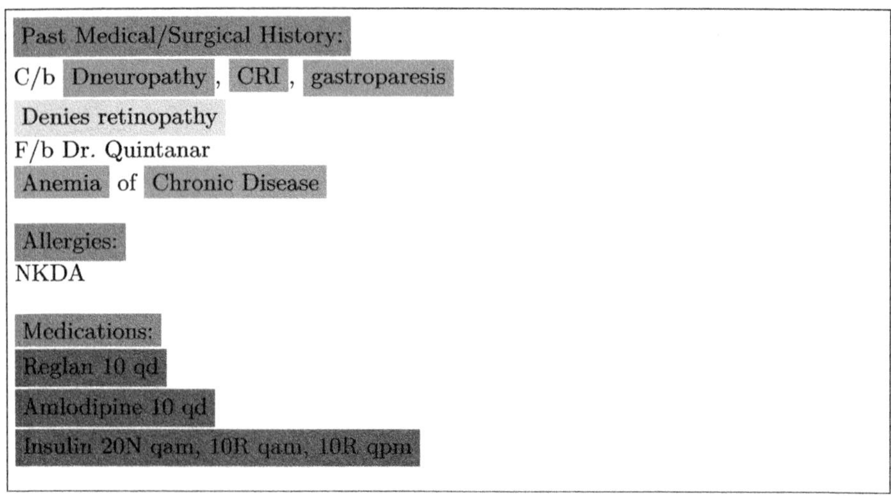

Fig. 6. Small excerpt of medication section from clinical note provided in the 2014 n2c2 track 2 on identifying risk factors for heart disease over time, annotated with the NLP component described in the methodology. (Color figure online)

4 Discussion

The proposed methodology was applied in the endocrinology medical field, in which we configured the most relevant protocols that we defined in discussion with endocrinologists from a Portuguese health institution. In this section we select and describe one of the configured protocols, how the system performed in the presented scenario, possible improvements during the treatment and existing system limitations, which are mainly focused on the text extraction process.

4.1 Use Case Overview

The proposed methodology was designed to be generalisable and improve clinical treatments without following the specific requirements for a given disease. However, we explored the potential of this proposal in the diabetes scenario as there is a lack of effective treatments in health institutions for patients with this disease, mainly due to insufficient exploitation of decision-making systems.

Hyperglycemia is a health condition characterised by abnormally high blood glucose, commonly due to a deficient insulin usage. Owing to the metabolic derangements of this clinical condition, regular monitoring and administration of the most effective treatment are major concerns for healthcare institutions. Inpatient hyperglycemia is an event that occurs frequently, with a rate of approximately 40% of all hospitalisations, therefore it is a metric that deserves special attention from health care institutions and public health services [14].

Basal-bolus insulin therapy is usually the recommended treatment to manage hyperglycemia in hospitalised diabetic patients [35]. However, this therapy is also associated with high rates of hypoglycemia, reaching values up to 32%, with the main reason for this occurrence being the meal insulin and food intake mismatch [34]. Therefore, it is possible to recognise that most of the adverse medication occasions and blunders happen when insulin is prescribed or administered. These hypoglycemia cases in non-intensive care unit settings are a concern as they have been linked with increased hospital complications, length of stay and mortality [17]. Several protocols have been proposed for glycemic administration to reduce these high rates [22]. However, these procedures are frequently available on paper and difficult to follow, hindering their regular use by non-trained professionals.

The proposed methodology aims to reduce this handicap by using a system to support the execution of the clinical protocols, that considers the information contained in clinical notes. The objective of the CDSS is to reduce calculation errors, misunderstood instructions and patient data analysis that influence the treatment decision. Therefore, we deployed the CDSS in a controlled environment and implemented some of the essential protocols being currently used at the hospitals to treat diabetes inpatients, namely:

- Diabetic inpatients [36]
- Hypoglycemia
- Surgical diabetic inpatient
- Continuous intravenous infusion [28]

4.2 Protocol Discussion

Diabetic patients have several base treatments defined depending on their clinical state. Different protocols exist, targeting hypoglycemic patients, hospitalised diabetic patients, diabetic surgical patients, diabetes in pregnant patients, ketoacidosis and hyperosmolar hyperglycemia syndrome in adults and children, among other more specific protocols. However, to provide a more in-depth description of our methodology, we describe the impact of the most common protocol which is used in hospitalised diabetic patients. This protocol is applied in type 2 diabetic inpatients and has two different stages: the admission stage where medication taken at home is converted to the medication used in the hospital; and then during the patient's stay after the initial set up.

The Total Daily Dosage (TDD) defines the amount of insulin that a patient must administer and is calculated based on the patient information. It is used as a reference for the basal or long-acting insulin dosages. However, when the patient is taking insulin before the admission, *i.e.* daily dosages at home, this information must be taken into account and protocols may need to be adjusted accordingly. Typically, this information is provided during the admission stage and is stored in clinical notes, which ends up not being adequately considered in the protocols.

Insulin taken by patients at home can contain a mixture of short and long-acting insulin in the same drug, and the percentages of each vary depending on the drug. Therefore, interpreting which drug and dosages are being taken during the day is essential to optimise TDD calculation. Table 1 presents the

Table 1. Percentage of long (LA) and short-acting (SA) insulins from the most common insulin products used by patients in a domestic setting.

Insulin products	LA insulin	SA insulin
Mixtard 30 Penfill	70%	30%
Insuman Comb 25	75%	25%
Humulin M3	70%	30%
NovoMix 30	70%	30%
Humalog Mix 25	75%	25%
Humalog Mix 50	50%	50%

most common insulin products that patients use at home. LA Insulin and SA Insulin columns represent the percentages of long and short-acting insulin in each product, respectively. Considering this information, it is possible to determine the total of both insulins being taken by the patient and split them as the protocol recommends.

In order to simplify the description of the system execution, the following example is provided:

Example: A patient is taking Mixtard 30 Penfill at home, 30 units before breakfast and 15 units before dinner. This insulin product contains 30% of short-acting and 70% of long-acting insulin as described in Table 1. Hence, this patient has a TDD of 45 units, more precisely 31,5 and 13,5 units of long and short-acting insulin, respectively. Based on the protocol, this patient needs to reduce the total amount of administered insulin, taking only $\frac{2}{3}$ of 31,5 units of long-acting insulin at breakfast during hospitalisation, and $\frac{2}{3}$ of the remaining daily dosage in short-acting insulin.

Moreover, this information is spread over patient diaries, product manuals and clinical guidelines. The system can gather all this information and, following the provided example, can also recognise that this patient is taking Mixtard 30 Penfill at home along with the respective dosages. This section describes some relevant aspects addressed by the proposed methodology. However, in addition to what has been previously described, the protocol also considers patient insulin resistance and the different sliding scales present in the protocol must be adjusted according to patient responses and their plasma glucose values.

4.3 Validation

Methodology validation was performed in a controlled environment using the dataset provided in the 2014 n2c2 track 2 on identifying risk factors for heart disease risk over time. The dataset consists of 1,304 clinical narratives from 296 diabetic patients and contains 2 to 5 records per patient. These narratives contain information about many heart disease risk factors, namely: diabetes, high blood pressure and cholesterol levels, obesity, coronary artery disease, smoking and medication [33]. Since these clinical narratives contain medical information on diabetes indicators and its respective medication, this dataset was considered suitable to validate our methodology.

From this dataset, we selected 25 patients whose notes contained more information to create some difficulties in the NLP methodologies (*e.g.* more redundant and less concise information). Additionally, we randomly added sentences indicating that the patient is taking insulin products at home, and following some criteria, we also added information about dosages that they administered during the day (before breakfast, lunch, dinner, meals or bedtime). Our system detected information on medication being taken by the patient for diabetes, namely the type of insulin (short and long-action can be identified in the clinical notes with R and N, respectively), and units which are important for computing the TDD.

Then, we manually simulated the physician work and protocol execution during treatments. Altogether, the proposed methodology produced positive results. However, we noticed that the system faced some complications in the clinical notes analysis stage. The system had issues when randomly inserted sentences were too complex, referencing past medication that is currently not being taken by the patient. However, we solved this issue by giving the physician the possibility to consult the clinical report in run-time, identifying and validating which were the sentences that originated that recommendation.

5 Conclusion

Clinical notes can be a major repository of relevant medical information, hence they have been a topic of much research throughout the past years. Similarly, the use of digital systems for decision-making and treatment guidance has also been a subject of much research. In this work we addressed an existing opportunity to enrich medical treatments by combining both topics, aiming to reduce existing gaps in treatment prescriptions.

The methodology herein proposed was integrated and validated with an open-source CDSS due to its autonomy and ease of development. However, the objective was to demonstrate the positive impact of combining these subjects and define a supporting approach. This methodology can be explored in the different decision-making features existent in the EHR systems available in the market.

We believe that automatically extracting patient information from physician notes, which are stored in free text, has the potential to improve treatment efficiency and reduce human errors. This work takes one step forward in the reuse of clinical notes to enhance the medical decision process in real time.

Acknowledgements. This work has received support from the EU/EFPIA Innovative Medicines Initiative 2 Joint Undertaking under grant agreement No 806968 and from the NETDIAMOND project (POCI-01-0145-FEDER-016385), co-funded by Centro 2020 program, Portugal 2020, European Union. João Figueira Silva and João Rafael Almeida are funded by the FCT - Foundation for Science and Technology (national funds) under the grants PD/BD/142878/2018 and SFRH/BD/147837/2019 respectively.

References

1. Almeida, J.R., Guimarães, J., Oliveira, J.L.: Simplifying the digitization of clinical protocols for diabetes management. In: 2018 IEEE 31st International Symposium on Computer-Based Medical Systems (CBMS), pp. 176–181. IEEE (2018)
2. Almeida, J.R., Oliveira, J.L.: GenericCDSS-a generic clinical decision support system. In: 2019 IEEE 32nd International Symposium on Computer-Based Medical Systems (CBMS), pp. 186–191. IEEE (2019)
3. Almeida, J.R., Matos, S.: Rule-based extraction of family history information from clinical notes. In: Proceedings of the 35th Annual ACM Symposium on Applied Computing, SAC 2020, pp. 670–675. Association for Computing Machinery, New York (2020). https://doi.org/10.1145/3341105.3374000
4. Almeida, J.R., Silva, J.F., Sierra, A.P., Matos, S., Oliveira, J.L.: Enhancing decision-making systems with relevant patient information by leveraging clinical notes. In: Proceedings of the 13th International Joint Conference on Biomedical Engineering Systems and Technologies, vol. 5 HEALTHINF: HEALTHINF, pp. 254–262. INSTICC, SciTePress (2020)
5. Antunes, R., Silva, J.F., Pereira, A., Matos, S.: Rule-based and machine learning hybrid system for patient cohort selection. In: Proceedings of the 12th International Joint Conference on Biomedical Engineering Systems and Technologies, vol. 2: HEALTHINF, pp. 59–67. INSTICC, SciTePress (2019). https://doi.org/10.5220/0007349300590067
6. Boxwala, A.A., et al.: GLIF3: a representation format for sharable computer-interpretable clinical practice guidelines. J. Biomed. Inform. **37**(3), 147–161 (2004)
7. Bright, T.J., et al.: Effect of clinical decision-support systems: a systematic review. Ann. Intern. Med. **157**(1), 29–43 (2012)
8. Cohen, R., Elhadad, M., Elhadad, N.: Redundancy in electronic health record corpora: analysis, impact on text mining performance and mitigation strategies. BMC Bioinform. **14**(10), 1–15 (2013). https://doi.org/10.1186/1471-2105-14-10
9. Costa, C.M.A.: Concepção, desenvolvimento e avaliação de um modelo integrado de acesso a registos clínicos electrónicos. Ph.D. thesis, University of Aveiro (2004). http://hdl.handle.net/10773/18802
10. HMS: 2018 n2c2 - Track 1: Cohort Selection for Clinical Trials (2018). https://portal.dbmi.hms.harvard.edu/projects/n2c2-t1/
11. HMS: 2019 n2c2 Shared-Task and Workshop, Track2: n2c2/OHNLP Track on Family History Extraction (2019). https://n2c2.dbmi.hms.harvard.edu/track2
12. HMS: 2019 n2c2 Shared-Task and Workshop, Track3: n2c2/UMass Track on Clinical Concept Normalization (2019). https://n2c2.dbmi.hms.harvard.edu/track3
13. Hripcsak, G., Albers, D.J.: Next-generation phenotyping of electronic health records. J. Am. Med. Inform. Assoc. **20**(1), 117–121 (2012). https://doi.org/10.1136/amiajnl-2012-001145
14. Inzucchi, S.E.: Management of hyperglycemia in the hospital setting. N. Engl. J. Med. **355**(18), 1903–1911 (2006)
15. Jensen, K., et al.: Analysis of free text in electronic health records for identification of cancer patient trajectories. Sci. Rep. **7**(46226), 1–12 (2017). https://doi.org/10.1038/srep46226
16. Katehakis, D.G., Tsiknakis, M.: Electronic health record. In: Wiley Encyclopedia of Biomedical Engineering. Wiley (2006). https://doi.org/10.1002/9780471740360.ebs1440

17. Kim, Y., Rajan, K.B., Sims, S.A., Wroblewski, K.E., Reutrakul, S.: Impact of glycemic variability and hypoglycemia on adverse hospital outcomes in non-critically ill patients. Diab. Res. Clin. Pract. **103**(3), 437–443 (2014)
18. Manning, C.D., Surdeanu, M., Bauer, J., Finkel, J., Bethard, S.J., McClosky, D.: The Stanford CoreNLP natural language processing toolkit. In: Association for Computational Linguistics (ACL) System Demonstrations, pp. 55–60 (2014). http://www.aclweb.org/anthology/P/P14/P14-5010
19. Matos, S.: Configurable web-services for biomedical document annotation. J. Cheminform. **10**(1), 68 (2018)
20. Miotto, R., Wang, F., Wang, S., Jiang, X., Dudley, J.T.: Deep learning for healthcare: review, opportunities and challenges. Brief. Bioinform. (2017). https://doi.org/10.1093/bib/bbx044
21. NCCIH: Clinical Practice Guidelines (2017). https://nccih.nih.gov/health/providers/clinicalpractice.htm
22. Neinstein, A., MacMaster, H.W., Sullivan, M.M., Rushakoff, R.: A detailed description of the implementation of inpatient insulin orders with a commercial electronic health record system. J. Diab. Sci. Technol. **8**(4), 641–651 (2014)
23. Nelson, S.J., Zeng, K., Kilbourne, J., Powell, T., Moore, R.: Normalized names for clinical drugs: RxNorm at 6 years. J. Am. Med. Inform. Assoc. **18**(4), 441 (2011). https://doi.org/10.1136/amiajnl-2011-000116
24. Neustein, A., Imambi, S.S., Rodrigues, M., Teixeira, A., Ferreira, L.: Application of text mining to biomedical knowledge extraction: analyzing clinical narratives and medical literature. In: Text Mining of Web-based Medical Content, pp. 3–32. De Gruyter (2014). https://doi.org/10.1515/9781614513902.3
25. O'Connor, P.J., et al.: Impact of electronic health record clinical decision support on diabetes care: a randomized trial. Ann. Fam. Med. **9**(1), 12–21 (2011). https://doi.org/10.1370/afm.1196
26. Pivovarov, R., Elhadad, N.: Automated methods for the summarization of electronic health records. J. Am. Med. Inform. Assoc. **22**(5), 938–947 (2015). https://doi.org/10.1093/jamia/ocv032
27. Sheikhalishahi, S., Miotto, R., Dudley, J.T., Lavelli, A., Rinaldi, F., Osmani, V.: Natural language processing of clinical notes on chronic diseases: systematic review. JMIR Med. Inform. **7**(2), e12239 (2019). https://doi.org/10.2196/12239. http://medinform.jmir.org/2019/2/e12239/
28. Shetty, S., Inzucchi, S., Goldberg, P., Cooper, D., Siegel, M., Honiden, S.: Adapting to the new consensus guidelines for managing hyperglycemia during critical illness: the updated Yale insulin infusion protocol. Endocr. Pract. **18**(3), 363–370 (2011)
29. Silva, J.F., Antunes, R., Almeida, J.R., Matos, S.: Clinical concept normalization on medical records using word embeddings and heuristics. In: 30th Medical Informatics Europe Conference, MIE (2020)
30. Singh, H., Giardina, T.D., Meyer, A.N.D., Forjuoh, S.N., Reis, M.D., Thomas, E.J.: Types and origins of diagnostic errors in primary care settings. JAMA Intern. Med. **173**(6), 418–425 (2013). https://doi.org/10.1001/jamainternmed.2013.2777
31. Stearns, M.Q., Price, C., Spackman, K.A., Wang, A.Y.: SNOMED clinical terms: overview of the development process and project status. In: Proceedings of the AMIA Symposium, pp. 662–666. American Medical Informatics Association, Washington (2001). https://www.ncbi.nlm.nih.gov/pmc/articles/PMC2243297/
32. Stewart, W.F., Shah, N.R., Selna, M.J., Paulus, R.A., Walker, J.M.: Bridging the inferential gap: the electronic health record and clinical evidence. Health Affairs **26**(Supplement 1), w181–w191 (2007). https://doi.org/10.1377/hlthaff.26.2.w181

33. Stubbs, A., Kotfila, C., Xu, H., Uzuner, Ö.: Identifying risk factors for heart disease over time: overview of 2014 i2b2/UTHealth shared task track 2. J. Biomed. Inform. **58**, S67–S77 (2015)
34. Umpierrez, G.E., et al.: Safety and efficacy of sitagliptin therapy for the inpatient management of general medicine and surgery patients with type 2 diabetes: a pilot, randomized, controlled study. Diab. Care **36**(11), 3430–3435 (2013)
35. Umpierrez, G.E., et al.: Management of hyperglycemia in hospitalized patients in non-critical care setting: an endocrine society clinical practice guideline. J. Clin. Endocrinol. Metab. **97**(1), 16–38 (2012)
36. Wexler, D.J., Shrader, P., Burns, S.M., Cagliero, E.: Effectiveness of a computerized insulin order template in general medical inpatients with type 2 diabetes: a cluster randomized trial. Diab. Care **33**(10), 2181–2183 (2010)
37. WHO: World Health Organization: International classification of diseases, 11th Revision (ICD-11) (2018). https://www.who.int/classifications/icd/en/

Mobile Marketing in Health: User Experience Guiding the Implementation of a Medical Booking Application

Tiago Fernandes and André Vasconcelos(✉)

INESC-ID, Instituto Superior Técnico, Universidade de Lisboa, Lisbon, Portugal
{tiago.f.b.fernandes, andre.vasconcelos}@tecnico.ulisboa.pt

Abstract. Mobile applications are, on average, faster than mobile websites, provide tailored content (according to the user preferences), and increase the user call to action (by providing notifications and instant updates), leading to an interactive user engagement. In the health care sector, it is also expected that medical appointments booking applications enlarge the accessibility of the health care services – providing broad access to the medical health professional CV and making available other patients reviews of the service. The research described in this paper presents an effort in the identification of the main uses for mobile marketing in the health sector, by describing four major use cases, namely: i) searching for an appointment, ii) booking a medical appointment, iii) history of the medical appointments, iv) alerts for future appointments, and v) mobile marketing. A mobile marketing app implementation is then described including i) the book medical appointment process, ii) the user onboarding, iii) the approach on prioritize search before login, iv) the mobile push notifications, and v) the user information logging. The results achieved are assessed and improved through an iterative testing approach, that provided important feedback to the development process. Additionally, user testing was performed in four scenarios. The mobile application developed present auspicious user experience results which promises a high adoption rate by real world users.

Keywords: Mobile health · Healthcare mobile application · Medical appointment booking · Mobile marketing · User experience

1 Introduction

Nowadays, people are becoming more proactive and more self-conscious when it comes to health. One way to make health services more available to the everyday user is to use modern technologies. Customers in most industries are already used to frictionless booking, whether that is getting a rideshare or booking a hotel.

Medical services applications (web platforms or mobile applications) are being used to increase accessibility of information about healthcare providers (e.g., preview the CV of a medical health professional, acquiring healthcare services, get other patients reviews of the service). There are already several examples of applications that

X. Ye et al. (Eds.): BIOSTEC 2020, CCIS 1400, pp. 541–564, 2021.
https://doi.org/10.1007/978-3-030-72379-8_27

help solving common problems as patient's transportation, or waiting lists for medical appointments, or providing consumer information about health services anywhere.

Although medical booking applications exist, most are specific of one heath care provider. Additionally, most applications are not built to a "mobile-first" approach, taking advantage of the mobile features as location sensor and the ability to start the interaction with the user.

This paper is focus on the development of a mobile application having mobile marketing as the main differentiating feature of it. This mobile application is expected to extend an online platform: MedClick (a medical care appointment booking service).

Mobile marketing supports the communication and promotion of offers to customers using a mobile medium [9]. The main difference to regular communication with the customers, is to not just wait for the customer to interact with the company but provide incentives to customers use or buy products or services considering each costumer specific needs.

The goal is to extend MedClick[1] platform. MedClick provides a one-stop platform to book a medical appointment, across multiple medical service providers. Patients can conveniently browse all available booking options, using different filtering criteria (e.g. date, location, price, insurance providers, customer reviews and recommendations). The research presented in this paper extends MedClick platform with mobile marketing features, provided in a mobile application. It is expected that the app pushes booking appointments to patients based on the location, medical history and recent searches.

The next section presents the background research, including i) an assessment of the major mobile development frameworks, ii) a review on mobile marketing, ii) a description on user experience approaches on mobile and iv) an analysis of mobile medical appointments booking applications. Section 3 describes the major use cases for the mobile marketing application. Section 4 presents the mobile app implementation process, which is assessed in Sect. 5. Finally, the conclusions and future work are described in Sect. 6.

2 Related Work

This section presents the background research performed, including the mobile development frameworks, the mobile marketing, the user experience guidelines and an assessment of medical appointment booking applications.

2.1 Frameworks

iOS and Android are the two dominant operating systems for mobile devices [1]. In order to ensure that mobile applications are available in these operating systems, one may code natively for both operating systems. However, this approach is time consuming and requires different programing skills (e.g. XCode for iOS and Android

[1] www.medclick.pt.

Studio for Android). Another approach is to use cross-platform development frameworks.

Cross-platform mobile application development frameworks have the goal of simplify the development of cross-platform mobile applications by reducing the development effort and the maintenance costs, therefore ensuring a shorter time-to-market - achieving the principle of “code once, deploy everywhere”.

Adobe PhoneGap. Adobe PhoneGap [2] is a development framework to build applications for mobile devices using CSS, HTML and JavaScript code and then deploy it to multiple mobile platforms without losing features of a native application. In order to achieve this, the framework provides an API (Application Programming Interface) to access the native operating system functionalities using JavaScript. The programmer codes the application logic using JavaScript and the PhoneGap API handles the communication with the native operating system. The core engine for PhoneGap is open source, under the Apache Cordova project [3]. The user interface layer of a PhoneGap application uses a web browser view that takes up to 100% of the screen.

Xamarin. Xamarin [4] is a cross platform development framework to build mobile applications using C#. The framework has two major platforms: Xamarin.iOS and Xamarin.Android. These are the C# object libraries that give developers access to iOS SDK (Software Development Kit) and the Android SDK, respectively. With these platforms the developer can share part of the codebase to create iOS and Android applications, however the visual aspects must be developed specifically for each operating system. There is also Xamarin.Forms, which gives the most development efficiency, enabling the developer to share almost 100% of the code and user interface between both operating systems, at the expense of application file size efficiency and performance.

XCode and Android Studio are required for the application compilation and, as the application grows, compilation time lasts longer.

React Native. React Native [5] is a JavaScript framework for developing mobile applications for iOS and Android. It is based on React, Facebook’s JavaScript library for building user interfaces, but instead of targeting the browser, it targets mobile platforms. React Native applications are written using a mixture of JavaScript and XML like markup, known as JSX. In order to behave like a native application, React Native invokes the native rendering APIs in Objective-C (for iOS) or Java (for Android). With this, the application will render using real mobile user interface components, not web views, and will look and feel like a native mobile application [6].

The easiest way to start a React Native project is to use the Expo toolchain [7]. It allows the programmer to start a project without installing or configuring any tools to build native code - no XCode or Android Studio installation required. In order to use system functionalities, Expo contains the Expo SDK, which is a native-and-JavaScript library which provides access to the device’s system functionality (the camera, contacts, local storage, and other hardware).

2.2 Mobile Marketing

"Mobile marketing refers to the two- or multi–way communication and promotion of an offer between a firm and its customers using a mobile medium, device, or technology" [8]. Mobile Marketing requires a mind shift in the communication with customers. Instead of waiting for the customer, companies should provide incentives to the customer to request the services provided [9]. In order to implement mobile marketing, services and products are presented to consumers considering time, location and each costumer specific needs and desires.

Location Based Services. These marketing campaigns work by giving the user promotions or information based on location [10]. For a clothing brand, for example, if the user decides to share its location to the application, the user could receive an alert when is near one of the brand stores, offering some kind of discount. Other example is for traffic or weather application, that can transmit information without the user having to search for it. These alerts can be received in the application via push notification, or SMS, or email.

Services Based on Personalized Information. These services act very similarly to the location-based ones but instead of relying on the user's location, they rely on the information about the user. Using the same example of a clothing store, if the company wants to do a promotion on a women's item, and they have information about the gender of its application users, they can send an alert just to the female audience about said promotion. This way companies do not reach all customer base but avoid annoying customers that most likely are not interested in some promotions.

Gamification. It is the use of game design elements to enhance non-game goods and services by increasing customer value and encouraging value-creating behaviors such as increasement of consumption, greater loyalty, engagement, or product advocacy. One example is discounts or free products a user can receive by using the brand application. It can be confused with loyalty programs, however gamification distinguishes itself by providing added social and motivational benefits through usage, like competing with friends for goals.

Referral Marketing. Relying on probably the oldest marketing strategy, word of mouth, referral marketing is the method of promoting products or services to new customers through existing customers. This works by giving current customers an incentive to invite more users to the platform/application/service. Referral programs are a good method to define consumer satisfaction. Major advantages of referral marketing programs as compared with traditional marketing programs include greater credibility of friend/family member recommendations over paid advertisements [11].

Onboarding. The concept of Onboarding comes from the human resources sphere and it is aimed at helping newcomers adapting to a new reality and getting comfortable with a new task.

In the context of mobile applications, user Onboarding is the process of providing instructions and highlighting key benefits and features of the application to the user, when the user launches the application for the first time, via a set of example screens. This process bases itself on the premise that users won't use your application if they don't understand it. This way the users feel quickly familiarized with the application and can find more easily the features they need. Another benefit is to improve application retention, which means users will continue to use the application over a certain period [12].

When working on user Onboarding, it is important to establish the most relevant features to the user because the information needs to be transmitted in the easiest and simplest way possible. Users don't like to spend much time learning how the product works before actually starting to interact with it. If the amount of information that the Onboarding tutorial tries to transmit to the user is too much, it will have the reverse result. In other words, it can make the user more confused.

Shareable Content. Having shareable content inside the application and using social networks is another way of marketing a mobile application, grow the brand user base and enhance engagement. Like Referral Marketing, it also consists in word of mouth, relying in the current users to promote and talk about the application to their friends and followers. However, the main difference is that the current user does not receive any incentive to share that content. Instead, the application relies on having such good user experience and such value to the users that they would want to recommend it to their closed ones and acquaintances.

App Store Rating. The App Store rating is essential in an application, as positive ratings and reviews can lead to more downloads because the opinion of other customers have a great impact on new users. Besides that, it gives the developer insight into real world usage that helps direct future updates. One way to increase the number of App Store ratings is to implement a nonintrusive way of asking the user for a review. The best way to obtain positive ratings is for the user to have a great overall experience when using the application, however, is also important to ask for feedback at appropriate times, preferably after the user has demonstrated engagement with the application. It is also important not to interrupt the user and only ask for feedback when the request makes sense. Lastly, the developer should not ask repeatedly for a review, because it may negatively influence the user opinion of the application.

2.3 User Experience

The user interface is one of the most relevant aspects of mobile application. When it comes to the mobile application user satisfaction, most technology firms turn towards the applications' User Interface (UI) and User Experience Design (UX). The user feelings when using the application are central for the its success.

User Testing. User testing is central for the success of most projects. Although the designer plays an important role in defining the UI, the UX is only best assessed through the interaction of the user (gathering insights from the users). This way it is possible to identify UX major flaws, before the application is being massively used by (real) costumers. User testing should be done early in the development cycle in order to find UX problems in early development stages.

Mobile Applications User Experience Design. Although there isn't a common definition of what is a good user experience, there are several principles that contribute to mobile apps have an adequate user experience.

Thus, designers are recommended to use the native operating system design guidelines, which present a set of usability guidelines (focus mainly on maintaining coherent interaction and presentation through applications over the whole platform). For iOS Apple's Human Interface Guidelines [13] and for Android Google's Material Design Guidelines [14] are the major guidelines to consider.

According to Apple, the iOS Guidelines differentiate themselves from other platforms in three primary themes: Clarity, Deference and Depth. The first one makes sure the application has legible text at every size, icons are precise and interface elements highlight in a subtle way the important and interactive content. The second one refers to fluid and simple interface to help the user interact with the content. Content should fill the entire screen while blur or translucency means there is more content to be revealed. The last one focus on depth, mainly with transitions when the user navigates through content. They also appeal to a consistent application, that implements familiar native interface elements, icons, text styles and uniform terminology, and keeping the user informed all times with feedback to every user action.

On the other hand, Google didn't create a design language only for its mobile operating system but for all its application across all platforms. This design language is called Material Design and it is meant to be a set of design principles that apply across device types and arbitrary software versions. In this Material Design world, the primary surface is a piece of paper, like a card, that can grow and shrink. Other pieces of paper can appear on the screen but always with transition. Material Design user interfaces exist in a 3D environment, achieving it by using light, surfaces and shadows. All elements move horizontally, vertically and at varying depth [15].

Respecting design guidelines is not enough. Always designing for the customer benefit is another important rule to follow. Therefore, the designer should prioritize features (instead of just adding features). Applications should be simple, with a refined experience around its core objectives, not putting too much information in the user interface. "Perfection is achieved, not when there is nothing more to add, but when there is nothing left to take away" [16].

2.4 Medical Appointments Booking Applications

There are several applications already available to the patients, that can schedule medical appointments. However, all have different features and characteristics. This analysis consists of the strong and weak points of each one, highlighting them in order to improve the solution proposed.

My CUF. My CUF [17] is an electronic health record portal for the private health care institution CUF. It gives its users an online members area that offer several functionalities and information about their history in CUF's clinics and hospitals. In this members' area, the user can schedule new appointments or exams, having the option to choose the health center, insurance plan, the specialty and the health professional. After selecting those options, if there are vacancies available, the user can choose the date of the appointment from a calendar screen with a weekly view. If not, it is presented a screen where it is asked the preferences of the patient for a booking request.

The portal also gives access to previous appointments and exams where the patient can see the report made by the health professional. Other functionalities include waiting times in all CUF's clinics and hospitals, a tab where the patient can see its medical prescriptions, a map to check where the nearby pharmacies are, a section to review previous appointments invoices. It also includes, in the home tab, links to the latest 3 articles of the "+Saúde", CUF's blog.

My CUF portal keeps track of the user history in the CUF's hospitals and clinics and in order to be accessible to users and patients of all age groups it has a feature to manage multiple accounts. In this feature, the user can add and manage any descendant so that they have a separate account with all the features while being under aged for example. Other option is to give a third party the ability to access multiple sections of the portal like booking appointments and exams, checking the patient history and review prescriptions or appointment invoices. This latter option is optimal to elderly patient or patients that are not comfortable in using new technologies but have a relative that can take care of those tasks for them.

The My CUF portal is available online as a web portal or as an iOS or Android application. All the functionalities are available in all platforms in a very similar user interface. This can be an advantage because the user sees the same design layout and has the same user experience whether on a computer or on a mobile device. However, this can lead to a bad user experience on mobile, mainly on iOS.

In both mobile operating systems guidelines, it is recommended to use bottom navigation bars to allow movement between primary destinations in an application [18, 19]. The reasoning behind this is that the bottom of the screen is the most comfortable area to reach with one-handed or one-thumb interactions; therefore the bottom is place to put important top level and frequently used actions, as: booking an appointment, exams and user profile. In spite of this, it is also common on Android to use a tab bar at the top of the screen, like the My CUF application uses, with "Facebook" being the most famous application to follow this (having different designs depending on the operating system, bottom bar on iOS and top bar on Android [20]). One of the reasons to have the top bar on Android is the software system buttons already on the bottom of the screen, which combined with the bottom navigation bar can make that part of the screen too dense and increase the chance of mistouch. So, this implantation may be familiar on Android but not as much on iOS, being this the reason, it can cause some confusion to longtime iOS users.

In 824 reviews on the Google Play Store it has a total score of 3.7 stars out of 5. On the Apple App Store the application has less ratings, 55, and it has a lower score of 3.0 stars out of 5. Most of the negative written reviews are about the login process because the user is forced to login each time the application is opened. There is an option to set a pin code or fingerprint authentication which makes sense for an application with sensible user data like this one, however, reviewers reported that this functionality is not working properly.

Zocdoc. Zocdoc [21] is an online medical care appointment booking service that provides an easy way to search for medical facilities and professionals based on location and specialty. It acts like the previously mentioned My CUF portal but with multiple medical care providers. In this service the patient can search for a medical appointment specifying the specialty, location, date and insurance. It is then presented a detailed list with the health professionals of the chosen specialty in the chosen location with appointments available starting from the date the user input in the previous screen. The user has the option to search through the days the health professionals have available, to get a map view of where the health professionals' medical facilities are and to filter even more the options, by gender, hours of availability, language, among others. When selecting a health professional, the application shows the user multiple time slots to book the appointment, where are the medical facilities of the health professional (the user can choose which one if there are more than one), patient written reviews of the health professional with separate ratings for waiting times and bedside manners, the health professional's statement, the languages spoken and the education of the health professional.

Besides the search functionality, the application also has a tab to check past and future appointments, a tab to view all the health professionals the patient had an appointment with, a settings tab and a well guide tab. In the latter one, the user is presented with a series of wellness recommendations like having an eye health exam every two years for example. This helps the user by keeping track of the dates of the required exams and reminding the user if a new exam or appointment is recommended.

Zocdoc service is available online as a web portal or as an iOS or Android application. It has all the functionalities available in all platforms but with interfaces that adapt to the system. In the web, the service adapts to the screen size, showing more or less content depending on the width and height of the browser window. In the iOS app it has a bottom navigation bar with the main functionalities as recommended by the operating system guidelines. In the Android app it uses the top tab bar, which can help to prevent mistouches in the lower part of the screen in phones that have system on-screen buttons. That's the main difference in the application between the two mobile operating systems, so the user should expect a native user experience in both.

With so much information presented in the web version it could be expected to have an overcomplicated mobile application. However, despite having all functionalities, Zocdoc achieves it in an intuitive, native and simple way, not damaging the mobile user experience.

In 6330 reviews on the Google Play Store it has a total score of 4.5 stars out of 5. On the Apple App Store the application has less ratings, 3200, but it has a higher score of 4.7 stars out of 5.

This means most users enjoy their experience while using the application and it meets their expectations.

Knok. Knok [22] is a platform, only accessible via a mobile application on Android and iOS, that lets its users schedule a medical appointment at their home. This allows the users to avoid the waiting rooms in a health center and transportation problems. Another very useful feature of this platform is the ability to choose the health professional for the appointment. When in need of medical attention, the patient sets its location on the application and it is presented with a list of the nearby health professionals. That was one of the main objectives of this platform, besides the easy booking of home health appointments. Users can then check the health professional's distance to the given location, price of the appointment, spoken languages, rating, professional experience, academic background and interests and choose accordingly to their needs.

The application has the same user interface in both iOS and Android, using a very simple and minimalistic design. The ease of use of the application extends to the interface, where most functions are on the lower part of the screen, facilitating the one-handed or one-thumb interactions improving the user experience on both platforms.

In 46 reviews on the Google Play Store it has a total score of 4.3 stars out of 5, with written reviews expressing how useful is the application. On the Apple App Store the application has less ratings, only 15, but it keeps the score in 4.2 stars out of 5. This means most users enjoy their experience while using the application and it meets their expectations.

Joaquim Chaves Saúde. Joaquim Chaves Saúde [23] is an electronic health record portal for the private health care institution Joaquim Chaves. It is very similar to the previously mentioned My CUF in terms of functionality. Its main functionalities are booking medical appointments, results of previous exams, medical history and information about Joaquim Chaves Clinics. The booking process starts by choosing the clinic to have an appointment. Just after selecting the clinic, the user is presented with a lot more options like insurance, specialty, type of appointment (subsection of specialty), the health professional and the date, with the option to choose which days of the week are preferred and at what time. In the next screen the user can book the appointment from a calendar with a weekly view.

There is information about the health professionals of the institution, however there is not a main tab for accessing it. To access it the user must go to the clinic's menu, choose a clinic and only there is presented an option to select a health professional. From there the patient can check the health professional's CV but there is no option to give a rating or review.

The Joaquim Chaves Saúde portal is available online as a web portal or as an iOS or Android application. However, not all functionalities are available in all platforms and the design is very different from the web portal to the mobile applications. Search and date filters are the main features of the web portal not presented on mobile. Besides the different design, not even the menu options are the same on the different platforms, and there are menus that are the same but have a different name. It is a good thing to be on all platforms possible in order to reach the highest number of users, however having such different designs of the same platform could be confusing to the user and not providing the best user experience.

In both mobile operating systems, the application looks the same, having some questionable design decisions like having a "hamburger button" on the right side of the screen to open the navigation drawer on the left [24].

In 49 reviews on the Google Play Store it has a total score of 3.1 stars out of 5. On the Apple App Store the application has less ratings, only 16, but it has a higher score of 3.6 stars out of 5. Users seem to give either 5 stars or 1 star which could mean that there are some critical bugs but when the application works users enjoy their experience.

Comparative Analysis. We present next a comparative analysis of the mobile medical appointments booking applications described before, highlighting the strong and weak points.

Table 1. Mobile medical appointments booking applications comparative analysis summary [15].

Functionalities	My CUF	Zocdoc	Knok	Joaquim Chaves Saúde
Medical Appointment Type	In provider	Multiple provider	At home/video	In provider
Health professional CV	Yes	Yes	No	Yes[a]
Rating	No	Yes	Yes	No
Insurance	Yes	Yes	Yes	Yes
Patient History	Yes	Yes	Yes[b]	Yes
Platforms	Web, iOS, Android	Web, iOS, Android	iOS, Android	Web, Android, iOS
Recommendation to users	Yes[c]	Yes	No	No

[a]Not working in the majority of health professionals
[b]There seems to be a section for it, but it shows just a blank page
[c]Not user specific, just general health articles

As described in Table 1 the service that reaches more people is Zocdoc [21], since it is not restricted to a single healthcare provider. Zocdoc provides all major functionalities and is available in every platform. Both My CUF [17] and Joaquim Chaves Saúde [23], the two services that only offer appointments in their own medical facilities, have the same main functionalities; the only difference is the recommendations made to its patients and the design of the applications and web portal.

3 Mobile Marketing in Health Use Cases

The objective of this paper is to create a mobile application for mobile marketing. This mobile application is an extension of the MedClick online platform, a medical appointment booking service.

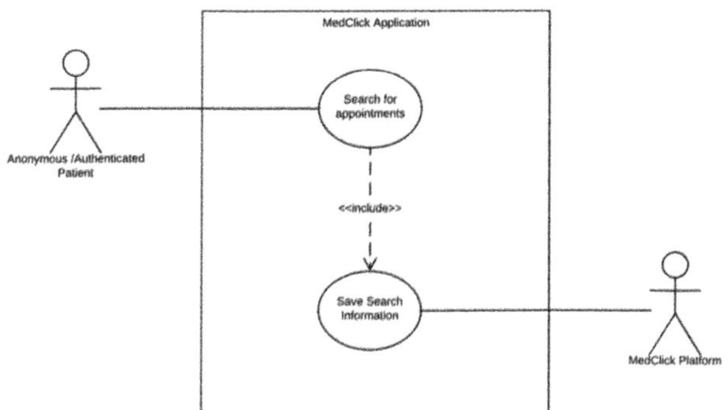

Fig. 1. Searching for Appointment Use Case [25].

MedClick is a web platform in which users schedule medical appointments based on the date, location, price, insurance providers and customer reviews. The mobile application is expected to integrate all the functionality of the web platform and enhance it with mobile marketing techniques. This adds value to the whole MedClick platform, that in this way can reach more users and in different devices, giving the user the ability to do the same task regardless of the device used. The approach proposed also takes advantage of the location sensors of mobile devices to support the medical appointment search process and in providing the user with useful push notifications.

The MedClick mobile application is expected to ensure the following major features:

- Searching for a medical appointment - The user, authenticated or not, can search for a medical appointment by specialty, location, date, health professional, price, insurance providers or customer reviews (see Fig. 1). It is not required authentication for this feature, to allow for a wider user base and for a better user experience, not having to login or sign up before exploring anything on the application.
- Booking a medical appointment – After reviewing all the previous point parameters, location, date, health professional, price, insurance providers and reviews, and selecting an available time slot for the appointment, the user is required to login or sign up in order to book the appointment (see Fig. 2).
- History of the medical appointments – The authenticated user can review all the previously attended appointments. This feature also includes the preview of the future appointments so that the user can keep track and cancel them if needed.
- Alerts for future appointments – The application should send a push notification to the user when the appointment date is close to make sure the user doesn't forget about it (Fig. 3).

- Mobile Marketing – Depending on the mobile marketing campaign available in the MedClick platform, the application sends a push notification to the user (Fig. 4).

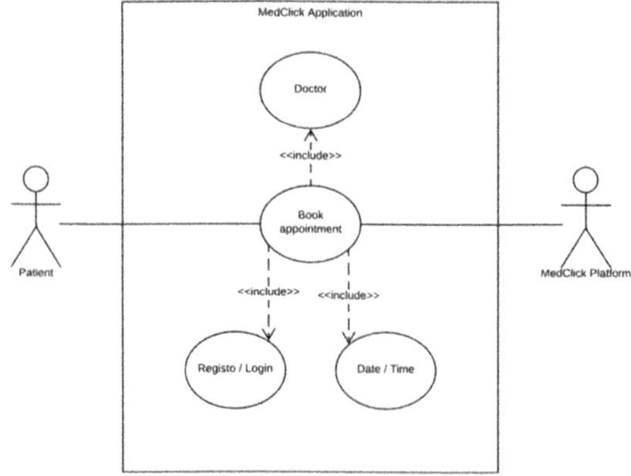

Fig. 2. Booking Medical Appointment Use Case [25].

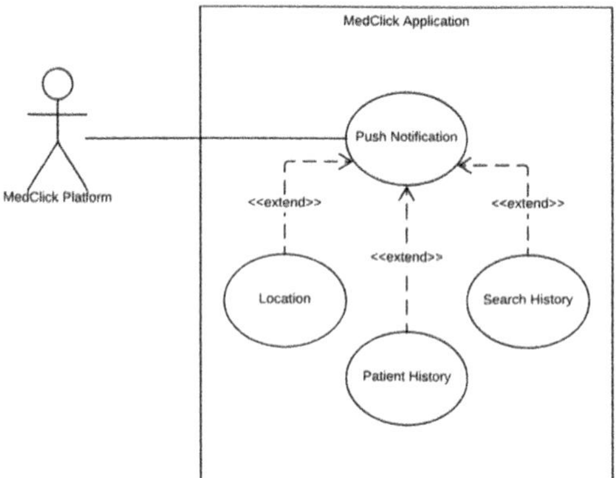

Fig. 3. Push Notification Use Case [25].

4 Mobile Marketing App

Based on the research made about cross platform mobile application frameworks, the framework chosen was the React Native with Expo toolchain[2]. With Native React it is possible to build a mobile application that is indistinguishable from a native mobile

[2] https://expo.io/.

application built using Swift or Java because it uses the same building blocks as regular iOS and Android applications. It will provide a superior user experience than hybrid applications. Additionally, from a development viewpoint, that is possible using just JavaScript code without the need to learn swift or C#. Features like hot reloading and simpler application deployment also support this decision.

After deciding about the development framework, the approach was to wireframe the application and all the functionalities before implementing them. Using wireframes, it was checked if the usability guidelines were being followed.

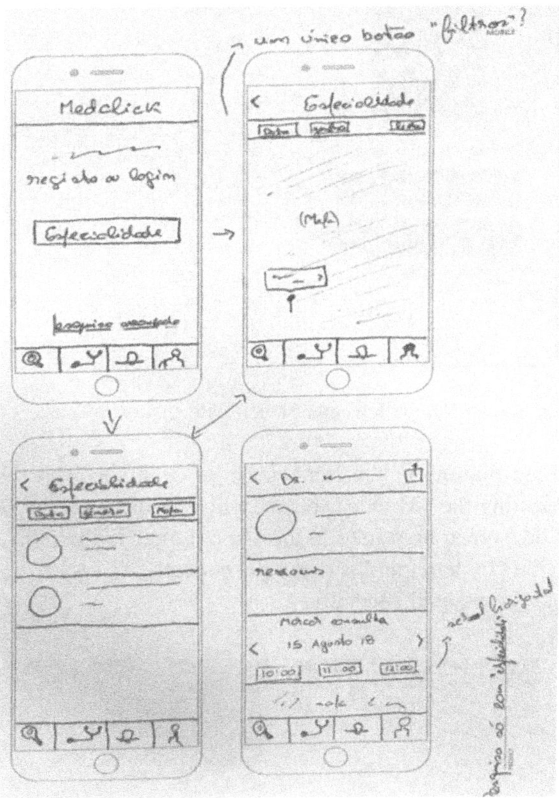

Fig. 4. Application wireframe example [25].

The next step was to start developing the application. The expo toolchain makes the initialization of the project a straightforward process. The command "expo init" gives several options to start the project. It was chosen a template with several example screens and tabs that were very similar to the design in the wireframes. After that it was a matter of developing screen by screen and feature by feature, testing them when implemented. These features include having an onboarding screen to introduce the user to the application, prioritizing most of the interaction with the application before login and sending push notifications to engage with the user.

4.1 Book Medical Appointment Process

The medical appointment process starts in the main screen of the application, as presented in Fig. 5. This screen provides users the suggestion to book a medical appointment.

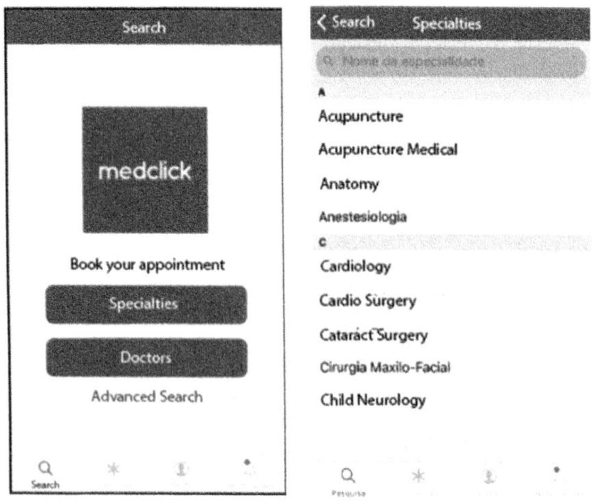

Fig. 5. Main Search Screen (on the left) and Screen with List of Specialties (on the right) [25].

Users have three options in this screen: choosing a specialty, choosing a health professional or selecting the advanced search option. If the specialty option is selected, users navigate to the screen presented in the same figure (in the right), a section list of the specialties divided by letter and sorted alphabetically. Users can also use the search bar to quickly find the wanted specialty.

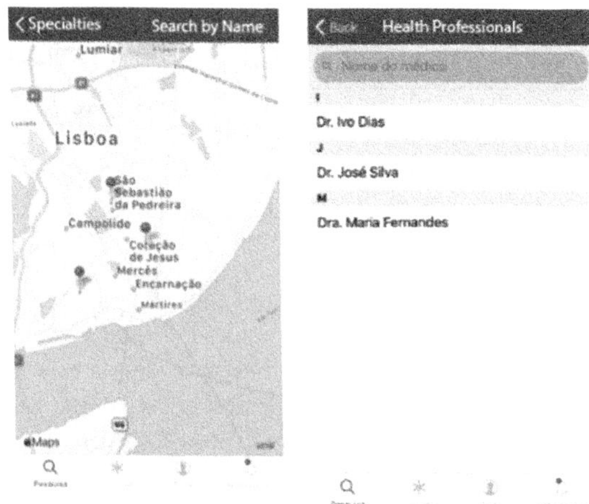

Fig. 6. Map Screen (on the left) and Screen with List of Health Professionals (on the right) [25].

The next screen presents a map that includes the locations of the healthcare providers that have medical services of the selected specialty (Fig. 6). In this screen users can tap on any map pin to select a healthcare provider or skip this step and choose the health professional by name.

In the main screen (Fig. 5), if users pressed the health Providers (Doctors) instead of the specialties, they would skip the list specialties screen and the map screen and navigate directly to the screen where they can choose the preferred health professional (Fig. 6).

After choosing the specialty, the health provider and the health professional, it is presented with a screen containing all the information about the health professional. In this screen, users can view the name of the health provider, contact, location, availabilities, map with providers, rating and curriculum (Fig. 7).

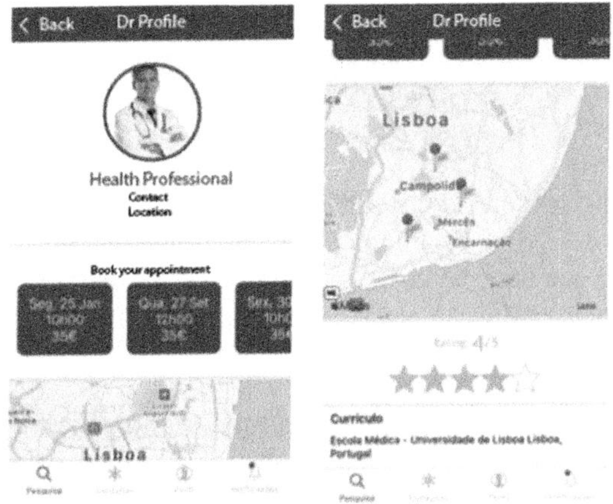

Fig. 7. Health Professional Information Screens [25].

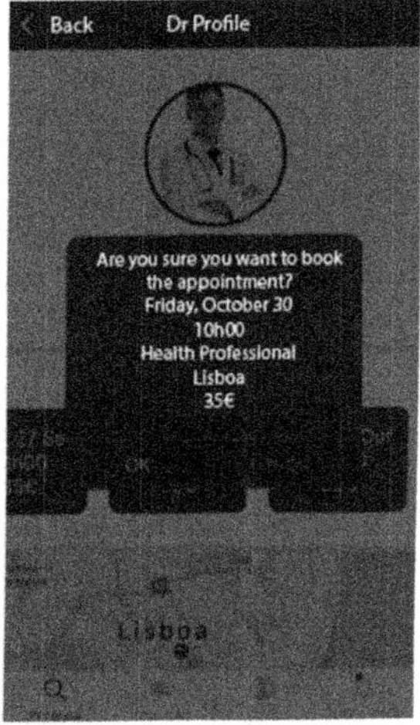

Fig. 8. Appointment Confirmation Alert [25].

When users select the desired date of the medical appointment, an alert appears on the screen to confirm all the choices made by the user (Fig. 8).

The next screen depends if the users are already logged in or not. If they are not logged in, a login screen is presented.

If the users are already logged in, they are redirected to the Appointments tab, where they can review all the past and future medical appointments booked through MedClick. An alert is shown letting the user know that the appointment is booked.

4.2 User Onboarding

Having an Onboarding screen is a very important aspect of the user experience of a mobile application. It gives users a quick and simple introduction in the first time they open the application, explaining its basic functionality. For this solution it was chosen a simple swipeable card interface with four cards in total, showing just one at a time. The four cards represent the four tabs of the application: Search, Appointments, Profile and Notifications. In each card, the name of the tab is a small description of that section, and contains information regarding what the users will find and can do in that section – see Fig. 9 and Fig. 10.

This way, even before interacting with the application, the users already know what to expect and where to find the functionality they are looking for. Only one card appears in the screen at a time, however it is possible to see part of the next card, giving users the idea that there are more cards to see and interact.

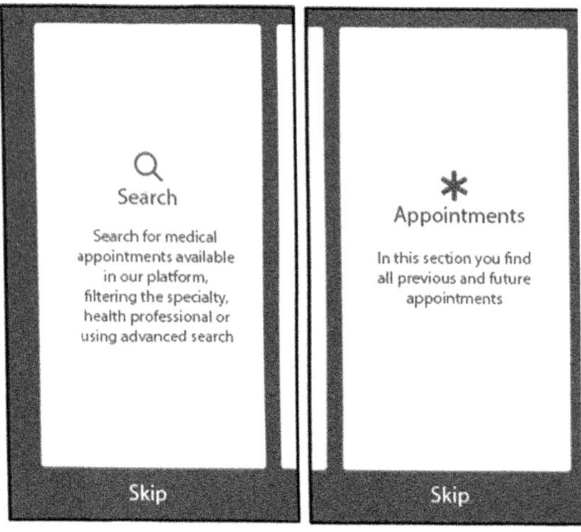

Fig. 9. Onboarding Screens (1/2) [25].

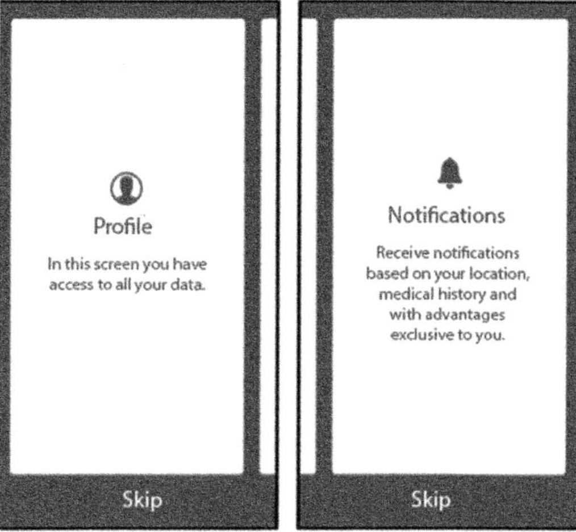

Fig. 10. Onboarding Screens (2/2) [25].

Below the cards there is an always visible button to skip this introduction screen. This gives users the chance to see all the cards or just ignore the tutorial all together, not making them lose time with something that they are not interested in.

4.3 Prioritize Search Before Login

All medical booking applications tested (see Sect. 2), apart from Zocdoc, request the user to login or register before even starting to use the application. This is a major obstacle to users because when they are expecting to start to interact with the application, and they must go through a tedious login or register process. MedClick mobile app has the goal of providing freedom to the user to search and use all the functionalities without the need to login or registration. This includes searching for an appointment, either by specialty or by health professional, searching the available healthcare providers and even receiving notifications based on the search history. This is achieved by creating a session linked to the device token, which can give the platform the ability to analyze the patients search history and notify them of a discounted appointment.

In the appointment tab and in the profile tab, when the user is not logged in, it is presented a simple button in the middle of the screen asking the user to login to access that information.

4.4 Mobile Notifications

One important aspect of the solution is the notifications functionality. There are several scenarios where a notification should be deployed to the application:

- When users enter a predetermined area, established by the MedClick platform, where it is available a mobile marketing campaign or some suggestion to the users of a certain location.

- All the search history of the users is saved on the MedClick platform, where it can then be analyzed to send suggestions of appointments and schedules based on that user's history. When this happens, a notification is sent to the user.
- To remind users of upcoming medical appointments. The application sends a push notification to the user when the appointment date is close to make sure the user did not forget about it.

For this to happen, when the user logs in the application, it sends to the server the token that identifies the device when receiving notifications, the ExpoPushToken. This token is then associated to the logged user. This way, anytime a notification is triggered to a specific user, the server knows to what device to send the notification (Fig. 11).

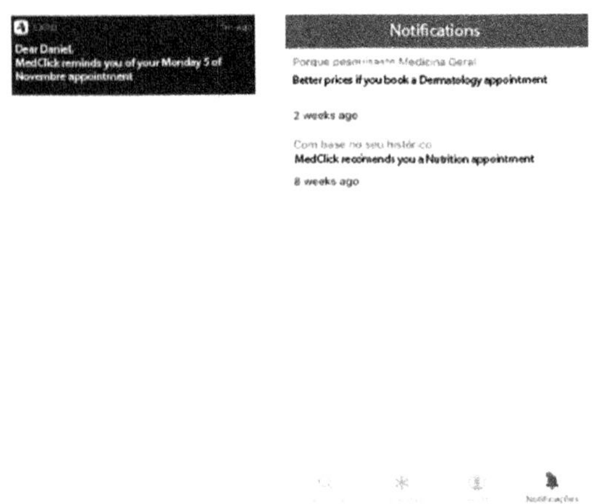

Fig. 11. Notification Screens [25].

4.5 User Information Logging

All the requests made by the application to the platform are saved in order keep track of the users' habits inside the application. This way it is possible for the users to receive notifications based on their search history, with suggestions for appointments or even discounted appointments.

5 Results Assessment

In this section it is described the iterative testing methodology and its contribution to the final solution. Then it is described the Focus Group Test Scenarios and its results. Finally, the limitations of the tests are discussed.

5.1 Iterative Testing Approach

The approach developed aim at having real users testing each iteration of the application. When testing, users will always have access to a feedback tab on the application where they can give feedback about the current screen. After concluding the testing process, it is presented a small questionnaire to the users with questions about their age, gender, profession and education. All this information is sent to the MedClick servers, as well as the users' location and information about the time spent on each screen of the application.

The test methodology was planned in order to receive real users' feedback and to improve the application in iterative steps. The first functionality tested was the book appointment process. The application was sent to several users. Some flaws were discovered very quickly. In the logs it was visible that some users were not completing the full testing process. Additionally, others were stuck on the same screen for a long period of time. There were also duplicated logs of users that reloaded the application and interacted again.

In total, in this short first iteration test, it was gathered data from 11 trustworthy tests, 8 male test users and 3 female test users, with an average age of 29,4 years. It was concluded that with these errors leading to such a small amount of data gathered, the testing approach should change and rely on focus group testing.

5.2 Focus Group Testing

After the first small iterative testing, it was decided to change the approach to a focus group testing, using a small group of people to test the application (in person), in this case, 18 people. Each person was given three test scenarios where he or she had to perform certain tasks in both the MedClick mobile application and in two other medical booking applications reviewed in Sect. 2, namely "My CUF" and "Joaquim Chaves Saúde" applications. These applications were chosen because they were the most similar ones to the proposed solution, in the Portuguese market.

To measure the impact of not having a login screen as the first interaction of the user with the application, users had to start each test without a logged session or any other preference in the application. Another reason for this was that neither My CUF nor Joaquim Chaves Saúde retain the user login after exiting the application. So, to make testing similar across all applications, login was needed in all scenarios.

Scenario 1 - Appointment Booking for a Health Professional. The first scenario given to the test users was to book an appointment for a specific health professional. This scenario assesses the impact of having a quick option to select the desired health professional and test the premise that if a patient wants to have a medical appointment with a specific health professional, all other parameters are not that relevant.

Table 2. Scenario 1 results [25].

Application	Average time to complete scenario	Standard deviation of average times
My CUF (Health Professional Maria de Vasconcelos)	≈1 m 25 s	≈18 s
Joaquim Chaves Saúde (Health Professional Maria de Fátima Miguel)	≈1 m 43 s	≈25 s
MedClick Mobile Application (Health Professional Maria Fernandes)	≈53 s	≈11 s

Most users had no problems in quickly identifying the search by health professional on the MedClick mobile application. This translated in Table 2 results, where users were in average more than 30 s quicker to complete the task comparing to the other two applications.

Another reason for these results were some bugs with the My CUF application that sometimes just loads blank screens and the user must go back and try to submit the request again for the process to continue.

Also, on the Joaquim Chaves Saúde application, even when choosing a specific health professional, the application requires users to select the type of appointment. This translated in an extra step users have to go through, most of times to select the only option presented, making this action completely unnecessary.

Lastly, one feedback received multiple times was to change the alert presented to after the login screen when login is needed. That way the last step before booking the appointment was confirming it.

Scenario 2 - Appointment Booking by Specialty. The second test scenario was to give users the task of booking another medical appointment but this time with the specialty as a main focus. All other parameters such as location, health professionals, date or others were completely optional and up to the user. This test assesses the impact of having the specialty parameter in the first step when trying to book a medical appointment (Table 3).

Table 3. Scenario 2 results [25].

Application	Average time to complete scenario	Standard deviation of average times
My CUF (Dermatology)	≈1 m 08 s	≈15 s
Joaquim Chaves Saúde (Dermatology)	≈1 m 11 s	≈18 s
MedClick Mobile Application (Dermatology)	≈1 m 04 s	≈14 s

In this test scenario, results were very similar across all applications, mainly because users had to go through every step when booking the appointment. This confirms the importance of having an option for the user to search directly for health professionals.

Scenario 3 – Past and Future Appointments. The third test scenario is simpler than scenario 1 and 2. It was given to the user the simple task of checking their past and future appointments. This scenario tests the utility of having a quick access to the patient's past and future appointments, accessing it via a main tab in the main screen of the application (Table 4).

Table 4. Scenario 3 results [25].

Application	Average time to complete scenario	Standard deviation of average times
My CUF	≈44 s	≈9 s
Joaquim Chaves Saúde	≈1 m 08 s	≈15 s
MedClick Mobile Application	≈38 s	≈8 s

The times referring My CUF and MedClick mobile application are mainly the time users spent logging in because both applications have the appointments tab quickly accessible and in an intuitive manner. The MedClick mobile application has a label below the icon on that tab, however numerous users pointed the lack of contrast making it difficult to read and quickly identify it. Several users were completely lost in the Joaquim Chaves Saúde application, because this tab does not have an intuitive name and many were looking in the appointments search section, confirming that having an option to search inside the tab with the past and future appointments is a good idea.

Scenario 4 – User Profile Information. The fourth and last test scenario is very similar to the third one. It is simply asked for users to review their profile information in the application (Table 5).

Table 5. Scenario 4 results [25].

Application	Average time to complete scenario	Standard deviation of average times
My CUF	≈42 s	≈13 s
Joaquim Chaves Saúde	≈46 s	≈14 s
MedClick Mobile Application	≈37 s	≈13 s

Once again, most of the time spent in this scenario was due to login, and in here most users had no problems finding the profile tab and completing the task. It should be noted that in a real-world scenario, MedClick mobile application saves the user login when closing the application, dramatically improving these times.

5.3 Limitations

In the iterative testing approach (presented in Sect. 5.1), user created errors resulting in false results, making hard to identify the causes of the real average time spent in each screen (bad user experience versus user disinterest).

On the other hand, the focus group test approach was important to overcome these limitations, but it has other limitations regarding the restricted audience.

The authors recommend that the app follows a soft-launch or pilot approach in order to enlarge the significance of the results. With a large number of users, it is expect to assess if the consumer prefers a web interface or a mobile app, if the mobile application brings new users to the platform and if they engage more with the platform (considering the marketing efforts).

6 Conclusions

The ability to provide services without human contact is mandatory for most industries. Currently, healthcare companies, to be "in business", must provide consumers the ability to book medical appointments anywhere, with any device.

This paper contributes to this subject by presenting a comprehensive background research, including i) an assessment of the major mobile development frameworks; ii) an review on mobile marketing; ii) a description on user experience approaches on mobile; and iv) an analysis of mobile medical appointments booking applications.

The research presented in this paper also describes the major uses for mobile marketing in the health sector, including i) searching for appointment, ii) booking a medical appointment, iii) history of the medical appointments, iv) alerts for future appointments, and v) mobile marketing.

The description of the implementation of a mobile marketing app, in the context of the health sector, is also presented by describing i) the book medical appointment process, ii) the user onboarding, iii) the approach on prioritize search before login, iv) the mobile notifications, and v) the user information logging.

The results achieved were assessed and improved through an iterative testing approach, that provided important feedback to the development process. Additionally, user testing was performed in four scenarios. The mobile application implemented presents above average user experience results that point to high adoption rates by real world users.

The authors suggest that, as future work, the application usability is assessed using an online survey, like the System Usability Scale (SUS) questionnaire. Another future research path is on assessing the impact of GDPR on mobile marketing use cases.

Considering the results presented in this paper, the authors expect that the further mobile marketing applications are deployed soon, and further functionalities are developed, with a relevant impact in the health sector process.

Acknowledgements. This work was supported by national funds through Fundação para a Ciência e a Tecnologia (FCT) with reference UID/CEC/50021/2019 and by the European Commission program H2020 under the grant agreement 822404 (project QualiChain).

References

1. GlobalStats StatCounter: Mobile Operating System Market Share Worldwide, December 2017–2019. https://gs.statcounter.com/os-market-share/mobile/worldwide. Accessed 28 Apr 2020
2. PhoneGap Homepage. https://phonegap.com/. Accessed 28 Apr 2020
3. Martinez, M., Lecomte, S.: Towards the quality improvement of cross-platform mobile applications. In: 2017 IEEE/ACM 4th International Conference on Mobile Soft-ware Engineering and Systems (MOBILESoft), Buenos Aires, pp. 184–188 (2017)
4. Xamarin Homepage. https://visualstudio.microsoft.com/xamarin/. Accessed 28 Apr 2020
5. React Native Homepage. https://facebook.github.io/react-native/. Accessed 28 Apr 2020
6. Asp, F.: A comparison of ionic 2 versus react native and android in terms of performance, by comparing the performance of applications (2018)
7. Expo Toolchain Homepage. https://expo.io. Accessed 28 Apr 2020
8. Shankar, V., Balasubramanian, S.: Mobile marketing: a synthesis and prognosis. J. Interact. Mark. **23**(2), 118–129 (2009)
9. Leppaniemi, M.: Mobile Marketing Communications in Consumer Markets. Oulin Yliopisto, Oulu (2008)
10. Gana, M., Toney, T., Kashif, H.: Consumers' value assessment on location-based service application as a mobile marketing tool. Int. J. Bus. Appl. Soc. Sci. **2**(3), 1–10 (2016)
11. Berman, B.: Referral marketing: harnessing the power of your customers. Bus. Horiz. **59**(1), 19–28 (2016)
12. Increase in Onboarding conversion, Localytics. https://info.localytics.com/hubfs/Case_Studies/Slice_Case_Study.pdf. Accessed 28 Apr 2020
13. Apple Developer Human Interface Guidelines. https://developer.apple.com/design/human-interface-guidelines/. Accessed 28 Apr 2020
14. Google's Material Design Guidelines. https://material.io/design/. Accessed 28 Apr 2020
15. Clifton, I.G.: Android User Interface Design: Implementing Material Design for Developers. Pearson Education, London (2015)
16. Saint-Exupéry, A., Galantière, L., Gilbert S.: 1943. Airman's Odyssey. Reynal & Hitchcock, New York (1984)
17. CUF Homepage. https://www.saudecuf.pt/. Accessed 28 Apr 2020
18. Apple Developer Human Interface Guidelines – Tabbars. https://developer.apple.com/design/human-interface-guidelines/ios/bars/tab-bars/. Accessed 28 Apr 2020
19. Google Design - Design from iOS to Android. https://design.google/library/design-ios-android-and-back-again/. Accessed 28 Apr 2020
20. Comparison between iOS and Android Applications. https://medium.com/@aoniwang/cross-platform-app-design-why-do-some-apps-look-different-on-ios-and-android-b75a1e3bf440. Accessed 28 Apr 2020
21. Zocdoc Homepage. https://www.zocdoc.com. Accessed 28 Apr 2020

22. Knok Healthcare Homepage. https://www.knokcare.com. Accessed 28 Apr 2020
23. Joaquim Chaves Saúde Homepage. https://www.jcs.pt/pt/home. Accessed 28 Apr 2020
24. Android Navigation Drawer. https://developer.android.com/training/implementing-navigation/nav-drawer/. Accessed 28 Apr 2020
25. Fernandes, T., Vasconcelos, A.: A user centred approach in the implementation of mobile marketing in health applications. In: Proceedings of the 14th International Conference on Health Informatics (HEALTHINF 2020), February 2020

Stochastic Workflow Modeling in a Surgical Ward: Towards Simulating and Predicting Patient Flow

Christoffer O. Back[1], Areti Manataki[4(✉)], Angelos Papanastasiou[3], and Ewen Harrison[2]

[1] Department of Computer Science, University of Copenhagen, Copenhagen, Denmark
back@di.ku.dk
[2] Usher Institute, University of Edinburgh, Edinburgh, U.K.
mail@ewenharrison.com
[3] Department of Mathematics and Statistics, University of Cyprus, Nicosia, Cyprus
apapan06@ucy.ac.cy
[4] School of Computer Science, University of St Andrews, St Andrews, U.K.
A.Manataki@st-andrews.ac.uk

Abstract. Intelligent systems play an increasingly central role in healthcare systems worldwide. Nonetheless, operational friction represents an obstacle to full utilization of scarce resources and improvement of service standards. In this paper we address the challenge of developing data-driven models of complex workflow systems - a prerequisite for harnessing intelligent technologies for workflow improvement. We present a proof-of-concept model parametrized using real-world data and constructed based on domain knowledge from the Royal Infirmary of Edinburgh, demonstrating how off-the-shelf process mining, machine learning and stochastic process modeling tools can be combined to build predictive models that capture complex control flow, constraints, policies and guidelines.

Keywords: Surgery · Surgical workflow · Bayesian network · Petri nets · Simulation · Data mining · Patient flow · Process mining

1 Introduction

Surgical care is a key component of healthcare systems worldwide, saving and improving thousands of lives every day. Over 10 million operations are performed each year in England [34], including high-risk cases and patients that require immediate life, limb or organ-saving interventions. Surgical care is also very costly, with more than $400 billion spent each year in the United States on operative procedures [1]. The number of people requiring surgery is rising every year, often leading to long waiting times that may put patients at risk.

Ensuring efficiency, timeliness and safety are crucial for providing high-quality service while controlling costs [16,26]. While many processes surrounding surgery are well structured, the dynamic nature of patient arrivals combined

X. Ye et al. (Eds.): BIOSTEC 2020, CCIS 1400, pp. 565–591, 2021.
https://doi.org/10.1007/978-3-030-72379-8_28

with the complexity of coordinating large numbers of specialized staff and facilities, means that delays and misalignments can have cascading effects leading to last-minute cancellations and under-utilization of expensive resources. There is, hence, an imperative need to improve surgical workflow. Some key questions here are: How can we improve overall surgical care performance in the most cost-effective way? How can we plan surgical care in a way that it is tailored to the individual patient?

There is a wealth of data being collected through hospital IT systems, which can be used towards answering these questions. This includes operating room management and usage data, electronic health records and surgery cancellation data. By adopting a process-based approach, one can make sense of such complex and big data and inform improvements in surgical care processes, including intelligent surgery planning, staff scheduling and workflow management.

This paper extends previous work [6] by presenting a preliminary investigation into stochastic workflow modeling and verification methods in surgical wards, with outset in a data set following patients from admission to discharge at the Royal Infirmary of Edinburgh in Scotland. With the aim of gaining a comprehensive understanding of surgical workflow, we use the data to investigate both *system-wide* surgical performance and *individual* patient flow. Results from these two types of modeling can be combined to enable personalised and efficient surgical scheduling.

In particular, we discuss how process mining methods can be used to gain insights regarding control-flow and temporal patterns in the surgical ward. Focusing on system-wide performance and recognizing the high level of uncertainty in the surgical department, we demonstrate how Stochastic Time Petri Nets can be used to effectively capture complex hospital policies and constraints. The choice of Stochastic Time Petri Nets allows for simulation of different scenarios, thus enabling what-if analysis. This is key for investigating different, and often competing, workflow improvement mechanisms. Focusing on individual patient flow, we propose the use of Bayesian Networks to predict patient-specific cycle times of individual surgical phases, from the time patients are sent for, through anesthesia and surgery, and until they leave recovery. Aside from their capacity to easily incorporate domain knowledge, Bayesian networks have the advantage that they can be queried in complex ways even with incomplete evidence, which is invaluable in the uncertain hospital environment. We present and compare three probabilistic models and we evaluate them w.r.t. to prediction accuracy. Crucially, we show that by incorporating a pre-processing step based on simple clustering of flows w.r.t. cycle times, we can improve the performance of our models noticeably.

The rest of the paper is structured as follows. In Sect. 2 we review existing literature. Our subsequent analysis of the data follows the classic data analytics workflow of *Describe* → *Diagnose* → *Predict*. In Sect. 3 we introduce the domain, the data set, and the data cleaning process. In Sect. 4, we present a descriptive analysis of the data set using process mining and standard statistical tools to identify control-flow and temporal patterns in the data. This informs the process of building system-wide simulation models and individual-patient predictive models, which we describe and evaluate in Sect. 5. In Sect. 6 we discuss our results and in Sect. 7 we conclude and discuss directions for future work.

2 Related Work

The modeling of surgical workflows has received a significant amount of attention by researchers, motivated by the prerogative to improve efficiency and resource utilisation while ensuring adherence to service standards.

Of particular interest for the present case study is the National Theatres Project in Scotland which outlines several areas for improvement that might be addressed by workflow optimization. This includes "appropriately increasing patient throughput, thereby using resources more productively and efficiently" by reducing unutilized (operating room) hours; reducing over/under-runs, late-starts, cancellations and delayed discharges; and avoiding unnecessary out-of-hours and nighttime procedures [32].

Previous research on modeling surgical ward processes varies greatly in terms of scope: from very fine-grained models of individual procedures to high-level models of treatment pathways well beyond the context of the surgical ward itself (e.g. from visit to a GP to follow-up evaluation and treatment). In their literature review on the topic [26] Laylis and Jannin identify a range of granularity. At the finest level are low-level physical movements such as tool usage patterns based on sensor data [4], phase detection [37], automatic identification of hand motions from video in [27] and [20]. Several investigations have been made into the modelling of Cholecystectomies, a highly standardized procedure [10–12,31].

In [36] the authors go beyond the modeling of the surgical procedure to include anesthesia and early recovery within the operating theatre, while [19] considers the patient flow from admission to recovery. Activities downstream from surgery, namely recovery in ICU wards can present a key bottleneck, as addressed in [5]. Extending the patient pathway further, follow-up post-surgery is incorporated in [21,28]. In general, however, most research appears to have focused primarily on either very low-level procedure or high-level treatment pathways. The patient flows we consider fall in between these levels of granularity.

The use of Bayesian networks to model stays in an emergency department is evaluated in [3]. In contrast to our approach, the view of patient flows is at a higher level of abstraction, and the main focus is the comparison of structure learning algorithms.

Modeling the duration of surgical procedures was investigated in [24,38] and we are able to report findings in line with these regarding the log-normal distribution of surgical times. Surgical duration was incorporated into sequencing and scheduling strategies in [16]. Stochastic balancing of bed capacity based on fluctuating demand patterns was explored in [15] and length of stay patterns in [5] while resource allocation and patient admission was addressed in [22].

More broadly, the problem of ensuring that systems fulfill a given set of specifications has been widely addressed in model checking and process mining research. The systems under consideration can range from electronic circuits and communication protocols [29,33], to business processes [14,23] and even biological systems [17].

We can verify whether a system satisfies a property or specification by means of state-space exploration [40] or rewrite rules [8], but often realistic models reach a level of complexity that precludes closed-form verification. This leaves simulation, essentially a random sampling of the model's state space, as a next best tool for verification and what-if analysis.

Incorporating desired constraints into a system model is straightforward [7], and allows for correct-by-construction plan generation, but also leads to state-space explosion. Advancements in seemingly unrelated areas such as robot motion [18] provide evidence that this approach to intelligent planning is feasible, even in complex domains.

3 Domain and Data Preparation

We were granted access to workflow data recorded at The Royal Infirmary of Edinburgh in connection with cases taking place from 2010 until 2018. The infirmary is Scotland's largest, with 900 beds and a 24-h accident and emergency department. The data at our disposal was recorded by the Operating Room Scheduling Office System (ORSOS), which is one component in the institution's overall IT-infrastructure.

Over 1700 types of procedures are recorded in the data set, about half of which are classified as emergency cases. Each treatment procedure is given a unique case ID, meaning that the same patient may be associated with multiple case IDs, even during the same stay for inpatients. Following patients' broader treatment patterns would be possible using this dataset, but lies beyond the scope and focus of this paper.

Data is entered manually by surgical support personnel, with the system requiring the entry of timestamps for each event in the patient flow. Figure 1 illustrates the proscribed sequence of events, along with an aggregation of activities into logical phases (pre-op, anesthesia, surgery, recovery).

The system attempts to enforce a strict linear ordering of events, though this can be overridden by personnel. If a timestamp is entered out of sequence, a warning is given, but can be entered upon confirmation. Staff are then sent a summary of anomalous cases for review at the end of the week.

Data Schema. In addition to timestamps for the 11 proscribed activities in a patient flow, 34 other attributes are recorded. Attributes of note include two different procedure coding schemes, case type (emergency/scheduled, day-case/inpatient), NCEPOD urgency classification[1], and the ASA patient condition rating.

---

[1] NCEPOD Classification of Intervention [30].

Some staffing details are also included, such as main and supervising surgeon and anesthetist, as well as the consultant assigned to the case. The source of admission (emergency room, etc.), as well as intended and actual destination following surgery (ICU, etc.) and crucially, the operating room number, are also included. Further details include the diabetic status of the patient, types of anesthetics administered, whether antibiotics were administered, and whether pre-session briefings and surgical pauses were held.

Cleaning and Preparation. A number of clearly anomalous entries are present in the dataset, comprising roughly 10% of the 38,728 entries. Due to the relatively small percentage of anomalies and the reasonably large dataset, we followed a precautionary principle and simply removed entire cases containing anomalous entries prior to further analysis and modeling. Table 1 provides an overview.

Duplicate entries may have been due to an attempt to correct a data entry error, but we are unable to determine which entry is reliable. The column *anaesthetic start time* was the only timestamp column to contain `NA` values. A larger number of cases have clearly anomalous values in the case date column, e.g. dates much too far in the past (year 1800) or future (year 3206).

Table 1. Anomalous cases removed prior to analysis. Originally published in [6].

Anomaly	Count	% of Total
Duplicate entries	58	0.15
Missing values	31	0.08
Dates out-of-range	475	1.23
Zero timestamps	3089	7.98
Bad ordering	443	1.44
Total	4096	10.58

4 Analysis

4.1 Control Flow Patterns

Based on input from domain experts, we were aware of the *de jure* workflow, which follows a simple linear flow of events as illustrated in Fig. 1. In addition to the anomalies discussed in Sect. 3, process mining techniques helped reveal further control-flow deviations, guiding the data cleaning process. In particular, we found dotted charts, directly-follows graphs and mined Petri Nets to be particularly informative.

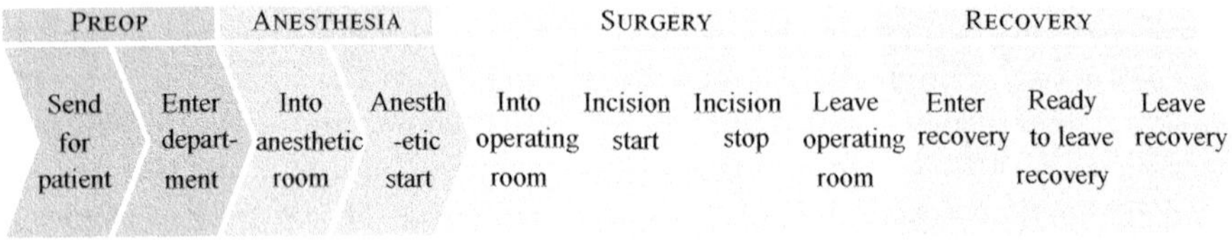

PREOP | ANESTHESIA | SURGERY | RECOVERY

Send for patient | Enter department | Into anesthetic room | Anesthetic start | Into operating room | Incision start | Incision stop | Leave operating room | Enter recovery | Ready to leave recovery | Leave recovery

Fig. 1. The *de jure* sequence of events recorded by the ORSOS system, representing the intended patient flow. Activities are linearly ordered, but can occur "simultaneously". That is, some activities (such as *Leave Operating Room*) can have the same timestamp as the "succeeding" activity (*Enter Recovery*), but should not occur after it. Originally published in [6].

Dotted Chart. One simple yet powerful tool for getting a quick, preliminary overview of process-related data is the dotted chart, which simply charts events w.r.t. case-id across time such that dots falling along a horizontal line represent events belonging to the same process instance (i.e. case).

Using the dotted chart in Fig. 2 we immediately identified a substantial gap in the dataset. Furthermore, we can see that some cases have events occurring many months, even years apart - almost certainly evidence of anomalous entries.

Directly-Follows Graph. Another simple visualization tool, directly-follows graphs consist of nodes and directed edges, where nodes represent the events in the log, and an edge exists between two nodes if there is at least one log trace where the source event is followed by the target event. Figure 3 shows the directly-follows graph obtained for our dataset, which includes node and edge frequencies. On one hand, the event frequencies on the graph confirmed that all events were included in each trace, in accordance with the *de jure* work-

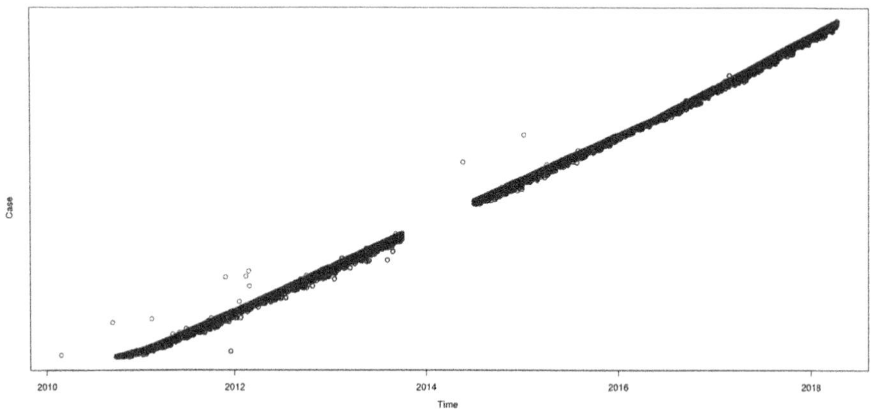

Fig. 2. A dotted chart showing all events in our dataset, arranged according to case id and timestamp. Originally published in [6].

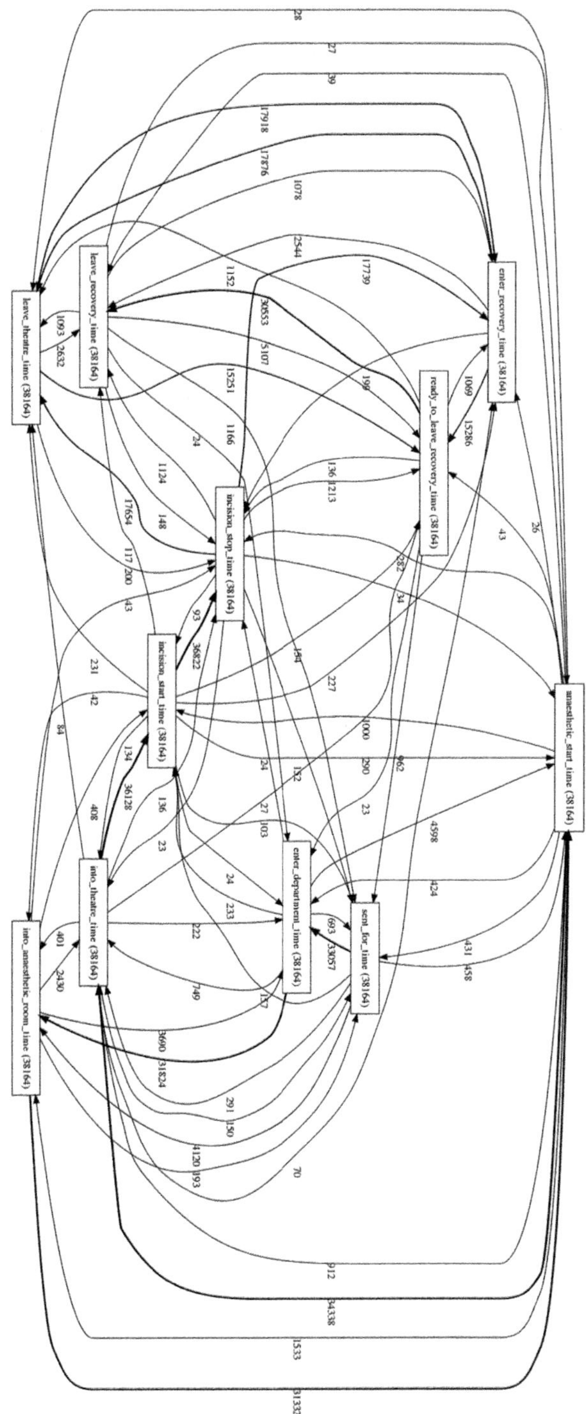

Fig. 3. Directly-follows graph indicating that nearly all possible pairwise event orderings occurred at least once in the data.

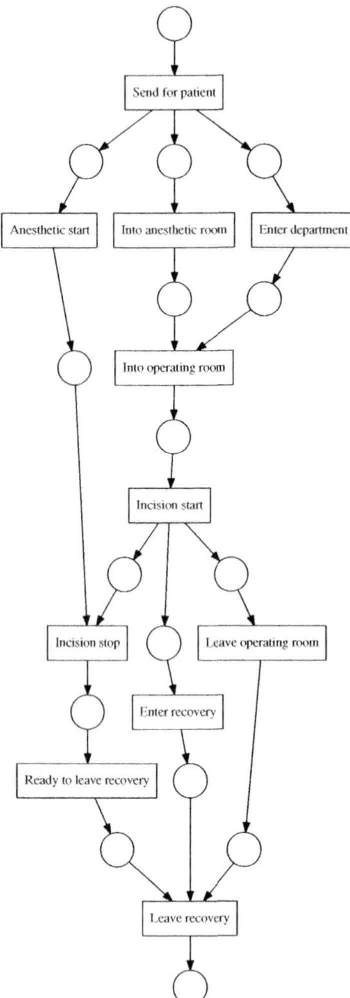

Fig. 4. Petri net generated by the Alpha miner on the top 20 trace variants. Originally published in [6].

flow. On the other hand, the graph indicated that nearly all possible pairwise event orderings occurred at least once in the data. This is inconsistent with the *de jure* workflow, and it includes several implausible event orderings. For example, there were a remarkable 154 traces where the last event in the *de jure* workflow, namely *leave_recovery_time*, occurs before the proscribed first event, namely *sent_for_time*.

Alpha Miner. For a more nuanced view of the control-flow evidenced by the event log, proper process mining algorithms can be used. The Alpha (α) miner was one of the first process mining algorithms developed, and though it has limitations regarding the variety of control constructs it is able to identify, for our purposes it provided interesting insights into course of events as evidenced by the data.

Figure 4 shows the result of running the SIMPLE version of the Alpha miner [2] from the `pm4py` package [9] on the top 20 sequence variants in the log. Mining on the entire log produces a flower model - a model which permits any behavior, in line with observation from the directly-follows graph in Fig. 3.

According to this model, several remarkable control patterns seem to be evidenced by the most frequently occurring sequence variants. For example, according to Fig. 4, *anesthetic_start* is not a precondition for *incision_start*. This observation led us to inquire with experts at the infirmary and to more closely investigate these cases in the dataset. Apparently, it was not uncommon for these two events to have exactly the same timestamp: a reflection, for example, of cases in which a surgeon administers a local anesthetic immediately prior to a minor surgery.

This observation gives rise to a further insight: nearly all process mining algorithms have a strong assumption of temporal monotonicity, i.e. events are strictly linearly ordered such that no two events share *exactly* the same timestamp. With the coarse level of temporal accuracy (1–5 min) in our dataset, exactly co-occurring events were common. In this sense, most process mining algorithms are unable to account for *true* concurrency in data.

4.2 Temporal Patterns

Beyond identifying anomalies in the data, there were few interesting control-flow patterns to identify at the level of patient flows, since they do in fact follow a (non-monotonic) linear process.

This left temporal patterns as the next obvious aspect to investigate, especially since both resource usage and service guidelines are largely temporally focused (e.g. target time to theatre, anesthetist availability).

Event Aggregation. In part due to large numbers of zero-duration cycle-times due to the phenomenon of co-occurring events, but also based on conversations with experts, we decided to group individual events into the four phases illustrated in Fig. 1. Aside from clearly representing logically meaningful phases, it was also clear that this aggregation smoothed out cycle-time distributions.

On one hand, this process of aggregation arguably *removes* valuable information that could inform our model, on the other, it constitutes a form of dimensionality reduction which helps control the complexity of our model and ultimately improves performance in the end.

Marginal Distributions. The simplest temporal pattern at the level of patient flows is the marginal distribution of cycle times across all patients regardless of procedure, condition, urgency, etc. Fitting a probability distribution to the empirical distributions of cycle time also constitutes the simplest possible predictive model, i.e. the maximum likelihood prediction based on the best-fit distribution.

In Table 2 we show the goodness-of-fit statistics (Kolmogorov-Smirnov criterion) for 7 types of distributions for both the individual events and events aggregated into phases. Those distributions best fit to the phase data are visually depicted.

In building the stochastic Petri net described in Sect. 5, we used these marginal distributions to parametrized transitions representing these phases. However, our modeling tool restricted the families of probability distributions to Exponential, Erlang and polynomials of exponentials. We illustrate our approximations to the best-fit distributions in Table 2 and give the exact parametrizations in Table 5.

Table 2. *Red*: Best fits for marginal distributions of cycle times, goodness-of-fit statistic used is the Kolmogorov-Smirnov criterion. *Blue*: distributions used for modelling, in which our tool restricted the choice of distributions to Erlang (pre-op) and polynomials of exponentials (remaining). Originally published in [6].

EVENT	Gaussian	Cauchy	Logistic	Log-Normal	Gamma	Weibull	Exponential	PLOT (Best fit for aggregate)
	GOODNESS-OF-FIT (KS)							
Send for patient	0.147	0.113	0.139	0.169	0.126	0.104	0.267	
Enter department	0.161	0.147	0.197	0.205	0.171	0.157	0.184	
Pre-op	0.094	0.087	0.123	0.127	0.09	**0.062**	0.24	0 20 40 60
Into anesthetic	0.226	0.166	0.168	0.153	0.133	0.15	0.19	
Anesthetic start	0.146	0.098	0.134	0.171	0.112	0.096	0.189	
Anesthetic	0.124	**0.077**	0.106	0.188	0.132	0.106	0.244	0 20 40 60 80 100
Into theatre	0.16	0.094	0.143	0.111	0.093	0.114	0.298	
Incision start	0.164	0.122	0.144	0.061	0.06	0.07	0.132	
Incision stop	0.187	0.145	0.168	0.111	0.144	0.128	0.25	
Surgery	0.16	0.11	0.134	**0.036**	0.071	0.087	0.193	0 100 200 300 400 500
Enter recovery	0.083	0.079	0.126	0.243	0.174	0.139	0.198	
Ready to leave	0.285	0.277	0.266	0.184	0.144	0.144	0.22	
Recovery	0.099	**0.083**	0.127	0.244	0.17	0.136	0.19	0 100 200 300

Mutual Information. To get an impression of which attributes might be informative independent variables in conditional distributions of cycle times, we calculated estimates of pairwise mutual information. Having an eye to identifying variables for inclusion in the Bayesian networks described in Sect. 5.2, we were interested in mutual information between all attributes.

As a measure of the expected decrease in uncertainty regarding the outcome of variable X upon learning the outcome of Y, mutual information is akin to standard correlation metrics, but well suited to hybrid (discrete/continuous) attributes and makes no assumption regarding normality or linearity.

Recalling the definition of the Shannon entropy of a random variable X as its expected information content, denoted $H[X]$, we can write mutual information directly as the decrease in entropy of X upon learning the outcome of Y. Formally, $I(X;Y) = H[X] - H[X|Y]$. Two completely independent variables will have mutual information of $H[X] - H[X] = 0$, while for two perfectly correlated variables it collapses to the entropy of the dependent variable $H[X] - 0 = H[X]$.

However, as an expected value (averaged over the sample space), it can hide that specific outcomes for a variable can have a high *pointwise mutual information* - which could be harnessed by a predictive model - yet disappear amongst many uninformative outcomes. For this reason we also manually explored conditional distributions for cycle times.

Conditional Cycle Time Distributions. Our investigation around the most informative features in the data set continued by exploring the conditional distributions of cycle times for the individual values attributes. By visualizing conditional distributions on the same plot, one gets a quick impression of whether an attribute is informative in this respect, or not. Even though this is a somewhat time-consuming, brute-force approach, exploring the data in this way turned out to be quite informative. This analysis played an important role for us in choosing which variables to include in the models we present in Sect. 5.2. Examples of some of the most informative attributes are presented in Fig. 5. For instance, one can see that the conditional cycle time distributions for surgery differ considerably based on ASA status, i.e. for normal healthy patients (ASA status 1), for patients with severe systemic disease that is a constant threat to life (ASA status 4) and for patients with non-assessed ASA status. The anesthetic cycle time distributions conditioned on source of admission also differ considerably, with patient cases coming from the High Dependency Unit spending longer on average in Anesthesia, compared to those coming from the Admissions Unit or some other source.

Principal Component Analysis and Patient Clusters. We explored the presence of groupings of patients in regards to duration by a combination of visual analysis, data transformation and clustering.

Judging by the original durations of the 4 phases of a patient's flow, there do not appear to be clear groupings of patients (Fig. 6a). However, after applying principal components analysis (PCA) and plotting the data w.r.t. the four principal components, clear groupings become apparent (Fig. 6b). Since PCA assumes normally distributed data, and since most durations more closely follow a log-normal distribution, the data was log-transformed prior to PCA transformation.

Afterwards, k-means clustering was used to discover grouping of patients. This derived attribute was added to the dataset and our predictive models, noticeably improving peformance. It should be noted that we retained all

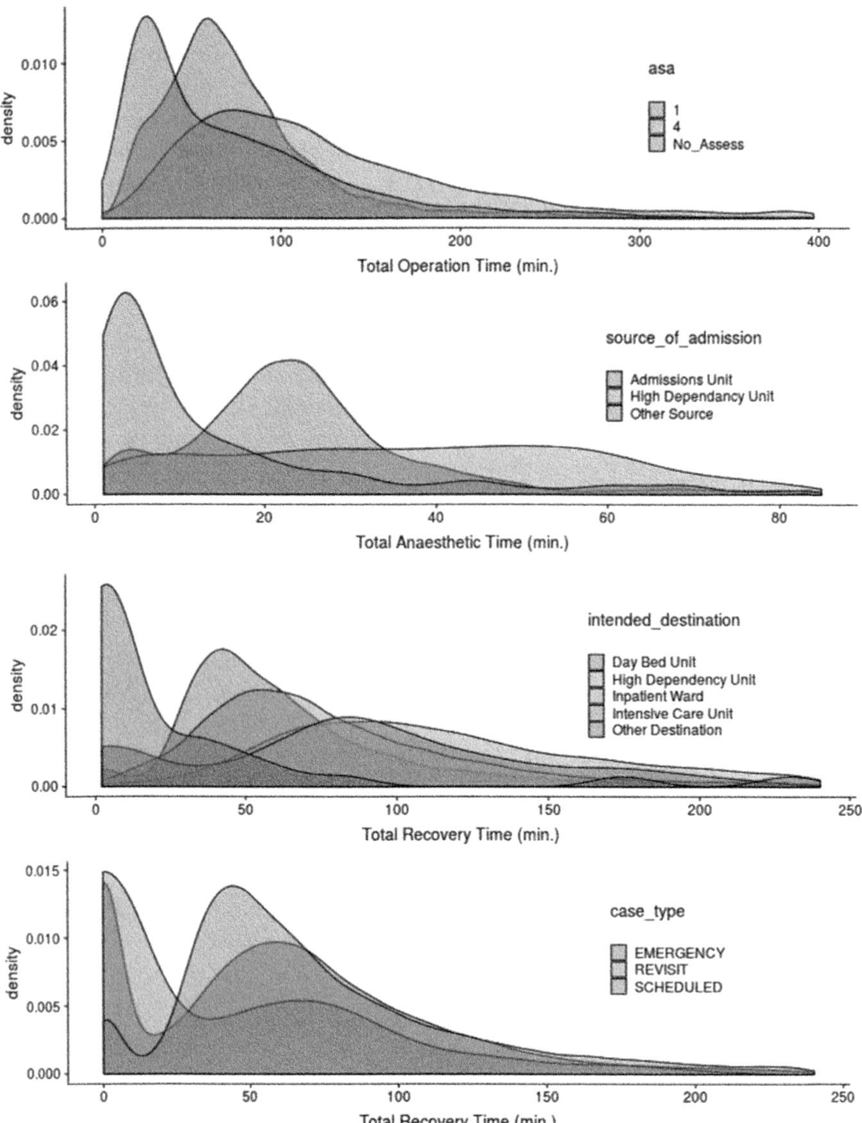

Fig. 5. Examples of conditional cycle time distributions. Top: conditioned on ASA status. Second from top: Source of Admission. Third from top: Intended Destination. Bottom: Case Type.

4 principal components, and thus employed PCA solely as a *transformation* rather than *dimensionality reduction* technique, as is common. This was due to the observation that removing those principal with lowest eigenvalues did not improve performance. This is not unexpected, considering the small number of dimensions.

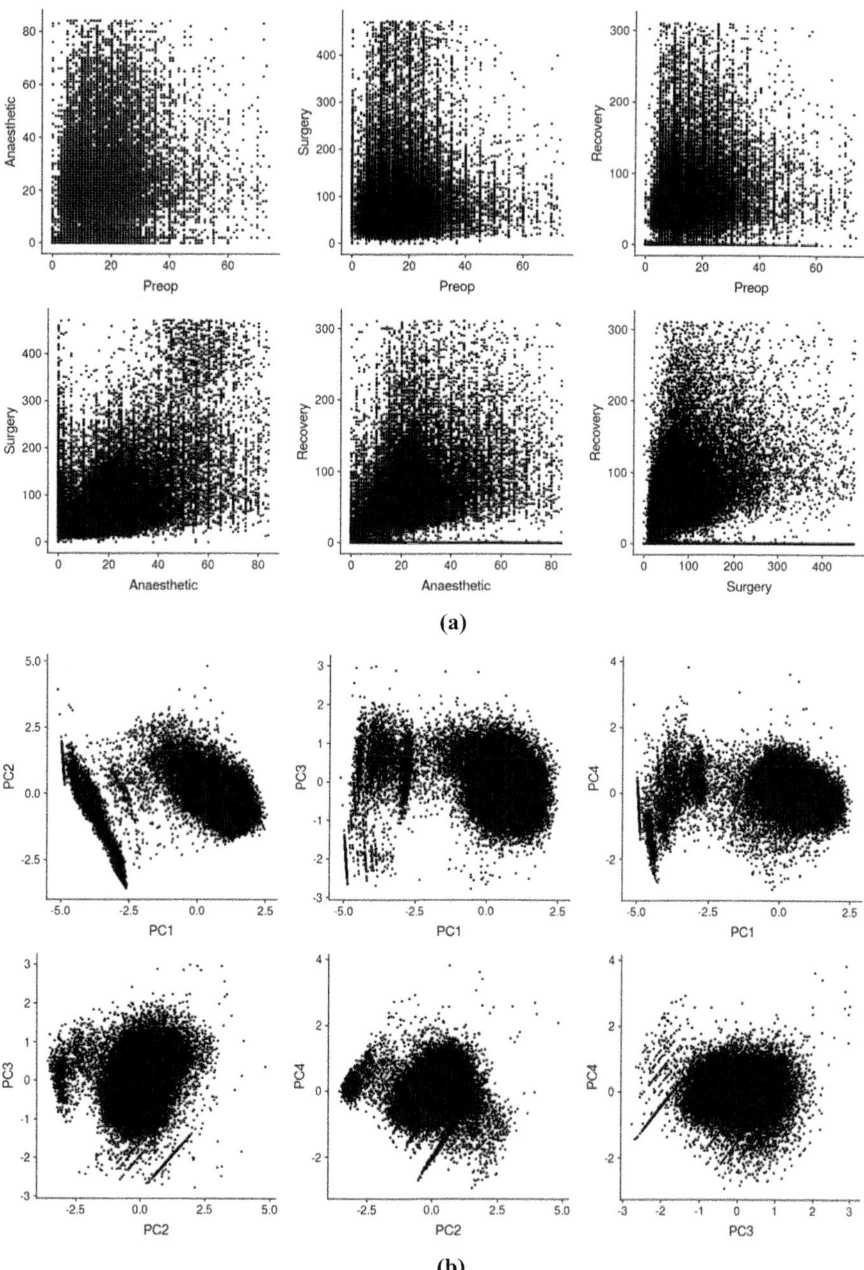

Fig. 6. **(a)** Raw durations of 4 phases plotted against each other. **(b)** Durations w.r.t. principal components. Data was log-transformed prior to PCA transformation.

4.3 Arrival Rates

Many of the aspects of patient flows we have considered so far concern patterns at the level of the individual patient. In order to model system-level dynamics it is crucial to consider how the system is affected by multiple processes competing for shared resources.

One key component in this analysis concerns the arrival of patients, in particular unplanned arrivals requiring immediate treatment, since this will affect and potentially interfere other patient flows. A clearly defined policy exists for the prioritisation of cases based on severity which can lead to cancellation of procedures.

A common assumption in performance modelling and queuing theory is that the number cases arriving for service within some interval follows a Poisson distribution. We found those cases arriving via the emergency room (unscheduled) did in fact follow a Poisson distribution remarkably well (Fig. 7) whereas scheduled cases did not. The latter is not so surprising since the arrival of scheduled cases is necessarily a non-random process and is adjusted to balance the arrival of emergency cases.

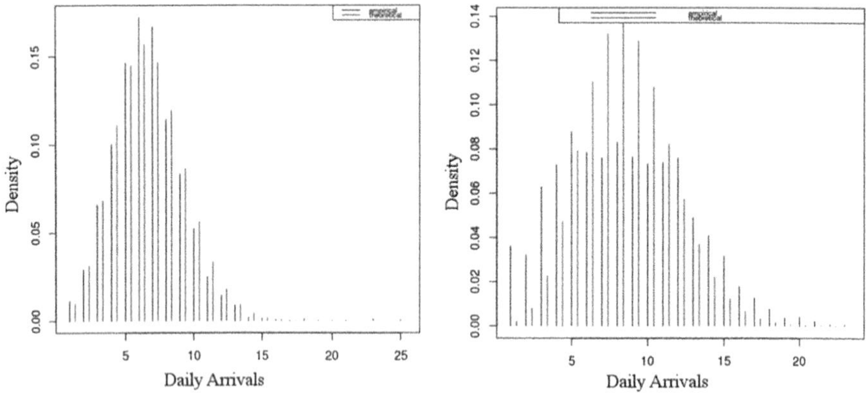

Fig. 7. Daily arrivals (black) along with best-fit Poisson distribution (red). *Left:* emergency cases. *Right:* scheduled cases. (Color figure online)

The close fit of daily emergency arrivals to a Poisson distribution allows us to accurately model the remaining stochastic transition in our model (the other representing marginal cycle times) using the closely related exponential distribution, which captures the corresponding distribution of inter-arrival times.

5 Modeling

5.1 Stochastic Time Petri Nets for System-Wide Simulation

To model the surgical workflow, we used Stochastic Time Petri Nets (STPN) which are essentially Petri nets in which the notion of time and uncertainty is incorporated by adding either a deterministic or a probabilistic delay for the firing of transitions. Specifically, transitions can be either immediate, deterministic or stochastic (Table 3). The model was implemented in ORIS API; a software tool for the modelling and evaluation of stochastic processes [13]. By using the functions provided by the ORIS tool we were able to evaluate the performance of the system by observing how different metrics change when we alternate some of its aspects.

Table 3. Overview of transition types in Stochastic Time Petri nets.

TRANSITION	REPRESENTATION	DESCRIPTION
Immediate	? condition	Fires immmediately if enabled, conflicts between competing enabled immediate transitions are resolved using priority ranking
Deterministic	5	Fires after a fixed amount of time upon becoming enabled
Stochastic	$\lambda e^{-\lambda x}$	Fires after a delay sampled from a probability distribution upon becoming enabled

Surgical Ward Workflow Description. The scenario that is considered for this study is the following: Emergency patients arrive in the hospital at a certain rate to receive treatment throughout the entire 24 h period (transition *arrival* in Fig. 8b) while elective ones are only allowed to arrive at the hospital during the working hours (uniform transition *arrival* in Fig. 8a with enabling function ?working_hours = 1). Emergency arrivals go through a checking procedure for the determination of the severity of their condition. For the current model we assume that about half of the cases do not require immediate intervention (uniform transitions *emergency_status* and *scheduled_status*). If it is decided that the operation must be performed immediately, the patient moves to the Preop room in order to get prepared for the operation (place *preop_room*). According to the NCEPOD urgency classification [30], target time to theater varies depending on the case. For the purposes of this study, only one type of emergency is considered, and the expected time to theater was set to 30 min. On the other hand, scheduled cases can be cancelled up to the time they are about to be placed under anaesthesia if there are no available resources (e.g. beds, surgeons, theaters) to continue the process (transitions *cancel_1,cancel_2*). This is not the case for emergency patients, however, who can move from phase to phase (pre-op, anesthesia, surgery, recovery) if the resources for the next part of the process are available. In this paper, we assume that a surgeon and an anesthetist is required for the surgery. Furthermore, the anesthetist is also required during anesthesia and recovery. Note that priority is given to emergency patients over scheduled

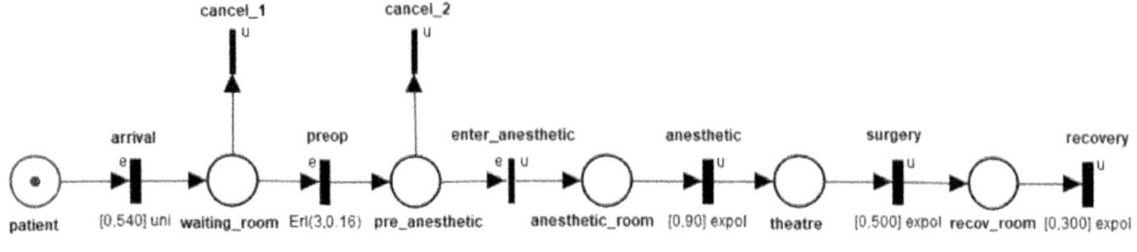

(a) Template for scheduled patient flow.

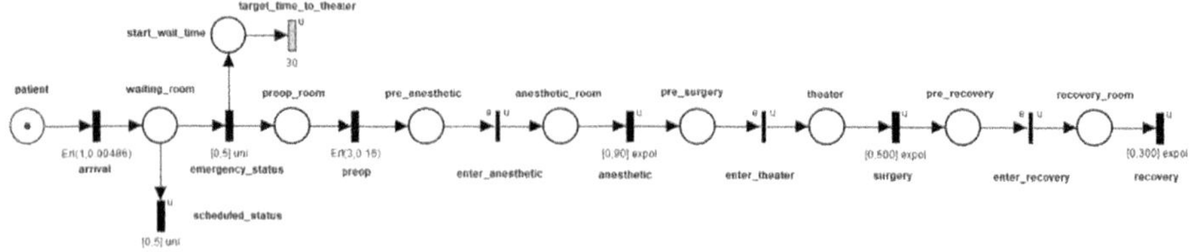

(b) Template for emergency patient flow.

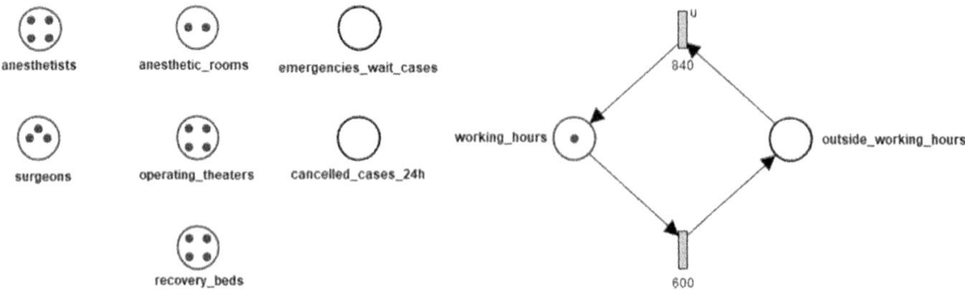

(c) Shared resources.

Fig. 8. Stochastic Time Petri Net used to model core aspects of patients flows.

ones when a decision has to be made regarding the entry to an operating theater or an anesthetic room. The duration of each phase (pre-op, anesthesia, surgery, recovery) is modelled using stochastic transitions with random firing rates following distributions that match our findings in Sect. 4 (Table 2). The properties of these transitions is shown in Table 5.

To account for cancellations and delays, two places were added in the STPN, namely *cancelled_cases_24h* and *emergencies_wait_cases*. In the former a token is added every time a scheduled case gets cancelled while in the latter a token is added whenever an emergency case is waiting for more than 30 min. Both places are reset to zero at the start of a working day. Prioritization and availability checking were incorporated in the model by setting the proper enabling functions and marking updates to transitions. For instance, the enabling function of the transition *enter_recovery* was set to *bed_available>0*. This property of the model prevents emergency patients to enter the recovery phase if there are no available beds. Table 4 illustrates some examples of how our STPN captures some other policies and guidelines.

Table 4. Simplified examples of some of the policies, guidelines and constraints for patient flows captured by our model, along with the fragment of the Petri net which captures this.

POLICY/GUIDELINE	PETRI NET FRAGMENT
Normal working hours are from 8-18	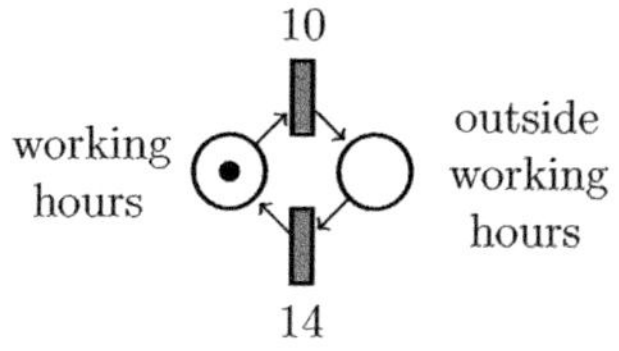 10 working hours / outside working hours 14
Non-emergency procedures should be handled within normal working hours	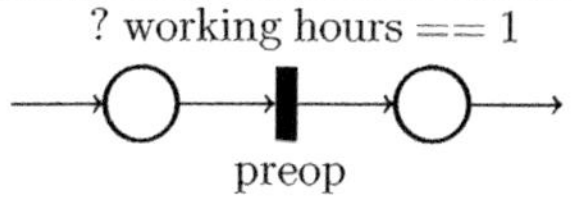 ? working hours == 1 preop
Scheduled cases can be cancelled all the way up to entering anesthetic room if all theatres are occupied by higher priority cases	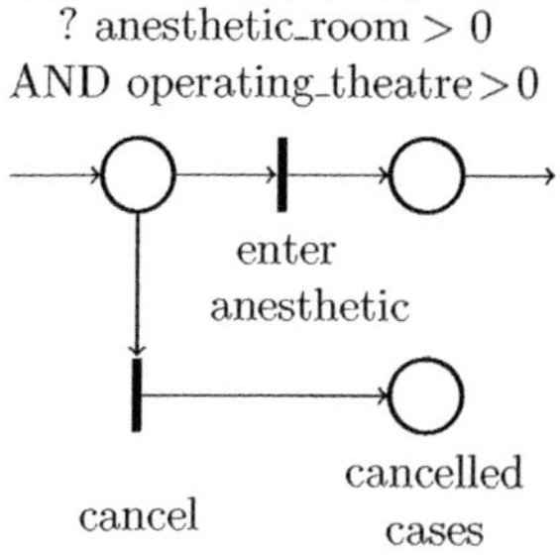 ? anesthetic_room > 0 AND operating_theatre>0 enter anesthetic cancel cancelled cases PRIORITY: enter anesthetic > cancel

Additional simplifying assumptions made for this first iteration of modeling include: that anesthetic rooms and operating theatres are completely independent, a constant number of resources are available within and outside working hours and only one type of recovery room is present whereas in reality different sections are present, such as ICU and high-dependency unit.

Figure 8c shows the basic outline of our model. Patient flows were modeled as individual workflow nets in order to capture constraint violations *for individual patients*. These workflow nets were then programmatically duplicated during simulations. Due to space limitations we are unable to elaborate all details of the model, particularly enabling/update functions and firing priorities, but the full model can be found online[2].

[2] http://www.github.com/apapan08.

Table 5. Fitted parameters for stochastic transitions. See Table 2 for a visualization.

Transition	Distribution	Parameters
Emergency arrivals	Exponential	$\lambda = 0.00487$
Preop	Erlang	$k = 3,\ \lambda = 0.16$
Anesthetic	Polynomial of exponentials	$1.5x^2e^{-0.11x}$ $-10xe^{-0.11x} + 30e^{-0.11x}$
Surgery	Polynomial of exponentials	$x^2e^{-0.0385x} + xe^{-0.0085x}$
Recovery	Polynomial of exponentials	$x^2e^{-0.05x} - 10xe^{-0.1x}$ $+ 150e^{-0.1x}$

Simulation. Using our model, we investigated different resource capacity scenarios (Table 6), with a focus on the ability of the system to fulfill two quality-of-service indicators:

- Number of scheduled cases cancelled in 24 timeframe
- Target time to theatre <30 min for emergency cases

These are properties that are straightforward to formalize and evaluate. In fact, any properties that can be formalized in an appropriate temporal logic such as LTL or MITL[3], which read similarly to natural language guidelines, can be evaluated. In addition to reporting the expected values for these QoS criteria, we included the expected resource availability over time. This helps us to identify when, and for which resources, potential bottlenecks arise. In a more sophisticated model, we would likely see more complex patterns resulting from interacting processes/resources.

Table 6. Resource capacity scenarios explored in simulations.

	Excess capacity	Sufficient capacity	Insufficient capacity
Scheduled cases/day	10	10	10
Anesthetists	10	8	4
Surgeons	8	5	3
Anesthetic rooms	8	4	2
Operating theatres	10	8	4
Recovery beds	12	6	4

We report results in terms of expected value[4] across 100 simulation runs of each scenario. That is, the number of cancelled cases or available operating

[3] Linear Temporal Logic, Metric Interval Temporal Logic.

[4] $E[X] = \sum x\ p(X = x)$.

theatres at a given time, averaged over simulation runs. With this simple model, the state of the system follows a consistent periodic fluctuation according to the working hours (Table 7). Realistically, however, greater fluctuations would be likely due to uneven patient inflows and staffing availability patterns over time.

5.2 Bayesian Nets for Individualised Prediction

In modeling cycle times in patient flows, our model in Table 2 considers only marginal distributions, i.e. cycle time estimates are identical for all patients. However, as we illustrated in Sect. 4.2, there clearly exist categories of patients with significant variations in cycle times.

Bayesian Nets are probabilistic graphical models that capture the structure of complex probability distributions. By exploiting conditional independence relations between variables, inference algorithms allow us to query the belief network in a flexible manner, even with only partial information [25]. In the present context, Bayesian nets allow us to take into account multiple attributes of a patient along with the partial completion of their treatment in order to make significantly more accurate and nuanced predictions regarding cycle time and other aspects, such as destination.

We present the results of two Bayesian networks in predicting cycle time, leaving as an important avenue of future research the integration of these predictive models into a more sophisticated process model which accounts individual patient attributes. Figure 9 illustrates that Bayesian networks can be integrated with Stochastic Petri net models to more accurately model transition distributions specifically.

The models were built and trained using algorithms implemented in the `bnlearn` package for the programming language R [35]. We used our own implementation of cross-validation, in part to avoid data snooping, and added simple smoothing procedures to account for undersampling.

Feature Selection. We evaluated two networks: a 10-variable model and a 22-variable extension of the first. The decision of which attributes to include was based in part on our exploration of conditional distributions in Sect. 4.2 and pairwise mutual information described in 4.2.

One feature of note is the *Cluster* node in both 10 and 22 variable models. This represents the patients groups identified in 4.2. Using simple k-means clustering, we experimented with identifying 5, 10, 15, and 20 patient clusters which proved moderately helpful in improving performance - in particular for predicting anesthetic cycle times using the 22-variable model.

Table 7. Simulation results for scenarios with (*top*) excess capacity, (*middle*) sufficient capacity, and (*bottom*) insufficient capacity averaged over 100 runs. Cancelled-Cases and Emergency-Delay represent failures to meet quality of service guidelines when the expected value exceeds 0. In other words: these are the system properties we are interested in verifying.

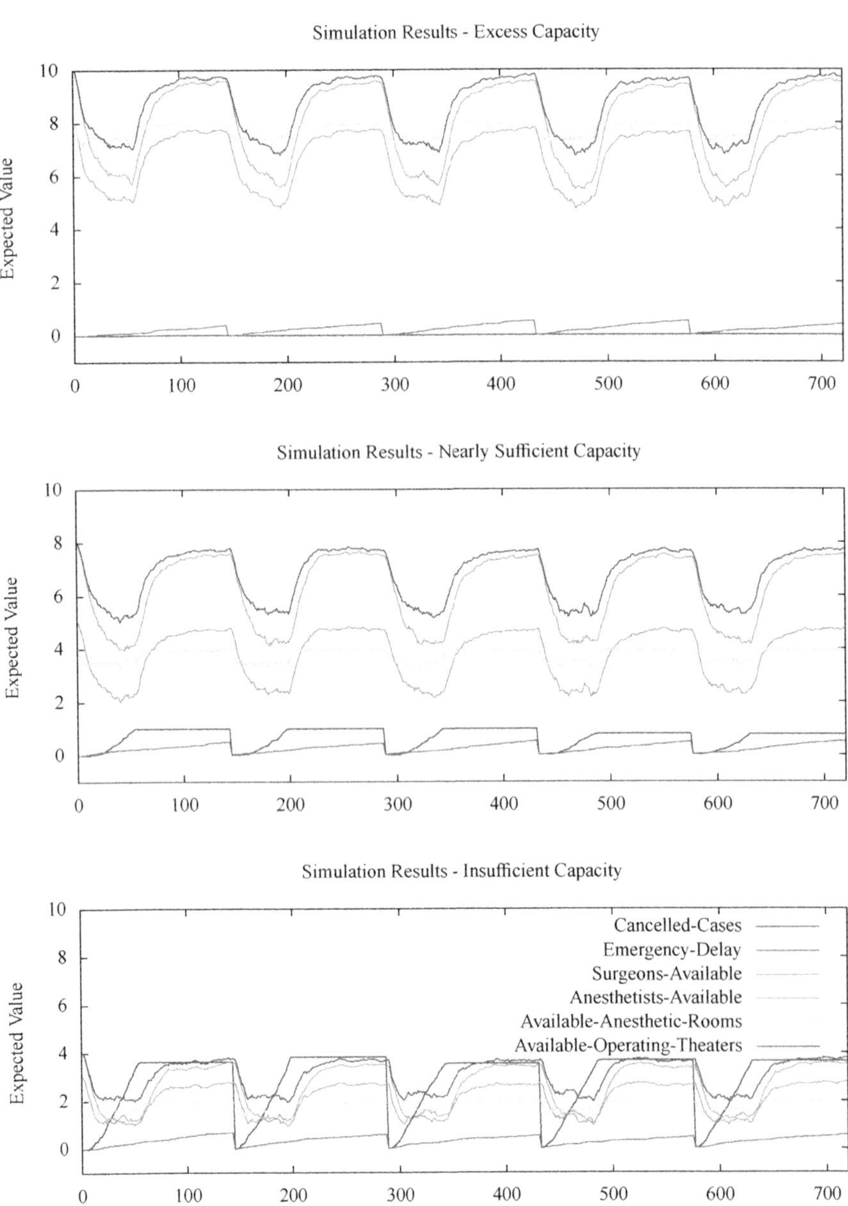

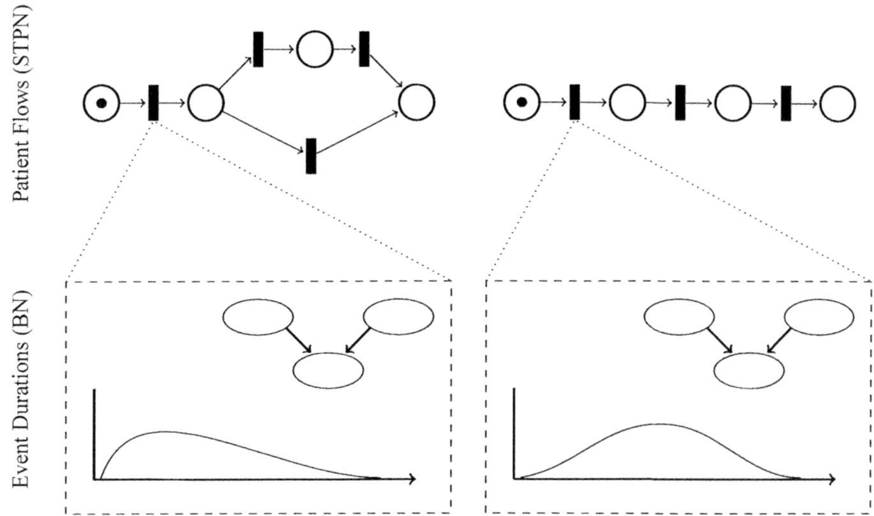

Fig. 9. Petri nets capture control-flow of a process, while Bayesian networks allow nuanced modelling of transition distributions based on case attributes. Integrating these two modelling perspectives is an important next step in developing data-driven, patient centric workflow models.

Structure Learning. There are two methods for constructing the graph structure of a Bayesian net: manually, based on expert knowledge; and automatically using structure learning algorithms. After several attempts at building nets manually, we found that automatically generated nets outperformed, despite sometimes finding odd connections between variables.

We employed the score-based structure learning algorithms hill-climbing and TABU structure-learning algorithms, using scoring functions Akaike and Bayesian Information Criterion (AIC/BIC). This choice was due to their computational tractability and suitability to the our hybrid dataset (continuous and discrete attributes). The 22 variable graph can be seen in Fig. 10.

Evaluation. Models were evaluated based on prediction of cycle times for the 4 phases of the surgical patient flow using 10-fold cross validation. We present mean *absolute* error in Fig. 11 for comprehensibility, but note that mean squared error results closely follow the same pattern. As a baseline for comparison, results are shown for the best-fit marginal distributions reported in Table 2.

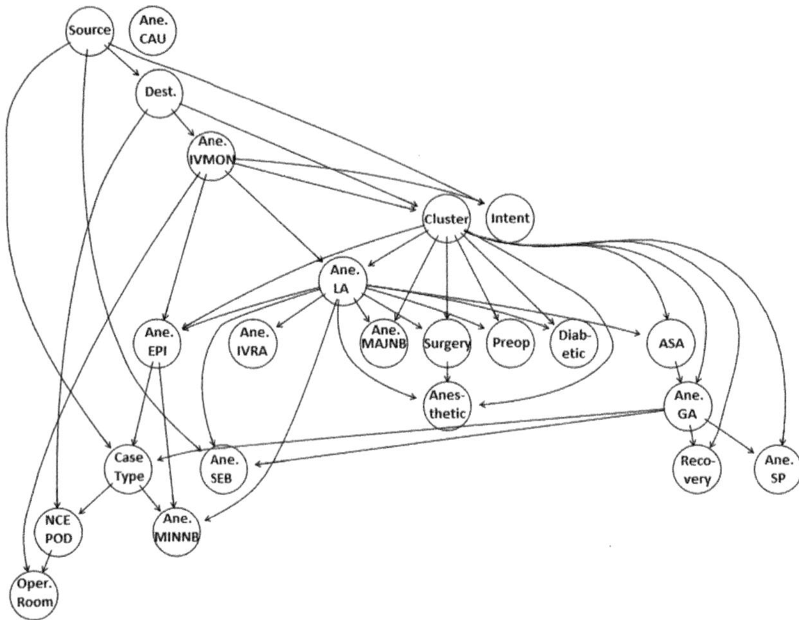

Fig. 10. A Bayesian belief network taking into account 22 attributes of a patient's treatment. Attributes prefixed by *Ane.* denote different types of anaesthetic. Note the central role of the latent *Cluster* attribute discovered in Sect. 4.2. Originally published in [6].

Avoiding Data Snooping. One pitfall that was important to avoid, in particular when modelling *partial executions* of patient flows, was that of inadvertent data snooping by including the *Cluster* attribute. When evaluating a model's predictive power on test data, the cluster should be consider an *unobserved variable.*

While intuitively obvious, this is a crucial methodological point, as including it would constitute a form of data snooping since the cluster itself is in fact derived from the target variables (cycle times). Nonetheless, the variable is able to play a role in the Bayesian network, despite being unobserved, via conditional dependencies between it, observed variables and unobserved target variables.

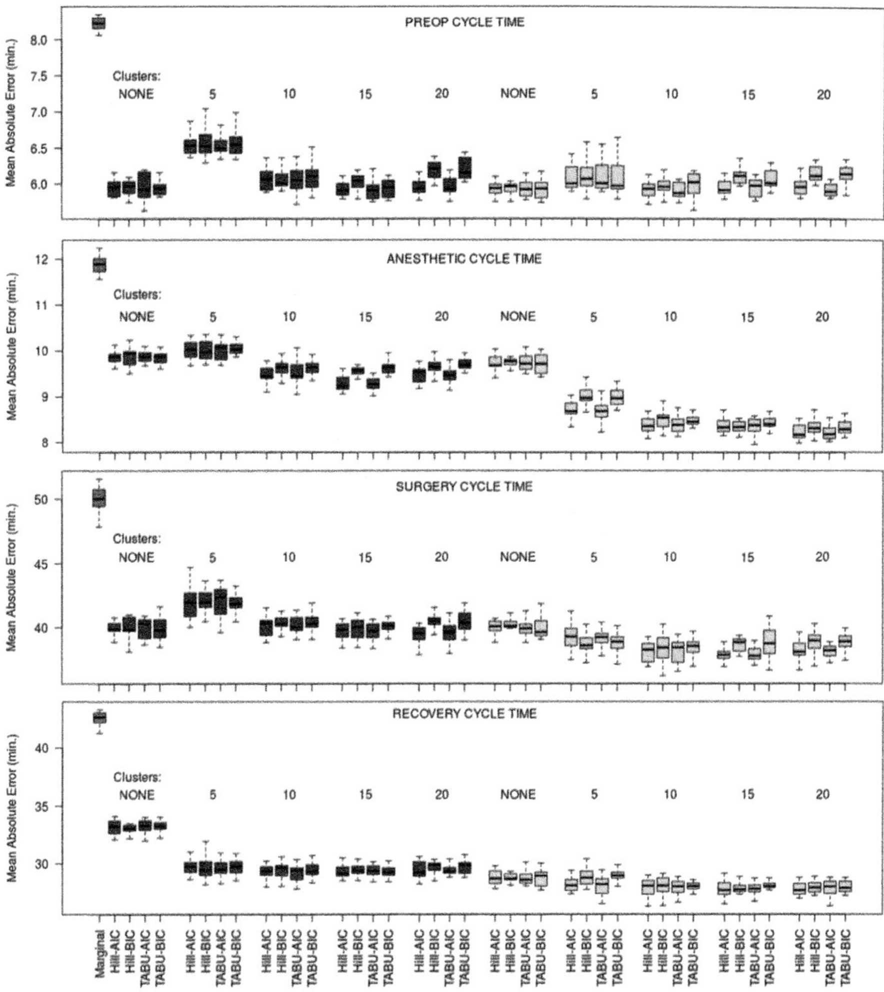

Fig. 11. Comparison of 40 different Bayesian net models using 10 (blue) and 22 (green) variables, but different structure learning algorithms. Results are based on 5 runs of 10-fold cross-validation for predicting cycle time of partially completed patient flows. As a baseline comparison, the simple best-fit marginal distribution (reported in Table 2) is shown in red. Originally published in [6]. (Color figure online)

6 Discussion

The case study presented in this paper has highlighted a number of challenges and lessons learnt that can be applied to other surgical workflow modeling projects, as well wider data-driven healthcare improvement initiatives. First, data quality assurance is key. One of the most immediate observations of our analysis was presence of a good deal of anomalous data. Process mining techniques proved to be useful for detecting outliers and identifying anomalies related to the control-flow.

Second, even though it seemed initially that there were no groupings of patients with regards to duration, PCA revealed latent patient categories in our data. Identifying these patient clusters improved Bayesian net prediction, even though interpreting what these categories mean is not straightforward.

Third, we showed that a reasonably accurate predictive model of event cycle times in the form of a simple Bayesian belief network can be built, which significantly outperforms simple marginal distribution fitting. The choice of Bayesian networks was motivated by their flexibility and interpretability, which is of great importance in safety-critical domains like healthcare. The ability to query these models suggests they would be a strong component of an intelligent probabilistic scheduling system in surgery.

Finally, Stochastic Time Petri Nets were found to be an appropriate formalism for capturing hospital policies and guidelines surrounding surgery, in particular regarding timing and resource requirements. Distinguishing between the workflows for emergency and scheduled cases was possible in a clear and transparent way, and incorporating case prioritization was straightforward. Even though the model presented in Sect. 5.1 is a simplified version of reality, it serves as proof-of-concept of how real-world data can be incorporated into a model that combines official procedures and guidelines with domain expert knowledge. Simulating different scenarios allowed us to test the limits of the system and to analyse the effect of varying resource allocation.

7 Conclusion and Future Work

In this paper, we presented a preliminary investigation into probabilistic workflow modeling, simulation and prediction methods in surgical wards. This is an important first step towards much-needed surgical care improvement. Our analysis is focused on key surgical phases, which is a level of granularity that has received less attention in existing literature.

Data-informed surgical care scheduling that takes into account individual patient characteristics, resource availability and hospital policies presents a promising approach to improving resource utilization, quality of care and, ultimately, patient and staff satisfaction. We have demonstrated the value of combining several data analysis paradigms, from mathematical modeling to process mining and machine learning, towards developing a model that effectively captures the complexity of surgical processes, while allowing for experimentation and insightful interrogation. This approach is applicable in other areas of the healthcare system, where under-utilization of expensive resources calls for precise scheduling to minimize costs and waiting times.

Our analysis considered both system-wide surgical performance (through Stochastic Time Petri Net modeling and simulation) and individual patient flow (through Bayesian Net cycle time prediction). In order to integrate the two in the future and incorporate Bayesian nets into Petri Net modeling, we propose the use of Bayesian Stochastic Petri Nets [39].

In the big data and precision medicine era, developing intelligent methods for dynamic and personalized scheduling in the surgical ward is a key research direction. Extending the work presented in this paper to incorporate more detailed information about the surgical ward is desirable, and would possibly require further domain knowledge and dimensionality reduction, so as to deal with the huge cardinality of some attributes. We also regard evaluation with domain experts as an important next step, ensuring that the recommendations of a future surgical scheduling system are understood and deemed useful by hospital staff.

Acknowledgements. We would like to thank Cameron Fairfield and Stephen Knight for their generous feedback regarding policies and on-the-ground practices at the Royal Infirmary of Edinburgh surgical ward.

References

1. Stahl, J.E., et al.: Reorganizing patient care and workflow in the operating room: a cost-effectiveness study. Surgery **139**(6), 717–728 (2006)
2. Van der Aalst, W.E.A.: Workflow mining: discovering process models from event logs. IEEE Trans. Knowl. Data Eng. **16**(9), 1128–1142 (2004)
3. Acid, S., et al.: A comparison of learning algorithms for Bayesian networks: a case study based on data from an emergency medical service. Artif. Intell. Med. **30**(3), 215–232 (2004)
4. Ahmadi, S.A., et al.: Motif discovery in or sensor data with application to surgical workflow analysis and activity detection. In: M2CAI workshop, MICCAI, London. Citeseer (2009)
5. Akkerman, R., Knip, M.: Reallocation of beds to reduce waiting time for cardiac surgery. Health Care Manage. Sci. **7**(2), 119–126 (2004)
6. Back, C.O., Manataki, A., Harrison, E.: Mining patient flow patterns in a surgical ward. In: HEALTHINF, pp. 273–283 (2020)
7. Baier, C., Katoen, J.P.: Principles of Model Checking. MIT press, Cambridge (2008)
8. Basin, D., Klaedtke, F., Müller, S., Zălinescu, E.: Monitoring metric first-order temporal properties. J. ACM **62**(2), 15:1–15:45 (2015)
9. Berti, A., et al.: Process mining for python (PM4Py): bridging the gap between process-and data science. In: ICPM Demo Track (CEUR 2374) (2019)
10. Blum, T., et al.: Workflow mining for visualization and analysis of surgeries. Int. J. Comput. Assist. Radiol. Surg. **3**(5), 379–386 (2008)
11. Bouarfa, L., et al.: Discovery of high-level tasks in the operating room. J. Biomed. Inform. **44**(3), 455–462 (2011)
12. Bouarfa, L., Dankelman, J.: Workflow mining and outlier detection from clinical activity logs. J. Biomed. Inform. **45**(6), 1185–1190 (2012)
13. Bucci, G., Carnevali, L., Ridi, L., Vicario, E.: Oris: a tool for modeling, verification and evaluation of real-time systems. Int. J. Softw. Tools Technol. Transfer **12**(5), 391–403 (2010)
14. Burattin, A., Maggi, F., Sperduti, A.: Conformance checking based on multi-perspective declarative process models. Exp. Syst. Appl. **65** (2015). https://doi.org/10.1016/j.eswa.2016.08.040
15. Cochran, J.K., Bharti, A.: Stochastic bed balancing of an obstetrics hospital. Health Care Manage. Sci. **9**(1), 31–45 (2006)

16. Denton, B., et al.: Optimization of surgery sequencing and scheduling decisions under uncertainty. Health Care Manage. Sci. **10**(1), 13–24 (2007)
17. Fages, F., Rizk, A.: From model-checking to temporal logic constraint solving. In: Gent, I.P. (ed.) CP 2009. LNCS, vol. 5732, pp. 319–334. Springer, Heidelberg (2009). https://doi.org/10.1007/978-3-642-04244-7_26
18. Fu, J., Topcu, U.: Computational methods for stochastic control with metric interval temporal logic specifications. In: 2015 54th IEEE Conference on Decision and Control (CDC), pp. 7440–7447. IEEE (2015)
19. Funkner, A.A., et al.: Towards evolutionary discovery of typical clinical pathways in electronic health records. Proc. Comput. Sci. **119**, 234–244 (2017)
20. Béjar Haro, B., Zappella, L., Vidal, R.: Surgical gesture classification from video data. In: Ayache, N., Delingette, H., Golland, P., Mori, K. (eds.) MICCAI 2012. LNCS, vol. 7510, pp. 34–41. Springer, Heidelberg (2012). https://doi.org/10.1007/978-3-642-33415-3_5
21. Huang, Z., et al.: Summarizing clinical pathways from event logs. J. Biomed. Inform. **46**(1), 111–127 (2013)
22. Hulshof, P.J.H., et al.: Tactical resource allocation and elective patient admission planning in care processes. Health Care Manage. Sci. **16**(2), 152–166 (2013)
23. Jimenez-Ramirez, A., Barba, I., Fernandez-Olivares, J., Del Valle, C., Weber, B.: Time prediction on multi-perspective declarative business processes. Knowl. Inf. Syst. **57**, 655–684 (2018). https://doi.org/10.1007/s10115-018-1180-3
24. Kayis, E., et al.: Improving prediction of surgery duration using operational and temporal factors. In: AMIA Annual Symposium Proceedings, vol. 2012, p. 456. American Medical Informatics Association (2012)
25. Koller, D., Friedman, N.: Probabilistic Graphical Models: Principles and Techniques. MIT press, Cambridge (2009)
26. Lalys, F., Jannin, P.: Surgical process modelling: a review. Int. J. Comput. Assist. Radiol. Surg. **9**(3), 495–511 (2014)
27. Lin, H.C., et al.: Towards automatic skill evaluation: detection and segmentation of robot-assisted surgical motions. Comput. Aided Surg. **11**(5), 220–230 (2006)
28. Mans, R., et al.: Mining processes in dentistry. In: Proceedings of the 2nd ACM SIGHIT International Health Informatics Symposium, pp. 379–388. ACM (2012)
29. Martina, S., Paolieri, M., Papini, T., Vicario, E.: Performance evaluation of Fischer's protocol through steady-state analysis of Markov regenerative processes. In: 2016 IEEE 24th International Symposium on Modeling, Analysis and Simulation of Computer and Telecommunication Systems (MASCOTS), pp. 355–360. IEEE (2016)
30. NCEPOD: NCEPOD classification of intervention. https://www.ncepod.org.uk/classification.html (2019). Accessed 22 Nov 2019
31. Neumuth, T., et al.: Analysis of surgical intervention populations using generic surgical process models. Int. J. Comput. Assist. Radiol. Surg. **6**(1), 59–71 (2011)
32. NHS Scotland: National theatres project report. https://www.isdscotland.org/Health-Topics/Quality-Indicators/National-Benchmarking-Project/National-Theatres-Project/ (2006). Accessed 22 Nov 2019
33. Paolieri, M., Horvath, A., Vicario, E.: Probabilistic model checking of regenerative concurrent systems. IEEE Trans. Softw. Eng. **42**(2), 153–169 (2015)
34. Royal College of Anaesthetists: Perioperative medicine: the pathway to better surgical care, London (2015)
35. Scutari, M.: Learning Bayesian Networks with the bnlearn R Package. J. Stat. Softw. **35**(3), 1–22 (2010). http://www.jstatsoft.org/v35/i03/

36. Stahl, J.E., et al.: Reorganizing patient care and workflow in the operating room: a cost-effectiveness study. Surgery **139**(6), 717–728 (2006)
37. Stauder, R., et al.: Random forests for phase detection in surgical workflow analysis. In: Stoyanov, D., Collins, D.L., Sakuma, I., Abolmaesumi, P., Jannin, P. (eds.) IPCAI 2014. LNCS, vol. 8498, pp. 148–157. Springer, Cham (2014). https://doi.org/10.1007/978-3-319-07521-1_16
38. Strum, D., et al.: Modeling the uncertainty of surgical procedure times: comparison of log-normal and normal models. Anesthesiology **92**(4), 1160–1167 (2000)
39. Taleb-Berrouane, M., Khan, F., Amyotte, P.: Bayesian stochastic petri nets (BSPN) - a new modelling tool for dynamic safety and reliability analysis. Reliab. Eng. Syst. Safety **193**, 106587 (2020)
40. Westergaard, M., Maggi, F.M.: Looking into the future: using timed automata to provide a priori advice about timed declarative process models. In: Meersman, R., et al. (eds.) OTM 2012. LNCS, vol. 7565, pp. 250–267. Springer, Heidelberg (2012). https://doi.org/10.1007/978-3-642-33606-5_16

Classification of Eating Behaviors in Unconstrained Environments

Kizito Nkurikiyeyezu[1](✉), Haruka Kamachi[1], Takumi Kondo[1], Archit Jain[2], Anna Yokokubo[1], and Guillaume Lopez[1]

[1] Wearable Environment and Information Systems Laboratory, Aoyama Gakuin University, 5 Chome-10-1 Fuchinobe, Chuo Ward, Sagamihara, Kanagawa 252-5258, Japan
kizito@wil-aoyama.jp

[2] Université Jean Monnet, 10 Rue Tréfilerie, 42100 Saint-Étienne, France
http://www.wil.it.aoyama.ac.jp

Abstract. Obesity and its numerous devastating consequences are on the rise globally. While widespread tactics to fight against obesity often focus on healthy eating, how the food is consumed is oftentimes overlooked even though convincing evidence attests that merely eating slowly and properly chewing one's meal significantly reduces obesity. This research introduces a method that recognizes common human actions during mealtime—namely, food chewing, food swallowing, drink swallowing, and talking. The proposed system is unobtrusive. It uses a cheap and small bone conduction microphone to collect intra-body sound and a smartphone that provides feedback in real-time. Our proposed approach achieves similar performances (Accuracy = 97.5%, Specificity = 98.0%, Precision = 83.8%, Recall = 91.7%, F_1 score = 87.2%, and MCC = 0.85) as those achieved by the most recent state of the art models even though our system uses modest machine learning models.

Keywords: Eating quantification · Chewing · Swallowing · Sound analysis · Activity recognition · Free-living conditions

1 Introduction

Healthy eating is often hailed as the most reliable method to fight against obesity. However, while a healthy diet certainly plays an influential role in weight loss, how the food is consumed is an often overlooked obesity-fighting mechanism. Indeed, accumulating evidence shows that merely eating slowly and properly chewing one's meal reduce obesity significantly. For instance, an up-to-date systematic review [25] on the topic concluded that inadequate mastication highly correlates with obesity. Likewise, a large scale study (N = 92,363 individuals) conducted between 2005 and 2013 found that those with slow eating habits had, among other numerous benefits, a lower BMI (22.3 ± 4.0), and a lower obesity rate (21.5%). In contrast, those with fast eating habits had a much higher BMI (25.0 ± 4.4) and a higher obesity rate (44.8%) [12].

X. Ye et al. (Eds.): BIOSTEC 2020, CCIS 1400, pp. 592–609, 2021.
https://doi.org/10.1007/978-3-030-72379-8_29

There exist diverse food intake monitoring mechanisms. The simplest strategies consist of manual self-reports. However, self-report is imprecise because it is biased and subjective [23,27]. The germane state of the art [2,24,26] proposes wearable devices as a more accurate alternative. Unlike manual mechanisms, wearable gadgets automatically monitor the dietary habits of the wearers; thus, they are immune to subjective bias. Moreover, they are more convenient and can provide real-time feedback to their users [26]. Although automatic food monitoring is still an open problem to solve [3,13,24], many solutions have been introduced and are extensively reviewed in e.g., [24,26]. For example, [3] proposed an earpiece that automatically monitors eating behavior in free-living conditions. Their system is based on an off-the-shelf contact microphone and has an $F_1 score$ that exceeds 77.5% for eating detection. Recently, [17] presented a framework for in-the-wild modeling of eating behavior using inertial measurement unit (IMU) signals that are recorded from smartphones. The proposed approach uses both convolutional and recurrent layers that are trained simultaneously. This model outperforms the state-of-the-art in detecting food bites ($F_1 score = 92.3\%$).

In our previous studies [14–16,20], we proposed a method that uses a cheap and small bone conduction microphone to automatically monitor eating behaviors. Our research was, however, restricted in scope. This paper extends the following improvements to our earlier research and to other existing relevant studies:

1) All experiments were conducted in free-living environments (e.g., at home when the subjects were eating with their families) to capture the complexity of the real-world.
2) There was no constraint on the type of food to eat and the participants were urged to have whatever they usually eat or drink.
3) The proposed approach recognizes five different eating activities (i.e., chewing, food swallowing, drink swallowing, talking and other noises).
4) The previous dataset was increased by 30% of new samples.
5) The proposed approach adds features engineering process, applies a less noisy oversampling method, adds features selection process, evaluates new classifiers, and provides more detailed evaluation metrics.
6) The proposed approach achieves comparable performance (Accuracy = 97.5%, Precision = 83.8%, Recall = 91.7%, Jaccard score = 0.89, Kappa score = 0.88, F_1 score = 87.2%, and Matthews Correlation Coefficient = 0.85) to those achieved by the most recent state of the art model proposed in [17] even though our proposed method uses much simpler machine learning models.

2 Methods

2.1 Data Collection

Sixteen subjects joined the experiments. All experiments were conducted in free-living environments to capture the complexity of the real-world. For instance, some experiments were recorded at home when the subjects were having supper

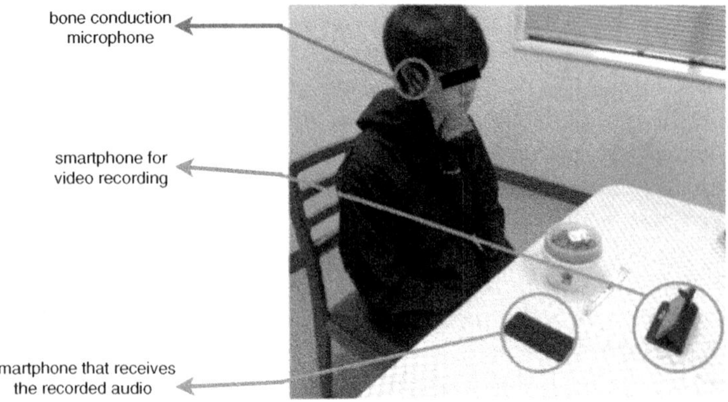

Fig. 1. Experimental setup of a typical dietary sound collection. The experiments were conducted in a free-living environment when the subjects dinned with e.g., their family. The dietary sounds were recorded using a bone conduction microphone. One smartphone was used to receive, via Bluetooth, the recorded dietary sounds. Another is used to record a video of the subject for data annotation purposes.

with their families. Others took place in a university cafeteria during lunch with colleagues. Additionally, there was no constraint on the type of food and the subjects were urged to have whatever they usually eat.

The dietary sounds were recorded ($Fs = 8$ kHz) using a commercial bone conduction microphone (Motorola Finiti HZ800 Bluetooth Headset, Motorola co. Ltd.) that is attached to a subject's ear. The microphone sends the recorded sounds to a smartphone via Bluetooth. The sounds are then saved for further analysis. At the same time, another smartphone records the subject's mouth and throat motion as shown in Fig. 1.

2.2 Audio Data Labeling

The collected dietary sounds are segmented and then labeled using Praat[1], a free software for speech analysis in phonetics that, among others things, allows speech labeling and segmentation. Labels were manually added by looking at the video which were recorded when the subjects were having their meals. The following five labels were added:

- *Chewing*—this label is assigned to any sound segment corresponding to when the subjects were crushing solid food with their teeth.
- *Food swallowing*—when the subjects swallow the chewed solid food but not when swallowing liquids.
- *Drink swallowing*—when the subjects swallow liquids but not solid foods.
- *Talking*—when the subjects are speaking.
- *Other sounds*—this label is assigned to sounds segments when other sounds other than the aforementioned are recorded.

[1] http://www.fon.hum.uva.nl/praat/.

2.3 Feature Computation

A total of 26 features (Table 1) were extracted from the recorded dietary sounds. The *chroma features* capture harmonic and melodic characteristics of music and they are robust to changes in timbre and instrumentation. They are also used for audio-matching. A chroma vector is a 12-element feature vector indicating how much energy is contained in each of the 12 pitch classes (C, C#, D, D#, E, F, F#, G, G#, A, A#, B). The 12-dimension chroma vector $v_c(t)$ is computed from a logarithmic Short-Time Fourier Transform (STFT) power spectrum $\psi_p(f,t)$ [8, 21] (Eq. (1)) and constitutes a compact representation of a sound [1].

Table 1. Summary of the extracted features [14].

Description	Number of features
Mean of chroma vector	1
Root mean square energy	1
Spectral centroid	1
Spectral bandwidth	1
Spectral roll off	1
Zero crossing rate	1
Mel-frequency cepstral coefficients	20

$$v_c(t) = \sum_{h=Oct_L}^{Oct_H} \int_{-\infty}^{\infty} BPF_{c,h}(f)\psi_p(f,t)df \tag{1}$$

$BPF_{c,h}(f)$ represents a band-pass filter (Eq. (3)) which passes the log-scale frequency $F_{c,h}$ (Eq. (2)) of pitch class c and is applied from low (Oct_L) to high (Oct_H) octaves.

$$F_{c,h} = 1200h + 100(c-1) \tag{2}$$

$$BPF_{c,h} = \frac{1}{2}\left\{1 - \frac{cos\left[2\pi\left(f - \left(F_{c,h} - 100\right)\right)\right]}{200}\right\} \tag{3}$$

The energy $E_s(t)$ of a continuous signal $x(t)$ and a discrete signal $x(n)$ corresponds to area under their squared magnitude (Eq. (4) and Eq. (5)). For audio signals, that roughly corresponds to the loudness of the signal.

$$E_s(t) = \int_{-\infty}^{\infty} |x(t)|^2 dt \tag{4}$$

$$E_s(t) = \sum_{n=-\infty}^{\infty} |x(n)^2| \tag{5}$$

The *Root Mean Square Energy (RMSE)* of an N samples discrete signal $s(n)$ is defined as the square root of the average of the sum of all samples n (Eq. (6)).

$$RMSE = \sqrt{\frac{1}{N}\sum_{N} |s(n)|^2} \tag{6}$$

The *spectral centroid (SC)* indicates which frequencies the energy of the spectrum is centered upon, i.e., it expresses where the center of gravity of the spectral energy resides [1] (Eq. (7)).

$$f_c = \frac{\sum_k S(k)f(k)}{\sum kS(k)} \tag{7}$$

where $S(k)$ is the spectral magnitude and $f(k)$ is the frequency at bin k.

The *Spectral bandwidth* (Eq. (8)) defines the order-p spectral bandwidth and is used to distinguish tonal sound from noise-like sounds [1].

$$f_b = \left(\sum_k S(k)\left(f(k) - f_c\right)^p\right)^{1/p} \tag{8}$$

where $S(k)$ is the spectral magnitude at frequency bin k, f(k) is the frequency at bin k, and f_c is the spectral centroid. When $p = 2$, this is like a weighted standard deviation.

The *Spectral roll-off* (Eq. (9)) of a point i is the frequency below which a specified percentile of the total spectral energy lies. It measures the skewness of the shape of the spectral [1,22] and can be used to differentiate voiced from unvoiced speech because the former has its energy concentrated in high-frequencies while the latter has more energy in its lower bands [22].

$$\sum_{k=b_1}^{i} s_k = K \sum_{k=b_1}^{b_2} s_k \tag{9}$$

where s_k is the spectral value at bin k, b_1 and b_2 are the band edges, in bins, over which to calculate the spectral spread. K is the percentage of total energy contained between b_1 and i.

Zero crossing rate (ZCR) (Fig. 2) indicates the number of times that a signal crosses the horizontal axis and it provides a rough estimate of the dominant frequency in the sound [1].

Mel frequency cepstral coefficients (MFCC) are popular feature for sound classification. MFCC take into account humans' perception of sound and model the sound's spectral energy distribution accordingly [5]. Indeed, it is reported

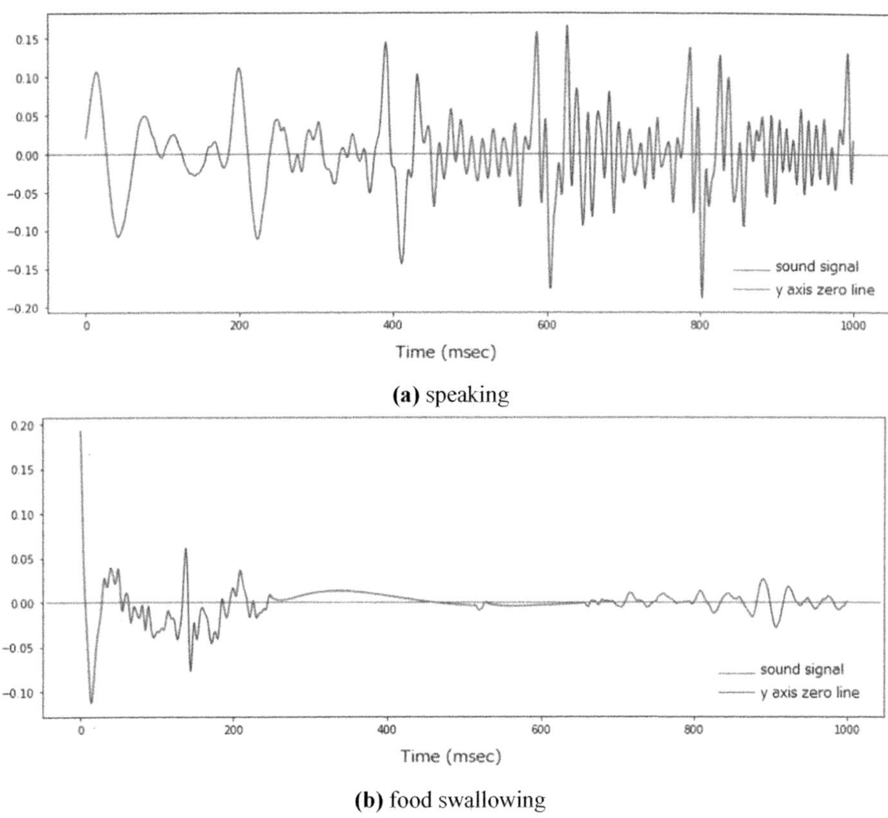

(a) speaking

(b) food swallowing

Fig. 2. A typical zero crossing rate of a talking and a swallowing sound [14].

that humans' perception of a frequency f in a sound follows a non-linear frequency scale [5,18]—the scale commonly known as the "mel" scale (Eq. (10))

$$f_{mel}(f) = 2595 log_{10} \left(1 + \frac{f}{700}\right) \tag{10}$$

The MFFC are fundamental acoustic feature for speech and speaker recognition applications [5] and are calculated as follows. First, a sound is windowed and split into frames $\{y(n)_{n=1}^{N}\}$. Next, an M point Discrete Fourier Transform (DFT) is used to compute the power spectrum $Y(k)$ of each frame $y(n)$ (Eq. (11)).

$$\left|Y(k)\right|^2 = \left|\sum_{n=1}^{M} y(n).e^{\left(\frac{-j2\pi.n.k}{M}\right)}\right| \tag{11}$$

Finally, the power spectrum $Y(k)$ is converted into logarithmic domain and used to calculate the MFFC coefficients C_m (Eq. (12)).

$$C_m = \sqrt{\frac{2}{Q}} \sum_{l=0}^{Q-1} log\Big[e(l+1)\Big] cos\left[\frac{m\pi}{Q}\Big(\frac{2l-1}{2}\Big)\right] \tag{12}$$

where $0 \leqslant m \leqslant R-1$, R being the desired number of ancestral features; and in our case, $R = 20$.

2.4 Feature Engineering

Two transformations was applied to the newly calculated dataset. The objective was to change the data distribution of of some features that were heavily skewed in order to potentially improve the performance of machine learning (ML) models. Box-Cox [4] and Yeo and Johnson [28] transformations were applied to the skewed features.

$$y(\lambda) = \begin{cases} \frac{y^\lambda - 1}{\lambda}, & \text{when } \lambda \neq 0 \\ log(y), & \text{when } \lambda = 0 \end{cases} \tag{13}$$

The Box-Cox transform (Eq. (13)) improves the properties of the data and results in a symmetric dataset with a Gaussian distribution. The Yeo and Johnson (Eq. (14)) transformation leads to similar benefits and, unlike the Box-Cox transform, can be applied to negative values.

$$y(\lambda) = \begin{cases} \frac{(y+1)^\lambda - 1}{\lambda}, & \text{when } \lambda \neq 0, \quad y \geqslant 0 \\ log(y+1), & \text{when } \lambda = 0, \quad y \geqslant 0 \\ \frac{(1-y)^{2-\lambda} - 1}{\lambda - 2}, & \text{when } \lambda \neq 2, \quad y < 0 \\ -log(1-y), & \text{when } \lambda = 2, \quad y < 0 \end{cases} \tag{14}$$

Additionally, new features (e.g., square, square root, cubit root, logarithms and inverse of each feature) were generate to improve the performance of the model.

2.5 Dataset Oversampling

The resulting dataset is intrinsically unbalanced (Table 2) because some dietary sounds are produced sporadically. For example, chewing generally takes a longer duration compared to drinking. Moreover, some people are fast eater while others eat slow and savor their meals.

When applying ML algorithms on imbalanced datasets, the resulting models tend to downplay the importance of the minority classes. This problem is addressed by oversampling the minority classes using the borderline-synthetic minority over-sampling technique (Borderline-SMOTE) [10]. This method is an extension to the synthetic minority over-sampling technique (SMOTE) [6]. For each minority class X_j, SMOTE select one random seed sample $X_j^{'}$ from its k nearest neighbors and a new synthetic sample X_{synth} is interpolated.

Table 2. Samples of each label in the dataset.

Label	Number of samples
Chewing	2001
Talking	554
Food swallowing	119
Drink swallowing	82
Other sounds	200

While the SMOTE method works well for many datasets, it creates noise that decrease the performance of many ML models. Indeed, during training, in attempt to achieve the best performance, most ML algorithms learn the boundary of each class as exactly as possible. Consequently, the samples at the borderline are prone to misclassifications compared to those far away from the boundary because they are located where different classes may overlap [10]. Consequently, the sample at the decision boundary needs a special treatment to avoid the potential misclassifications. Unlike SMOTE—which oversamples all samples of the minority classes—the Borderline-SMOTE oversamples only the samples of the minority classes that are located on the boundary of the decision boundary.

Prior to applying the oversampling method, 25% of the samples in the dataset was randomly selected and reserved for testing the performance of the ML models. The remaining 75%, the training set, was oversampled using the Borderline-SMOTE and used to train various predictive ML models.

2.6 Feature Selection

The feature engineering resulted in a total 958 features. There is a need to reduce this number to minimize overfitting and to avoid the curse of dimensionality. The following feature selection approaches were applied in a sequence. First, we removed features with unique values. These features would be practically useless for any ML model because they have a zero variance. Second, we removed the features that have a zero predictive importance, i.e., these features, have no information gain according to a gradient boosting machine (GBM) learning model. We also remove any features in the 5% lowest feature importance. Third, we remove highly correlated features. We computed the correlation between features and removed one feature of each pair whose correlation coefficient $c > 0.9$. Finally, a recursive feature elimination (RFE) [9] is used to rank and select the most optimum number of features.

2.7 Model Training and Evaluation

A Tree-based pipeline optimization mechanism [19] was used to optimize (e.g., feature selection and hyperparameter tuning) the ML pipeline and to maximize the classification accuracy. Four auspicious pipelines based on an Extreme Gradient Boosting[2], a K-nearest Neighbors[3], a Random Forest[4] and Light Gradient Boosting Machine[5] models were evaluated. Two types of models were trained. The first model was trained on the original dataset before re-sampling and the second model was trained on the oversampled dataset. In all cases, the result reported in this study are based on the performance of the models when validated on the test set that was set aside before any oversampling.

3 Results and Discussion

Table 3 compares the performance of the models trained on the oversampled dataset and tested on the reserved unaltered (i.e., non-resampled) test samples. Although all the models performed quite well, the *RandomForest* model slightly outperformed others. All the performance reported henceforth are based on the performance of the *RandomForest* pipeline. On the contrary—and as expected—the models trained on the non-resampled dataset performed poorly (Table 4) compared to the models trained on the oversampled dataset (Table 5).

The models trained on the non-resampled dataset have adequate performance in predicting when the subjects were chewing or talking but have very poor performance in predicting when the subjects were swallowing drinks or when they were swallowing food (Table 4). On the contrary, although the model trained on the oversampled dataset sometimes confused food and drink swallowing for chewing (Fig. 4), in general, it consistently performed well ($specificity >$ $94.0\%, miss\ rate < 17\%$ and $F_1 > 74.0\%$, and $MCC > 0.76$) in distinguishing all classes (Table 5).

		Predicted values	
		FALSE	TRUE
Actual values	FALSE	True Negatives (TN)	False Positives (FP)
	TRUE	False Negatives (FN)	True Positives (TP)

Fig. 3. Confusion matrix.

The performance of a model on an imbalanced dataset is normally evaluated in terms of its confusion matrix (Fig. 3). To test the performance of a classification model that is trained on an imbalanced dataset, the *accuracy* (Eq. (15))

[2] $XGB(colsample\_bytree = 0.5, \gamma = 0.7, depth = 4, subsample = 0.4)$.
[3] $KNeighbors(k\_neighbors = 14, weights =$ "distance").
[4] $RandomForest(depth = 24, max\_features =$ "log_2").
[5] $LGBM(colsample\_bytree = 0.7, depth = 32, num\_leaves = 70, \alpha = 0.5)$.

Table 3. Performance of the models trained on the oversampled dataset.

	XGBoost	KNeighbors	RandomForest	LGBM
Accuracy	97.29	96.32	97.56	97.62
Balanced accuracy	90.19	89.16	91.69	90.12
$F_\beta(\beta = 0.5)$	0.83	0.79	0.85	0.84
$F_\beta(\beta = 1)$	85.47	82.64	87.27	86.37
Jaccard-score	0.88	0.84	0.89	0.89
Geometric mean	94.69	92.78	95.18	95.04
Precision	81.95	78.10	83.83	83.41
Recall	90.19	89.16	91.69	90.12
Specificity	97.88	97.12	98.08	98.02
Matthews correlation coefficient	0.83	0.79	0.85	0.84

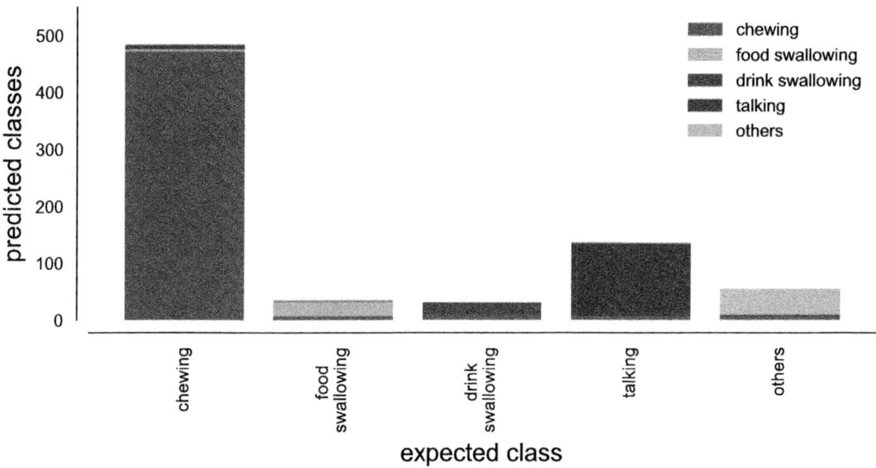

Fig. 4. Dietary sounds class labels prediction error. The model performs well in segregating the various dietary sounds labels. Nevertheless, it occasionally confuses food and drink swallowing for food chewing.

is usually deceitful because it gives equal weight to false positives (FP) and false negatives (FN) [11]. On the contrary, a balanced accuracy (Eq. (16)) gives equal weight to FP and FN by computing the average of positive class instances that are correctly predicted and that of negative instances that are correctly classified.

$$accuracy = \frac{TP + TN}{TP + FP + TN + FN} \tag{15}$$

$$balanced\, accuracy = \frac{TP}{2(TP + FN)} + \frac{TN}{2(TN + FP)} \tag{16}$$

Table 4. Performance of the model trained on the non-resampled dataset.

	Chewing	Food swallowing	Drink swallowing	Talking	Other sounds
Sensitivity	97.60	3.33	4.76	82.61	38.00
Specificity	64.02	99.58	100.00	98.17	97.68
Precision	85.02	25.00	100.00	91.20	54.29
Miss Rate	2.40	96.67	95.24	17.39	62.00
Accuracy	86.74	95.67	97.29	95.26	93.64
$F_\beta(\beta = 1)$	90.88	5.88	9.09	86.69	44.71
Matthews correlation coefficient	0.69	0.08	0.22	0.84	0.42

In Table 3, one must note that, while the accuracy is high ($accuracy = 97.56\%$), the balanced accuracy is relatively lower ($accuracy = 91.69\%$), which implies that the model performs modestly compared to what what an *accuracy* alone would have suggested.

Table 5. Performance of the model trained on the oversampled dataset.

	Chewing	Food swallowing	Drink swallowing	Talking	Other sounds
Sensitivity	94.40	86.67	90.48	94.93	92.00
Specificity	95.40	98.87	98.61	98.67	98.84
Precision	97.72	76.47	65.52	94.24	85.19
Miss rate	5.60	13.33	9.52	5.07	8.00
Accuracy	94.72	98.38	98.38	97.97	98.38
$F_\beta(\beta = 1)$	96.03	81.25	76.00	94.58	88.46
Matthews correlation coefficient	0.88	0.81	0.76	0.93	0.88

The strong performance of the model trained on the oversampled dataset is further attested by its Receiver Operating Characteristic (ROC) and its Area Under the Curve (Fig. 5). The ROC evaluates the trade-offs between the model's sensitivity and its specificity. It computes the model's performance at various error rates and helps assess the percentage of samples that will be properly predicted for a given *FP/(TN+FP)*. Figure 5a shows that the model trained on the non-resampled dataset performs poorly because many positive and negative instances are incorrectly classified. It is important to note that some classes are misclassified more than others. For instance, the model predicts reasonably well when the subjects were talking and chewing but the model achieves a much lower performance in predicting when the subjects were swallowing drinks. On the contrary, as shown in Fig. 5b, the model trained on the oversampled dataset performs much better: most of the positive instances are correctly predicted and very few negative instances are misclassified. Furthermore, this model has a high performance for all classes. The AUC represents the area under the entire ROC curve. A perfect classifier would correctly classify all positive instances and misclassifies no negative instances. Consequently, its AUC = 1. On the contrary, the

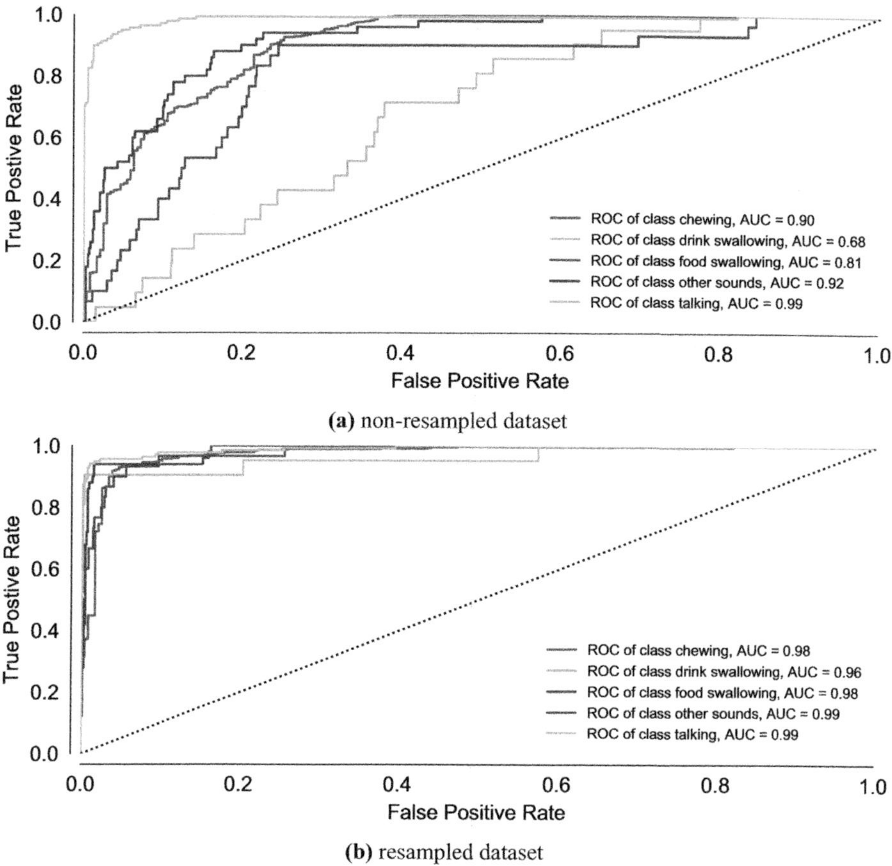

(a) non-resampled dataset

(b) resampled dataset

Fig. 5. Trade-off between the model's sensitivity and specificity. The dotted line represents the performance of a classifier that generates predictions uniformly at random. The area under the curve (AUC) expresses the relationship between false positives and true positives. The model performed very well because it achieved a high AUC. It also has few false positives and predicted many true positives.

worst classifier would incorrectly misclassify all positive and negative instances and would be represented with a single point $P = (1, 0)$ with an AUC$=0$. The model trained on the oversampled dataset has much better performance because its $AUC > 0.98$ for all classes.

The models also achieved relatively high precision and high recall. The precision (Eq. (17)) evaluates how often the samples that were predicted as positive were actually positive. The recall (Eq. (18)) estimates how many times positive samples were predicted as positive.

$$precision = \frac{TP}{TP + FP} \tag{17}$$

$$recall = \frac{TP}{TP + FN} \tag{18}$$

In short, the recall measures how many proper predictions the model makes while the precision estimates the pertinence of the predictions. For imbalanced datasets, the most optimum model would achieve a high recall without shrinking its precision [11]. These two objectives, however, are often antagonistic because increasing TP of the minority classes also increases its number of FP, which reduces the precision. Figure 6 shows the trade-offs between recall and precision. A perfect model ($area = 1.0$) would be made of two lines: a horizontal line $y = 1$ and a vertical line $x = 1$. Conversely, a poor classifier would only achieve a high recall only if its precision is low. Figure 6 highlights the performance of the oversampled model compared to that of the non-resampled model. Indeed, the former (Fig. 6b) has a higher area and its curves are steepest when their recalls are closer to 1.0. On the contrary, the latter (Fig. 6a) has much lower areas, and for some classes (e.g.,food swallowing and drink swallowing) the performance is worse than a random classifier.

The F_β score (Eq. (19)) expresses the performance of a given classifier in terms of the compromise between the classifier's recall and its precision [11].

$$\begin{aligned} F_\beta &= (1 + \beta^2) \cdot \frac{precision \cdot recall}{(\beta^2 \cdot precision) + recall} \\ &= \frac{(1 + \beta^2) \cdot TP}{(1 + \beta^2) \cdot TP + \beta^2 \cdot FN + FP} \end{aligned} \tag{19}$$

When $\beta = 0$, the F_β score would only consider the precision. A $\beta > 1$ gives more weight to recall over precision. In this study, $F_\beta(\beta = 0.5)$ and $F_\beta(\beta = 1)$ are considered. The former gives emphasizes precision over recall. The later gives an equal balance between the two. As shown in Table 3, Table 4 and Table 5, the model trained on the oversampled dataset outperformed the one trained on the original dataset.

The Jaccard score (Eq. (20)) estimates the fraction of elements that are shared between two sets A and B. It is a ration between the number of times a given value occurs in both A and B to the total number of distinct items in A and B.

$$\begin{aligned} J(A, B) &= \frac{|A \cap B|}{|A \cup B|} \\ &= \frac{|A \cap B|}{|A| + |B| - |A \cap B|} \end{aligned} \tag{20}$$

where $\cap$ represent an intersection, $\cup$ denotes a union, and $||$ stands for the number of elements of the set. Consequently, in our case, it estimates the performance of the classifiers by comparing the predicted labels to the expected label. A perfect classifier would achieve a $Jaccard\,score = 1$. As shown in Table 3, the predicted labels are 89% similar to the expected labels.

Unlike the other model evaluation measures, the Matthews Correlation Coefficient (MCC) (Eq. (21)) evaluates the performance of a classifier in terms of

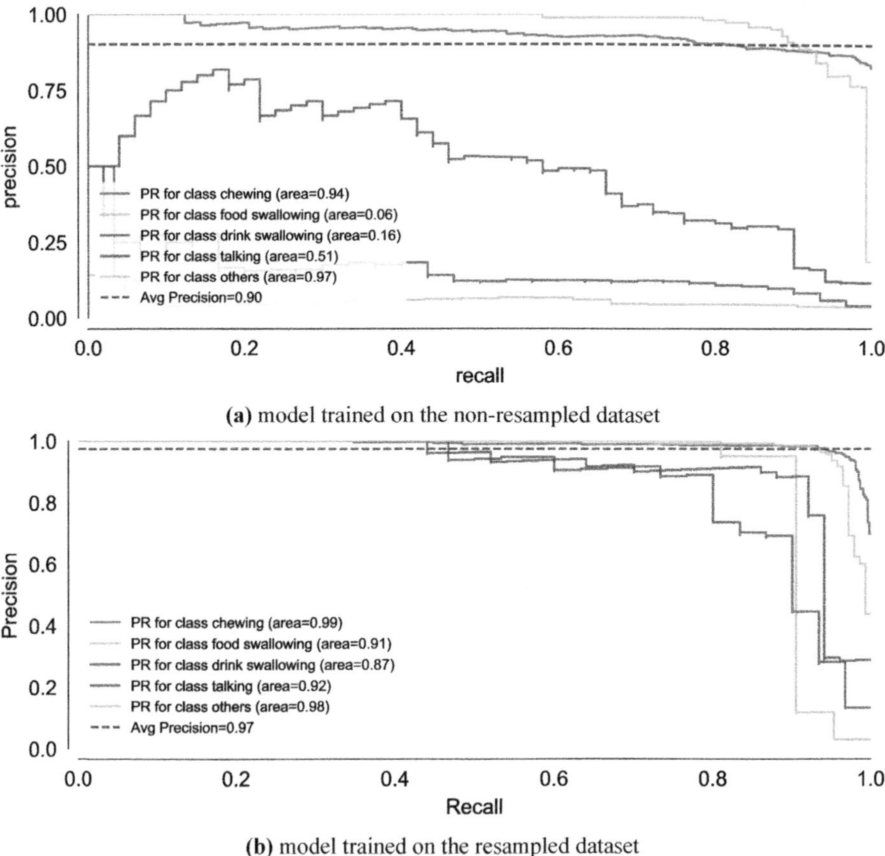

(a) model trained on the non-resampled dataset

(b) model trained on the resampled dataset

Fig. 6. Trade-offs between the recall and precision. The model trained on the non-resampled dataset has a much lower performance (e.g., low area) compared to model trained on the oversampled dataset. The latter has higher area and its curves are steepest when their respective recalls curves are closed to 1.0.

the four sections of the confusion matrix (i.e., in terms of TP, FP, TN and FP).

$$\frac{c \times s - \sum_{k}^{K} p_k \times t_k}{\sqrt{\left(s^2 - \sum_{k}^{K} p_k^2\right) - \left(s^2 - \sum_{k}^{K} t_k^2\right)}} \tag{21}$$

with:

c the total number of sample correctly predicted
s the total number of samples
t_k the number of time a class k truly occurred
p_k the number of time class k was predicted

Compared to other model evaluation metrics, the MCC is more reliable because it produces a high score only when the model has good performances in all the four categories of the confusion matrix and is considered a good evaluation metrics even for imbalanced classes [7]. A mediocre classier has MCC values that range between -1 and 0 while a perfect classifier has a $MCC = +1$. Table 3 and Table 5 show that the models trained on the oversampled dataset have a good performance ($MCC = 0.85$). However, the model achieved the best performance when predicting the *talking* classes ($MCC = 0.93$) but blunders when predicting the *drink swallowing* classes ($MCC = 0.76$). On the contrary, the model trained on the non-resampled dataset has poor performance (Table 4), especially when predicting the *drink swallowing* classes ($MCC = 0.22$).

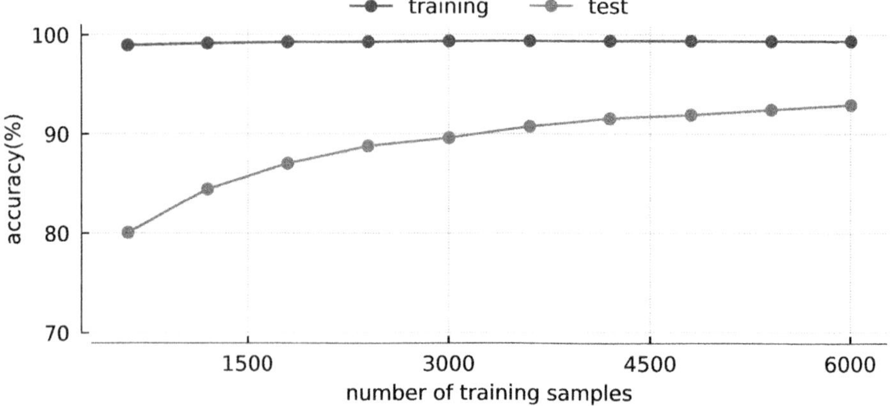

Fig. 7. Training and test score versus the number of training samples. The solid line indicates the mean value while the shaded area represents the standard deviation. Both the training and the test score exhibit a low variability; thus, the model has a low bias and a low variance. However, the test score improves with more training samples, which implies that more training samples might lead to a better performance.

Finally, Fig. 7 shows the performance of the model with respect to the increase in the training samples. With much fewer samples, there is a large gap between the performance of the training and the test set. This may implies that the model has a high variance and is over-fitting. On the contrary, increasing the training sample closes the gap. However, with the available training samples, the training and the test score have not converged together, which implies that more training samples might lead to a better performance.

4 Conclusion

Predominant methods for fighting against obesity focus on healthy eating but often ignore the importance of slowly eating and properly chewing in fighting against obesity. This research proposed a method that recognizes common human actions during mealtime (i.e., food chewing, food swallowing, drink swallowing, and talking). The proposed approach uses a cheap wearable bone conduction microphone that records intra-body sounds that are produced when a person eats. We conducted experiments on 16 subjects. All experiments were conducted in free-living environments to capture the complexity of the real-world. For instance, some dietary sounds were recorded at home when the subjects were having supper with their families. Others were collected in a university cafeteria during lunch with colleagues. Additionally, there was no constraint on the type of food and the subjects were urged to have whatever they usually eat. We trained and tested machine learning models on the obtained dataset and found that the proposed approach achieves similar performances as that of the most recent state of the art models ($accuracy = 97.5\%$, $precision = 83.8\%$, $recall = 91.7\%$, $Jaccard\ score = 0.89$, $Kappa\ score = 0.88$, $F_1\ score = 87.2\%$ and $MCC = 0.85$) even though our system uses modest machine learning models. Nevertheless, while the model generally performs well in distinguishing the various mealtime activities, it sometimes confused food and drink swallowing for chewing.

References

1. Alías, F., Socoró, J., Sevillano, X.: A Review of physical and perceptual feature extraction techniques for speech, music and environmental sounds. Appl. Sci. **6**(5), 143 (2016). https://doi.org/10.3390/app6050143
2. Amft, O., Troster, G.: On-body sensing solutions for automatic dietary monitoring. IEEE Pervasive Comput. **8**(2), 62–70 (2009). https://doi.org/10.1109/MPRV.2009.32
3. Bi, S., et al.: Auracle: detecting eating episodes with an ear-mounted sensor. In: Proceedings of the ACM on Interactive, Mobile, Wearable and Ubiquitous Technologies, vol. 2, no. 3, pp. 1–27, September 2018. https://doi.org/10.1145/3264902
4. Box, G.E.P., Cox, D.R.: An analysis of transformations. J. Roy. Stat. Soc.: Series B (Methodol.) **26**(2), 211–243 (1964). https://doi.org/10.1111/j.2517-6161.1964.tb00553.x
5. Chakroborty, S., Roy, A., Saha, G.: Fusion of a complementary feature set with MFCC for improved closed set text-independent speaker identification. In: 2006 IEEE International Conference on Industrial Technology, pp. 387–390. IEEE (2006). https://doi.org/10.1109/ICIT.2006.372388
6. Chawla, N.V., Bowyer, K.W., Hall, L.O., Kegelmeyer, W.P.: SMOTE: synthetic minority over-sampling technique. J. Artif. Intell. Res. **16**, 321–357 (2002). https://doi.org/10.1613/jair.953
7. Chicco, D., Jurman, G.: The advantages of the Matthews correlation coefficient (MCC) over F1 score and accuracy in binary classification evaluation. BMC Genomics **21**(1), 6 (2020). https://doi.org/10.1186/s12864-019-6413-7
8. Goto, M.: SmartMusicKIOSK: music listening station with chorus-search function. In: Proceedings of the 16th Annual ACM Symposium on User Interface Software and Technology - UIST 2003, vol. 5, pp. 31–40. ACM Press, New York (2003). https://doi.org/10.1145/964696.964700, http://portal.acm.org/citation.cfm?doid=964696.964700
9. Guyon, I., Weston, J., Barnhill, S., Vapnik, V.: Gene selection for cancer classification using support vector machines. Mach. Learn. **46**(1–3), 389–422 (2002). https://doi.org/10.1023/A:1012487302797

10. Han, H., Wang, W.Y., Mao, B.H.: Borderline-SMOTE: a new over-sampling method in imbalanced data sets learning. Adv. Intell. Syst. Comput. **683**, 878–887 (2005). https://doi.org/10.1007/11538059_91
11. He, H., Ma, Y.: Imbalanced Learning: Foundations, Algorithms, and Applications. Wiley-IEEE Press, July 2013
12. Hurst, Y., Fukuda, H.: Effects of changes in eating speed on obesity in patients with diabetes: a secondary analysis of longitudinal health check-up data. BMJ Open **8**(1), e019589 (2018). https://doi.org/10.1136/bmjopen-2017-019589
13. Hussain, G., Javed, K., Cho, J., Yi, J.: Food intake detection and classification using a necklace-type piezoelectric wearable sensor system. IEICE Trans. Inf. Syst. **101**(11), 2795–2807 (2018). https://doi.org/10.1587/transinf.2018EDP7076
14. Jain, A., Kondo, T., Kamachi, H., Yokokubo, A., Lopez, G.: Detailed classification of meal-related activities from eating sound collected in free living conditions. In: Proceedings of the 13th International Joint Conference on Biomedical Engineering Systems and Technologies - Vol. 5: HEALTHINF, pp. 284–291. INSTICC, SCITEPRESS, February 2020. https://doi.org/10.5220/0009187502840291
15. Kondo, T., Kamachi, H., Ishii, S., Yokokubo, A., Lopez, G.: Robust classification of eating sound collected in natural meal environment. In: Proceedings of the 2019 ACM International Joint Conference on Pervasive and Ubiquitous Computing and Proceedings of the 2019 ACM International Symposium on Wearable Computers - UbiComp/ISWC 2019, pp. 105–108. ACM Press, New York, September 2019. https://doi.org/10.1145/3341162.3343780
16. Kondo, T., Shiro, H., Yokokubo, A., Lopez, G.: Optimized classification model for efficient recognition of meal-related activities in daily life meal environment. In: 2019 Joint 8th International Conference on Informatics, Electronics & Vision (ICIEV) and 2019 3rd International Conference on Imaging, Vision & Pattern Recognition (icIVPR), pp. 146–151. IEEE, May 2019. https://doi.org/10.1109/ICIEV.2019.8858526, https://ieeexplore.ieee.org/document/8858526/
17. Kyritsis, K., Diou, C., Delopoulos, A.: A data driven end-to-end approach for in-the-wild monitoring of eating behavior using smartwatches. IEEE J. Biomed. Health Inform. 1 (2020). https://doi.org/10.1109/JBHI.2020.2984907
18. de Lara, J.R.C., et al.: A method of automatic speaker recognition using cepstral features and vectorial quantization. In: Sanfeliu, A., Cortés, M.L. (eds.) CIARP 2005. LNCS, vol. 3773, pp. 146–153. Springer, Heidelberg (2005). https://doi.org/10.1007/11578079_16
19. Le, T.T., Fu, W., Moore, J.H.: Scaling tree-based automated machine learning to biomedical big data with a feature set selector. Bioinformatics **36**(1), 250–256 (2020). https://doi.org/10.1093/bioinformatics/btz470
20. Lopez, G., Mitsui, H., Ohara, J., Yokokubo, A.: Effect of feedback medium for real-time mastication awareness increase using wearable sensors. In: Proceedings of the 12th International Joint Conference on Biomedical Engineering Systems and Technologies, pp. 442–449, no. Biostec. SCITEPRESS - Science and Technology Publications (2019). https://doi.org/10.5220/0007569804420449
21. Mellina, A., Sentinelli, A., Marfia, G., Roccetti, M.: AREEB: automatic refrain extraction for thumbnail. In: 2012 IEEE Consumer Communications and Networking Conference (CCNC), no. Mi, pp. 472–476. IEEE, January 2012. https://doi.org/10.1109/CCNC.2012.6181003
22. Scheirer, E., Slaney, M.: Construction and evaluation of a robust multifeature speech/music discriminator. In: 1997 IEEE International Conference on Acoustics, Speech, and Signal Processing, vol. 2, pp. 1331–1334. IEEE Comput. Soc. Press (1801). https://doi.org/10.1109/ICASSP.1997.596192

23. Schoeller, D.A.: Limitations in the assessment of dietary energy intake by self-report. Metabolism **44**(SUPPL. 2), 18–22 (1995). https://doi.org/10.1016/0026-0495(95)90204-X
24. Selamat, N.A., Ali, S.H.M.: Automatic food intake monitoring based on chewing activity: a survey. IEEE Access **8**, 48846–48869 (2020). https://doi.org/10.1109/ACCESS.2020.2978260
25. Tada, A., Miura, H.: Association of mastication and factors affecting masticatory function with obesity in adults: a systematic review. BMC Oral Health **18**(1), 76 (2018). https://doi.org/10.1186/s12903-018-0525-3
26. Vu, T., Lin, F., Alshurafa, N., Xu, W.: Wearable food intake monitoring technologies: a comprehensive review. Computers **6**(1), 1–28 (2017). https://doi.org/10.3390/computers6010004
27. Westerterp, K.R., Goris, A.H.: Validity of the assessment of dietary intake: problems of misreporting. Curr. Opinion Clin. Nutr. Metab. Care **5**(5), 489–493 (2002). https://doi.org/10.1097/00075197-200209000-00006
28. Yeo, I.K.: A new family of power transformations to improve normality or symmetry. Biometrika **87**(4), 954–959 (2000). https://doi.org/10.1093/biomet/87.4.954

Author Index

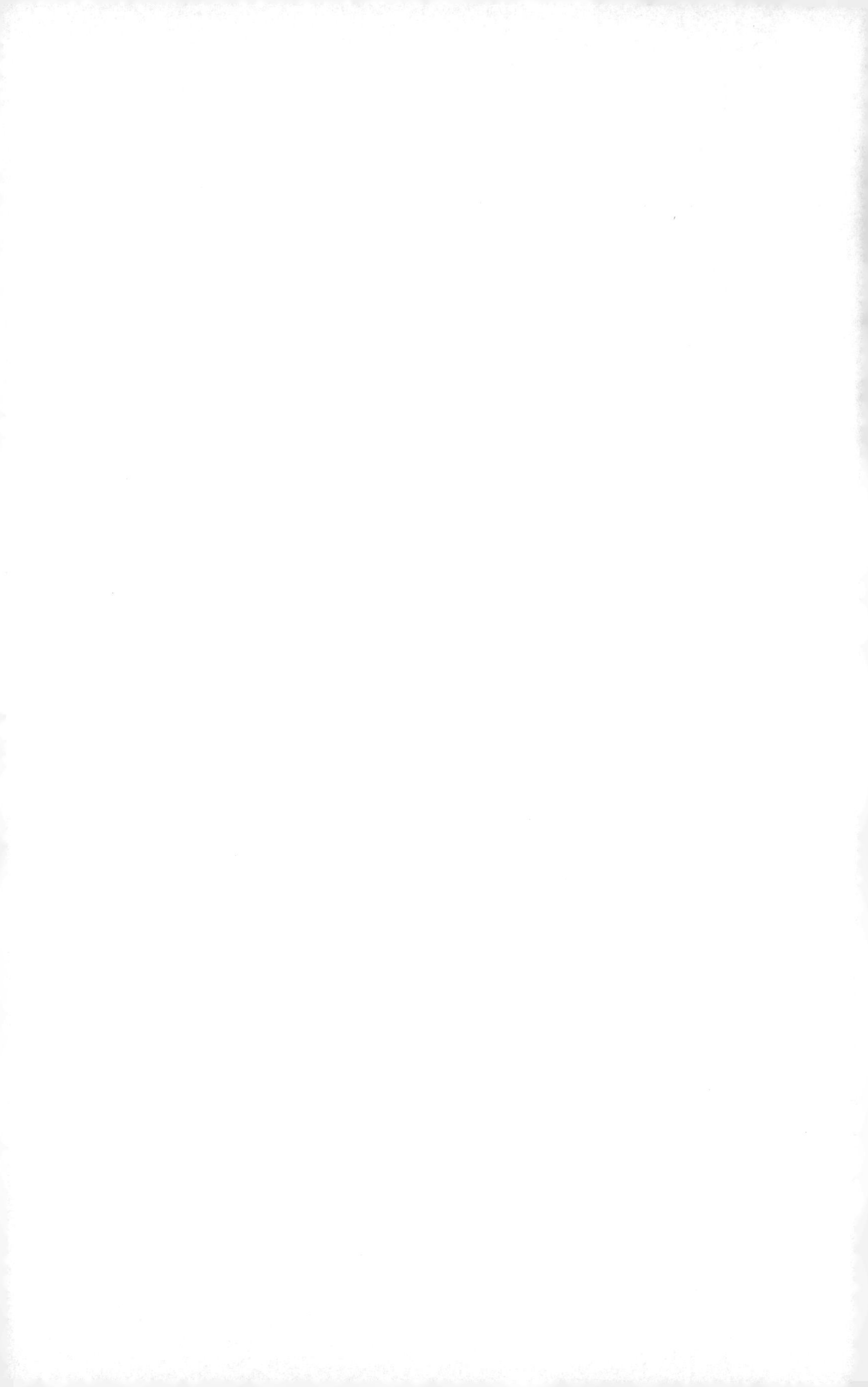

Printed by Printforce, the Netherlands